Transient Ischemic Attack and Stroke

Diagnosis, Investigation, and Treatment

Second Edition

The second edition of *Transient Ischemic Attack and Stroke* covers the clinical background and management of the full clinical spectrum of cerebrovascular disease, from TIA to vascular dementia, in a compact but evidence-based format, making it a comprehensive primer in stroke medicine. Accurate diagnosis and appropriate investigation and management have a major impact on patient outcomes in cerebrovascular disease, such as the effect of urgent antithrombotic treatment on early recurrent stroke after TIA and minor stroke, the effect of interventions such as thrombectomy and hemicraniectomy in major acute stroke, and the effect of stroke units and organized stroke care.

Written by a leading team of clinicians and researchers in the field, this book will be essential to neurologists, geriatricians, stroke physicians, allied health workers, and all others with an interest in stroke.

Gary K. K. Lau is Clinical Research Fellow at the Centre for Prevention of Stroke and Dementia, Nuffield Department of Clinical Neurosciences, University of Oxford.

Sarah T. Pendlebury is Associate Professor in Medicine and Old Age Neuroscience at the Centre for Prevention of Stroke and Dementia, Nuffield Department of Clinical Neurosciences, University of Oxford.

Peter M. Rothwell is Action Research Professor of Neurology at the University of Oxford and the Director at the Centre for Prevention of Stroke and Dementia, Nuffield Department of Clinical Neurosciences, University of Oxford.

T0177133

Transient Ischemic Attack and Stroke

Diagnosis, Investigation, and Treatment

Second Edition

Gary K. K. Lau
Sarah T. Pendlebury
Peter M. Rothwell

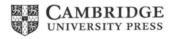

CAMBRIDGE
UNIVERSITY PRESS

University Printing House, Cambridge CB2 8BS, United Kingdom

One Liberty Plaza, 20th Floor, New York, NY 10006, USA

477 Williamstown Road, Port Melbourne, VIC 3207, Australia

314–321, 3rd Floor, Plot 3, Splendor Forum, Jasola District Centre, New Delhi – 110025, India

103 Penang Road, #05-06/07, Visioncrest Commercial, Singapore 238467

Cambridge University Press is part of the University of Cambridge.

It furthers the University's mission by disseminating knowledge in the pursuit of
education, learning, and research at the highest international levels of excellence.

www.cambridge.org
Information on this title: www.cambridge.org/9781107485358
DOI: 10.1017/9781316161609

© Gary Lau, Sarah Pendlebury, and Peter Rothwell 2018

This publication is in copyright. Subject to statutory exception
and to the provisions of relevant collective licensing agreements,
no reproduction of any part may take place without the written
permission of Cambridge University Press.

First published 2018
Reprinted 2021

Printed in the United Kingdom by Print on Demand, World Wide

A catalogue record for this publication is available from the British Library.

Library of Congress Cataloging-in-Publication Data
Names: Pendlebury, Sarah T., author. | Rothwell, Peter M., author. | Lau, Gary K. K., 1984– author.
Title: Transient ischemic attack and stroke : diagnosis, investigation and treatment / Sarah T. Pendlebury,
Peter M. Rothwell, Gary K.K. Lau.
Description: Second edition. | Cambridge ; New York, NY : Cambridge University Press, 2018. | Includes
bibliographical references and index.
Identifiers: LCCN 2017058250 | ISBN 9781107485358 (paperback : alk. paper)
Subjects: | MESH: Ischemic Attack, Transient – diagnosis | Stroke – diagnosis | Ischemic Attack,
Transient – therapy | Stroke – therapy
Classification: LCC RC388.5 | NLM WL 356 | DDC 616.8/1–dc23
LC record available at https://lccn.loc.gov/2017058250

ISBN 978-1-107-48535-8 Paperback

Cambridge University Press has no responsibility for the persistence or accuracy of
URLs for external or third-party internet websites referred to in this publication
and does not guarantee that any content on such websites is, or will remain,
accurate or appropriate.

Every effort has been made in preparing this book to provide accurate and up-to-date information that is in
accord with accepted standards and practice at the time of publication. Although case histories are drawn
from actual cases, every effort has been made to disguise the identities of the individuals involved.
Nevertheless, the authors, editors, and publishers can make no warranties that the information contained
herein is totally free from error, not least because clinical standards are constantly changing through
research and regulation. The authors, editors, and publishers therefore disclaim all liability for direct or
consequential damages resulting from the use of material contained in this book. Readers are strongly
advised to pay careful attention to information provided by the manufacturer of any drugs or equipment
that they plan to use.

Contents

Preface to the Second Edition

As predicted by Charles Warlow in his *Foreword* to the first edition of this book, advances in the field of cerebrovascular diseases have continued at pace during the 9 years since the first edition was written. Changes in clinical practice continue to come mainly from multicenter randomized clinical trials and well-designed cohort studies, particularly with better phenotyping of patients.

We now know, for example, that about 90% of the global stroke burden is attributable to modifiable risk factors and is therefore potentially preventable. We are also beginning to understand how novel non-Mendelian genetic variants also account for some of the unexplained susceptibility of stroke. We now have a better sense of who will and who won't benefit from existing treatments and also a number of new treatment strategies. For example, the benefit of tissue plasminogen activator in treatment of acute ischemic stroke patients presenting within 4.5 hours of symptom onset is now well established regardless of age and stroke severity. Endovascular treatment is now able to extend the time window of treating selected patients with acute ischemic stroke of the anterior circulation due to large vessel occlusion to 6 hours. In a subset of individuals with significant ischemic penumbra identified by appropriate neuroimaging, time window for endovascular treatment can even be extended to up to 24 hours. Non-vitamin K antagonist oral anticoagulants were not available when the first edition of this book was written but have since been shown to be effective and are now widely used in clinical practice. Patent foramen ovale closure has also recently been confirmed to be beneficial in a selected subset of individuals with stroke. The important contribution of vascular factors to dementia is increasingly recognized together with the impact of cerebrovascular events on both acute and longer-term cognitive decline.

These advances (and many more) in the field of cerebrovascular diseases have been summarized in this updated second edition. We hope you will enjoy reading this new edition as much as we have enjoyed updating it.

Epidemiology

In order to understand the clinical management of transient ischemic attacks (TIAs) and stroke, to plan clinical services or to design randomized controlled trials, and to measure the overall impact of treatments, it is important to understand the epidemiology of stroke.

Definitions of Transient Ischemic Attack and Stroke

A stroke is defined as rapidly developing clinical symptoms and/or signs of focal, and at times global (applied to patients in deep coma and to those with subarachnoid hemorrhage), loss of brain function, with symptoms lasting more than 24 hours or leading to death, with no apparent cause other than that of vascular origin (Hatano 1976). Conventionally, a TIA is distinguished from stroke on the basis of an arbitrary 24-hour cutoff for resolution of symptoms (Box 1.1). Hence a TIA is defined as an acute loss of focal brain or monocular function with symptoms lasting less than 24 hours and that is thought to be caused by inadequate cerebral or ocular blood supply as a result of arterial thrombosis, low flow, or embolism associated with arterial, cardiac, or hematological disease (Hatano 1976).

Since the early part of the twentieth century, a variety of definitions of TIA have been used (Table 1.1). However, the definition given in Box 1.1 has recently been challenged since the 24-hour time limit is arbitrary rather than being based on clinical, imaging, or pathological criteria. The 24-hour cutoff does not reflect the fact that the majority of TIAs last for less than 60 minutes, nor does it indicate a lack of infarction on brain imaging. Some TIAs are associated with radiological evidence of cerebral infarction, but there is poor correlation between clinical and imaging findings (Table 1.2). An alternative, but controversial (Easton *et al.* 2004), definition for TIA has been proposed as comprising a transient episode of neurological dysfunction caused by focal brain or retinal ischemia without evidence of acute infarction on brain imaging (Albers *et al.* 2002). The proposed new definition for TIA has the problem that brain imaging does not correlate particularly well with pathological

---

BOX 1.1 Definitions of Transient Ischemic Attack and Stroke as Used in This Book

Transient Ischemic Attack An acute loss of focal brain or monocular function with symptoms lasting less than 24 hours and that is thought to be caused by inadequate cerebral or ocular blood supply as a result of arterial thrombosis, low flow, or embolism associated with arterial, cardiac, or hematological disease (Hatano 1976).

Stroke Rapidly developing clinical symptoms and/or signs of focal, and at times global (applied to patients in deep coma and to those with subarachnoid hemorrhage), loss of brain function, with symptoms lasting more than 24 hours or leading to death, with no apparent cause other than that of vascular origin (Hatano 1976).

Table 1.1 History of the definition of transient ischemic attack

Year	Description
1914 Hunt (1914)	Characterized "the role of the carotid arteries in the causation of vascular lesions of the brain" and described "attacks of threatened hemiplegia and cerebral intermittent claudication"
1954 CM Fisher at the *First and Second Conferences on Cerebral Vascular Diseases*, Princeton, USA	Described "transient ischemic attacks . . . which may last from a few seconds up to several hours, the most common duration being a few seconds up to 5 or 10 minutes"
1961 CM Fisher at the *Third Conference on Cerebral Vascular Diseases*	TIA described as "the occurrence of single or multiple episodes of cerebral dysfunction lasting no longer than one hour and clearing without significant residuum"
1964 Acheson and Hutchinson (1964)	Series of patients with "transient cerebral ischemia" defined as "duration of attack less than an hour"
1964 Marshall (1964)	Series of 180 patients with TIAs defined as "of less than 24-hours duration"
1975 Advisory Council for National Institute of Neurological and Communicative Disorders and Stroke (1975)	TIA defined as lasting "no longer than a day (24-hours)," although typically lasting from 2 to 15 minutes
1976 World Health Organization bulletin (Hatano 1976)	TIA defined as lasting less than 24 hours
2002 for the TIA Working Group (Albers *et al.* 2002)	TIA definition proposed based on absence of infarction on brain scanning and a 1-hour time window

Note: TIA, transient ischemic attack.

infarction: brain imaging may be normal in clinically definite stroke, silent infarction may occur, and imaging sensitivity is highly dependent on both imaging method and area of the brain being examined. Moreover, there is uncertainty regarding the pathological correlates of imaging changes such as diffusion-weighted magnetic resonance imaging (DWI) hyper-intensity (Chapters 10 and 11) and leukoaraiosis, and as imaging technology advances, what is defined as TIA will change. The definition of TIA used throughout this book is, therefore, the conventional one based on symptoms or signs lasting less than 24 hours.

Anything that causes a TIA may, if more severe or prolonged, cause a stroke (Sempere *et al.* 1998). There are many non-vascular conditions that may cause symptoms suggestive of TIA or stroke, and these are referred to in this book as "TIA mimics" or "stroke mimics." The separation of TIA from stroke on the basis of a 24-hour time limit is useful since the differential diagnosis of the two syndromes is different to some extent (i.e., the spectrum of TIA mimics differs from that of stroke mimics).

Given the common mechanisms underlying TIA and stroke, the investigation of patients with these syndromes is similar. However, in TIA and minor stroke, the emphasis is on rapid identification and treatment of the underlying cause in order to prevent a recurrent

Table 1.2 Advantages and disadvantages of conventional and imaging-based definitions of transient ischemic attack

Definition	Advantages	Disadvantages
Conventional definition	Diagnosis can be made at assessment (provided that symptoms have resolved) either prior to imaging or in centers where imaging is unavailable	Diagnosis based on an arbitrary cut-point of no physiological or prognostic significance
	Comparisons with previous studies using conventional definition possible	Diagnosis based on patient recall, which may vary with time
		Diagnosis cannot be made with certainty within 24 hours in a patient with resolving (but persistent) symptoms
Imaging-based definition	Based on pathophysiological endpoint and emphasizes prognostic importance of cerebral infarction	Diagnosis based on interpretation of imaging, which is likely to vary between individuals and centers; also, sensitivity of imaging techniques is likely to increase with time with developments in computed tomography and magnetic resonance technology
	Majority of transient ischemic attacks last less than 60 minutes	Pathophysiological significance of changes on new imaging techniques not fully understood
	Encourages use of neurodiagnostic investigations	Classification of events lasting more than 1 hour without infarction unclear
	Consistent with the distinction between unstable angina and myocardial infarction	Diagnosis cannot be made in centers where no imaging is available

and possibly more severe event, whereas in severe stroke, the initial emphasis of investigation is on targeting treatment to minimize subsequent deficit. Therefore, in this book, we have considered TIA and minor stroke separately from severe stroke to reflect the difference in clinical approach to minor versus more severe cerebrovascular events.

There is no accepted definition for what constitutes "minor" stroke. This distinction between minor and major stroke is sometimes based on a score on the National Institutes of Health Stroke Scale (NIHSS) at assessment of ≤ 3 (Wityk *et al.* 1994) or a score of ≤ 2 on the modified Rankin Scale (mRS) at 1 month. Such distinctions are problematic because the NIHSS score will vary with time after the stroke and the mRS at 1 month may increase if a minor stroke is followed by a major stroke. We take the pragmatic view that minor stroke includes those strokes mild enough for patients to be seen in an emergency outpatient setting or to be sent home after initial assessment and treatment in the hospital.

Approximately 85% of all first-ever strokes are ischemic; 10% are caused by primary intracerebral hemorrhage, and approximately 5% are from subarachnoid hemorrhage (Rothwell *et al.* 2004). Within ischemic stroke, 25% are caused by large artery disease, 25% by small vessel disease, 20% by cardiac embolism, 5% by other rarer causes, and the remaining 25% are of undetermined etiology. Ischemic stroke may also be classified by anatomical location, using simple clinical features, as total anterior circulation stroke, partial anterior circulation stroke, lacunar stroke, and posterior circulation stroke. This is of some help in identifying the likely underlying pathology and gives information as to prognosis (Chapter 9).

The Burden of Transient Ischemic Attack and Stroke

Data from the Global Burden of Diseases, Injuries, and Risk Factors Study (GBD), one of the most comprehensive observational epidemiological studies to date, estimated the absolute numbers of people with first stroke in 119 countries (58 high-income, 61 low- and middle-income) to be 16.9 million in 2010 (Feigin *et al.* 2014). More than 38% of new strokes (50% in high-income and 32% in low- and middle-income countries) were in people aged 75 years and older. In the UK alone, there were about 150,000 new strokes in 2010 (Feigin *et al.* 2014), making it by far the most common neurological disorder (MacDonald *et al.* 2000) (Table 1.3). The Framingham Study estimated 1 in 6 men and 1 in 5 women may suffer from a stroke if they lived to be 75 years old (Seshadri *et al.* 2006). Stroke is the second most common cause of death worldwide (Lozano *et al.* 2012). However, mortality data underestimate the true burden of stroke since, in contrast to coronary heart disease and cancer, the major burden of stroke is chronic disability rather than death (Wolfe 2000), and in 2010, GBD noted 102 million disability-adjusted life-years (DALYs) were lost due to stroke (Feigin *et al.* 2014).

Stroke is the third-leading cause of premature death and disability, and approximately a third of stroke survivors are functionally dependent at 1 year (Murray et al. 2012; MacDonald *et al.* 2000). Stroke also causes secondary medical problems, including dementia, depression, epilepsy, falls, and fractures. Globally, with an increasing number of people with stroke (ischemic and hemorrhagic), stroke-related deaths, and DALYs lost due to stroke, the burden of stroke is increasing (Krishnamurthi *et al.* 2013; Feigin *et al.* 2014). This will probably increase further, unless there are substantial decreases in age- and sex-specific incidence (Rothwell *et al.* 2004). Furthermore, while ischemic stroke is the main pathological stroke subtype, the burden of hemorrhagic stroke (mortality-to-incidence ratio and DALYs lost) is much higher (Krishnamurthi *et al.* 2013).

In the UK, the treatment of and productivity lost arising from stroke result in total society costs of approximately £9 billion per year, accounting for about 6% of the total National Health Service (NHS) and Social Services expenditure (Rothwell 2001; Saka *et al.* 2009). However, a significant bulk of the global stroke burden is borne by low- and middle-income countries, due partially to a disproportionate higher incidence of hemorrhagic stroke in these countries (Krishnamurthi *et al.* 2013).

Additionally, TIAs are also common, and it is estimated that 54,000 TIAs occur each year in England (Giles and Rothwell 2007). By definition, TIA causes transient symptoms only and, therefore, has no long-term sequelae per se. However, the importance of TIA lies in the high early risk of stroke and the longer-term risk of other vascular disease. Indeed, it has been estimated that approximately 20% of strokes are preceded by TIA (Rothwell and Warlow 2005).

Table 1.3 Comparative incidence and prevalence rates of common neurological conditions measured in a population-based study of approximately 100,000 people registered with 13 general practices in London, UK, and conducted between 1995 and 1996

Condition	Incidence rate (95% CI)[a]	Prevalence rate (95% CI)[a]
First TIA or stroke[b]	2.05 (1.83–2.30)	
Second TIA or stroke[b]	0.42 (0.33–0.55)	
Intracranial hemorrhage	0.10 (0.05–0.17)	0.5 (0.2–0.8)
Any stroke		9 (8–11)
Epilepsy[c]	0.46 (0.36–0.60)	4 (4–5)
First seizure	0.11 (0.07–0.18)	
Primary CNS tumor	0.10 (0.05–0.18)	
Parkinson's disease	0.09 (0.12–0.27)	2 (1–3)
Shingles	1.40 (1.04–1.84)	
Bacterial infection of CNS	0.07 (0.04–0.13)	1 (0.8–2.0)
Multiple sclerosis	0.07 (0.04–0.11)	2 (2–3)
Myasthenia gravis	0.03 (0.008–0.070)	
Guillain-Barré syndrome	0.03 (0.01–0.06)	
Motor neuron disease	0.02 (0.003–0.050)	0.1 (0.01–0.30)

Notes: CI, confidence interval; TIA, transient ischemic attack; CNS, central nervous system.
[a] Age- and sex-adjusted rates per 1,000 population.
[b] Includes ischemic and hemorrhagic stroke.
[c] Two or more unprovoked seizures.
Source: From MacDonald *et al.* (2000).

Understanding of the epidemiology of stroke has lagged behind that of coronary heart disease because of a lack of research funding for stroke (Rothwell 2001; Pendlebury *et al.* 2004; Pendlebury 2007) and because stroke is a much more heterogeneous disorder. Separate assessment of the different stroke subtypes should ideally be made in epidemiological studies of stroke. Stroke subtype identification was often not possible in early studies because of a lack of brain and vascular imaging, and it remains problematic today because of the frequent difficulty in ascribing a cause for a given stroke even when imaging is available. The epidemiology of TIA is more challenging even than stroke since patients with TIAs are more heterogeneous and present to a variety of different clinical services, if they present to medical attention at all. Furthermore, reliable diagnosis of TIA requires early and expert clinical assessment (there is no diagnostic test for TIA), making epidemiological studies labor intensive and costly.

Mortality

Stroke mortality rises rapidly with age (Rothwell *et al.* 2005). The increase in mortality in the elderly is mainly a result of the steep rise in the incidence of stroke with age but also, to a lesser extent, reflects the increase in case fatality in older patients. In other words, older people are more likely to have a stroke (incidence), and if they do have one, it is more likely to be fatal (case fatality). GBD estimated that in 2010, there were 5.9 million stroke deaths, 71% of which occurred in low- and middle-income countries (Feigin *et al.* 2014). Mortality-to-incidence ratio was 0.35 (0.32 in high-income countries and 0.36 in low- and middle-income countries). Although the overall age-adjusted mortality rate reduced by 25% (37%, 95% CI, 31–41% in high-income countries and 20%, 95% CI, 15–30% in low-income and middle-income countries) during 1990–2010, the absolute numbers of stroke-related deaths increased by 26%, much of which was accounted for by patients aged 75 years and older. Age-standardized rates of stroke mortality in people aged 75 years and older in low- and middle-income countries exceeded mortality rates by a third compared to those of high-income countries of the same age group and by more than twofold in those younger than 75. When stratified by geographical region, mortality-to-incidence ratios of stroke decreased in all GBD regions, with the exception of south Asia, eastern Europe, and high-income Asia Pacific, where they remained largely unchanged (Feigin *et al.* 2014).

Mortality-to-incidence ratios decreased for both ischemic (21%, 95% CI, 10–27%) and hemorrhagic (27%, 95% CI, 19–35%) stroke in high-income countries during 1990–2010. While mortality-to-incidence ratio also decreased for hemorrhagic stroke in low- and middle-income countries (36%, 95% CI, 16–49%), this was not significant for ischemic stroke (16%, 95% CI, –5 to 37%) (Krishnamurthi *et al.* 2013).

Incidence, Prevalence, and Time Trends

The incidence of new cases of first-ever TIA or stroke can only be reliably assessed in prospective population-based studies (Sudlow and Warlow 1996; Feigin *et al.* 2003; Rothwell *et al.* 2004) since hospital-based studies are subject to referral bias (Table 1.4). One of the most comprehensive population-based studies of stroke and TIA incidence is the Oxford Vascular Study (OXVASC), which has near-complete case ascertainment of all patients, irrespective of age, in a population of 93,000 defined by registration with nine general practices in Oxfordshire, UK (Coull *et al.* 2004). This is in contrast to previous studies, such as the MONICA project and the Framingham study, which had an age cutoff at 65 or 75 years or relied on voluntary participation.

The OXVASC study showed that the annual incidence of stroke in the UK in the first few years of this century, including subarachnoid hemorrhage, was 2.3/1,000 and the incidence of TIA was 0.5/1,000 (Rothwell *et al.* 2005), with about a quarter of events occurring in those under the age of 65 and about half in those above the age of 75 (Fig. 1.1). The incidence of cerebrovascular events in OXVASC was similar to that of acute coronary vascular events in the same population during the same period (Fig. 1.2), with a similar age distribution (Rothwell *et al.* 2005). Incidence rates, however, measure first-ever-in-a-lifetime definite events only and exclude possible, recurrent, and suspected events and so do not represent the true burden of a condition. This is especially true for TIA, where a significant proportion of cases referred to a TIA service have alternative, non-vascular conditions. Thus consequently, although the annual incidence of definite, first-ever-in-a-lifetime TIA in OXVASC was 0.5/1,000, the rate of definite or possible, incident or recurrent TIA was 1.1/1,000, and the rate of all referrals to a TIA clinic including all TIAs, suspected events with non-vascular causes and minor strokes was 3.0/1,000 (Giles and Rothwell 2007) (Table 1.5).

Table 1.4 Population- and hospital-based incidence studies

Study type	Description	Advantages	Disadvantages
Population-based	Multiple overlapping, prospective methods of case ascertainment used to identify all individuals with condition of interest from a predefined population; includes searches of both primary and secondary care and databases of diagnostic tests and death certification/ mortality statistics	More accurate measurement of incidence through minimizing referral bias: individuals who are not managed in the hospital are included, particularly elderly, those with mild conditions, and fatal events occurring outside the hospital	Time consuming and resource intensive
		Results of studies conducted in different populations and over different time periods can be directly compared (after statistical adjustment for age and sex)	Patients with the condition but who do not seek medical attention or who are misdiagnosed in primary care not included
		Representative of the requirements of an entire population	Mortality statistics are not collected reliably
Hospital-based	Methods of case ascertainment used to identify all cases that are referred, admitted, managed, or discharged from a hospital setting from a predefined population	Less time consuming and less resource intensive	Prone to referral bias; outpatient attendance variably included and events managed only in the community not included
	Typically, hospital-based databases only searched	Representative of the requirements for hospital services	Liable to inaccuracies of diagnostic coding
			Patients transferred between departments or hospitals either not identified or double counted
			Referral rates to the hospital vary geographically and over time; comparison between studies, therefore less reliable

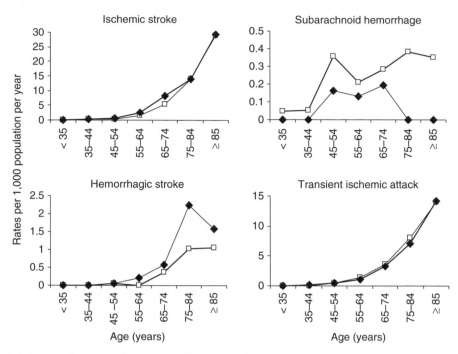

Fig. 1.1 Age-specific rates of all events for different types of acute cerebrovascular event in men (diamonds) and women (open squares) in Oxfordshire from 2002 to 2005 (Rothwell *et al.* 2005).

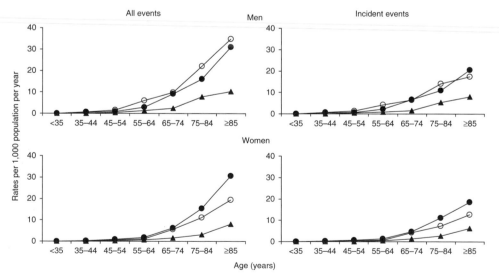

Fig. 1.2 Age-specific rates of all events and of incident events for stroke (i.e., not including transient ischemic attack; closed circles), myocardial infarction and sudden cardiac death combined (i.e., not including unstable angina; open circles), and acute peripheral vascular events (triangles) in men and women in Oxfordshire from 2002 to 2005 (Rothwell *et al.* 2005).

Table 1.5 Incidence rates of transient ischemic attack and stroke according to stringency of definition applied and previous cerebrovascular disease measured in OXVASC (2002–2005)

Category of event	Incidence rate (95% CI)[a]
TIA, incident only	
Definite	0.47 (0.39–0.56)
Definite and probable[b]	0.59 (0.5–0.68)
TIA, incident and recurrent	
Definite	0.82 (0.72–0.94)
Definite and probable[b]	0.95 (0.84–1.07)
All definite, probable, and suspected TIA (including all referrals to a TIA service with an eventual non-neurovascular diagnosis)	2.06 (1.89–2.23)
Stroke,[c] incident only	
Definite and probable	1.39 (1.25–1.54)
Stroke,[c] incident and recurrent	
Definite and probable	1.85 (1.70–2.02)
All definite, probable and suspected (including all referrals to the hospital of suspected stroke with an eventual non-neurovascular diagnosis)	2.29 (1.89–2.23)

Notes: CI, confidence interval; TIA, transient ischemic attack.
[a] Unadjusted rate per 1,000 population.
[b] Probable TIA defined as any transient symptoms lasting less than 24 hours of likely (but not certain) vascular etiology that was felt to justify secondary prevention treatment.
[c] Stroke includes ischemic and primary intracerebral hemorrhage but not subarachnoid hemorrhage.
Source: From Giles and Rothwell (2007).

Stroke prevalence is the total number of people with stroke in a population at a given time and is usually measured by cross-sectional surveys (Box 1.2). It is a function of stroke incidence and survival and, therefore, varies over time and between populations with differing age and sex structures. In the UK, the point prevalence of stroke was 507 (95% confidence interval [CI], 302–781) per 100,000 people in 1990 and 573 (95% CI, 339–899) per 100,000 people in 2010 (Feigin *et al.* 2014). Measuring TIA prevalence is methodologically more challenging because it is difficult to confirm, without direct patient assessment, whether transient neurological symptoms reported in a population survey are of vascular origin. Accurate data are, therefore, lacking, but a large telephone survey of randomly selected households in the USA reported a prevalence of physician-diagnosed TIA of 23/1,000 while a further 32/1,000 recalled symptoms consistent with TIA that had not been reported to medical attention (Johnston *et al.* 2003).

A reduction in stroke and TIA incidence since the late 1980s would be expected, given that randomized trials have shown several interventions to be effective in the primary and secondary prevention of stroke. The most recent studies of time trends in stroke incidence from GBD 2010 showed that from 1990 to 2010, the age-standardized incidence of stroke significantly decreased by 12% (95% CI, 6–17) in high-income countries but increased by

---

BOX 1.2 Definitions of Incidence and Prevalence

Incidence Rate The number of new cases of a condition per unit time per unit of population at risk. Usually expressed as the number of new cases per 1,000 or 100,000 population at risk per year.

Adjusted/Standardized Incidence Rates Overall incidence rates depend critically on the age and sex structure of the population studied. For example, a relatively old population may have a higher mortality rate than a younger population even if, age for age, the rates are similar. Incidence rates from different populations are, therefore, often compared following adjustment or standardization by applying age- and sex-specific rates to a "standard" population.

Prevalence Rate The total number of cases of a condition per unit of population at risk at a given time. Usually expressed as a percentage or the total number of cases per 1,000 or 100,000 population at risk.

12% (95% CI, –3 to 22%) in low- and middle-income countries (Feigin *et al.* 2014). When analyses were stratified by stroke subtype, incidence of ischemic and hemorrhagic stroke reduced by 13% (95% CI, 6–18%) and 19% (95% CI, 1–15%) respectively in high-income countries. In contrast, in low- and middle-income countries, ischemic stroke incidence increased non-significantly by 6% (95% CI, –7 to 32%) while hemorrhagic stroke incidence increased by 22% (95% CI, 5–30%) (Krishnamurthi *et al.* 2013). Similarly, between the periods 1981–1984 and 2002–2004, a 40% reduction in the incidence of fatal and disabling stroke was found in Oxfordshire, UK (Rothwell *et al.* 2004), although this reduction was less marked in the oldest old (Fig. 1.3). High-quality population-based studies of time trends in TIA and minor stroke are lacking. However, moderate rises in TIA incidence were reported in Oxfordshire, UK, between the periods 1981–1984 and 2002–2004 (Fig. 1.3) (Rothwell *et al.* 2004) and in Novosibirsk, Russia, between the periods 1987–1988 and 1996–1997 (Feigin *et al.* 2000), but no significant change in TIA incidence was found in Dijon, France, between 1985 and 1994 (Lemesle *et al.* 1999).

It is difficult to find a single explanation for the differences in change in incidence of major stroke in recent years in countries of different income levels and a contemporaneous stabilization or increase in the rates of TIA. Reductions in stroke incidence and mortality in high-income countries are likely related to better preventive strategies leading to a decline in the prevalence of causative risk factors, increased recognition of stroke symptoms leading to earlier medical advice sought, and better acute treatment and rehabilitation strategies (Murray *et al.* 2003; Wald and Law 2003). Increases in stroke incidence in low- and middle-income countries are likely to be more complex and may be related to a number of factors. Childhood mortality has substantially reduced and diseases related to infection and malnutrition have been replaced by non-communicable diseases such as stroke. Industrialization and urbanization have also led to an increase in smoking rates, and changes in nutritional quality of foods with increasing use of processed foods have resulted in an increased intake of salt and fat. Rises in TIA incidence are likely to reflect changes in public health awareness and behavior, with people now being more likely to seek medical attention for transient neurological symptoms.

Racial and Social Factors

There are racial and social differences in susceptibility to stroke and TIA (Forouhi and Satter 2006) and in the incidence of the various stroke subtypes (Fig. 1.4). Some of these

(a)

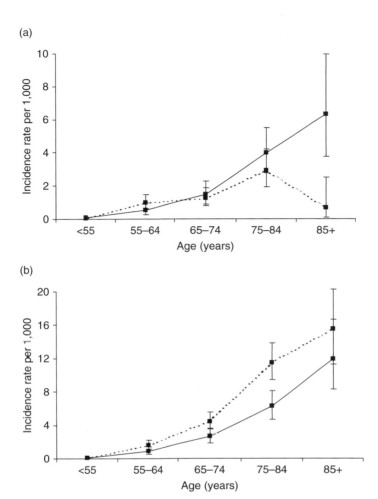

(b)

Fig. 1.3 The age-specific incidence of transient ischemic attack (a) and major disabling stroke (b) in Oxfordshire in 1981–1984 (the Oxford Community Stroke Project [OCSP], – – -) and 2002–2004 (the Oxford Vascular Study [OXVASC] —) (Rothwell *et al.* 2004).

racial differences are partly caused by differences in risk factor prevalence: hypertension and diabetes mellitus are more common in blacks, and coronary heart disease is more common in whites, for example (Sacco 2001). Other differences are not properly understood, such as the much higher proportion of stroke caused by intracerebral hemorrhage in Southeast Asia and the Far East than in Western countries (Krishnamurthi *et al.* 2013) and the higher prevalence of intracranial atherosclerosis in Black populations and Asians than in Western countries (Feldmann *et al.* 1990; Leung *et al.* 1993; Sacco *et al.* 1995; Wityk *et al.* 1996).

Black Populations The burden of stroke is higher in Blacks than Whites for both ischemic, particularly small vessel stroke, and hemorrhagic stroke (Woo *et al.* 1999; Schneider *et al.* 2004; Pandey and Gorelick 2005; White *et al.* 2005; Wolfe *et al.* 2006a, b). This pattern may be related in part to a higher prevalence of hypertension and diabetes mellitus (Gillum 1999;

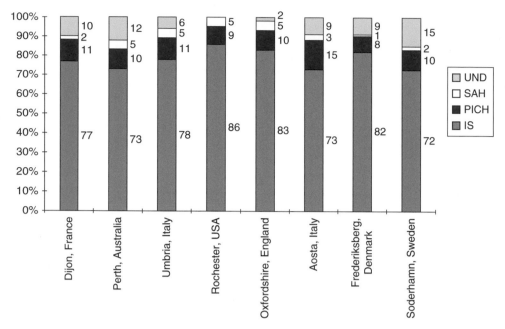

Fig. 1.4 The proportions of first-ever-in-a-lifetime strokes caused by ischemic stroke (IS), primary intracerebral hemorrhage (PICH), and subarachnoid hemorrhage (SAH) and of undetermined cause (UND) in "ideal" incidence studies. Numbers indicate the percentage estimates (Sudlow and Warlow 1997).

Sacco 2001). Intracranial large artery occlusive vascular disease also appears to be more common in Blacks than in Whites (Sacco *et al.* 1995; Wityk *et al.* 1996; Lynch and Gorelick 2000). In the single relevant study, rates of TIA were found to be higher in Blacks than Whites (Kleindorfer *et al.* 2005).

Maori and Pacific Islands People in New Zealand have a higher stroke incidence than Europeans, perhaps owing to differences in risk factors and health-related behaviors (Bonita *et al.* 1997; Feigin *et al.* 2006).

Chinese Stroke, particularly primary intracerebral hemorrhage, is more common in China than in Western countries (Krishnamurthi *et al.* 2013), which is probably attributable to the high prevalence of hypertension and smoking (Hu *et al.* 2012). There is also less extracranial but more intracranial arterial disease (Feldmann *et al.* 1990; Leung *et al.* 1993; Sacco *et al.* 1995; Wityk *et al.* 1996).

South Asian Populations People of South Asian origin in the UK have a high prevalence of coronary heart disease and stroke, central obesity (as evidenced by high waist-to-hip ratio), insulin resistance, non-insulin-dependent (type 2) diabetes, and hypertension (Cappuccio 1997; Kain *et al.* 2002; Bhopal *et al.* 2005). This increase in vascular risk seems to be a result partly of genetic susceptibility, such as high serum lipoprotein A levels, and partly of dietary- and lifestyle-induced changes in lipid levels.

Deprivation In the UK, both stroke incidence and poor outcome after stroke are greater in areas of socioeconomic disadvantage (Kaplan and Keil 1993; Avendaño *et al.* 2004). This is partly because poverty is associated with adverse health behaviors and risk factors such as smoking (Hart *et al.* 2000a). There is also evidence that poor maternal and infant health and poor nutrition are associated with an increased risk of stroke and stroke-related mortality in later life (Barker 1995; Martyn *et al.* 1996; Hankey 2012). However, the adverse effect of socioeconomic deprivation also appears to be cumulative throughout life (Davey Smith *et al.* 1997; Hart *et al.* 2000b).

Seasonal and Diurnal Variation

In most studies, both stroke mortality and hospital admission rates are higher in winter than in summer (Douglas *et al.* 1991; Pan *et al.* 1995; Feigin and Wiebers 1997). This seasonal variation might be explained by the complications of stroke being more likely to occur in the winter (e.g., pneumonia) and cannot simply be assumed to reflect stroke incidence. Where incidence has been measured in the community, there is little seasonal variation, at least in temperate climates, although primary intracerebral hemorrhage is somewhat more likely in the winter months and on cold days (Rothwell *et al.* 1996; Jakovljevic *et al.* 1996).

Stroke occurs most frequently in the hour or two after waking in the morning, but whether this applies to all subtypes of stroke is difficult to say because of the relatively small proportion of intracranial hemorrhages in most studies (Kelly-Hayes *et al.* 1995; Elliott 1998). Subarachnoid hemorrhage is very unlikely to occur during sleep and, in general, is most likely to occur during strenuous activities (Wroe *et al.* 1992). There are no equivalent data for TIA, although provisional results from OXVASC suggest that incidence also shows diurnal variation, and apparent TIA incidence falls slightly on the weekend, possibly because patients are less likely to present to medical attention (Giles *et al.* 2006).

References

Acheson J, Hutchinson EC (1964). Observations on the natural history of transient cerebral ischaemia. *Lancet* **ii**:871–874.

Advisory Council for the National Institute of Neurological and Communicative Disorders and Stroke (1975). A classification and outline of cerebrovascular diseases. II. *Stroke* 6:564–616.

Albers GW, Caplan LR, Easton JD *et al.* (2002). Transient ischemic attack: Proposal for a new definition. *New England Journal of Medicine* 347:1713–1716

Avendaño M, Kunst AE, Huisman M *et al.* (2004). Educational level and stroke mortality. A comparison of 10 European populations during the 1990s. *Stroke* 35:432–437

Barker DJP (1995). Fetal origins of coronary heart disease. *British Medical Journal* 311:171–174

Bhopal R, Fischbacher C, Vartiainen E *et al.* (2005). Predicted and observed cardiovascular disease in South Asians: Application of FINRISK, Framingham and SCORE models to Newcastle Heart Project data. *Journal of Public Health* 27:93–100

Bonita R, Broad JB, Beaglehole R (1997). Ethnic differences in stroke incidence and case fatality in Auckland New Zealand. *Stroke* 28:758–761

Cappuccio FP (1997). Ethnicity and cardiovascular risk: Variations in people of African ancestry and South Asian origin. *Journal of Human Hypertension* 11:571–576

Coull AJ, Lovett JK, Rothwell PM *et al.* (2004). Population based study of early risk of stroke after transient ischaemic attack or minor stroke: Implications for public education and organisation of services. *British Medical Journal* 328:326

Davey Smith G, Hart C, Blane D *et al.* (1997). Lifetime socioeconomic position and mortality:

Prospective observational study. *British Medical Journal* 314:547–552

Douglas AS, Allan TM, Rawles JM (1991). Composition of seasonality of disease. *Scottish Medical Journal* 36:76–82

Easton JD, Albers GW, Caplan LR *et al.* (2004). Discussion: Reconsideration of TIA terminology and definitions. *Neurology* 62:S29–S34

Elliott WJ (1998). Circadian variation in the timing of stroke onset: A meta-analysis. *Stroke* 29:992–996

Feigin VL, Wiebers DO (1997). Environmental factors and stroke: A selective review. *Journal of Stroke and Cerebrovascular Diseases* 6:108–113

Feigin VL, Shishkin SV, Tzirkin GM *et al.* (2000). A population-based study of transient ischemic attack incidence in Novosibirsk, Russia, 1987–1988 and 1996–1997. *Stroke* 31:9–13

Feigin VL, Shishkin SV, Tzirkin GM *et al.* (2003). A population-based study of transient ischemic attack incidence in Novosibirsk, Russia 1987–1988 and 1996–1997. *Stroke* 31:9–13

Feigin VL, Carter K, Hackett M *et al.* (2006). Ethnic disparities in incidence of stroke subtypes: Auckland Regional Community Stroke Study 2002–2003. *Lancet Neurology* 5:130–139

Feigin VL, Forouzanfar MH, Krishnamurthi R *et al.* (2014). Global and regional burden of stroke during 1990–2010: Findings from the Global Burden of Disease Study 2010. *Lancet* 383:245–255

Feldmann E, Daneault N, Kwan E *et al.* (1990). Chinese–white differences in the distribution of occlusive cerebrovascular disease. *Neurology* 40:1541–1545

Forouhi NG, Sattar N (2006). CVD risk factors and ethnicity: A homogeneous relationship? *Atherosclerosis Supplement* 7:11–19

Giles MF, Rothwell PM (2007). Substantial underestimation of the need for outpatient services for TIA and minor stroke. *Age Ageing* 36:676–680

Giles MF, Flossman E, Rothwell PM (2006). Patient behaviour immediately after transient ischemic attack according to clinical characteristics, perception of the event, and predicted risk of stroke. *Stroke* 37:1254–1260

Gillum RF (1999). Risk factors for stroke in blacks: A critical review. *American Journal of Epidemiology* 150:1266–1274

Hankey GJ (2012). Nutrition and the risk of stroke. *Lancet Neurology* 11:66–81

Hart CL, Hole DJ, Davey Smith G (2000a). Influence of socioeconomic circumstances in early and later life on stroke risk among men in a Scottish cohort study. *Stroke* 31:2093–2097

Hart CL, Hole DJ, Davey Smith G (2000b). The contribution of risk factors to stroke differentials by socioeconomic position in adulthood: The Renfrew/Paisley study. *American Journal of Public Health* 90:1788–1791

Hatano S (1976). Experience from a multicentre stroke register: A preliminary report. *Bulletin WHO* 54:541–553

Hu SS, Kong LZ, Gao RL *et al.* (2012). Outline of the report on cardiovascular disease in China, 2010. *Biomedical and Environmental Sciences* 25:251–256

Hunt JR (1914). The role of the carotid arteries in the causation of vascular lesions of the brain, with remarks on certain special features of symptomatology. *American Journal of Medical Science* 147:704

Jakovljevic D, Salomaa V, Sivenius J *et al.* (1996). Seasonal variation in the occurrence of stroke in a Finnish adult population. The FINMONICA Stroke Register. *Stroke* 27:1774–1779

Johnston SC, Fayad PB, Gorelick PB *et al.* (2003). Prevalence and knowledge of transient ischemic attack among US adults. *Neurology* 60:1429–1434

Kain K, Catto AJ, Young J *et al.* (2002). Increased fibrinogen, von Willebrand factor and tissue plasminogen activator levels in insulin resistant South Asian patients with ischaemic stroke. *Atherosclerosis* 163:371–376

Kaplan GA, Keil JE (1993). Socioeconomic factors and cardiovascular disease: A review of the literature. *Circulation* 88:1973–1998

Kelly-Hayes M, Wolf PA, Kase CS *et al.* (1995). Temporal patterns of stroke onset. The Framingham Study. *Stroke* 26:1343–1347

Kleindorfer D, Panagos P, Pancioli A *et al.* (2005). Incidence and short-term prognosis of transient ischemic attack in a population-based study. *Stroke* 36:720–723

Krishnamurthi RV, Feigin VL, Forouzanfar MH *et al.* (2013). Global and regional burden of first-ever ischemic and hemorrhagic stroke during 1990–2010: Findings from the Global Burden of Disease Study 2010. *Lancet Global Health* **1**: e259–281

Lemesle M, Milan C, Faivre J *et al.* (1999). Incidence trends of ischemic stroke and transient ischemic attacks in a well-defined French population from 1985 through 1994. *Stroke* **30**:371–377

Leung SY, Ng THK, Yuen ST *et al.* (1993). Pattern of cerebral atherosclerosis in Hong Kong Chinese: severity in intracranial and extracranial vessels. *Stroke* **24**:779–786

Lozano R, Naghavi M, Foreman *et al.* (2012). Global and regional mortality from 235 causes of death for 20 age groups in 1990 and 2010: A systematic analysis for the Global Burden of Disease Study 2010. *Lancet* **380**:2095–2128

Lynch GF, Gorelick PB (2000). Stroke in African Americans. *Neurology Clinic* **18**:273–290

MacDonald BK, Cockerell OC, Sander JWAS *et al.* (2000). The incidence and lifetime prevalence of neurological disorders in a prospective community-based study in the UK. *Brain* **123**:665–676

Marshall J (1964). The natural history of transient ischaemic cerebro-vascular attacks. *Quarterly Journal of Medicine* **33**:309–324.

Martyn CN, Barker DJP, Osmond C (1996). Mothers' pelvic size, fetal growth and death from stroke and coronary heart disease in men in the UK. *Lancet* **348**:1264–1268

Murray CJL, Vos T, Lozano R *et al.* (2012). Disability-adjusted life years (DALYs) for 291 diseases and injuries in 21 regions, 1990–2010: A systematic analysis for the Global Burden of Disease Study 2010. *Lancet* **380**:2197–2223

Murray CJL, Lauer JA, Hutubessy RCW *et al.* (2003). Effectiveness and costs on interventions to lower systolic blood pressure: A global and regional analysis on reduction of cardiovascular risk. *Lancet* **361**:717–725

Pan WH, Li LA, Tsai MJ (1995). Temperature extremes and mortality from coronary heart disease and cerebral infarction in elderly Chinese. *Lancet* **345**:353–355

Pandey DK, Gorelick PB (2005). Epidemiology of stroke in African Americans and Hispanic Americans. *Medical Clinics of North America* **89**:739–752

Pendlebury ST (2007). Worldwide under-funding of stroke research. *International Journal of Stroke* **2**:80–84

Pendlebury ST, Rothwell PM, Algra A *et al.* (2004). Underfunding of stroke research: A Europe-wide problem. *Stroke* **35**:2368–2371

Rothwell PM (2001). The high cost of not funding stroke research: A comparison with heart disease and cancer. *Lancet* **19**:1612–1616

Rothwell PM, Warlow CP (2005). Timing of transient ischaemic attacks preceding ischaemic stroke. *Neurology* **64**:817–820

Rothwell PM, Wroe SJ, Slattery J *et al.* (1996). Is stroke incidence related to season or temperature? *Lancet* **347**:934–936

Rothwell PM, Coull AJ, Giles MF *et al.* (2004). Change in stroke incidence, mortality, case-fatality, severity and risk factors in Oxfordshire, UK from 1981 to 2004 (Oxford Vascular Study). *Lancet* **363**:1925–1933

Rothwell PM, Coull AJ, Silver LE *et al.* (2005). Population-based study of event-rate, incidence, case fatality and mortality for all acute vascular events in all arterial territories (Oxford Vascular Study). *Lancet* **366**:1773–1783

Sacco RL (2001). Newer risk factors for stroke. *Neurology* **57**:S31–S34

Sacco RL, Kargman DE, Gu Q *et al.* (1995). Race-ethnicity and determinants of intracranial atherosclerotic cerebral infarction. The Northern Manhattan Stroke Study. *Stroke* **26**:14–20

Saka O, McGuire A, Wolfe C (2009). Cost of stroke in the United Kingdom. *Age and Ageing* **38**:27–32

Schneider AT, Kissela B, Woo D *et al.* (2004). Ischemic stroke subtypes: a population-based study of incidence rates among blacks and whites. *Stroke* **35**:1552–1556

Sempere AP, Duarte J, Cabezas C *et al.* (1998). Aetiopathogenesis of transient ischaemic attacks and minor ischaemic strokes: a community-based study in Segovia, Spain. *Stroke* **29**:40–45

Seshadri S, Belser A, Kelly-Hayes M *et al.* (2006). The lifetime risk of stroke: estimates from the Framingham Study. *Stroke* **37**:345–350

Sudlow CLM, Warlow CP (1996). Comparing stroke incidence worldwide. What makes the studies comparable? *Stroke* **27**:550–558

Sudlow CLM, Warlow CP (1997). Comparable studies of the incidence of stroke and its pathological types – results from an international collaboration. *Stroke* **28**:491–499

Wald NJ, Law MR (2003). A strategy to reduce cardiovascular disease by more than 80%. *British Medical Journal* **326**:1419

White H, Boden-Albala B, Wang C *et al.* (2005). Ischemic stroke subtype incidence among whites, blacks and Hispanics: the Northern Manhattan Study. *Circulation* **111**:1327–1331

Wityk RJ, Pessin MS, Kaplan RF *et al.* (1994). Serial assessment of acute stroke using the NIH Stroke Scale. *Stroke* **25**:362–365.

Wityk RJ, Lehman D, Klag M *et al.* (1996). Race and sex differences in the distribution of cerebral atherosclerosis. *Stroke* **27**:1974–1980

Wolfe CDA (2000). The impact of stroke. *British Medical Bulletin* **56**:275–286

Wolfe CD, Corbin DO, Smeeton NC *et al.* (2006a). Estimation of the risk of stroke in black populations in Barbados and South London. *Stroke* **37**:1986–1990

Wolfe CD, Corbin DO, Smeeton NC *et al.* (2006b). Poststroke survival for black-Caribbean populations in Barbados and South London. *Stroke* **37**:1991–1996

Woo D, Gebel J, Miller R *et al.* (1999). Incidence rates of first-ever ischemic stroke subtypes among blacks: A population-based study. *Stroke* **30**:2517–2522

Wroe SJ, Sandercock P, Bamford J *et al.* (1992). Diurnal variation in the incidence of stroke: the Oxfordshire Community Stroke Project. *British Medical Journal* **304**:155–157

Risk Factors

This chapter outlines the major known risk factors for TIA and stroke. Knowledge of these risk factors is necessary in order to understand the etiology of TIA and stroke, to predict risk, and to develop effective preventive strategies.

There are many more data on risk factors for acute coronary events than for ischemic stroke (Bhatia and Rothwell 2005) because of more intensive investigation in routine clinical practice and because heart disease receives much higher levels of research funding than stroke (Rothwell 2001; Pendlebury 2007).

The main risk factors for ischemic stroke are listed in Box 2.1. There are probably few qualitative differences between risk factors for ischemic stroke and coronary heart disease, but there are quantitative differences. Smoking, raised plasma cholesterol, and male sex are stronger risk factors for myocardial infarction, while hypertension is a stronger risk factor for stroke (Endres *et al.* 2011). The tendency for epidemiologists to lump all types of stroke together might explain some of the quantitative differences between risk factors for stroke and coronary heart disease. For example, it is possible that strokes associated with large artery disease have a more similar risk factor profile to coronary heart disease than cardioembolic stroke. To date, differences in risk factor relationships with the different stroke subtypes are unclear (Schulz and Rothwell 2003; Jackson and Sudlow 2005). The prevalence of various demographic and risk factors for different stroke subtypes in the Oxford Vascular Study are shown in Table 2.1.

Non-Modifiable Risk Factors

Age

Age is the strongest risk factor for ischemic stroke of all subtypes and for primary intracerebral hemorrhage, but it is less important for subarachnoid hemorrhage (Bamford *et al.* 1990; Rothwell *et al.* 2005). Overall stroke incidence at age 75–84 is approximately 25 times higher than at age 45–54 (see Fig. 1.2).

Sex and Sex Hormones

Stroke is slightly more common in men than in women (see Fig. 1.2), although the male excess is less marked than in coronary heart disease and peripheral arterial disease (Rothwell *et al.* 2005; Reeves *et al.* 2008). This excess of vascular events in men has been attributed to differences in endogenous sex hormones, in particular estrogen. In animal models, for example, female rodents with middle cerebral artery occlusion had smaller stroke volumes than males, whereas ovariectomized rodents had similar stroke volumes to males (McCullough *et al.* 2001). Estrogen improves endothelial function, decreases cerebral

---

BOX 2.1 Risk Factors for Ischemic Stroke

Factors associated with an increased risk of vascular disease

Increasing age	Sex hormones – hormonal contraception / hormone replacement therapy
Male sex	Substance abuse
Hypertension, high blood pressure variability	Excess alcohol consumption
Cigarette smoking	Migraine
Insulin resistance and diabetes mellitus	Chronic kidney disease
Blood lipids – high total cholesterol, apolipoprotein (Apo) B / ApoA1 ratio	Chronic inflammation
Atrial fibrillation	Recent infection[a]
Diet – low in fruits, vegetables or whole grains; high in sodium or sugar	Raised hematocrit
High body mass index	Raise white blood cell count
Obstructive sleep apnea	Hyperhomocystenemia
Physical inactivity	Raised von Willebrand factor[a]
Family history of stroke	Increasing plasma fibrinogen[a]
Air pollution – ambient fine particulate matter (PM$_{2.5}$) and household pollution from solid fuels	Raised factor VII coagulant activity[a]
Psychosocial – stress, depression, job strain, long working hours	Raised tissue plasminogen activator antigen[a]
Social deprivation	Low blood fibrinolytic activity[a]

Evidence of preexisting vascular disease

Transient ischemic attacks	Cardiac failure
Cervical arterial bruit and stenosis	Left ventricular hypertrophy
Myocardial infarction/angina	Peripheral vascular disease

[a] Possible association with stroke.

---

vascular tone, and increases cerebral blood flow, while testosterone has opposite effects (Krause *et al.* 2006).

With menopause, there is a significant decline in estrogen levels with relative androgen excess, which is accompanied by a doubling in stroke risk in the decade after menopause (Lisabeth and Bushnell 2012). These changes in endogenous hormone levels are associated with an increase in total cholesterol, LDL-cholesterol, and apolipoprotein B within 1 year of the last menstrual period (Matthews *et al.* 2009), possibly accounting for the marked increase in stroke risk after menopause. Clinical trials on exogenous oral estrogen with or without progesterone in post-menopausal women have been disappointing, however, and

Table 2.1 Demographics and risk factor prevalence in incident strokes in OXVASC

	Prevalence (%)		
	IS[a]	PICH[b]	SAH[b]
Mean age	74.9	75.3	54.8
Male (%)	48.6	50.0	30.3
Previous acute coronary syndrome	11.5	15.4	3.0
Previous acute peripheral vascular event	2.9	3.8	0.0
History of hypertension	56.3	59.6	24.2
Diabetes mellitus	10.1	0.0	3.0
Hypercholesterolemia	20.1	14.3	6.1
Atrial fibrillation	18.2	15.4	0.0
Current smoker	17.2	15.4	24.2

Notes: IS, ischemic stroke; PICH, primary intracerebral hemorrhage; SAH, subarachnoid hemorrhage.
[a] Three-year data from 2002 to 2005.
[b] Five-year data from 2002 to 2007.
Sources: From Rothwell et al. (2004a) and Lovelock et al. (2007).

meta-analysis of existing trials has shown that hormone replacement therapy is associated with a 32% increased risk of stroke and twofold increased risk of venous thromboembolic events (Sare et al. 2008). Similarly, exogenous high-dose estrogen given to elderly men with prostatic cancer increases their risk of vascular death (Byar and Corle 1988).

It is postulated that an increased risk of stroke and venous thromboembolic events with hormone replacement therapy may be related to the route (oral versus transdermal), dose and timing of estrogen administration after onset of menopausal symptoms (Lisabeth and Bushnell 2012). Transdermal estrogen appears to be safer than oral estrogen with respect to stroke risk because it is not metabolized via the liver and hence does not result in an increase in clotting factors and inflammatory markers seen with oral replacement (Hemelaar et al. 2008; Renoux et al. 2010). However, the Kronos Early Estrogen Prevention Study did not show any significant differences in carotid intima-media thickness or coronary artery calcium score progression in patients who were randomized to having oral versus transdermal route of estrogen (Harman et al. 2014). Increasing dosages of estrogen have also been associated with higher risks of TIA or ischemic stroke (Grodstein et al. 2000; Renoux et al. 2010). Timing of hormonal therapy after menopausal symptoms is also important as estrogen replacement at physiological concentrations may have beneficial effects on endothelial dysfunction during the early stages of atherosclerosis, but in patients with established disease, estrogen may be harmful by promoting progression and instability of atherosclerotic plaque (Mendelsohn and Karas 2005). Oral estrogen is associated with a lower risk of carotid intima-media thickness progression if initiated within 6 years of menopause but not if initiated 10 or more years after menopause (Hodis et al. 2016).

However, risk of stroke does not differ in individuals on estrogen alone or on combined estrogen plus progestin (Renoux *et al.* 2010).

Oral contraceptives increase the risk of ischemic stroke (the risk is less for hemorrhagic stroke), but the increased risk is small for low-dose estrogen preparations unless there are associated factors such as migraine or cigarette smoking (Chang *et al.* 1999; Bousser and Kittner 2000; Donaghy *et al.* 2002).

Genetics

The genetics of sporadic and familial stroke are further discussed in Chapter 3.

Modifiable Risk Factors

Recent large studies on modifiable risk factors of stroke – e.g., Global Burden of Disease Study 2013 (Feigin *et al.* 2016) and INTERSTROKE (O'Donnell *et al.* 2016) – have demonstrated that approximately 90% of the global stroke burden is attributable to modifiable risk factors. These include (1) hypertension; (2) poor diet (high in sodium; low in fruits, vegetables, and whole grains); (3) obesity (high body mass index and waist-to-hip ratio); (4) smoking; (5) dyslipidemia (high total cholesterol and apolipoprotein [Apo] B / ApoA1 ratio); (6) atrial fibrillation; (7) air pollution (ambient particulate matter pollution and household air pollution from solid fuels); (8) high fasting blood glucose; (9) low physical activity; (10) excess alcohol consumption; and (11) psychosocial factors (stress and depression).

Blood Pressure

Hypertension is the most important treatable risk factor for stroke with a population attributable risk of about 48% (Endres *et al.* 2011; O'Donnell *et al.* 2016). Increasing blood pressure is strongly associated with subsequent stroke risk (Gil-Nunez and Vivancos-Mora 2005; Goldstein and Hankey 2006), and stroke mortality rises steeply, more marked in the young than in the old, with increasing systolic blood pressure (Kearney *et al.* 2005) (Fig. 2.1). The relationship between usual diastolic blood pressure and stroke is "log–linear" throughout the normal range, with no evidence of a threshold below which the risk becomes stable (Rodgers *et al.* 1996). Stroke incidence doubles with each 7.5 mmHg increase in usual diastolic blood pressure in Western populations and with each 5.0 mmHg in Japanese and Chinese populations (MacMahon *et al.* 1990; Eastern Stroke and Coronary Heart Disease Collaborative Research Group 1998; Lewington *et al.* 2002). Visit-to-visit variability in systolic blood pressure and maximum systolic blood pressure are also strong predictors of stroke, independent of mean systolic blood pressure (Rothwell *et al.* 2010).

The strength of the association between blood pressure and stroke is attenuated with increasing age, although the absolute risk of stroke in the elderly is far higher than in the young (Lewington *et al.* 2002). Nevertheless, hypertension is still a risk factor in the very elderly, although it is weaker because stroke may be associated with low blood pressure owing to cardiac failure and other comorbid conditions (Birns *et al.* 2005). Moreover, in patients with bilateral severe carotid stenosis or occlusion, stroke risk is higher at low blood pressures, suggesting that aggressive blood pressure lowering may be harmful in this group (Rothwell *et al.* 2003). The relationship with systolic blood pressure is similar and possibly

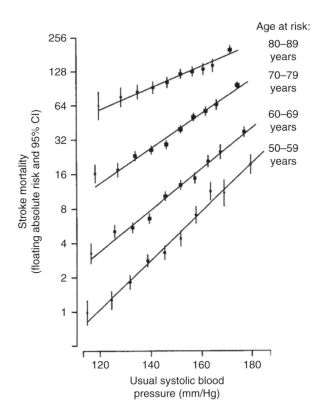

Age at risk:

80–89 years

70–79 years

60–69 years

50–59 years

Fig. 2.1 Stroke mortality by usual systolic blood pressure and age showing a steep rise in mortality with rising blood pressure and that the rate of risk increase with change in blood pressure is greater in the young than in the old (from Kearney *et al.* 2005). CI, confidence interval.

stronger than with diastolic blood pressure (Keli *et al.* 1992), and even "isolated" systolic hypertension is associated with increased risk (Sagie *et al.* 1993; Petrovitch *et al.* 1995; Lewington *et al.* 2002). Hypertension is more common in stroke patients from black than from white populations (Sacco 2001).

Cigarette Smoking

Cigarette smoking is associated with ischemic stroke, with a relative risk of approximately 2. There is a dose–response relationship, and males and females are equally affected (Shah *et al.* 2010). Smoking has been related to the extent of carotid disease on arterial angiography (Homer *et al.* 1991), on ultrasound (Fine-Edelstein *et al.* 1994; Howard *et al.* 1998), and in identical twins discordant for smoking (Haapanen *et al.* 1989). The evidence for a link between cigarette smoking and primary intracerebral hemorrhage is less clear (Shah *et al.* 2010). However, smoking remains one of the most important risk factors for subarachnoid hemorrhage (Feigin *et al.* 2005). Environmental smoke similarly increases the risk of stroke (Shah *et al.* 2010). In light smokers (<20 cigarettes / day), risk of stroke reduces to a level that is similar to non-smokers at around 5 years after smoking cessation (Wannamethee *et al.* 1995). Although use of electronic cigarettes is becoming more popular, epidemiological data on stroke risk due to use of electronic cigarettes are lacking. Recent animal studies utilizing mouse models have shown that electronic cigarettes may be no safer than tobacco smoking and may pose a similar, if not higher, risk for severe strokes (Sifat *et al.* 2017).

Diabetes Mellitus and Insulin Resistance

Diabetes doubles the risk of ischemic stroke (Tuomilehto and Rastenyte 1999; Wannamethee *et al.* 1999; Rothwell 2005), and the risk of fatal stroke is higher in those with a higher glycosylated hemoglobin (HbA1c) at diagnosis (Stevens *et al.* 2004). There is a high prevalence of diabetes in stroke patients from black populations (Sacco 2001). It should be noted that any studies linking diabetes with stroke mortality data will exaggerate the association because diabetics who have a stroke are more likely to die of it than non-diabetics (Jorgensen *et al.* 1994). Randomized trials have shown that diabetic treatment with insulin or sulfonylureas decreases progression of carotid intima-media thickness and reduces the risk of microvascular and macrovascular complications of diabetes (UK Prospective Diabetes Study [UKPDS] Group 1998; Diabetes Control and Complications Trial/Epidemiology of Diabetes Interventions and Complications Research Group 2003, 2005).

Individuals with insulin resistance without diabetes are similarly at increased risk of ischemic stroke (Rundek *et al.* 2010). Pioglitazone reduces the risk of recurrent stroke and myocardial infarction in TIA/ischemic stroke patients with insulin resistance (Kernan *et al.* 2016).

Blood Lipids

Increasing levels of total plasma cholesterol and low density lipoprotein cholesterol, and to a lesser extent decreasing levels of high density lipoprotein cholesterol, are strong risk factors for coronary heart disease, whereas blood triglyceride levels are less predictive. Reduction of plasma cholesterol by 1 mmol/L reduces the relative risk of coronary events by at least a third (Lewington and Clarke 2005), with little diminution of benefit in the elderly (Clarke *et al.* 2002; Huxley *et al.* 2002; Baigent *et al.* 2005). The relationship between blood lipids and stroke is much weaker, but there is some evidence that cholesterol is negatively associated with intracranial hemorrhage, which obscures the weak positive association with ischemic stroke in studies where stroke subtype is not characterized (Prospective Studies Collaboration 1995; Eastern Stroke and Coronary Heart Disease Collaborative Research Group 1998; Koren-Morag *et al.* 2002; Zhang *et al.* 2003).

Data from the Heart Protection Study of cholesterol lowering in patients with known vascular disease or diabetes have shown that such therapy reduces the risk of stroke on follow-up, but it did not show a reduction in recurrent stroke (Heart Protection Study Collaborative Group 2002; Collins *et al.* 2004), possibly because of lack of differentiation of stroke subtype or the fact that patients were at low risk of stroke recurrence since the incident strokes occurred on average 4.6 years before the study onset. However, the Stroke Prevention by Aggressive Reduction in Cholesterol Levels (SPARCL) trial showed that atorvastatin in patients who had had a stroke or TIA within 1 to 6 months before study entry did reduce overall stroke risk (Amarenco *et al.* 2006), although there was a significant increase in risk of intracerebral hemorrhage on statin treatment (Chapter 24). Interestingly, the same trend had been found in the Heart Protection Study in the 3,280 patients with previous stroke or TIA (Collins *et al.* 2004), in whom simvastatin 40 mg also increased the risk of hemorrhagic stroke, although this risk was not seen in meta-analyses of primary prevention trials (Amarenco and Labreuche 2009). Thus, the randomized evidence does suggest that there is a causal association between plasma low density lipoprotein cholesterol and risk of ischemic stroke, but more work is required to determine the cause of the increase in risk of hemorrhagic stroke.

Atrial Fibrillation

Non-rheumatic atrial fibrillation is by far the most common cause of cardioembolic stroke but cannot cause more than one-fifth of all ischemic strokes since it is present in this proportion of patients who have an ischemic stroke (Sandercock et al. 1992; Schulz and Rothwell 2003; Rothwell et al. 2004a); this excludes the very elderly, where its prevalence is highest (Yiin et al. 2014). The average absolute risk of stroke in patients without prior stroke who have non-rheumatic atrial fibrillation and are not taking anticoagulation drugs is approximately 4% per year, five to six times greater than in those in sinus rhythm (Hart et al. 1999; Wolf et al. 1991; Lip 2005); the risk is much higher again in patients with rheumatic atrial fibrillation.

The stroke risk associated with atrial fibrillation in an individual patient is higher in the presence of a previous embolic event, increasing age, hypertension, diabetes, left ventricular dysfunction, or an enlarged left atrium (Stroke Prevention in Atrial Fibrillation Investigators 1992, 1995; Atrial Fibrillation Investigators 1994, 1998; di Pasquale et al. 1995; Lip and Boos 2006). At least 10 similar stroke risk stratification schemes for atrial fibrillation have been published (Lip and Boos 2006; Nattel and Opie 2006; Lip et al. 2010). The best validated of these, the CHA_2DS_2-VASc Score, attributes 1 point each for age 65–74, female sex, congestive heart failure, hypertension, vascular disease, and diabetes history and 2 points for age ≥75 years and history of prior stroke, TIA, or thromboembolism (Chapter 24). Patients with a CHA_2DS_2-VASc score of 0 have a stroke risk of 0.2% per year and a stroke, TIA, or systemic embolism risk of 0.3% per year (Friberg et al. 2012), while those with a maximum score of 9 have a yearly stroke risk of 12.2% and 17.4% risk of stroke, TIA, or systemic embolism (Friberg et al. 2012) (Chapter 14).

Paroxysmal atrial fibrillation carries the same stroke risk as persistent atrial fibrillation (Lip and Hee 2001; Saxonhouse and Curtis 2003) and should be treated similarly. There is no evidence that conversion to sinus rhythm followed by pharmacotherapy to try to maintain such rhythm is superior to rate control in terms of mortality and stroke risk (Segal et al. 2001; Blackshear and Safford 2003; Hart et al. 2003).

Some of the association between atrial fibrillation and stroke must be coincidental because atrial fibrillation can be caused by coronary and hypertensive heart disease, both of which may be associated with atheromatous disease or primary intracerebral hemorrhage. Although anticoagulation markedly reduces the risk of first or recurrent stroke, this is not necessarily evidence for causality because this treatment may be working in other ways, such as by inhibiting artery-to-artery embolism, although trials of warfarin in secondary prevention of stroke in sinus rhythm have shown no benefit over aspirin (Chapter 24).

Cardioembolism

Apart from atrial fibrillation, there are many other causes of cardioembolic stroke including prosthetic heart valves and patent foramen ovale (see Chapter 6).

Obesity and the Metabolic Syndrome

Any relationship between obesity and stroke is likely to be confounded by the positive association of obesity with hypertension, diabetes, hypercholesterolemia, and lack of exercise and the negative association with smoking and concurrent illness. Nevertheless, stroke is more common in the obese, and abdominal obesity appears to be an independent predictor of stroke (Suk *et al.* 2003). The constellation of metabolic abnormalities including central obesity, decreased high density lipoprotein, elevated triglycerides, elevated blood pressure, and impaired glucose tolerance is known as the metabolic syndrome and is associated with a threefold increase risk of type 2 diabetes and a twofold increase in cardiovascular risk (Eckel *et al.* 2005; Grundy *et al.* 2005).

Metabolic syndrome is thought to be the main driver for the modern-day epidemic of diabetes and vascular disease. As well as primary prevention of acute vascular events in patients with the metabolic syndrome (Eckel *et al.* 2005; Grundy *et al.* 2005), an additional aim should be prevention of progression to frank diabetes. Both lifestyle modification with diet and exercise (Tuomilehto *et al.* 2001; Diabetes Prevention Program Research Group 2002) and treatment with angiotensin-converting enzyme inhibitors or angiotensin antagonists (Yusuf *et al.* 2000; Dahlof *et al.* 2002; Julius *et al.* 2004) have been shown to be effective in reducing progression to diabetes in patients with the metabolic syndrome.

Diet

Relating various dietary constituents to the risk of vascular disease is difficult since observational data are likely to be biased. As noted previously, there is good evidence that dietary and lifestyle modification can improve vascular risk in patients with the metabolic syndrome, but randomized trials of dietary interventions, including fish oil supplementation and vitamin supplementation, have generally been disappointing (Steinberg 1995; Stephens 1997; GISSI-Prevenzione Investigators 1999; Leppala *et al.* 2000; Yusuf *et al.* 2000; Heart Protection Study Collaborative Group 2002; Hooper *et al.* 2004, 2008).

A higher sodium intake is associated with an increased risk of stroke (Aburto *et al.* 2013), and a reduction in salt intake reduces blood pressure in both normotensive and hypertensive individuals (He and MacGregor 2004). However, it remains unclear whether reducing sodium intake lowers stroke risk (Adler *et al.* 2014). In contrast, a high intake of potassium may reduce stroke risk (Khaw and Barrett-Connor 1987; Whelton *et al.* 1997).

Compared to individuals with less than three servings of fruit and vegetables a day, those with three to five servings per day are at 11% lower risk of stroke, and those who have more than five servings per day are at 26% lower risk of stroke (He *et al.* 2006). An increased fish intake is also associated with a lower risk of stroke, in particular ischemic stroke (He *et al.* 2004). The Mediterranean diet supplemented with extra-virgin oil or nuts has also been shown to reduce the incidence of major cardiovascular events, including stroke (Estruch *et al.* 2013).

Exercise

A systematic review of 23 studies found that moderate and high levels of physical activity are associated with reduced risk of all stroke (Lee *et al.* 2003). This reduced risk is thought to be related to lower body weight, blood pressure, blood viscosity, fibrinogen concentration, and better lipid profiles.

Alcohol

A systematic review of thirty-five observational studies indicated that heavy (> 5 units/day) alcohol consumption increases the relative risk of stroke by 1.6 (95% confidence interval [CI], 1.4–1.9), particularly hemorrhagic stroke (relative risk, 2.18; 95% CI, 1.5–3.2) (Reynolds *et al.* 2003). Moderate consumption of alcohol appears to lower stroke risk by comparison with abstention (Reynolds *et al.* 2003; Elkind *et al.* 2006). Binge drinking is also independently associated with stroke (Sundell *et al.* 2008).

Recreational Drug Use

Recreational drugs may cause stroke due to a number of different mechanisms. Sympathomimetics such as amphetamines may result in a sudden rise in blood pressure resulting in intracerebral hemorrhage (Westover *et al.* 2007). Cocaine is a potent vasoconstrictor and has been associated with both ischemic and hemorrhagic stroke (Westover *et al.* 2007). Cannabis is also a potent vasoactive agent and has been associated with ischemic stroke secondary to reversible multifocal intracranial stenosis, a variant of reversible cerebral vasoconstriction syndrome (Wolff *et al.* 2013). Recreational drugs such as amphetamine, cocaine, and cannabis as well as non-recreational drugs that have vasoactive effects have also been associated with reversible cerebral vasoconstriction syndrome (Ducros 2012).

Intravenous injection of recreational drugs may be accompanied by injection of air and talcum powder, resulting in embolic strokes. Bacteria may also be injected, causing right-sided valvular infective endocarditis and strokes due to septic emboli. Agents administered subcutaneously may be associated with vasculitis due to toxic or hypersensitivity reactions.

Obstructive Sleep Apnea

Obstructive sleep apnea increases the risk of stroke, including wake-up stroke (Hsieh *et al.* 2012), independent of body habitus, hypertension, and other cardiovascular risk factors (Yaggi *et al.* 2005). Possible mechanisms include acute hemodynamic changes during apneic episodes, decreased cerebral blood flow, paradoxical embolization, hypercoagulability, hypoxia-related cerebral ischemia, and increased arterial stiffness and sympathetic tone (Yaggi et *al.* 2005).

Renal Disease

An impaired glomerular filtration rate and proteinuria are risk factors of both ischemic and hemorrhagic stroke, independent of age, sex, and cardiovascular risk factors (Ninomiya *et al.* 2009; Lee *et al.* 2010; Gutiérrez *et al.* 2012; Toyoda *et al.* 2014). Besides shared risk factors (age, hypertension, diabetes, hyperlipidemia, and smoking), patients with renal impairment are also susceptible to stroke due to raised levels of inflammatory and thrombogenic markers, increased oxidative stress, and sympathetic nerve overactivity (Toyoda *et al.* 2014). In more severe cases of renal failure with uremia, patients have an accumulation of uremic toxins and are also anemic and malnourished as well as having various electrolyte disorders (e.g., calcium and phosphate abnormalities) (Toyoda *et al.* 2014). These factors would result in endothelial dysfunction, vascular calcification, and arteriosclerosis, further increasing the risk of stroke (Toyoda *et al.* 2014).

Hemostatic Variables

Despite much effort, very few consistent associations have been found between coagulation parameters, fibrinolytic activity, platelet behavior, and risk of stroke (Markus and Hambley 1998; Sacco 2001). Although there is a relationship between increasing plasma fibrinogen and stroke (Rothwell et al. 2004b; Danesh et al. 2005), it is attenuated by adjusting for cigarette smoking and other confounding variables such as infections and social class (Brunner et al. 1996; Lowe et al. 1997). Raised plasma factor VII coagulant activity, raised tissue plasminogen activator antigen, low blood fibrinolytic activity, and raised von Willebrand factor are risk factors for coronary heart disease and perhaps also for stroke (Meade et al. 1993; Qizilbash et al. 1997; Macko et al. 1999).

Hematocrit

Although cerebral blood flow is strongly related to hematocrit, any effect of increasing hematocrit on risk of stroke or type of stroke is weak and confounded by cigarette smoking, blood pressure, and plasma fibrinogen (Welin et al. 1987). However, raised hematocrit does seem to be associated with an increased case fatality in ischemic stroke (Allport et al. 2005).

Infections and Inflammation

Both chronic and acute infection have been implicated in the development and stability of atheromatous plaques (Danesh et al. 1997). Although patients with periodontal disease have been associated with ischemic stroke (Grau et al. 2004), observational epidemiological studies of infections in general (Grau et al. 1998), together with serological evidence of specific infectious agents (e.g., Chlamydia pneumoniae, Helicobacter pylori, and cytomegalovirus), have not shown convincing evidence of a relationship with stroke or coronary heart disease (Markus and Mendall 1998; Danesh et al. 1999, 2000; Fagerberg et al. 1999; Glader et al. 1999; Strachan et al. 1999; Danesh et al. 2003; Ngeh et al. 2003). Randomized trials using clarithromycin to eliminate chlamydia infection in patients with stable coronary artery disease resulted in a higher risk of cardiovascular mortality in the treatment arm (Jespersen et al. 2006).

Homocysteinemia

There is an association between the rare inborn recessive condition of homocysteinemia and arterial and venous thrombosis, and observational data link coronary heart disease, stroke, and venous thromboembolism with increasing plasma homocysteine (Wald et al. 2002, 2004). This led to trials of folic acid and pyridoxine supplementation to lower homocysteine levels (Hankey 2002; Hankey and Eikelboom 2005). Results from such trials have so far been disappointing: the Vitamin Intervention for Stroke Prevention Study (VISP) and the Norwegian Vitamin Trial (NORVIT) (Toole et al. 2004; Bonaa et al. 2006) trials showed no treatment effect on recurrent stroke, coronary events, or deaths. Preliminary results from the Study of Vitamins to Prevent Stroke (VITATOPS) trial have shown no evidence of reduced levels of inflammation, endothelial dysfunction, or the hypercoagulability postulated to be increased by elevated homocysteine levels in patients with previous TIA or stroke treated with folic acid, vitamin B_{12}, and vitamin B_6 (Dusitanond et al. 2005). However, a recent systematic review of all randomized trials of homocysteine lowering does suggest a modest reduction in stroke risk (Wang et al. 2007).

Non-Stroke Vascular Disease

Coronary heart disease is associated with ischemic stroke in postmortem (Stemmermann *et al.* 1984), twin (Brass *et al.* 1996), case–control (Feigin *et al.* 1998), and cohort studies (Harmsen *et al.* 1990; Shaper *et al.* 1991; Wolf *et al.* 1991; Touzé *et al.* 2006) as are electrocardiographic abnormalities, cardiac failure, left ventricular hypertrophy, claudication, and asymptomatic peripheral vascular disease (Leys *et al.* 2006).

Abdominal aortic aneurysms occur in about 10–20% of patients with cerebrovascular disease, but it is not known if people with aneurysms have more strokes or other vascular events compared with people without aneurysms (Hollander *et al.* 2003; Leys *et al.* 2006).

Other Possible Associations

Innumerable other risk factors have been linked with coronary heart disease, and to a lesser extent stroke, but data are sparse, and there is probably a lot of confounding.

References

Aburto NJ, Ziolkovska A, Hooper L *et al.* (2013). Effect of lower sodium intake on health: Systematic review and meta-analyses. *British Medical Journal* 346:f1326

Adler AJ, Taylor F, Martin N *et al.* (2014). Reduced dietary salt for the prevention of cardiovascular disease. *Cochrane Database of Systematic Reviews* 12:CD009217

Allport LE, Parsons MW, Butcher KS *et al.* (2005). Elevated hematocrit is associated with reduced reperfusion and tissue survival in acute stroke. *Neurology* 65:1382–1387

Amarenco P, Bogousslavsky J, Callahan A III *et al.* (2006). High-dose atorvastatin after stroke or transient ischemic attack. *New England Journal of Medicine* 355:549–559

Amarenco P, Labreuche J (2009). Lipid management in the prevention of stroke: Review and updated meta-analysis of statins for stroke prevention. *Lancet Neurology* 8:453–463

Atrial Fibrillation Investigators (1994). Risk factors for stroke and efficacy of antithrombotic therapy in atrial fibrillation. *Archives of Internal Medicine* 154:1449–1457

Atrial Fibrillation Investigators (1998). Echocardiographic predictors of stroke in patients with atrial fibrillation. *Archives of Internal Medicine* 158:1316–1320

Baigent C, Keech A, Kearney PM *et al.* (2005). Efficacy and safety of cholesterol-lowering treatment: Prospective meta-analysis of data from 90 056 participants in 14 randomized trials of statins. *Lancet* 66:1267–1278

Bamford J, Sandercock PAG, Dennis M *et al.* (1990). A prospective study of acute cerebrovascular disease in the community: The Oxfordshire Community Stroke Project 1981–86. 2. Incidence, case fatality rates and overall outcome at one year of cerebral infarction, primary intracerebral and subarachnoid haemorrhage. *Journal of Neurology, Neurosurgery and Psychiatry* 53:16–22

Bhatia M, Rothwell PM (2005). A systematic comparison of the published data available on risk factors for stroke, compared with risk factors for coronary heart disease. *Cerebrovascular Diseases* 20:180–186

Birns J, Markus H, Kalra L (2005). Blood pressure reduction for vascular risk: Is there a price to be paid? *Stroke* 36:1308–1313

Blackshear JL, Safford RE (2003). AFFIRM and RACE trials: Implications for the management of atrial fibrillation. *Cardiology Electrophysiology Review* 7:366–369

Bonaa KH, Njlstad I, Ueland PM *et al.* (2006). Homocysteine lowering and cardiovascular events after acute myocardial infarction. *New England Journal of Medicine* 354:1578–1588

Bousser MG, Kittner SJ (2000). Oral contraceptives and stroke. *Cephalagia* 20:183–189

Brass LM, Hartigan PM, Page WF *et al.* (1996). Importance of cerebrovascular disease in studies of myocardial infarction. *Stroke* 27:1173–1176

Brunner E, Davey Smith G, Marmot M et al. (1996). Childhood social circumstances and psychosocial and behavioural factors as determinants of plasma fibrinogen. Lancet 347:1008–1013

Byar DP, Corle DK (1988). Hormone therapy for prostate cancer: Results of the Veterans Administration Cooperative Urological Research Group Studies. NCI Monographs 7:165–170

Chang CL, Donaghy M, Poulter N et al. (1999). Migraine and stroke in young women: Case–control study. British Medical Journal 318:13–18

Clarke R, Lewington S, Youngman L et al. (2002). Underestimation of the importance of blood pressure and cholesterol for coronary heart disease mortality in old age. European Heart Journal 23:286–293

Collins R, Armitage J, Parish S et al. (2004). Effects of cholesterol-lowering with simvastatin on stroke and other major vascular events in 20 536 people with cerebrovascular disease or other high-risk conditions. Lancet 363:757–767

Dahlof B, Devereux RB, Kjeldsen SE et al. (2002). Cardiovascular morbidity and mortality in Losartan Intervention For End Point Reduction in Hypertension (LIFE) study: A randomized trial against atenolol. Lancet 359:995–1003

Danesh J, Collins R, Peto R (1997). Chronic infections and coronary heart disease: Is there a link? Lancet 350:430–436

Danesh J, Youngman L, Clark S et al. (1999). Helicobacter pylori infection and early onset myocardial infarction: Case–control and sibling pairs study. British Medical Journal 319:1157–1162

Danesh J, Whincup P, Walker M et al. (2000). Chlamydia pneumoniae IgG titres and coronary heart disease: Prospective study and meta-analysis. British Medical Journal 321:208–213

Danesh J, Whincup P, Walker M (2003). Chlamydia pneumoniae IgA titres and coronary heart disease: Prospective study and meta-analysis. European Heart Journal 24:881

Danesh J, Lewington S, Thompson SG et al. (2005). Plasma fibrinogen level and the risk of major cardiovascular diseases and non-vascular mortality: An individual participant meta-analysis. Journal of American Medical Association 294:1799–1809

Diabetes Control and Complications Trial/ Epidemiology of Diabetes Interventions and Complications Research Group (2003). Intensive diabetes therapy and carotid intima-media thickness in type I diabetes mellitus. New England Journal of Medicine 346:393–403

Diabetes Control and Complications Trial/ Epidemiology of Diabetes Interventions and Complications Research Group (2005). Intensive diabetes treatment and cardiovascular disease in patients with type I diabetes. New England Journal of Medicine 353:2643–2653

Diabetes Prevention Program Research Group (2002). Reduction in the incidence of type 2 diabetes with lifestyle intervention or metformin. New England Journal of Medicine 346:393–403

di Pasquale G, Urbinati S, Pinelli G (1995). New echocardiographic markers of embolic risk in atrial fibrillation. Cerebrovascular Diseases 5:315–322

Donaghy M, Chang CL, Poulter N et al. (2002). European Collaborators of the World Health Organization Collaborative Study of Cardiovascular Disease and Steroid Hormone Contraception. Duration, frequency, recency, and type of migraine and the risk of ischemic stroke in women of childbearing age. Journal of Neurology, Neurosurgery and Psychiatry 73:747–750

Ducros A (2012). Reversible cerebral vasoconstriction syndrome. Lancet Neurology 11:906–917

Dusitanond P, Eikelboom JW, Hankey GJ et al. (2005). Homocysteine-lowering treatment with folic acid, cobalamin and pyridoxine does not reduce blood markers of inflammation, endothelial dysfunction or hypercoagulability in patients with previous transient ischemic attack or stroke: A randomized substudy of the VITATOPS trial. Stroke 36:144–146

Eastern Stroke and Coronary Heart Disease Collaborative Research Group (1998). Blood pressure, cholesterol and stroke in Eastern Asia. Lancet 352:1801–1807

Eckel RH, Grundy SM, Zimmet PZ (2005). The metabolic syndrome. *Lancet* **365**: 1415–1428

Elkind MS, Sciacca R, Boden-Albala B *et al.* (2006). Moderate alcohol consumption reduces risk of ischemic stroke: The Northern Manhattan Study. *Stroke* **37**:13–19

Endres M, Heuschmann PU, Laufs U *et al.* (2011). Primary prevention of stroke: Blood pressure, lipids, and heart failure. *European Heart Journal* **32**:545–552

Estruch R, Ros E, Salas-Salvadó J *et al.* (2013). Primary prevention of cardiovascular disease with a Mediterranean diet. *New England Journal of Medicine* **368**:1279–1290

Fagerberg B, Gnarpe J, Gnarpe H *et al.* (1999). *Chlamydia pneumoniae* but not cytomegalovirus antibodies are associated with future risk of stroke and cardiovascular disease: A prospective study in middle-aged to elderly men with treated hypertension. *Stroke* **30**:299–305

Feigin VL, Wiebers DO, Nikitin YP *et al.* (1998). Risk factors for ischemic stroke in a Russian community: A population-based case–control study. *Stroke* **29**:34–39

Feigin VL, Rinkel GJ, Lawes CM *et al.* (2005). Risk factors for subarachnoid hemorrhage: An updated systematic review of epidemiological studies. *Stroke* **36**:2773–2780

Feigin VL, Roth GA, Naghavi *et al.* (2016). Global burden of stroke and risk factors in 188 countries, during 1990–2013: A systematic analysis for the Global Burden of Disease Study 2013. *Lancet Neurology* **15**:913–924

Fine-Edelstein JS, Wolf PA, O'Leary *et al.* (1994). Precursors of extracranial carotid atherosclerosis in the Framingham Study. *Neurology* **44**:1046–1050

Friberg L, Rosenqvist M, Lip GY *et al.* (2012). Evaluation of risk stratification schemes for ischaemic stroke and bleeding in 182678 patients with atrial fibrillation: The Swedish Atrial Fibrillation cohort study. *European Heart Journal* **33**:1500–1510

Gil-Nunez AC, Vivancos-Mora J (2005). Blood pressure as a risk factor for stroke and the impact of antihypertensive treatment. *Cerebrovascular Diseases* **20**:40–52

GISSI-Prevenzione Investigators (1999). Dietary supplementation with n-3 polyunsaturated fatty acids and vitamin E after myocardial infarction: Results of the GISSI-Prevenzione trial. *Lancet* **354**:447–455

Glader CA, Stegmayr B, Boman J *et al.* (1999). *Chlamydia pneumoniae* antibodies and high lipoprotein (a) levels do not predict ischemic cerebral infarctions: Results from a nested case–control study in northern Sweden. *Stroke* **30**:2013–2018

Goldstein LB, Hankey GJ (2006). Advances in primary stroke prevention. *Stroke* **37**:317–319

Grau AJ, Buggle F, Becher H *et al.* (1998). Recent bacterial and viral infection is a risk factor for cerebrovascular ischemia: Clinical and biochemical studies. *Neurology* **50**:196–203

Grau AJ, Becher H, Ziegler CM *et al.* (2004). Periodontal disease as a risk factor for ischemic stroke. *Stroke* **35**:396–501

Grodstein F, Manson JE, Colditz GA *et al.* (2000). A prospective, observational study of postmenopausal hormone therapy and primary prevention of cardiovascular disease. *Annals of Internal Medicine* **133**:922–941

Grundy SM, Cleeman JI, Daniels SR *et al.* (2005). Diagnosis and management of the metabolic syndrome: An American Heart Association/ National Heart Lung and Blood Institute Scientific Statement. *Circulation* **112**:2735–2752

Gutiérrez OM, Judd SE, Muntner P *et al.* (2012). Racial differences in albuminuria, kidney function, and risk of stroke. *Neurology* **79**:1686–1692

Haapanen A, Koskenvuo M, Kaprio J *et al.* (1989). Carotid arteriosclerosis in identical twins discordant for cigarette smoking. *Circulation* **80**:10–16

Hankey GJ (2002). Is homocysteine a causal and treatable risk factor for vascular diseases of the brain (cognitive impairment and stroke). *Annals of Neurology* **51**:279–281

Hankey GJ, Eikelboom JW (2005). Homocysteine and stroke. *Lancet* **365**:194–196

Harman SM, Black DM, Naftolin F *et al.* (2014). Arterial imaging outcomes and cardiovascular risk factors in recently menopausal women: A randomized trial. *Annals of Internal Medicine* **161**:249–260

Harmsen P, Rosengren A, Tsipogiannia A *et al.* (1990). Risk factors for stroke in middle-aged men in Goteborg Sweden. *Stroke* 21:223–229

Hart RG, Benavente O, McBride R *et al.* (1999). Antithrombotic therapy to prevent stroke in patients with atrial fibrillation: A meta-analysis. *Annals of Internal Medicine* 131:492–501

Hart RG, Halperin JL, Pearce, LA *et al.* (2003). Lessons from the Stroke Prevention in Atrial Fibrillation trials. *Annals of Internal Medicine* 138:831–838

He FJ, MacGregor GA (2004). The effect of longer-term modest salt reduction on blood pressure. *Cochrane Database of Systematic Reviews* 1:CD004937

He FJ, Nowson CA, MacGregor GA (2006). Fruit and vegetable consumption and stroke: Meta-analysis of cohort studies. *Lancet* 367:320–326

He K, Song Y, Daviglus ML *et al.* (2004). Fish consumption and incidence of stroke: A meta-analysis of cohort studies. *Stroke* 35:1538–1542

Heart Protection Study Collaborative Group (2002). MRC/BHF Heart Protection Study of cholesterol lowering with simvastatin in 20 536 high-risk individuals: A randomized placebo-controlled trial. *Lancet* 360:7–22

Hemelaar M, van der Mooren M, Rad M *et al.* (2008). Effects of non-oral postmenopausal hormone therapy on markers of cardiovascular risk: A systematic review. *Fertility and Sterility* 90:642–672

Hodis HN, Mack WJ, Henderson VW *et al.* (2016). Vascular effects of early versus late postmenopausal treatment with estradiol. *New England Journal of Medicine* 374:1221–1231

Hollander M, Hak AE, Koudstaal PJ *et al.* (2003). Comparison between measures of atherosclerosis and risk of stroke: The Rotterdam Study. *Stroke* 34:2367–2372

Homer D, Ingall TJ, Baker HL *et al.* (1991). Serum lipids and lipoproteins are less powerful predictors of extracranial carotid artery atherosclerosis than are cigarette smoking and hypertension. *Mayo Clinic Proceedings* 66:259–267

Hooper L, Capps N, Clements G *et al.* (2004). Foods or supplements rich in omega-3 fatty acids for preventing cardiovascular disease in patients with ischemic heart disease. *Cochrane Database of Systematic Reviews* 4:CD003177

Hooper L, Capps N, Clements G *et al.* (2008). Anti-oxidant foods or supplements for preventing cardiovascular disease. *Cochrane Database of Systematic Reviews* 3:CD001558

Howard G, Wagenknecht LE, Burke GL *et al.* (1998). Cigarette smoking and progression of atherosclerosis: The Atherosclerosis Risk in Communities (ARIC) Study. *Journal of the American Medical Association* 279:119–124

Hsieh SW, Lai CL, Liu CK *et al.* (2012). Obstructive sleep apnea liked to wake-up strokes. *Journal of Neurology* 259:1433–1439

Huxley R, Lewington S, Clarke R (2002). Cholesterol, coronary heart disease and stroke: A review of published evidence from observational studies and randomized controlled trials. *Seminars in Vascular Medicine* 2:315–323

Jackson C, Sudlow C (2005). Are lacunar strokes really different? A systematic review of differences in risk factor profiles between lacunar and non-lacunar infarcts. *Stroke* 36:891–901

Jespersen CM, Als-Nielsen B, Damgaard M *et al.* (2006). Randomized placebo controlled multicentre trial to assess short term clarithromycin for patients with stable coronary heart disease: CLARICOR trial. *British Medical Journal* 332:22–27

Jorgensen HS, Nakayama H, Raaschou HO *et al.* (1994). Stroke in patients with diabetes. The Copenhagen Stroke Study. *Stroke* 25:1977–1984

Julius S, Kjeldsen SE, Weber M *et al.* (2004). Outcomes in hypertensive patients at high cardiovascular risk, treated with regimens based on valsartan or amlodipine: The VALUE randomized trail. *Lancet* 363:2022–2031

Kearney PM, Welton M, Reynolds K *et al.* (2005). Global burden of hypertension: Analysis of worldwide data. *Lancet* 365:217–223

Keli S, Bloemberg B, Kromhout D (1992). Predictive value of repeated systolic blood pressure measurements for stroke risk. The Zutphen Study. *Stroke* 23:347–351

Kernan WN, Viscoli CM, Furie KL *et al.* (2016). Pioglitazone after ischemic stroke or transient ischemic attack. *New England Journal of Medicine* **374**:1321–1331

Khaw KT, Barrett-Connor E (1987). Dietary potassium and stroke-associated mortality. A 12-year prospective population study. *New England Journal of Medicine* **316**:235–240

Koren-Morag N, Tanne D, Graff E *et al.* (2002). Low and high density lipoprotein, cholesterol and ischemic cerebrovascular disease. The Bezafibrate Infarction Prevention Registry. *Archives of International Medicine* **162**:993–999

Krause DN, Duckles SP, Pelligrino DA (2006). Influence of sex steroid hormones on cerebrovascular function. *Journal of Applied Physiology* **101**:1252–1261

Lee CD, Folsom AR, Blair SN (2003). Physical activity and stroke risk. A meta-analysis. *Stroke* **34**:2475–2482

Lee M, Saver JL, Chang KH *et al.* (2010). Low glomerular filtration rate and risk of stroke: Meta-analysis. *British Medical Journal* **341**:c4249

Leppala JM, Virtamo J, Fogelholm R *et al.* (2000). Controlled trial of alpha-tocopherol and beta-carotene supplements on stroke incidence and mortality in male smokers. *Arteriosclerosis, Thrombosis and Vascular Biology* **20**:230–235

Lewington S, Clarke R (2005). Combined effects of systolic blood pressure and total cholesterol on cardiovascular disease risk. *Circulation* **112**:3373–3374

Lewington S, Clarke R, Qizilbash N *et al.* (2002). Age-specific relevance of usual blood pressure to vascular mortality: A meta-analysis of individual data for one million adults in 61 prospective studies. *Lancet* **360**:1903–1913

Leys D, Woimant F, Ferrieres J *et al.* (2006). Detection and management of associated atherothrombotic locations in patients with a recent atherothrombotic ischemic stroke: Results of the DETECT survey. *Cerebrovascular Diseases* **21**:60–66

Lip GY (2005). Atrial fibrillation (recent onset). *Clinical Evidence* **14**:71–89

Lip GY, Boos CJ (2006). Antithrombotic treatment in atrial fibrillation. *Heart* **92**:155–161

Lip GY, Hee FL (2001). Paroxysmal atrial fibrillation. *Quarterly Journal of Medicine* **94**:665–678

Lip GY, Nieuwlaat R, Pisters R *et al.* (2010). Refining clinical risk stratification for predicting stroke and thromboembolism in atrial fibrillation using a novel risk factor-based approach: the euro heart survey on atrial fibrillation. *Chest* **137**:263–272

Lisabeth L, Bushnell C (2012). Stroke risk in women: The role of menopause and hormone therapy. *Lancet Neurology* **11**:82–91

Lovelock CE, Molyneux AJ, Rothwell PM for the Oxford Vascular Study (2007). Change in incidence and aetiology of intracerebral haemorrhage in Oxfordshire, UK, between 1981 and 2006: A population-based study. *Lancet Neurology* **6**:487–493

Lowe GDO, Lee AJ, Rumley A *et al.* (1997). Blood viscosity and risk of cardiovascular events: The Edinburgh Artery Study. *British Journal of Haematology* **96**:168–173

MacMahon S, Peto R, Cutler J *et al.* (1990). Blood pressure, stroke and coronary heart disease. Part 1. Prolonged differences in blood pressure: Prospective observational studies corrected for the regression dilution bias. *Lancet* **335**:765–774

Macko RF, Kittner SJ, Epstein A *et al.* (1999). Elevated tissue plasminogen activator, antigen and stroke risk. The Stroke Prevention in Young Women Study. *Stroke* **30**:7–11

Markus HS, Hambley H (1998). Neurology and the blood: Haematological abnormalities in ischemic stroke. *Journal of Neurology, Neurosurgery and Psychiatry* **64**:150–159

Markus HS, Mendall MA (1998). Helicobacter pylori infection: A risk factor for ischemic cerebrovascular disease and carotid atheroma. *Journal of Neurology, Neurosurgery and Psychiatry* **64**:104–107

Matthews K, Crawford S, Chae C *et al.* (2009). Are changes in cardiovascular disease risk factors in midlife women due to chronological aging or to the menopausal transition? *Journal of the American College of Cardiology* **54**:2366–2373

McCullough LD, Alkayed NJ, Traystman RJ *et al.* (2001). Postischemic estrogen reduces hypoperfusion and secondary ischemic after experimental stroke. *Stroke* **32**:796–802

Meade TW, Ruddock V, Stirling Y *et al.* (1993). Fibrinolytic activity, clotting factors and long-term incidence of ischemic heart disease in the Northwick Park Heart Study. *Lancet* **342**:1076–1079

Mendelsohn M, Karas R (2005). Molecular and cellular basis of cardiovascular genetic differences. *Science* **308**:1583–1587

Nattel S, Opie L (2006). Controversies in atrial fibrillation. *Lancet* **367**:262–272

Ngeh J, Gupta S, Goodbourn C *et al.* (2003). *Chlamydia pneumoniae* in elderly patients with stroke (C-PEPS): A case–control study on the seroprevalence of *Chlamydia pneumoniae* in elderly patients with acute cerebrovascular disease. *Cerebrovascular Diseases* **15**:11–16

Ninomiya T, Perkovic V, Verdon C *et al.* (2009). Proteinuria and stroke: a meta-analysis of cohort studies. *American Journal of Kidney Diseases* **53**:417–425

O'Donnell MJ, Chin SL, Rangarajan S *et al.* (2016). Global and regional effects of potentially modifiable risk factors associated with acute stroke in 32 countries (INTERSTROKE): A case-control study. *Lancet* **388**:761–775

Pendlebury ST (2007). Worldwide under-funding of stroke research. *International Journal of Stroke* **2**:80–84

Petrovitch H, Curb D, Bloom-Marcus E (1995). Isolated systolic hypertension and risk of stroke in Japanese-American men. *Stroke* **26**:25–29

Prospective Studies Collaboration (1995). Cholesterol, diastolic blood pressure and stroke: 13 000 strokes in 450 000 people in 45 prospective cohorts. *Lancet* **346**:1647–1653

Qizilbash N, Duffy S, Prentice CRM *et al.* (1997). Von Willebrand factor and risk of ischemic stroke. *Neurology* **49**:1552–1556

Reeves MJ, Bushnell CD, Howard G *et al.* (2008). Sex differences in stroke: epidemiology, clinical presentation, medical care, and outcomes. *Lancet Neurology* **7**:915–926

Renoux C, Dell'aniello S, Garbe E *et al.* (2010). Transdermal and oral hormone replacement therapy and the risk of stroke: A nested case-control study. *British Medical Journal* **340**: c2519

Reynolds K, Lewis B, Nolen JD *et al.* (2003). Alcohol consumption and risk of stroke: A meta-analysis. *Journal of the American Medical Association* **289**:579–588

Rodgers A, MacMahon S, Gamble G *et al.* (1996). Blood pressure and risk of stroke in patients with cerebrovascular disease. *British Medical Journal* **313**:147

Rothwell PM (2001). The high cost of not funding stroke research: A comparison with heart disease and cancer. *Lancet* **19**:1612–1616

Rothwell PM (2005). Prevention of stroke in patients with diabetes mellitus and the metabolic syndrome. *Cerebrovascular Diseases* **1**:24–34

Rothwell PM, Howard SC, Spence D (2003). Relationship between blood pressure and stroke risk in patients with symptomatic carotid occlusive disease. *Stroke* **34**:2583–2590

Rothwell PM, Coull AJ, Giles MF *et al.* (2004a). Change in stroke incidence, mortality, case-fatality, severity and risk factors in Oxfordshire, UK from 1981 to 2004 (Oxford Vascular Study). *Lancet* **363**:1925–1933

Rothwell PM, Howard SC, Power DA *et al.* (2004b). Fibrinogen and risk of ischemic stroke and coronary events in 5183 patients with transient ischemic attack and minor ischemic stroke. *Stroke* **35**:2300–2305

Rothwell PM, Coull AJ, Silver LE *et al.* (2005). Population-based study of event-rate, incidence, case fatality and mortality for all acute vascular events in all arterial territories (Oxford Vascular Study). *Lancet* **366**:1773–1783

Rothwell PM, Howard SC, Dolan E *et al.* (2010). Prognostic significance of visit-to-visit variability, maximum systolic blood pressure, and episodic hypertension. *Lancet* **375**:895–905

Rundek T, Gardener H, Xu Q *et al.* (2010). Insulin resistance and risk of ischemic stroke among nondiabetic individuals from the northern Manhattan study. *Archives of Neurology* **67**:1195–1200

Sacco RL (2001). Newer risk factors for stroke. *Neurology* **57**:S31–S34

Sagie A, Larson MG, Levy D (1993). The natural history of borderline isolated systolic hypertension. *New England Journal of Medicine* **329**:1912–1917

Sandercock PAG, Bamford J, Dennis M *et al.* (1992). Atrial fibrillation and stroke: Frequency in different stroke types and influence on early and long term prognosis. The Oxfordshire

Community Stroke Project. *British Medical Journal* **305**:1460–1465

Sare GM, Gray LJ, Bath PM (2008). Association between hormone replacement therapy and subsequent arterial and venous vascular events: A meta-analysis. *European Heart Journal* **29**:2031–2041

Saxonhouse SJ, Curtis AB (2003). Risks and benefits of rate control versus maintenance of sinus rhythm. *American Journal of Cardiology* **91**:27D–32D

Schulz UG, Rothwell PM (2003). Differences in vascular risk factors between aetiological subtypes of ischemic stroke in population-based incidence studies. *Stroke* **34**:2050–2059

Segal JB, McNamara RL, Miller MR *et al.* (2001). Anticoagulants or antiplatelet therapy for non-rheumatic atrial fibrillation and flutter. *Cochrane Database Systematic Reviews* **1**: CD001938

Shah RS, Cole JW (2010). Smoking and stroke: The more you smoke the more you stroke. *Expert Review of Cardiovascular Therapy* **8**:917–932

Shaper AG, Phillips AN, Pocock SJ *et al.* (1991). Risk factors for stroke in middle-aged British men. *British Medical Journal* **302**:1111–1115

Sifat AE, Vaidya B, Villalba H *et al.* (2017). E-cigarette exposure alters brain glucose utilization and stroke outcome. Abstract at International Stroke Conference 2017

Steinberg D (1995). Clinical trials of antioxidants in atherosclerosis: Are we doing the right thing? *Lancet* **346**:36–38

Stemmermann GN, Hayashi T, Resch JA *et al.* (1984). Risk factors related to ischemic and hemorrhagic cerebrovascular disease at autopsy: The Honolulu Heart Study. *Stroke* **15**:23–28

Stephens N (1997). Anti-oxidant therapy for ischemic heart disease: Where do we stand? *Lancet* **349**:1710–1711

Stevens RJ, Coleman RL, Adler AI *et al.* (2004). Risk factors for myocardial infarction, case fatality and stroke case fatality in type 2 diabetes: UKPDS 66. *Diabetes Care* **27**:201–207

Strachan DP, Carrington D, Mendall MA *et al.* (1999). Relation of *Chlamydia pneumoniae* serology to mortality and incidence of ischemic heart disease over 13 years in the Caerphilly

Prospective Heart Disease Study. *British Medical Journal* **318**:1035–1039

Stroke Prevention in Atrial Fibrillation Investigators (1992). Predictors of thromboembolism in atrial fibrillation: II Echocardiographic features of patients at risk. *Annals of Internal Medicine* **116**:6–12

Stroke Prevention in Atrial Fibrillation Investigators (1995). Risk factors for thromboembolism during aspirin therapy in patients with atrial fibrillation: The Stroke Prevention in Atrial Fibrillation Study. *Journal of Stroke and Cerebrovascular Disease* **5**:147–157

Suk SH, Sacco RL, Boden-Albala B *et al.* (2003). Abdominal obesity and risk of ischemic stroke: The Northern Manhattan Stroke Study. *Stroke* **34**:1586–1592

Sundell L, Salomaa V, Vartiainen E *et al.* (2008). Increased stroke risk is related to a binge drinking habit. *Stroke* **39**:3179–3184

Toole JF, Malinow MR, Chambless LE *et al.* (2004). Lowering homocysteine in patients with ischemic stroke to prevent recurrent stroke, myocardial infarction and death: The Vitamin Intervention for Stroke Prevention (VISP) randomized controlled trial. *Journal of the American Medical Association* **291**:565–575

Touzé E, Warlow CP, Rothwell PM (2006). Risk of coronary and other nonstroke vascular death in relation to the presence and extent of atherosclerotic disease at the carotid bifurcation. *Stroke* **37**:2904–2909

Toyoda K, Ninomiya T (2014). Stroke and cerebrovascular diseases in patients with chronic kidney disease. *Lancet Neurology* **13**:823–833

Tuomilehto J, Rastenyte D (1999). Diabetes and glucose intolerance as risk factors for stroke. *Journal of Cardiovascular Risk* **6**:241–249

Tuomilehto J, Lindstrom J, Erikkson JG *et al.* (2001). Prevention of type 2 diabetes mellitus by changes in lifestyle among subjects with impaired glucose tolerance. *New England Journal of Medicine* **344**:1343–1350

UK Prospective Diabetes Study (UKPDS) Group (1998). Intensive blood-glucose control with sulphonylureas or insulin, compared with conventional treatment and risk of complications in patients with type 2 diabetes (UKPDS 33). *Lancet* **352**:837–853

Wald DS, Law M, Morris JK (2002). Homocysteine and cardiovascular disease: Evidence on causality from a meta-analysis. *British Medical Journal* 325:1202–1206

Wald DS, Law M, Morris JK (2004). The dose–response relationship between serum homocysteine and cardiovascular disease: Implications for treatment and screening. *European Journal of Cardiovascular Prevention and Rehabilitation* 11:250–253

Wang X, Qin X, Demirtas H et al. (2007). Efficacy of folic acid supplementation in stroke prevention: A meta-analysis. *Lancet* 369:1876–1882

Wannamethee SG, Shaper AG, Whincup PH (1995). Smoking cessation and the risk of stroke in middle-aged men. *Journal of American Medical Association* 274:155–160

Wannamethee SG, Perry IJ, Shaper AG (1999). Non-fasting serum glucose and insulin concentrations and the risk of stroke. *Stroke* 30:1780–1786

Welin L, Svardsudd K, Wilhelmsen L et al. (1987). Analysis of risk factors for stroke in a cohort of men born in 1913. *New England Journal of Medicine* 317:521–526

Westover AN, McBride S, Haley RW. (2007). Stroke in young adults who abuse amphetamines or cocaine: A population-based study of hospitalized patients. *Archives of General Psychiatry* 64:495–502

Whelton PK, He J, Cutler JA et al. (1997). Effects of oral potassium on blood pressure: Meta-analysis of randomized controlled clinical trials. *Journal of the American Medical Association* 277:1624–1632

Wolf PA, D'Agostino RB, Belanger AJ et al. (1991). Probability of stroke: A risk profile from the Framingham Study. *Stroke* 22:312–318

Wolff V, Armspach JP, Lauer V et al. (2013). Cannabis-related stroke: Myth or reality? *Stroke* 44:558–563

Yaggi HK, Concato J, Kernan WN et al. (2005). Obstructive sleep apnea as a risk factor for stroke and death. *New England Journal of Medicine* 353:2034–2041

Yiin GS, Howard DP, Paul NL et al. (2014). Age-specific incidence, outcome, cost, and projected future burden of atrial fibrillation-related embolic vascular events: A population-based study. *Circulation* 130:1236–1244

Yusuf S, Phil D, Sleight DM et al. (2000). Effects of an angiotensin-coverting-enzyme inhibitor ramipril on cardiovascular events in high-risk patients. *New England Journal of Medicine* 342:145–153

Zhang X, Patel A, Horibe H et al. (2003). Cholesterol coronary heart disease and stroke in the Asia Pacific region. *International Journal of Epidemiology* 32:563–572

Chapter 3

Genetics

Advances in techniques of genetic investigation have allowed researchers to begin to understand the role of genetic factors both in sporadic stroke and in single gene disorders. Although genetic investigations still have a relatively limited role in routine clinical practice, it is important that clinicians are aware of the relevance of family history of vascular disease to the management of patients with TIA and stroke and of the common hereditary forms of cerebrovascular disease.

Genetic Risk Factors for "Sporadic" Stroke

The contribution of genetic factors to stroke risk in populations has been difficult to establish, as is the case for coronary heart disease (Alberts 1991), and it is made more difficult by the fact that stroke is a heterogeneous clinical syndrome with numerous underlying pathologies and that many of the risk factors for stroke have strong genetic components. Reliable interpretation of published family history studies is undermined by major heterogeneity, insufficient detail, and potential publication and reporting bias, with much stronger associations in smaller and less methodologically rigorous studies (Flossmann et al. 2004). Few studies consider the number of affected and unaffected relatives or phenotyped strokes in detail, and the majority of studies do not adjust associations for intermediate phenotypes (Flossmann et al. 2005). No twin study and only a minority of family history studies have differentiated between ischemic and hemorrhagic stroke in the proband. There are very few data on the influence of family history on stroke severity and no data on stroke recovery. Generally, genetic influences are stronger in patients with a relatively early age of stroke onset, and a family history of stroke confers a higher risk of stroke if onset was before 70 years of age (Schulz et al. 2004).

Based on the assumption that at least some of the risk of apparently sporadic stroke is genetic, large numbers of studies using different methodologies have been carried out in an attempt to identify the genes involved (Falcone et al. 2014) (Table 3.1). However, it seems likely that the genetic component of stroke risk is modest and that many, indeed probably hundreds of, genes are involved, each one contributing only a small increased risk. Cohorts so far have generally not been large enough to reliably detect the sort of small effects that might realistically be expected and have had other methodological limitations, including poor choice of controls in case–control studies, inadequate distinction between the different pathological types and subtypes of stroke for which genetic influences may differ, failure to replicate positive results in an independent and adequately sized study, and testing of multiple genetic or subgroup hypotheses with no adjustment of p values for declaring statistical significance (Dichgans and Markus 2005; Sudlow et al. 2006). However, in recent years, large international collaborations such as the International Stroke Genetics

Table 3.1 Summary of different methods of identifying genetic risk factors for stroke

	Description	Advantages	Disadvantages
Candidate gene study	A molecular variant in a gene that is functionally relevant to the disease of interest is first identified. The role of the gene in conferring risk for that disease is then studied using a case–control or cohort method	Large number of potential genes available for study	Genes of interest must be identified a priori, and novel genes are not identified. A positive association does not prove causation but represents close linkage between the gene of interest and a nearby disease-causing locus
Linkage study	Analysis of pedigree by the tracking of a gene through a family by following the inheritance of a (closely associated) gene or trait. If genes are linked by residing on the same chromosome, there would be a greater association than if the genes were not linked	Polygenic disorders can be studied	Because stroke is a disease of middle and old age, identification of living, affected relatives is difficult
Genome-wide association study (GWAS)	Aims to identify common genetic variants (those that account for >5% of the allele frequency) associated with the outcome of interest. Variations in single nucleotide polymorphisms (SNPs) throughout the genome are analyzed and compared between individuals with and without a disease. Genetic variations that are more frequent in those with the disease are then considered pointers to the disease-causing locus	Huge numbers of genes can be studied at the same time in a "hypothesis-free" approach without making any assumptions about the underlying biological mechanisms involved	Multiple associations are identified, which invariably include many false positives. This, however, can be overcome by increasing the threshold of declaring significance to p of 5×10^{-8}, which corresponds to a Bonferroni correction of 1 million tests

Consortium (ISGC) has been established, and via pooling data from cohorts worldwide, further studies such as the METASTROKE collaboration and National Institute of Neurological Disorders and Stroke (NINDS) Stroke Genetics Network (SiGN) studies were launched (Traylor *et al.* 2012; Meschia *et al.* 2013; NINDS SiGN and ISGC 2016). Using genome-wide data, these studies have estimated the hereditability of stroke to be ~38% for ischemic stroke (~40% for stroke due to large artery atherosclerosis, ~33% due to cardioembolism, and ~16% due to small vessel disease) and ~29% for intracerebral hemorrhage (~48% for lobar intracerebral hemorrhage and ~30% for non-lobar intracerebral hemorrhage) (Bevan *et al.* 2012; Devan *et al.* 2013). These collaborations have also been successful in identifying a number of novel genetic variants affecting risk of stroke, some of which are summarized in Tables 3.2 and 3.3.

Candidate Gene Studies

Prior to the launch of the human genome project, most genetic studies have been candidate gene studies, in which the frequency of different genotypes at a specific locus or loci within a gene or genes thought likely to be in some way connected with stroke risk are compared between stroke cases and stroke-free controls. Candidate genes have generally been selected on the basis of their known or presumed involvement in the control of factors or pathways likely to influence stroke risk: blood pressure, lipid metabolism, inflammation, coagulation, homocysteine metabolism, and so on (Hassan and Markus 2000; Casas *et al.* 2004). Rigorous meta-analyses of candidate gene studies, in both stroke and other vascular diseases such as coronary heart disease, have highlighted various methodological problems, particularly the inadequate size of studies (Keavney *et al.* 2000; Wheeler *et al.* 2004; Sudlow *et al.* 2006). Large numbers of candidate gene studies have together identified a handful of genes that, on the basis of results from meta-analyses, seem likely to influence risk of ischemic stroke modestly. These genes include those encoding factor V Leiden, methylenetetrahydrofolate reductase, prothrombin, and angiotensin-converting enzyme (Casas *et al.* 2004, 2006).

Linkage Studies

As yet, there have been far fewer stroke genetics studies that use more traditional genetic study designs, based on collecting information and DNA from related individuals with and without the disease of interest. This is at least partly because family members of stroke patients are often no longer alive, and so obtaining information and samples for DNA extraction from large enough numbers of relatives is challenging (Hassan *et al.* 2002). The Icelandic deCODE group identified two candidate genes for ischemic stroke, encoding the enzymes phosphodiesterase-4D and arachidonate 5-lipoxygenase-activating protein (ALOX5AP; Gulcher *et al.* 2005). There is still some debate, however, about their influence in non-Icelandic populations, since their effect on ischemic stroke risk has been confirmed in only a few replication studies (Gulcher *et al.* 2006; Rosand *et al.* 2006).

Genome-Wide Association Studies (GWAS)

The combination of technological developments allowing rapid genotyping at multiple loci, the attraction of non-hypothesis-driven genetic studies, and the recognized limitations of traditional linkage approaches have led to an increasing interest in GWAS, where multiple polymorphisms across the genome are genotyped and compared in cases and controls,

Table 3.2 Genetic variants affecting risk of ischemic stroke in a non-Mendelian manner

Ischemic stroke	SNP with strongest association	Chromosome	Gene	Risk allele	Risk allele frequency	Odds ratio (95% CI)	Mechanism	References
Cardioembolic	rs2200733	4q25	*PITX2*	G	~21%	1.37 (1.30–1.45)	*PITX2* encodes a transcriptional activator that plays a part in the development of the sinoatrial node and in regulation of ion channels that modulate cardiac conduction	Gudbjartsson *et al.* 2007; Gretarsdottir *et al.* 2008; Lemmens *et al.* 2010; Lubitz *et al.* 2010; NINDS SiGN and ISGC 2016
	rs7193343	16q22	*ZFHX3*	A	~19%	1.17 (1.11–1.23)	*ZFHX3* encodes transcription factor ATBF1, but the mechanism linking this locus to atrial fibrillation/cardio-embolic stroke is uncertain	Gudbjartsson *et al.* 2009; NINDS SiGN and ISGC 2016
	rs505922	9q34	*ABO*	A	~19%	1.09 (1.02–1.16)	*ABO* gene variants have been associated with factor VIII and von Willebrand factor levels, suggesting a role of the *ABO* gene in the coagulation pathway	Williams *et al.* 2013; NINDS SiGN and ISGC 2016
Large artery atherosclerosis	rs11984041	7p21	*HDAC9*	A	~16%	1.24 (1.15–1.33)	*HDAC9* is expressed in vascular smooth muscle cells and endothelium of large arteries. It encodes histone deacetylase. The mechanisms of HDAC9 genetic polymorphisms in causing	Bellenguez *et al.* 2012; NINDS SiGN and ISGC 2016

Category	SNP	Locus	Gene	Allele	Frequency	OR (95% CI)	Mechanism	Reference
							large artery atherosclerosis uncertain but may be due to *HDAC9* mediated increased vascular smooth muscle cell proliferation	NINDS SiGN and ISGC 2016
	rs12122341	1p13	*TSPAN2*	G	~25%	1.19 (1.12–1.26)	*TSPAN2* is highly expressed in arterial tissue and blood cells and encodes tetraspanin-2, which plays a role in cell development and growth	NINDS SiGN and ISGC 2016
	rs556621	6p21	*SUPT3H/ CDC5L*	A	~33%	1.21 (1.12–1.28)	Uncertain	Holliday *et al.* 2012; NINDS SiGN and ISGC 2016
	rs2383207	9p21	*CDKN2B-AS1*			1.15 (1.08–1.23)	Uncertain	NINDS SiGN and ISGC 2016
	rs505922	9q34	*ABO*	A	~19%	1.15 (1.07–1.24)	*ABO* gene variants have been associated with factor VIII and von Willebrand factor levels, suggesting a role of the *ABO* gene in the coagulation pathway	Williams *et al.* 2013; NINDS SiGN and ISGC 2016
Small vessel disease	rs12204590	6p25	*FOXF2*	A	~21%	1.08 (1.05–1.12)	*FOXF2* is expressed in brain pericytes and encodes a transcription factor FOXF2, which plays a role in cerebral vascular wall morphogenesis and function	Neurology Working Group of CHARGE Consortium; NINDS SiGN and ISGC 2016

Table 3.2 (cont.)

Ischemic stroke	SNP with strongest association	Chromosome	Gene	Risk allele	Risk allele frequency	Odds ratio (95% CI)	Mechanism	References
	rs10744777	12q24	ALDH2	T	~66%	1.17 (1.11–1.23)	ALDH2 encodes aldehyde dehydrogenase, which has a major role in aldehyde detoxication in mitochondria and attenuates or ablates neuronal mitochondrial damage. ALDH2 is also involved in the regulation of cardiovascular hemostasis	Guo et al. 2013; NINDS SiGN and ISGC 2016

Notes: NINDS, National Institute of Neurological Disorders and Stroke; SiGN, Stroke Genetics Network; ISGC, International Stroke Genetics Consortium; CHARGE, Cohorts for Heart and Aging Research in Genomic Epidemiology
Sources: NINDS SiGN and ISGC (2016) and Boehme et al. (2017).

Table 3.3 Genetic variants affecting risk of intracerebral hemorrhage in a non-Mendelian manner

	SNP with strongest association	Chromosome	Gene	Risk allele	Risk allele frequency	Odds ratio (95% CI)	Mechanism	References
Lobar	rs429358/ rs7412	19q13	*APOE*	ε2	7%	1.82 (1.50–2.23)	*APOE* encodes apolipoprotein E. The ε2 risk allele promotes structural vasculopathic changes in amyloid-laden vessels, making them prone to rupture	Biffi *et al.* 2010
	rs429358/ rs7412	19q13	*APOE*	ε4	12%	2.20 (1.85–2.63)	*APOE* encodes apolipoprotein E. The ε4 risk allele promotes vascular amyloid deposition	Biffi *et al.* 2010
Non-lobar	rs2984613	1q22	*PMF1/ SLC25A44*	C	32%	1.33 (1.22–1.46)	PMF1 codes for polyamine-modulated factor 1, a protein needed for chromosome alignment and segregation and kinetochore formation during mitosis, while *SLC25A44* codes for a mitochondrial carrier protein. Mitochondrial dysfunction may result in intracerebral hemorrhage	Woo *et al.* 2014
Lobar and non-lobar	1355C→T; 1612C→G	13q34	*COL4A1*	T; G	<1%	—		Weng *et al.* 2012

Table 3.3 (cont.)

SNP with strongest association	Chromosome	Gene	Risk allele	Risk allele frequency	Odds ratio (95% CI)	Mechanism	References
3448C→A; 5068G→A; 3368A→G	13q34	COL4A2	A; A; G	<1%	—	COL4A2 encodes collagen type IV α2 protein. Mutations of COL4A2 results in impaired secretion of both collage type IV α1 and α2, hence resulting in cytotoxicity and an increased risk of intracerebral hemorrhage	Jeanne et al. 2012

Sources: NINDS SiGN and ISGC (2016) and Boehme *et al.* (2017).

looking for loci where significant differences may suggest genetic influences on disease risk. The ISGC have pooled together a number of cohorts that have used GWAS and have, successfully discovered a number of novel genetic variants affecting stroke risk (see Tables 3.2 and 3.3) (Neurology Working Group of the Cohorts for Heart and Aging Research in Genomic Epidemiology [CHARGE] Consortium; SiGN; ISGC 2016).

Association with Intermediate Phenotypes (Endophenotypes)

A number of genetic studies of so-called intermediate phenotypes, markers of predisposition to stroke or other vascular diseases, which can be measured in large numbers of subjects both with and without vascular risk factors or disease, have been performed over the years. These intermediate phenotypes include carotid intima media thickness and leukoaraiosis as measured or graded on computed tomography (CT) scans or magnetic resonance imaging (MRI) of the brain and candidate gene, linkage, and GWA studies have been used (Humphries and Morgan 2004; Dichgans and Markus 2005; French *et al.* 2014).

Monogenetic (Mendelian) Stroke Syndromes

A few strokes are clearly "familial" with a simple Mendelian pattern of inheritance of the underlying cause (Table 3.4). Some of these genetic causes of stroke are described in the following section.

Cerebral Autosomal Dominant Arteriopathy with Subcortical Infarcts and Leukoencephalopathy

Cerebral autosomal dominant arteriopathy with subcortical infarcts and leukoencephalopathy (CADASIL) is an autosomal dominant syndrome characterized by recurrent small vessel ischemic stroke in middle age and subcortical dementia with pseudobulbar palsy, usually in the absence of vascular risk factors (Singhal *et al.* 2004). Mood disturbance and migraine with aura often precede the strokes, but there is considerable phenotypic variation (Dichgans *et al.* 1998). Death usually occurs in the sixth or seventh decade. Brain MRI is always abnormal in symptomatic patients, and often in asymptomatic subjects too, and shows widespread focal, diffuse, and confluent white matter changes (Fig. 3.1), particularly in the periventricular and subcortical regions (Chabriat *et al.* 1995, 1998; Hutchinson *et al.* 1995; Dichgans *et al.* 1998). Changes at the temporal poles, the external capsule, and the corpus callosum are characteristic.

The disease has been reported from many parts of the world, and there are now more than 500 families described. The prevalence of genetically proven disease in the west of Scotland has been reported to be 1.98 per 100,000 adults, and the probable mutation prevalence was estimated to be 4.14 (95% CI, 3.04–5.53) per 100,000 adults (Razvi *et al.* 2005).

The underlying small vessel arteriopathy is distinct from arteriosclerotic and amyloid angiopathy and can be found in skin and muscle biopsies as well as in the leptomeningeal and perforating arteries of the brain (Jung *et al.* 1995). There is concentric thickening of the arterial walls with extensive deposition of eosinphilic granular material in the media and internal elastic membrane (Fig. 3.1).

The genetic locus is on chromosome 19q12 (Tournier-Lasserve *et al.* 1993). The deleterious mutations in the human equivalent of the mouse *Notch3* gene were found to be the causative gene for CADASIL (Dichgans *et al.* 1996; Joutel *et al.* 1996).

Table 3.4 Mendelian (single-gene) disorders that include stroke in their phenotypic manifestations

Ischemic stroke	Inheritance	Gene	Stroke mechanism	Associated clinical features	Diagnostic test
CADASIL	Autosomal dominant	NOTCH3	Small-vessel disease	Migraine with aura	Mutational screening, skin biopsy
CADASIL	Autosomal recessive	HTRA1	Small-vessel disease	Premature baldness; severe low back pain; spondylosis deformans or disk herniation	Mutational analysis
Fabry's disease	X-linked	GAL	Large-artery disease and small-vessel disease	Angiokeratoma; neuropathic pain; acroparesthesia; hypohydrosis; corneal opacities; cataract; renal and cardiac failure	α-galactosidase activity, mutational screening
MELAS	Maternal	mtDNA	Complex (microvascular and neuronal factors)	Developmental delay; sensorineural hearing loss; short stature; seizures; episodic vomiting; diabetes; migraine-like headache; cognitive decline	Muscle biopsy, mutational analysis of mtDNA
Sickle-cell disease	Autosomal recessive	HBB	Large-artery disease, small-vessel disease, hemodynamic insufficiency	Pain crises; bacterial infection; vaso-occlusive crises; pulmonary and abdominal crises; anemia; myelopathy; seizure	Peripheral blood smear, electrophoresis, mutational analysis
Homocystinuria	Autosomal recessive	CBS and others	Large-artery disease, cardioembolism, small-vessel disease, arterial dissection	Mental retardation; atraumatic dislocation of lenses; skeletal abnormalities (Marfan-like); premature atherosclerosis; thromboembolic events	Urine analysis, measurement of concentrations of homocysteine and methionine in plasma (mutational analysis)

	Inheritance	Gene	Clinical features	Diagnosis
Marfan's syndrome	Autosomal dominant	FBN1	Cardioembolism and arterial dissection	Pectus carinatum or excavatum; upper-to-lower-segment ratio <0.86, or arm-span-to-height ratio >1.5; scoliosis >20%; ectopia lentis; dilation or dissection of the ascending aorta; lumbosacral dural ectasia	Clinical diagnosis, mutational screening
Ehlers-Danlos syndrome type IV	Autosomal dominant	COL3A1	Arterial dissection	Easy bruising; thin skin with visible veins; characteristic facial features; rupture of arteries, uterus, or intestines	Biochemical studies, mutational screening
Pseudoxanthoma elasticum	Autosomal recessive	ABCC6	Large-artery disease and small-vessel disease	Skin changes (increased elasticity and yellow-orange popular lesions); ocular changes (angioid streaks); hypertension	Skin biopsy, mutational screening
Intracerebral hemorrhage				
Familial cerebral amyloid angiopathy	Autosomal dominant	APP	Rupture of cortical cerebral small vessels	Cerebral lobar macrohemorrhages and microhemorrhages; white-matter lesions; cognitive impairment	Brain biopsy, mutational screening
COL4A1-related intracerebral hemorrhage	Autosomal dominant	COL4A1	Rupture of cortical and subcortical cerebral small vessels	Infantile hemiparesis; congenital porencephaly; white-matter lesions; cerebral macrohemorrhages and microhemorrhages (lobar and non-lobar); transient ischemic attacks	Clinical diagnosis, mutational screening

CADASIL=cerebral autosomal dominant arteriopathy with subcortical infarcts and leukoencephalopathy. CARASIL=cerebral autosomal recessive arteriopathy with subcortical infarcts and leukoencephalopathy. MELAS=mitochondrial myopathy, encephalopathy, lactic acidosis, and stroke. mtDNA=mitochondrial DNA. Reprinted from *The Lancet Neurology*, Vol. number 13, GJ Falcone *et al.* Current concepts and clinical applications of stroke genetics, Page number 408, Copyright (2014), with permission from Elsevier.

(a) (c)

(b)

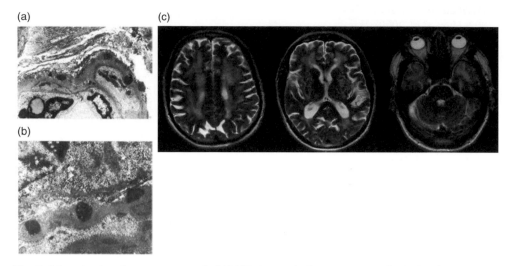

Fig. 3.1 Investigations from a patient with CADASIL (see text). Electron micrographs (a, b) of muscle show thickening of the basal lamina of the small blood vessels and the presence of dense eosinophilic material; magnetic resonance brain imaging shows widespread periventricular and subcortical leukoaraiosis with involvement of bilateral temporal poles as well as multiple enlarged basal ganglia perivascular spaces (c).

The *Notch3* gene is involved in mediating signal transduction between neighboring cells. In contrast to other *Notch* genes, which are ubiquitously expressed, *Notch3* is mainly expressed in vascular smooth muscle cells. *Notch3* has a role in arterial development (Monet-Lepretre *et al.* 2009), arteries from transgenic mice show a diminished flow-induced dilatation, and the pressure-induced myogenic tone is significantly increased in their arteries compared with those in wild-type mice (Dubroca *et al.* 2005). Approximately 70% of the characterized mutations so far cluster in exons 3 and 4 (Joutel *et al.* 1997). At present, there appears to be no genotype–phenotype correlation. The vast majority of known patients are members of affected families, but de novo mutations have been reported, and so CADASIL can affect patients without a family history (Joutel *et al.* 2000).

The diagnosis should be considered in patients under 70 years of age who present with symptoms of subcortical cerebrovascular disease especially if they occur without classical risk factors but with an appropriate family history. The characteristic changes on MRI, which is the most useful and sensitive screening tool, are apparent in all symptomatic and a large number of asymptomatic patients. The diagnosis is confirmed in the majority of patients by screening for mutations, particularly in exons 3 and 4. The search for rarer mutations, however, is very costly and not usually carried out except for research. A useful alternative is to search for granular osmiophilic material in skin biopsies, although this can also be normal (Ebke *et al.* 1997).

Cerebral Autosomal Recessive Arteriopathy with Subcortical Infarcts and Leukoencephalopathy

Cerebral autosomal recessive arteriopathy with subcortical infarcts and leukoencephalopathy (CARASIL) is a much rarer condition compared with CADASIL and has been described in only about fifty patients to date, mainly in Japan and China (Yanagawa *et al.* 2002; Hara *et al.* 2009). It is due to mutations in the *HTRA1* gene, inherited in an autosomal recessive manner. The *HTRA1* gene codes for the HTRA1 enzyme, and mutations in the *HTRA1* gene result in ineffective regulation of TGF-ß signaling, the downstream consequences of which include cerebral small vessel arteriopathy (Yanagawa *et al.* 2002; Hara *et al.* 2009).

Hereditary Dyslipidemias

Hereditary dyslipidemias such as familial hypercholesterolemia, type II and type IV hyperlipidemia, and Tangiers' disease predispose to premature large vessel atherosclerosis and hence stroke (Meschia 2003; Hutter *et al.* 2004).

Connective Tissue Disease

Several inherited connective tissue disorders increase the risk of arterial dissection and other vascular abnormalities, including aneurysms and vaso-occlusive disease.

Fabry's Disease

Fabry's disease is an X-linked disorder causing deficiency of α-galactosidase, which leads to an accumulation of glycosphingolipids in vascular endothelial and other cells. The associated cerebrovascular disorder is mainly ischemic stroke, but intracerebral hemorrhage and subarachnoid hemorrhage can also occur. Approximately two-thirds of the infarcts involve the vertebrobasilar territory. Strokes usually occur from the third decade onward. Systemic non-vascular features of the phenotype include angiokeratomata, painful acroparesthesia, and renal failure. The frequency of previously unknown Fabry's disease in patients with cryptogenic stroke under the age of 55 has been reported to be up to 5% (Rolfs *et al.* 2005).

Cardiac Disorders

Hypertrophic cardiomyopathy is frequently autosomal dominant with incomplete penetrance. Mutations in several genes encoding structural muscle proteins have been found (Franz *et al.* 2001). Approximately 20% of those with dilated cardiomyopathy have familial disease, with autosomal dominant, recessive, X-linked, and mitochondrial inheritance seen (Franz *et al.* 2001). Most cardiomyopathies predispose to arrhythmia, but there are also a number of primary cardiac arrhythmias, including the long QT syndromes of Jervell, Lange, and Nielsen, which are autosomal recessive; and the Romano Ward, which is autosomal dominant. A variety of mutations in sodium and potassium channels have been implicated (Viskin and Long 1999). There are also reports of familial atrial fibrillation (Brugada *et al.* 1997). Atrial myxoma (Chapter 6) is associated with a high risk of embolization and stroke and can be familial, particularly in younger patents and in men (Carney 1985).

Hematological Disorders

Various genetic blood disorders including sickle cell anemia and familial thrombophilias (Chapter 2) are associated with stroke.

Familial Cerebral Amyloid Angiopathy

Cerebral amyloid angiopathy (CAA) is an organ-specific form of amyloid-ß protein deposition (Aß40) in small and medium-sized arteries, and less commonly capillaries, of the cerebral cortex and leptomeninges (Attems *et al.* 2011). Although the majority of cases are sporadic and mainly affect the elderly (Charidimou *et al.* 2012) (Chapter 7), hereditary forms of CAA also exist (majority autosomal dominant), and several genetic mutations have been identified including those in the *APP* (encodes amyloid-ß protein precursor), presenilin, and cystatin C genes (Yamada 2015). Individuals with CAA often present with multiple, recurrent lobar hemorrhages (Charidimou *et al.* 2012) but may also present with transient focal neurological episodes (also known as amyloid spells) (Charidimou *et al.* 2013) and cognitive impairment (Case *et al.* 2016; Fotiadis *et al.* 2016) (Chapter 7).

COL4A1-Related Intracerebral Hemorrhage

Mutations in the *COL4A1* gene cause intracerebral hemorrhage, inherited by an autosomal dominant manner. *COL4A1* encodes the α1 chain of type IV collagen, which forms the basement membrane of all tissues including blood vessels and hence is crucial in contributing to the strength of tissues. Patients with rare mutations of this gene may present with perinatal or adult onset intracerebral hemorrhage, porencephaly, and small vessel disease, with neuroimaging demonstrating microbleeds, lacunes, and leukoaraiosis (Gould *et al.* 2006; van der Knaap *et al.* 2006; Vahedi *et al.* 2007).

Genetic Variations Affecting Risk of Common Stroke Syndromes (Non-Mendelian Inheritance)

In recent years, a number of common genetic variants identified via candidate gene analysis and GWAS have been shown to be associated with an increased risk of various ischemic stroke subtypes and intracerebral hemorrhage. Many of these discoveries were only made possible through the pooling of samples from multiple cohorts such as via the ISGC. Some of the recently described genetic variants that affect one's risk of ischemic and hemorrhagic stroke are tabulated in Tables 3.2 and 3.3 (Falcone *et al.* 2014; NINDS SiGN and ISGC 2016; Boehme *et al.* 2017).

References

Alberts MJ (1991). Genetic aspects of cerebrovascular disease. *Stroke* **22**:276–280

Attems J, Jellinger K, Thal DR *et al.* (2011). Review: Sporadic cerebral amyloid angiopathy. *Neuropathology and Applied Neurobiology* **37**:75–93

Bellenguez C, Bevan S, Gschwendtner A *et al.* (2012). Genome-wide association study identifies a variant in HDAC9 associated with large vessel ischemic stroke. *Nature Genetics* **44**:328–333

Bevan S, Traylor M, Adib-Samii P *et al.* (2012). Genetic heritability of ischemic stroke and the contribution of previously reported candidate gene and genomewide associations. *Stroke* **43**:3161–3167

Biffi A, Sonni A, Anderson CD *et al.* (2010). Variants at APOE influence risk of deep and lobar intracerebral hemorrhage. *Annals of Neurology* **68**:934–943

Boehme AK, Esenwa C, Elkind MSV (2017). Stroke risk factors, genetics and prevention. *Circulation Research* **120**:472–495

Brugada R, Tapscott T, Czernuszewicz GZ *et al.* (1997). Identification of a genetic locus for familial atrial fibrillation. *New England Journal of Medicine* **336**:905–911

Carney JA (1985). Differences between nonfamilial and familial cardiac myxoma. *American Journal of Surgery and Pathology* 9:53–55

Casas JP, Hingorani AD, Bautista LE *et al.* (2004). Meta-analysis of genetic studies in ischemic stroke: Thirty-two genes involving approximately 18 000 cases and 58 000 controls. *Archives of Neurology* 61:1652–1661

Casas JP, Cavalleri GL, Bautista LE *et al.* (2006). Endothelial nitric oxide synthase gene polymorphisms and cardiovascular disease: A HuGE review. *American Journal of Epidemiology* 164:921–935

Case NF, Charlton A, Zwiers A *et al.* (2016). Cerebral amyloid angiopathy is associated with executive dysfunction and mild cognitive impairment. *Stroke* 47:2010–2016

Chabriat H, Vahedi K, Iba-Zizen MT *et al.* (1995). Clinical spectrum of CADASIL: A study of 7 families. *Lancet* 346:934–939

Chabriat H, Levy C, Taillia H *et al.* (1998). Patterns of MRI lesions in CADASIL. *Neurology* 51:452–457

Charidimou A, Gang Q, Werring DJ (2012). Sporadic cerebral amyloid angiopathy revisited: recent insights into pathophysiology and clinical spectrum. *Journal of Neurology, Neurosurgery and Psychiatry* 83:124–137

Charidimou A, Baron JC, Werring DJ (2013). Transient focal neurological episodes, cerebral amyloid angiopathy, and intracerebral hemorrhage risk: Looking beyond TIAs. *International Journal of Stroke* 8:105–108

Devan WJ, Falcone GJ, Anderson CD *et al.* (2013). Heritability estimates identify a substantial contribution to risk and outcome of intracerebral hemorrhage. *Stroke* 44:1578–1583

Dichgans M, Markus HS (2005). Genetic association studies in stroke: Methodological issues and proposed standard criteria. *Stroke* 36:2027–2031

Dichgans M, Mayer M, Müller-Myhsok B *et al.* (1996). Identification of a key recombinant narrows the CADASIL gene region to 8 cM and argues against allelism of CADASIL and familial hemiplegic migraine. *Genomics* 32:151–154

Dichgans M, Mayer M, Uttner I *et al.* (1998). The phenotypic spectrum of CADASIL: Clinical findings in 102 cases. *Annals of Neurology* 44:731–739

Dubroca C, Lacombe P, Domenga V *et al.* (2005). Impaired vascular mechanotransduction in a transgenic mouse model of CADASIL arteriopathy. *Stroke* 36:113–117

Ebke M, Dichgans M, Bergmann M *et al.* (1997). CADASIL: Skin biopsy allows diagnosis in early stages. *Acta Neurology Scandinavica* 95:351–357

Falcone GJ, Malik R, Dichgans M *et al.* (2014). Current concepts and clinical applications of stroke genetics. *Lancet Neurology* 13:405–418

Flossmann E, Schulz UG, Rothwell PM (2004). Systematic review of methods and results of studies of the genetic epidemiology of ischemic stroke. *Stroke* 35:212–227

Flossmann E, Schulz UG, Rothwell PM (2005). Potential confounding by intermediate phenotypes in studies of the genetics of ischaemic stroke. *Cerebrovascular Diseases* 19:1–10

Fotiadis P, van Rooden S, van der Grond J *et al.* (2016). Cortical atrophy in patients with cerebral amyloid angiopathy: A case-control study. *Lancet Neurology* 15:811–819

Franz WM, Muller OJ, Katus HA (2001). Cardiomyopathies: From genetics to the prospect of treatment. *Lancet* 358:1627–1637

French CR, Seshadri S, Destefano AL *et al.* (2014). Mutation of FOXC1 and PITX2 induces cerebral small-vessel disease. *Journal of Clinical Investigation* 124:4877–4881

Gould DB, Phalan FC, van Mil SE *et al.* (2006). Role of COL4A1 in small-vessel disease and hemorrhagic stroke. *New England Journal of Medicine* 354:1489–1496

Gretarsdottir S, Thorleifsson G, Manolescu A *et al.* (2008). Risk variants for atrial fibrillation on chromosome 4q25 associate with ischemic stroke. *Annals of Neurology* 64:402–409

Gudbjartsson DF, Arnar DO, Helgadottir A *et al.* (2007). Variants conferring risk of atrial fibrillation on chromosome 4q25. *Nature* 448:353–357

Gudbjartsson DF, Holm H, Gretarsdottir S *et al.* (2009). A sequence variant in ZFHX3 on 16q22 associates with atrial fibrillation and ischemic stroke. *Nature Genetics* **41**:876–878

Gulcher JR, Gretarsdottir S, Helgadottir A *et al.* (2005). Genes contributing to risk for common forms of stroke. *Trends in Molecular Medicine* **11**:217–224

Gulcher JR, Kong A, Gretarsdottir S *et al.* (2006). Reply to "Many hypotheses but no replication for the association between PDE4D and stroke." *Nature Genetics* **38**:1092–1093

Guo JM, Liu AJ, Zang P *et al.* (2013). ALDH2 protects against stroke by clearing 4-HNE. *Cell Research* **23**:915–930

Hara K, Shiga A, Fukutake T (2009). Association of HTRA1 mutations and familial ischemic cerebral small-vessel disease. *New England Journal of Medicine* **360**:1729–1739

Hassan A, Markus HS (2000). Genetics and ischaemic stroke. *Brain* **123**:1784–1812

Hassan A, Sham PC, Markus HS (2002). Planning genetic studies in human stroke: sample size estimates based on family history data. *Neurology* **58**:1483–1488

Holliday EG, Maguire JM, Evans TJ *et al.* (2012). Common variants at 6p21.1 are associated with large artery atherosclerotic stroke. *Nature Genetics* **44**:1147–1151

Humphries SE, Morgan L (2004). Genetic risk factors for stroke and carotid atherosclerosis: Insights into pathophysiology from candidate gene approaches. *Lancet Neurology* **3**:227–235

Hutchinson M, O'Riordan J, Javed M *et al.* (1995). Familial hemiplegic migraine and autosomal dominant ateriopathy with leukoencephalopathy (CADASIL). *Annals of Neurology* **38**:817–824

Hutter CM, Austin MA, Humphries SE (2004). Familial hypercholesterolemia, peripheral arterial disease and stroke: A HuGE minireview. *American Journal of Epidemiology* **160**:430–435

Jeanne M, Labelle-Dumais C, Jorgensen J *et al.* (2012). COL4A2 mutations impair COL4A1 and COL4A2 secretion and cause hemorrhagic stroke. *American Journal of Human Genetics* **90**:91–101

Joutel A, Corpechot C, Ducros A *et al.* (1996). Notch3 mutations in CADASIL, a hereditary adult-onset condition causing stroke and dementia. *Nature* **383**:707–710

Joutel A, Vahedi K, Corpechot C *et al.* (1997). Strong clustering and stereotyped nature of Notch3 mutations in CADASIL patients. *Lancet* **350**:1511–1515

Joutel A, Dodick DD, Parisi JE *et al.* (2000). De novo mutation in the Notch3 gene causing CADASIL. *Annals of Neurology* **47**:388–391

Jung HH, Bassetti C, Tournier-Lasserve E *et al.* (1995). Cerebral autosomal dominant arteriopathy with subcortical infarcts and leukoencephalopathy: A clinicopathological and genetic study of a Swiss family. *Journal of Neurology, Neurosurgery and Psychiatry* **59**:138–143

Keavney B, McKenzie C, Parish S *et al.* (2000). Large-scale test of hypothesised associations between the angiotensin-converting-enzyme, insertion/deletion polymorphism and myocardial infarction in about 5000 cases and 6000 controls. International Studies of Infarct Survival (ISIS) Collaborators. *Lancet* **355**:434–442

Lemmens R, Buysschaert I, Geelen V *et al.* (2010). The association of the 4q25 susceptibility variant for atrial fibrillation with stroke is limited to stroke of cardioembolic etiology. *Stroke* **41**:1850–1857

Lubitz SA, Sinner MF, Lunetta KL *et al.* (2010). Independent susceptibility markers for atrial fibrillation on chromosome 4q25. *Circulation* **122**:976–984

Meschia JF (2003). Familial hypercholesterolemia: Stroke and the broader perspective. *Stroke* **34**:22–25

Meschia JF, Arnett DK, Ay H *et al.* (2013). Stroke Genetics Network (SiGN) study: Design and rationale for a genome-wide association study of ischemic stroke subtypes. *Stroke* **44**:2694–2702

Monet-Lepretre M, Bardot B, Lemaire B *et al.* (2009). Distinct phenotypic and functional features of CADASIL mutations in the Notch3 ligand binding domain. *Brain* **132**:1601–1612

Neurology Working Group of the Cohorts for Heart and Aging Research in Genomic Epidemiology (CHARGE) Consortium; Stroke Genetics Network (SiGN); International Stroke

Genetics Consortium (ISGC) (2016). Identification of additional risk loci for stroke and small vessel disease: A meta-analysis of genome-wide association studies. *Lancet Neurology* 15:695–707

NINDS Stroke Genetics Network (SiGN) and International Stroke Genetics Consortium (ISGC) (2016). Loci associated with ischemic stroke and its subtypes (SiGN): A genome-wide association study. *Lancet Neurology* 15:174–184

Razvi SS M, Davidson R, Bone I *et al.* (2005). The prevalence of cerebral autosomal dominant arteriopathy with subcortical infarcts and leucoencephalopathy (CADASIL) in the west of Scotland. *Journal of Neurology, Neurosurgery and Psychiatry* 76:739–741

Rolfs A, Bottcher T, Zschiesche M *et al.* (2005). Prevalence of Fabry disease in patients with cryptogenic stroke: A prospective study. *Lancet* 366:1794–1796

Rosand J, Bayley N, Rost N *et al.* (2006). Many hypotheses but no replication for the association between PDE4D and stroke. *Nature Genetics* 38:1091–1092

Schulz UG, Flossman E, Rothwell PM (2004). Heritability of ischemic stroke in relation to age, vascular risk factors and subtypes of incident stroke in population-based studies. *Stroke* 35:819–824

Singhal S, Bevan S, Barrick T *et al.* (2004). The influence of genetic and cardiovascular risk factors on the CADASIL phenotype. *Brain* 127:2031–2038

Sudlow C, Martinez Gonzalez NA, Kim J *et al.* (2006). Does apolipoprotein E genotype influence the risk of ischemic stroke, intracerebral hemorrhage, or subarachnoid hemorrhage? Systematic review and meta-analyses of 31 studies among 5961 cases and 17 965 controls. *Stroke* 37:364–370

Tournier-Lasserve E, Joutel A, Melki J *et al.* (1993). Cerebral autosomal dominant arteriopathy with subcortical infarcts and leukoencephalopathy maps to chromosome 19q12. *Nature Genetics* 3:256–259

Traylor M, Farrall M, Holliday EG *et al.* (2012). Genetic risk factors for ischemic stroke and its subtypes (the METASTROKE Collaboration): A meta-analysis of genome-wide association studies. *Lancet Neurology* 11:951–962

Vahedi K, Boukobza M, Massin P *et al.* (2007). Clinical and brain MRI follow-up study of a family with COL4A1 mutation. *Neurology* 69:1564–1568

van der Knaap MS, Smit LME, Barkhof F *et al.* (2006). Neonatal porencephaly and adult stroke related to mutations in collage IV A1. *Annals of Neurology* 59:504–511

Viskin S, Long QT (1999). Syndromes and torsade de pointes. *Lancet* 354:1625–1633

Weng WC, Sonni A, Labelle-Dumais C *et al.* (2012). COL4A1 mutations in patients with sporadic late-onset intracerebral hemorrhage. *Annals of Neurology* 71:470–477

Wheeler JG, Keavney BD, Watkins H *et al.* (2004). Four paraoxonase gene polymorphisms in 11 212 cases of coronary heart disease and 12 786 controls: Meta-analysis of 43 studies. *Lancet* 363:689–695

Williams FM, Carter AM, Hysi PG *et al.* (2013). Ischemic stroke is associated with the ABO locus: the EuroCLOT study. *Annals of Neurology* 73:16–31

Woo D, Falcone GJ, Devan WJ *et al.* (2014). Meta-analyses of genome-wide association studies identifies 1q22 as a susceptibility locus for intracerebral hemorrhage. *American Journal of Human Genetics* 94:511–521

Yamada M (2015). Cerebral amyloid angiopathy: emerging concepts. *Journal of Stroke* 17:17–30

Yanagawa S, Ito N, Arima K *et al.* (2002). Cerebral autosomal recessive arteriopathy with subcortical infarcts and leukoencephalopathy. *Neurology* 58:817–820

Anatomy and Physiology

Knowledge of the anatomy of the blood supply of the brain is often helpful in understanding the etiology and mechanisms of TIA and stroke, which enables accurate targeting of acute treatment and secondary prevention. An awareness of the mechanisms underpinning the regulation of cerebral blood flow allows the clinician to identify patients at risk of stroke and assess the possible effects of treatments.

The Anatomy of the Cerebral Circulation

The brain makes up only 2% of the total body weight, but when the body is at rest, it receives 20% of the cardiac output and consumes about 20% of the total inspired oxygen. The anterior two-thirds of the brain is supplied by the two internal carotid arteries, and the posterior third of the brain by the two vertebral arteries (Fig. 4.1). These four arteries anastomose at the base of the brain to form the circle of Willis (Fig. 4.2).

The detailed anatomy of the cerebral circulation is well described by Sheldon (1981). There is individual variation in arterial anatomy and thus in the territories of supply of the various major arteries, which can be asymmetrical and may change over time, depending on obstruction to vessel flow and the availability of functional collaterals (van der Zwan *et al.* 1992, Hartkamp *et al.* 1999) (Fig. 4.3). Developmental anomalies of the major cerebral vessels include:

- inequality in size of the two vertebral arteries.
- a combined origin of the left common carotid and innominate arteries.
- the right common carotid artery arising from the aortic arch.
- the left vertebral artery arising directly from the aorta.
- hypoplasia or absence of the proximal part of one anterior cerebral artery so that blood flow to both anterior cerebral arteries comes from one internal carotid artery.
- hypoplasia or absence of the anterior communicating artery.
- hypoplasia or absence of one or both posterior communicating artery(ies).
- hypoplasia or absence of one or both proximal posterior cerebral artery(ies) (P1 segment) such that blood flow to the posterior cerebral artery is predominantly from the internal carotid artery (fetal origin of the posterior cerebral artery).
- a persistent trigeminal artery joining the internal carotid artery to the basilar artery.
- a paired or fenestrated basilar artery.

The **internal carotid artery** starts as the carotid sinus at the bifurcation of the **common carotid artery** at the level of the thyroid cartilage. It runs up the neck, without any branches, to the base of the skull where it passes through the foramen lacerum to enter the carotid canal of the petrous bone. It then runs through the cavernous sinus in an

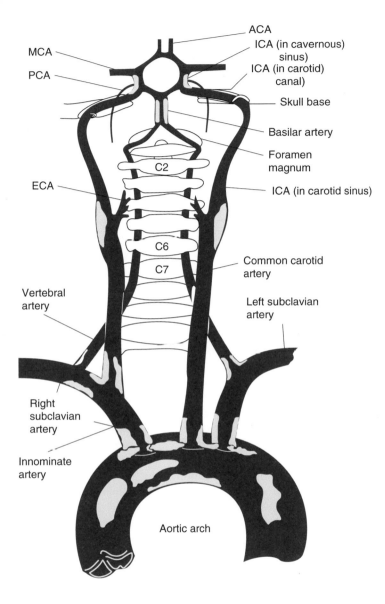

ACA

ICA (in cavernous) sinus)

ICA (in carotid) canal)

MCA

PCA

Skull base

Basilar artery

Foramen magnum

C2

ECA

ICA (in carotid sinus)

C6

C7

Common carotid artery

Vertebral artery

Left subclavian artery

Right subclavian artery

Innominate artery

Aortic arch

Fig. 4.1 The anatomy of the arterial circulation to the brain. Gray indentations into the arterial lumen represent sites at which atherothrombosis is particularly common. ACA, anterior cerebral artery; ECA, external carotid artery; ICA, internal carotid artery; MCA, middle cerebral artery; PCA, posterior cerebral artery.

S-shaped curve (the carotid siphon), pierces the dura, and exits just medial to the anterior clinoid process. It then bifurcates into the anterior cerebral artery and the larger middle cerebral artery.

The **external carotid artery** also starts at the bifurcation. Branches supply the jaw, face, scalp, neck, and meninges via the superficial temporal, facial, and occipital arteries.

The **ophthalmic artery** is the first major branch of the internal carotid artery and arises in the cavernous sinus. It passes through the optic foramen to supply the eye and other structures in the orbit.

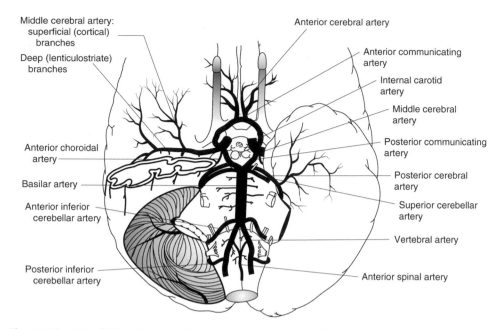

Fig. 4.2 The circle of Willis at the base of the brain as seen from below. There is considerable anatomical variation, and this figure represents one of the more common arrangements.

The **posterior communicating artery** is the next artery to arise from the internal carotid artery and passes back to join the first part of the posterior cerebral artery, so contributing to the circle of Willis. Tiny branches supply the adjacent optic chiasm, optic tract, hypothalamus, thalamus, and midbrain.

The **anterior choroidal artery** arises from the last section of the internal carotid artery, just beyond the posterior communicating artery origin, and supplies the optic tract, internal capsule, medial parts of the basal ganglia, medial part of the temporal lobe, thalamus, lateral geniculate body, proximal optic radiation, and midbrain. Occasionally it arises from the proximal middle cerebral artery or posterior communicating artery. Minor twiglets from the distal internal carotid artery contribute blood to the pituitary gland, optic chiasm, and nearby structures, including the meninges.

The **anterior cerebral artery** passes horizontally and medially to enter the interhemispheric fissure. It then anastomoses with its counterpart of the opposite side via the **anterior communicating artery**, curves up around the genu of the corpus callosum, and supplies the anterior and medial parts of the cerebral hemisphere. Small branches also supply parts of the optic nerve and chiasm, hypothalamus, anterior basal ganglia, and internal capsule.

The **middle cerebral artery** enters the Sylvian fissure and divides into two to four branches, which supply the lateral parts of the cerebral hemisphere. From its main trunk, a medial and lateral group of tiny lenticulostriate arteries and arterioles pass upward to penetrate the base of the brain and supply the basal ganglia and internal capsule (Marinkovic *et al.* 1985). Some of these small penetrating vessels extend up into the white matter of the corona radiata in the centrum semiovale toward the small medullary perforating branches of the cortical arteries coming down from above.

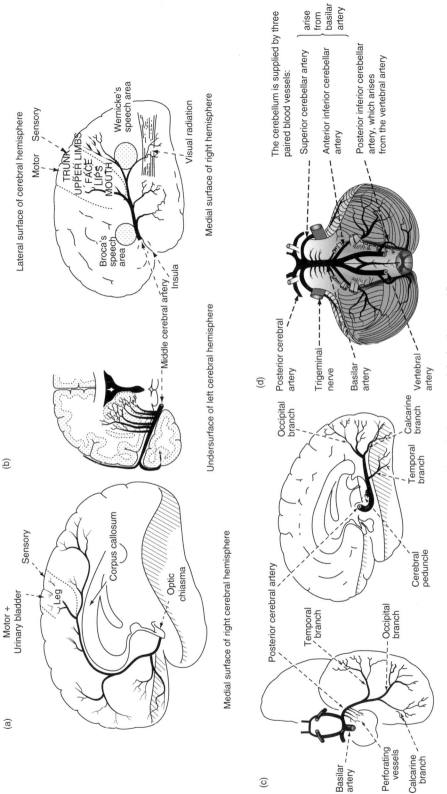

Fig. 4.3 Brain areas supplied by the anterior (a), middle (b), and posterior (c) cerebral arteries and the basilar artery (d).

(a)

Medial surface of right cerebral hemisphere

Motor +
Urinary bladder
Sensory
Leg
Corpus callosum
Optic
chiasma

(b)

Lateral surface of cerebral hemisphere

Motor   Sensory
TRUNK
UPPER LIMBS
FACE
LIPS
MOUTH
Wernicke's
speech area

Broca's
speech
area

Medial surface of right hemisphere

Visual radiation

Undersurface of left cerebral hemisphere

Middle cerebral artery

Insula

(c)

Posterior cerebral artery

Temporal
branch

Occipital
branch

Basilar
artery

Perforating
vessels

Calcarine
branch

Occipital
branch

Calcarine
branch

Temporal
branch

Cerebral
peduncle

(d)

The cerebellum is supplied by three
paired blood vessels:

Superior cerebellar artery
Anterior inferior cerebellar
artery
} arise
from
basilar
artery

Posterior inferior cerebellar
artery, which arises
from the vertebral artery

Posterior cerebral
artery

Trigeminal
nerve

Basilar
artery

Vertebral
artery

The **vertebral artery** arises from the proximal subclavian artery and ascends to pass through the transverse foramina of the sixth to second cervical vertebrae, giving off small muscular branches on the way. It then passes posteriorly around the articular process of the atlas to enter the skull through the foramen magnum. It unites with the opposite vertebral artery on the ventral surface of the brainstem at the pontomedullary junction to form the basilar artery. Branches to the meninges arise at the foramen magnum. The vertebral artery gives rise to the anterior and posterior spinal arteries; the posterior inferior cerebellar artery, which supplies the inferior vermis and inferior and posterior surfaces of the cerebellar hemispheres and brainstem; and the small penetrating arteries to the medulla.

The **basilar artery** ascends ventral to the pons to the ponto–midbrain junction in the interpeduncular cistern, where it divides into the two posterior cerebral arteries. Numerous small branches penetrate the brainstem and cerebellum. The basilar artery also gives rise to the anterior inferior cerebellar artery, which supplies the rostral cerebellum, brainstem, and inner ear; and the superior cerebellar artery, which supplies the brainstem, superior half of the cerebellar hemisphere, vermis, and dentate nucleus.

The **posterior cerebral artery** encircles the midbrain close to the oculomotor nerve at the level of the tentorium and supplies the inferior part of the temporal lobe and the occipital lobe (Marinkovic *et al.* 1987). Many small perforating arteries arise from the proximal portion of the posterior cerebral artery to supply the midbrain, thalamus, hypothalamus, and geniculate bodies. Sometimes a single perforating artery (artery of Percheron) supplies the medial part of both thalami and/or both sides of the midbrain. In approximately 15% of individuals, the posterior cerebral artery is a direct continuation of the posterior communicating artery, its main blood supply then coming from the internal carotid artery rather than the basilar artery (fetal origin of the posterior cerebral artery).

The meninges is supplied by branches of the external carotid artery, internal carotid artery, and vertebral arteries. The most prominent branches of the external carotid artery are the middle meningeal artery and tributaries of the ascending pharyngeal and occipital arteries. Most of the branches from the internal carotid artery arise near the cavernous sinus and from the ophthalmic artery in the orbit. Branches from the vertebral artery arise at the foramen magnum. There are numerous meningeal anastomoses between these small arteries.

The scalp is supplied by branches of the external carotid artery, particularly the superficial temporal, occipital, and posterior auricular arteries. Above the orbit, there is a contribution from terminal branches of the ophthalmic artery. There is a rich anastomotic network between the various arteries of the scalp.

Collateral Blood Supply to the Brain

The collateral blood supply to the brain is described by Liebeskind (2003). Common sites of collateral blood supply to and within the brain are:

- circle of Willis between anterior and posterior cerebral arteries.
- leptomeningeal anastomoses between surface of brain and anterior, middle, and posterior cerebral arteries.
- muscular branches of the vertebral artery in the neck.
- orbital anastomoses between branches of the external carotid and ophthalmic arteries.
- dural anastomoses between meningeal and internal, external, and vertebral arteries.
- choroidal anastomoses between internal carotid and posterior cerebral arteries.

Normally, the internal carotid artery provides blood to the anterior two-thirds of the ipsilateral cerebral hemisphere and the posterior circulation is supplied by the vertebral, basilar, and posterior cerebral arteries. Collateral channels may develop in response to occlusion of one or more of the intracerebral vessels, particularly if flow limitation is gradual rather than sudden. Unlike the normal cerebral blood supply, the functional capacity of the collateral blood supply to respond to changes in perfusion pressure is limited. Collateral blood flow may develop through various mechanisms in different areas.

The Circle of Willis

This is formed by the proximal part of the two anterior cerebral arteries connected by the anterior communicating artery and the proximal part of the two posterior cerebral arteries, which are connected to the distal internal carotid arteries by the posterior communicating arteries. However, approximately 50% of patients have one or more hypoplastic or absent segments, usually one of the communicating arteries, and atheroma may limit the potential for collateral flow (Fig. 4.2).

Leptomeningeal Anastomoses

These may develop on the surface of the brain between cortical branches of the anterior, middle, and posterior cerebral arteries and, to a lesser extent, between pial branches of the cerebellar arteries.

Muscular Branches of the Vertebral Artery in the Neck

At positions distal to a vertebral obstruction, these muscular branches may receive blood retrogradely from occipital and ascending pharyngeal branches of the external carotid artery or from the deep and ascending cervical arteries. In addition, anastomoses can develop between branches of the subclavian artery and external carotid artery when the common carotid artery is obstructed.

Around the Orbit

Branches of the external carotid artery can anastomose with branches of the ophthalmic artery if the internal carotid artery is severely stenosed or obstructed. Collateral flow from the external carotid artery into the orbit then passes retrogradely through the ophthalmic artery to fill the carotid siphon, middle cerebral artery, and anterior cerebral artery. Sometimes flow may even reach the posterior cerebral artery and vertebrobasilar system.

Dural Anastomoses

These can develop between meningeal branches of the internal carotid artery, external carotid artery, and vertebral arteries. Occasionally, small dural anastomoses develop between cortical, leptomeningeal, and dural arteries.

Parenchymal Anastomoses

These occasionally develop in the pre-capillary bed of the perforating arteries at the base of the brain supplying the basal ganglia.

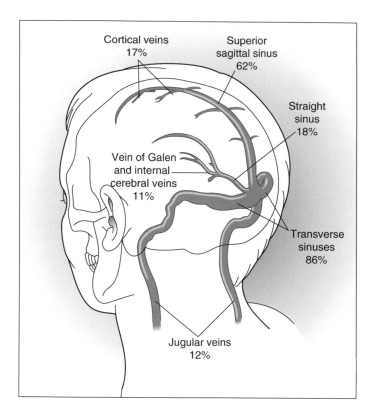

Fig. 4.4 Schematic diagram of the anatomy of the venous drainage of the brain. The frequencies of thrombosis in the various sinuses are given as percentages (see Chapter 29). In most patients, thrombosis occurs in more than one sinus (Stam 2005).

The Anterior Choroidal Artery

This branch of the internal carotid artery can anastomose with the posterior choroidal artery, a branch of the posterior cerebral artery.

Venous Drainage

The venous anatomy is very variable. Venous blood flows centrally via the deep cerebral veins and peripherally via the superficial cerebral veins into the dural venous sinuses, which lie between the outer and meningeal inner layer of the dura and drain into the internal jugular veins (Stam 2005) (Fig. 4.4). The cerebral veins do not have valves and are thin walled, and the blood flow is often in the same direction as in neighboring arteries. There are numerous venous connections between the cerebral veins and the dural sinuses, the venous system of the meninges, skull, scalp, and nasal sinuses, allowing infection or thrombus to propagate between these vessels.

The Regulation of Cerebral Blood Flow

Knowledge of cerebral blood flow regulation, and the relationship between cerebral blood flow and cerebral metabolism, has had a major influence on the understanding of the pathophysiology of impaired perfusion reserve and acute ischemic stroke (Frackowiak 1986; Marchal *et al.* 1996; Baron 2001; Rutgers *et al.* 2004).

Cerebral blood flow in normal humans is approximately 50 ml/min per 100 g brain. Using positron emission tomography (PET) (Frackowiak *et al.* 1980), it has been shown that cerebral blood flow, cerebral blood volume, and cerebral energy metabolism, measured as cerebral metabolic rate of oxygen ($CMRO_2$) or glucose (CMRglu), are all coupled and higher in gray than in white matter. This means that the oxygen extraction fraction is similar (approximately one-third) throughout the brain (Leenders *et al.* 1990). Therefore, in a normal resting human brain, cerebral blood volume is a reliable reflection of function or $CMRO_2$. There is a gradual fall of cerebral blood flow, cerebral blood volume, CMRglu, and $CMRO_2$ with age, but they remain coupled so that the oxygen extraction fraction remains more or less constant (Blesa *et al.* 1997).

Cerebral Blood Flow and Blood Gas Tensions

Cerebral blood flow is very susceptible to small changes in arterial partial pressure of carbon dioxide ($PaCO_2$): an acute rise of 1 mmHg causes an immediate increase in cerebral blood flow of approximately 5% through dilatation of cerebral resistance vessels. In chronic respiratory failure, however, adaptation occurs so that cerebral blood flow is normal despite hypercapnia. Modest changes in arterial oxygen tension do not affect cerebral blood flow, but when the PaO_2 falls below about 50 mmHg and oxygen saturation starts falling, there is a fall in cerebral vascular resistance and cerebral blood flow rises (Brown *et al.* 1985). Increasing PaO_2 above the normal level has little effect on cerebral blood flow.

Cerebral Blood Flow and Brain Function

Increasing regional functional activity of the brain, for instance in the motor cortex contralateral to voluntary hand movements, increases regional metabolic activity in the same area (Lassen *et al.* 1977; Geisler *et al.* 2006). The increasing $CMRO_2$ and CMRglu are achieved not by increasing oxygen extraction fraction or the glucose extraction fraction but by rapid (over seconds) local vasodilatation of the cerebral resistance vessels, increase in cerebral blood volume, and, therefore, increase in cerebral blood flow. Conversely, low functional and metabolic demand, as occurs in a cerebral infarction, is associated with a low cerebral blood flow.

Cerebral Blood Flow, Perfusion Pressure, and Autoregulation

Cerebral blood flow depends on cerebral perfusion pressure and cerebrovascular resistance. The perfusion pressure is the difference between systemic arterial pressure at the base of the brain when in the recumbent position and the venous pressure at exit from the subarachnoid space, the latter being approximated by the intracranial pressure. Cerebral perfusion pressure divided by cerebral blood flow gives the cerebrovascular resistance. In normal humans, cerebral blood flow remains almost constant when the mean systemic blood pressure is between approximately 50 and 170 mmHg, which, under normal circumstances, when the intracranial venous pressure is negligible, is the same as the cerebral perfusion pressure. This homeostatic mechanism to maintain a constant cerebral blood flow in the face of changes in cerebral perfusion pressure is known as autoregulation (Reed and Devous 1985; Powers 1993). Autoregulation is less effective in the elderly, and so postural hypotension is more likely to be symptomatic (Wollner *et al.* 1979; Parry *et al.* 2006).

Within the autoregulatory range, as cerebral perfusion pressure falls, there is within seconds, vasodilatation of the small cerebral resistance vessels, a fall in cerebrovascular resistance, and a rise in cerebral blood volume. As a result, cerebral blood flow remains constant (Aaslid *et al.* 1989). If vasodilatation is maximal and cerebral perfusion pressure continues to fall owing to a drop in systemic blood pressure or an increase in intracranial pressure, cerebral blood flow starts to decline as the cerebral perfusion reserve is exhausted. However, metabolic activity is maintained by increasing oxygen extraction fraction: this is "misery" perfusion or oligemia. Eventually, the oxygen extraction fraction is maximal, and with further cerebral perfusion pressure reduction, metabolic activity is reduced, $CMRO_2$ starts to fall, and metabolism becomes limited by perfusion. This is what is normally meant by ischemia; the perfusion reserve is exhausted, and flow is inadequate to meet the metabolic demands of the tissues. At this point, the patient becomes symptomatic with non-focal neurological features such as faintness if the whole brain is involved or focal neurological features such as hemiparesis if only part of the brain is involved.

If the perfusion pressure rises above the autoregulatory range, where compensatory vasoconstriction and cerebral perfusion pressure are maximal, then hyperemia occurs followed by vasogenic edema, raised intracranial pressure, and the clinical syndrome of hypertensive encephalopathy.

Cerebral Perfusion Reserve

It follows from the above that the ratio of cerebral blood flow to cerebral blood volume is a measure of cerebral perfusion reserve (Schumann *et al.* 1998). Below a ratio of approximately 6.0, even if cerebral blood flow is still normal, vasodilatation and cerebral blood volume are maximal and the reserve is exhausted, as shown by a rising oxygen extraction fraction on PET.

Chronically impaired perfusion reserve tends to occur when one or both internal carotid arteries are stenosed by at least 50% of the luminal diameter (Brice *et al.* 1964; DeWeese *et al.* 1970; Schroeder 1988) or are occluded, and the collateral circulation is inadequate (Powers *et al.* 1987; Kluytmans *et al.* 1999). In this situation, the brain is vulnerable to any further fall in cerebral perfusion pressure, and cerebral metabolism is beginning to become impaired, with the appearance of structural abnormalities on MRI (van der Grond *et al.* 1996; Isaka *et al.* 1997; Derdeyn *et al.* 1999).

Indirect assessment of perfusion reserve can be achieved by using transcranial Doppler ultrasound, single-photon emission CT, PET, dynamic CT, or functional MRI to measure cerebral blood flow response to hypercapnia during carbon dioxide inhalation or breath holding or after intravenous acetazolamide, a carbonic anhydrase inhibitor (Arigoni *et al.* 2000; Kikuchi *et al.* 2001; Shiogai *et al.* 2002, 2003; Shiino *et al.* 2003). However, there is uncertainty about how these various tests should be standardized and how to define "normality", given that a continuous variable is being measured. It should be noted that indirect methods of measuring perfusion reserve are inaccurate when the normal relationships between cerebral blood flow, cerebral blood volume, oxygen extraction fraction, and vascular reactivity break down, as they may well do in a newly ischemic or infarcted brain.

Impaired perfusion reserve is associated with an increased likelihood of recurrent stroke (Yamauchi *et al.* 1996), prior ischemic events in patients with carotid occlusion

(Derdeyn *et al.* 1999, 2005), presence of silent brain infarction, and increased likelihood of need for carotid shunting in carotid endarterectomy (Kim *et al.* 2000). Extracranial to intracranial bypass surgery has been shown to improve cerebral perfusion reserve in patients with large vessel occlusive disease (Schmiedek *et al.* 1994; Grubb *et al.* 1998). However, randomized controlled trials have failed to show a clinical benefit of extracranial-intracranial bypass surgery (EC/IC Bypass Study Group 1985; Powers *et al.* 2011), and hence extracranial-intracranial bypass surgery is not routinely recommended for secondary stroke prevention in current international guidelines (Kernan *et al.* 2014). Medical treatment with angiotensin-converting enzyme inhibitors has also been shown to increase cerebral perfusion reserve in patients with previous minor stroke (Hatazawa *et al.* 2004).

Cerebral Blood Flow, Hypertension, and Stroke

In chronically hypertensive patients, the autoregulatory range is shifted upward so that cerebral blood flow starts falling and ischemic symptoms occur at a higher systemic blood pressure than normal (Strandgaard and Paulson 1992), but autoregulation appears otherwise to be maintained (Traon *et al.* 2002) except in malignant hypertension (Immink *et al.* 2004). The upward shift of autoregulation appears to return toward normal when hypertension is treated. Conversely, hypertensive encephalopathy is more likely to occur in acute hypertension when the upper limit of autoregulation is still normal, such as occurs in eclampsia.

Autoregulation is impaired or abolished in damaged areas of brain, and then cerebral blood flow becomes "pressure passive" and follows perfusion pressure. Both static and dynamic cerebral autoregulation are impaired in patients with stroke (Strandgaard and Paulson 1992; Eames *et al.* 2002; Georgiadis *et al.* 2002; Novak *et al.* 2003), but treatment of hypertension with angiotensin-converting enzyme inhibitors and angiotensin II receptor antagonists subacutely after stroke appears to lower systemic pressure without compromising cerebral blood flow (Paulson and Waldemar 1990; Moriwaki *et al.* 2004; Nazir *et al.* 2004).

References

Aaslid R, Lindegaard KF, Sorteberg W *et al.* (1989). Cerebral autoregulation dynamics in humans. *Stroke* 20:45–52

Arigoni M, Kneifel S, Fandino J *et al.* (2000). Simplified quantitative determination of cerebral perfusion reserve with H₂(15)O PET and acetazolamide. *European Journal of Nuclear Medicine* 27:1557–1563

Baron JC (2001). Perfusion thresholds in human cerebral ischemia: Historical perspective and therapeutic implications. *Cerebrovascular Diseases* 11:2–8

Blesa R, Mohr E, Miletich RS *et al.* (1997). Changes in cerebral glucose metabolism with normal aging. *European Journal of Neurology* 4:8–14

Brice JG, Dowsett DJ, Lowe RD (1964). Haemodynamic effects of carotid artery stenosis. *British Medical Journal* ii:1363–1366

Brown MM, Wade JP, Marshall J (1985). Fundamental importance of arterial oxygen content in the regulation of cerebral blood flow in man. *Brain* 108:81–93

Derdeyn CP, Grubb RL Jr., Powers WJ (1999). Cerebral hemodynamic impairment: Methods of measurement and association with stroke risk. *Neurology* 53:251–259

Derdeyn CP, Grubb RL Jr., Powers WJ (2005). Indications for cerebral revascularization for patients with atherosclerotic carotid occlusion. *Skull Base* 15:7–14

DeWeese JA, May AG, Lipchik EO *et al.* (1970). Anatomic and haemodynamic correlations in carotid artery stenosis. *Stroke* 1:149–157

Eames PJ, Blake MJ, Dawson SL *et al.* (2002). Dynamic cerebral autoregulation and beat to beat blood pressure control are impaired in acute ischaemic stroke. *Journal of Neurology, Neurosurgery and Psychiatry* 72:467–472

EC/IC Bypass Study Group (1985). Failure of extracranial-intracranial arterial bypass to reduce the risk of ischemic stroke: Results of an international randomized trial. *New England Journal of Medicine* **313**:1191–1200

Frackowiak RSJ (1986). PET scanning: Can it help resolve management issues in cerebral ischaemic disease? *Stroke* **17**:803–807

Frackowiak RSJ, Jones T, Lenzi GL et al. (1980). Regional cerebral oxygen utilization and blood flow in normal man using oxygen-15 and positron emission tomography. *Acta Neurologica Scandinavica* **62**:336–344

Geisler BS, Brandhoff F, Fiehler J et al. (2006). Blood-oxygen-level-dependent MRI allows metabolic description of tissue at risk in acute stroke patients. *Stroke* **37**:1778–1784

Georgiadis D, Schwarz S, Cencetti S et al. (2002). Noninvasive monitoring of hypertensive breakthrough of cerebral autoregulation in a patient with acute ischemic stroke. *Cerebrovascular Diseases* **14**:129–132

Grubb RL Jr., Derdeyn CP, Fritsch SM et al. (1998). Importance of hemodynamic factors in the prognosis of symptomatic carotid occlusion. *JAMA* **280**:1055–1060

Hartkamp MJ, van der Grond J, van Everdingen KJ et al. (1999). Circle of Willis collateral flow investigated by magnetic resonance angiography. *Stroke* **30**:2671–2678

Hatazawa J, Shimosegawa E, Osaki Y et al. (2004). Long-term angiotensin-converting enzyme inhibitor perindopril therapy improves cerebral perfusion reserve in patients with previous minor stroke. *Stroke* **35**:2117–2122

Immink RV, van den Born BJ, van Montfrans GA et al. (2004). Impaired cerebral autoregulation in patients with malignant hypertension. *Circulation* **110**:2241–2245

Isaka Y, Nagano K, Narita M et al. (1997). High signal intensity of T_2-weighted magnetic resonance imaging and cerebral hemodynamic reserve in carotid occlusive disease. *Stroke* **28**:354–357

Kernan KN, Ovbiagele B, Black HR et al. (2014). Guidelines for the prevention of stroke in patients with stroke and transient ischemic attack: A guideline for healthcare professionals from the American Heart Association/America Stroke Association. *Stroke* **45**:2160–2236

Kikuchi K, Murase K, Miki H et al. (2001). Measurement of cerebral hemodynamics with perfusion-weighted MR imaging: Comparison with pre- and post-acetazolamide ^{133}Xe-SPECT in occlusive carotid disease. *American Journal of Neuroradiology* **22**:248–254

Kim JS, Moon DH, Kim GE et al. (2000). Acetazolamide stress brain-perfusion SPECT predicts the need for carotid shunting during carotid endarterectomy. *Journal of Nuclear Medicine* **41**:1836–1841

Kluytmans M, van der Grond, KJ, van Everdingen KJ et al. (1999). Cerebral hemodynamics in relation to patterns of collateral flow. *Stroke* **30**:1432–1439

Lassen NA, Roland PE, Larsen B et al. (1977). Mapping of human cerebral functions: A study of the regional cerebral blood flow pattern during rest its reproducibility and the activations seen during basic sensory and motor functions. *Acta Neurology Scandinavica* **64**:262–263

Leenders KL, Perani D, Lammertsma AA et al. (1990). Cerebral blood flow, blood volume and oxygen utilisation. Normal values and effect of age. *Brain* **113**:27–47

Liebeskind DS (2003). Collateral circulation. *Stroke* **34**:2279–2284

Marchal G, Beaudouin V, Rioux P et al. (1996). Prolonged persistence of substantial volumes of potentially viable brain tissue after stroke. A correlative PET–CT study with voxel-based data analysis. *Stroke* **27**:599–606

Marinkovic SV, Milisavljevic MM, Kovacevic MS et al. (1985). Perforating branches of the middle cerebral artery. Micro-anatomy and clinical significance of their intracerebral segments. *Stroke* **16**:1022–1029

Marinkovic SV, Milisavljevic MM, Lolic-Draganic V et al. (1987). Distribution of the occipital branches of the posterior cerebral artery. Correlation with occipital lobe infarcts. *Stroke* **18**:728–732

Moriwaki H, Uno H, Nagakane Y et al. (2004). Losartan, an angiotensin II (AT1) receptor antagonist, preserves cerebral blood flow in hypertensive patients with a history of stroke. *Journal of Human Hypertension* 18:693–699

Nazir FS, Overell JR, Bolster A *et al.* (2004). The effect of losartan on global and focal cerebral perfusion and on renal function in hypertensives in mild early ischaemic stroke. *Journal of Hypertension* 22:989–995

Novak V, Chowdhary A, Farrar B *et al.* (2003). Altered cerebral vasoregulation in hypertension and stroke. *Neurology* 60:1657–1663

Parry SW, Steen N, Baptist M *et al.* (2006). Cerebral autoregulation is impaired in cardioinhibitory carotid sinus syndrome. *Heart* 92:792–797

Paulson OB, Waldemar G (1990). ACE inhibitors and cerebral blood flow. *Journal of Human Hypertension* 4(Suppl 4):69–72

Powers WJ (1993). Acute hypertension after stroke: The scientific basis for treatment decisions. *Neurology* 43:461–467

Powers WJ, Press GA, Grubb RL *et al.* (1987). The effect of haemodynamically significant carotid artery disease on the haemodynamic status of the cerebral circulation. *Annals of Internal Medicine* 106:27–34

Powers WJ, Clarke WR, Grubb RL Jr *et al.* (2011). Extracranial-intracranial bypass surgery for stroke prevention in hemodynamic cerebral ischemia: The Carotid Occlusion Surgery Study randomized trial. *JAMA* 306:1983–1992

Reed G, Devous M (1985). South-western Internal Medicine Conference: Cerebral blood flow autoregulation and hypertension. *American Journal of Medical Science* 289:37–44

Rutgers DR, Klijn CJ, Kappelle LJ *et al.* (2004). Recurrent stroke in patients with symptomatic carotid artery occlusion is associated with high-volume flow to the brain and increased collateral circulation. *Stroke* 35:1345–1349

Schroeder T (1988). Haemodynamic significance of internal carotid artery disease. *Acta Neurologica Scandinavica* 77:353–372

Schmiedek P, Piepgras A, Leinsinger G *et al.* (1994). Improvement of cerebrovascular reserve capacity by EC-IC arterial bypass surgery in patients with ICA occlusion and hemodynamic cerebral ischaemia. *Journal of Neurosurgery* 81:236–244

Schumann P, Touzani O, Young AR *et al.* (1998). Evaluation of the ratio of cerebral blood flow to cerebral blood volume as an index of local cerebral perfusion pressure. *Brain* 121:1369–1379

Sheldon JJ (1981). *Blood Vessels of the Scalp and Brain.* Oak Ridge, NJ: CIBA Pharmaceutical Corporation.

Shiino A, Morita Y, Tsuji A *et al.* (2003). Estimation of cerebral perfusion reserve by blood oxygenation level-dependent imaging: Comparison with single-photon emission computed tomography. *Journal of Cerebral Blood Flow and Metabolism* 23:121–135

Shiogai T, Uebo C, Makino M *et al.* (2002). Acetazolamide vasoreactivity in vascular dementia and persistent vegetative state evaluated by transcranial harmonic perfusion imaging and Doppler sonography. *Annals of the New York Academy of Sciences* 977:445–453

Shiogai T, Koshimura M, Murata Y *et al.* (2003). Acetazolamide vasoreactivity evaluated by transcranial harmonic perfusion imaging: Relationship with transcranial Doppler sonography and dynamic CT. *Acta Neurochirurgia Supplement* 86:57–62

Stam J (2005). Thrombosis of the cerebral veins and sinuses. *New England Journal of Medicine* 352:1791–1798

Strandgaard S, Paulson OB (1992). Regulation of cerebral blood flow in health and disease. *Journal of Cardiovascular Pharmacology* 19: S89–S93

Traon AP, Costes-Salon MC, Galinier M *et al.* (2002). Dynamics of cerebral blood flow autoregulation in hypertensive patients. *Journal of Neurology Science* 195:139–144

van der Grond J, Eikelboom BC, Mali WP (1996). Flow-related anaerobic metabolic changes in patients with severe stenosis of the internal carotid artery. *Stroke* 27:2026–2032

van der Zwan A, Hillen B, Tulleken CAF *et al.* (1992). Variability of the territories of the major cerebral arteries. *Journal of Neurosurgery* 77:927–940

Wollner L, McCarthy ST, Soper NDW *et al.* (1979). Failure of cerebral autoregulation as a cause of brain dysfunction in the elderly. *British Medical Journal* **1**:1117–1118

Yamauchi H, Fukuyama H, Nagahama Y *et al.* (1996). Evidence of misery perfusion and risk for recurrent stroke in major cerebral arterial occlusive diseases from PET. *Journal of Neurology, Neurosurgery and Psychiatry* **61**:18–25

Pathophysiology of Acute Cerebral Ischemia

The brain normally derives its energy from the oxidative metabolism of glucose. Because there are negligible stores of glucose in the brain, when cerebral blood flow falls and the brain becomes ischemic, a series of neurophysiological and functional changes occur at various thresholds of flow before cell death (infarction). The degree of cell damage depends on not only the depth of ischemia but also its duration and the availability of collateral circulation (Liebeskind 2003; Zemke *et al.* 2004; Harukuni and Bhardwaj 2006). Different mechanisms are responsible for reversible loss of cellular function and for irreversible cell death, and there are also differences between the mechanisms that cause death of neurons, glia, and endothelial cells and perhaps between cells in white versus gray matter.

Mechanisms of Cerebral Ischemia

When cerebral blood flow falls below approximately 20 ml/min per 100 g brain, the oxygen extraction fraction becomes maximal and the cerebral metabolic rate of oxygen begins to fall, resulting in ischemia (Wise *et al.* 1983). The electroencephalograph readings flatten, evoked responses disappear, and neurological signs appear. In fact, a high oxygen extraction fraction is only seen early after acute ischemic stroke, in the first day or so, and functional recovery is still possible if flow is restored. Although the exact cellular pathways of ischemia and infarction are not fully described in humans, four overlapping mechanisms are at work: excitotoxicity, depolarization, inflammation, and apoptosis (Table 5.1). Excitotoxicity and depolarization are processes that occur within minutes and hours of an ischemic insult, while inflammation and apoptosis occur within hours and days. The clinical significance of these different mechanisms lies in the potential to design therapies that intervene at different levels in cellular pathways, thereby preventing or delaying damage to neuronal cells and increasing the potential for recovery (neuroprotection), although developments so far have been disappointing (Chamorro *et al.* 2016).

Excitotoxicity

Focal impairment of cerebral blood flow restricts the delivery of oxygen and glucose, with resultant disruption of cellular oxidative phosphorylation and energy production. Membranes become rapidly depolarized and extracellular glutamate accumulates by movement across electrical gradients, compounded by disturbance of synaptic reuptake processes. Extracellular glutamate binds to and activates various membrane receptors, most importantly NMDA (N-methyl-D-aspartate) and AMPA (α-amino-3-

Table 5.1 Summary of the principle mechanisms of cerebral ischemic damage

Mechanisms	Events
Excitotoxicity	Membrane depolarization in response to disrupted cellular oxidative and energy production processes leading to damaging activity of secondary messengers
Depolarization	Local depolarization caused by focal hypoxia decompensates already threatened metabolism in penumbra and propagates ischemic damage
Inflammation	Injury mediated by enzymic (proteases and collagenases), cellular (neutrophils and macrophages), and vascular processes
Apoptosis	Programmed or ordered cell death mediated by caspase enzymes

hydroxy-5-methyl-4-isooxazolepropionate), which open transmembrane channels permeable to cations including sodium, potassium, calcium, and hydrogen. Water follows passively as the influx of sodium and chloride ions exceeds the efflux of potassium ions, and the resulting edema has deleterious effects locally and distantly through mass effect.

An intracellular increase in the secondary messenger calcium initiates a series of damaging cytoplasmic and nuclear events (Bano and Nicotera 2007). Proteolytic enzymes are activated, which degrade cytoskeleton proteins such as actin and spectrin. Free radical species are generated by activated cyclooxygenase and phospholipase enzymes, and these overwhelm endogenous scavenging mechanisms and cause lipid peroxidation and membrane damage as well as triggering inflammation and apoptosis. These cellular pathways and resultant damage are particularly important in the mitochondria (Back *et al.* 2004; Warner *et al.* 2004; Zemke *et al.* 2004).

Depolarization

In the core of the ischemic region, cells undergo anoxic depolarization with the release of potassium ions and glutamate and never repolarize. However, depolarization can be induced in nearby neurons by the resultant increase in extracellular potassium and glutamate, and sometimes repolarization can occur at the expense of further energy consumption. Repetitive de- and repolarization around ischemic areas is thought to further decompensate metabolism in the penumbra and propagate local ischemia (Hossmann 2006).

Inflammation

Intracellular calcium ions and free radicals trigger the expression of a range of pro-inflammatory genes, leading to the production of inflammatory mediators such as interleukin-1b, tumor necrosis factor, and platelet-activating factor by injured brain cells. Adhesion molecules on endothelial cell surfaces are also induced, leading to the accumulation and movement of neutrophils into the brain parenchyma (Zheng and Yenari 2004). This process can cause further damage through processes in the vasculature (local vasoconstriction and platelet activation), at the cellular level (protease and collagenase production), and by initiation of cell signaling (macrophage recruitment and microglial activation).

Apoptosis

Apoptosis is programmed cell death and differs from necrosis in that it results in minimal inflammation and release of genetic material. Although necrosis is the predominant process that follows acute ischemia, apoptosis is important after more minor injury, particularly within the ischemic penumbra. Apoptosis is executed by the production, activation, and action of caspases, which are protein-cleaving enzymes that dismantle cytoskeleton proteins and enzymes responsible for cellular repair (Zhang *et al.* 2004). Neurons are particularly susceptible to caspase-mediated cell death after cerebral ischemia, as demonstrated by the reduction in infarct size by caspase inhibitors in experimental models.

The Ischemic Penumbra and the Therapeutic Time Window

Around acutely infarcted brain, there is an ischemic penumbra (Astrup *et al.* 1981). Here the blood flow is low, function impaired, and the oxygen extraction fraction high. In other words, there is viable tissue with misery perfusion where the needs of the tissue are not being met. The tissue may die or recover, depending on the speed and extent of restoration of blood flow. This concept opens up the possibility of a therapeutic time window during which restoration of flow or neuronal protection from ischemic damage might prevent both immediate cell death and the recruitment of neurons for apoptosis (see Chapter 21).

PET studies in humans have demonstrated that about one-third of the ultimately infarcted tissue identified by late CT is in areas where, within hours of stroke onset, there had been potentially viable "penumbral" tissue (Marchal *et al.* 1996a). However, it is still not clear for how long this penumbral region persists in a potentially viable state, although time periods as long as 18 hours have been suggested, and it appears that some recovery is possible if flow is restored (Lassen *et al.* 1991; Furlan *et al.* 1996). Accurate information about the ischemic penumbra, and any areas of luxury perfusion, requires PET, which is not practical in the routine management of acute ischemic stroke. Diffusion-weighted and perfusion MRI (Baird *et al.* 1997; Barber *et al.* 1998a) and dynamic CT have been proposed to delineate the penumbra, and recent studies utilizing these techniques have successfully shown that the time window for treatment of ischemic stroke could be extended (Goyal *et al.* 2013; Albers et al. 2018; Nogueira et al. 2018) (Chapter 11).

Recanalization and Reperfusion

Spontaneous recanalization, at least of middle cerebral artery occlusion, occurs in up to two-thirds of patients within a week of stroke onset, many in the first 48 hours (Fieschi *et al.* 1989; Kaps *et al.* 1992; Zanette *et al.* 1995; Arnold *et al.* 2005). In general, the functional outcomes and final infarct size are both better with recanalization and reperfusion, and even with early hyperperfusion, than if the middle cerebral artery remains occluded (Wardlaw *et al.* 1993; Marchal *et al.* 1996b; Barber *et al.* 1998b).

During or following a cerebrovascular event, some brain areas may show relative or absolute hyperemia owing to good collateral flow, reperfusion after an occluded artery has been reopened, and/or inflammation and vasodilatation in response to hypercapnia. In hyperemic areas, oxygen extraction fraction is low and there is luxury perfusion, indicating

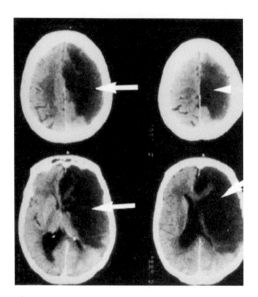

Fig. 5.1 Brain CT images showing a large hypodense (arrows) edematous cerebral infarct in the distribution of the middle cerebral artery, with midline shift. Such large infarcts cause herniation of the cingulate gyrus under the falx cerebri; of the ispsilateral uncus under the tentorium to compress the oculomotor nerve, posterior cerebral artery, and brainstem; and of the contralateral cerebral peduncle to cause ipsilateral hemiparesis.

that flow is in excess of metabolic requirements, perhaps because the tissue has been irreversibly damaged.

Ischemic Cerebral Edema

Cerebral ischemia causes not only reversible and then irreversible loss of brain function but also cerebral edema (Symon *et al.* 1979; Hossman 1983). Ischemic edema is partly "cytotoxic" and partly "vasogenic". Cytotoxic edema starts early, within minutes of stroke onset, and affects the gray more than the white matter, where damaged cell membranes allow intracellular water to accumulate. Vasogenic edema, which starts rather later, within hours of stroke onset, affects the white matter more, where the damaged blood–brain barrier allows plasma constituents to enter the extracellular space. Ischemic cerebral edema reaches its maximum in 2 to 4 days and then subsides over a week or 2 weeks.

Cerebral edema not only increases local hydrostatic pressure and compromises blood flow further but also causes mass effect, brain shift, and eventually brain herniation (Fig. 5.1). Death in the first week after cerebral infarction is often a result of these mass effects.

Diaschisis

Acute or chronic cerebral injury may cause effects in remote areas of brain (Meyer *et al.* 1993), so-called diaschisis, by reducing neuronal inputs and metabolic activity: in the contralateral cerebellum and ipsilateral internal capsule, thalamus, and basal ganglia after cortical lesions; in the ipsilateral cortex following internal capsule and thalamic lesions; and in the contralateral hemisphere. The functional consequences of diaschisis are not clear (Bowler *et al.* 1995).

Pathophysiology of Acute Intracerebral Hemorrhage

The events following intracerebral hemorrhage have been most intensively studied for the most common type: rupture of one or more deep perforating arteries. The extravasated blood causes disruption of white matter tracts and irreversible damage to neurons in the deep nuclei or the cortex. The resultant increase in intracranial pressure may threaten other parts of the brain, particularly when the intracranial pressure reaches levels of the same order of magnitude as the arterial pressure, bringing the cerebral perfusion pressure close to zero (Rosand *et al.* 2002). Direct mechanical compression of the brain tissue surrounding the hematoma and, to some extent, vasoconstrictor and pro-inflammatory substances in extravasated blood also lead to impaired blood supply (Castillo *et al.* 2002; Butcher *et al.* 2004). Cellular ischemia leads to further swelling from edema (Gebel *et al.* 2002; Siddique *et al.* 2002), which is initially cytotoxic and later vasogenic.

Hydrocephalus may be an additional space-occupying factor. This complication is especially likely to occur with cerebellar hematomas, but a large hematoma in the region of the basal ganglia may also cause enlargement of the ventricular system by rupture into the third ventricle or through dilatation of the opposite lateral ventricle, with midline shift and obstruction of the third ventricle, while the ipsilateral ventricle is compressed. The zone of ischemia around the hematoma may swell through systemic factors such as hypotension or hypoxia. Often there is also loss of cerebral autoregulation in the vasculature supplying the region of the hematoma. Some perifocal ischemic damage occurs at the time of bleeding and cannot be prevented, but it is uncertain whether the vicious cycle of ongoing ischemia causing steadily increasing pressure can be interrupted in its early stages.

References

Albers GW, Marks MP, Kemp S *et al.* (2018). Thrombectomy for stroke at 6 to 16 hours with selection by perfusion imaging. *New England Journal of Medicine* doi:10.1056/NEJMoa1713973 [Epub ahead of print]

Arnold M, Nedeltchev K, Remonda L *et al.* (2005). Recanalisation of middle cerebral artery occlusion after intra-arterial thrombolysis: Different recanalisation grading systems and clinical functional outcome. *Journal of Neurology, Neurosurgery Psychiatry* 76:1373–1376

Astrup J, Siesjo BK, Symon L (1981). Thresholds in cerebral ischaemia. The ischaemic penumbra. *Stroke* 12:723–725

Back T, Hemmen T, Schuler OG (2004). Lesion evolution in cerebral ischemia. *Journal of Neurology* 251:388–397

Baird AE, Benfield A, Schlaug G *et al.* (1997). Enlargement of human cerebral ischaemic lesion volumes measured by diffusion-weighted magnetic resonance imaging. *Annals of Neurology* 41:581–589

Bano D, Nicotera P (2007). Ca^{2+} signals and neuronal death in brain ischemia. *Stroke* 38 (Suppl 2):674–676

Barber PA, Darby DG, Desmond PM *et al.* (1998a). Prediction of stroke outcome with echoplanar perfusion- and diffusion-weighted MRI. *Neurology* 51:418–426

Barber PA, Davis SM, Infeld B *et al.* (1998b). Spontaneous reperfusion after ischaemic stroke is associated with improved outcome. *Stroke* 29:2522–2528

Bowler JV, Wade JP H, Jones BE *et al.* (1995). Contribution of diaschisis to the clinical deficit in human cerebral infarction. *Stroke* 26:1000–1006

Butcher KS, Baird T, MacGregor L *et al.* (2004). Perihematomal edema in primary intracerebral hemorrhage is plasma derived. *Stroke* 35:1879–1885

Castillo J, Dávalos A, Alvarez-Sabín J *et al.* (2002). Molecular signatures of brain injury after intracerebral hemorrhage. *Neurology* 58:624–629

Chamorro A, Dirnagl U, Urra X et al. (2016). Neuroprotection in acute stroke: Targeting excitotoxicity, oxidative and nitrosative stress, and inflammation. Lancet Neurology 15:869–881

Fieschi C, Argentino C, Lenzi GL et al. (1989). Clinical and instrumental evaluation of patients with ischaemic stroke within the first six hours. Journal of Neurological Sciences 91:311–322

Furlan M, Marchal G, Viader F et al. (1996). Spontaneous neurological recovery after stroke and the fate of the ischaemic penumbra. Annals of Neurology 40:216–226

Gebel JM Jr., Jauch EC, Brott TG et al. (2002). Natural history of perihematomal edema in patients with hyperacute spontaneous intracerebral hemorrhage. Stroke 33:2631–2635

Goyal M, Menon BK, Derdeyn CP (2013). Perfusion imaging in acute ischemic stroke: Let us improve the science before changing clinical practice. Radiology 266:16–21

Harukuni I, Bhardwaj A (2006). Mechanisms of brain injury after global cerebral ischemia. Neurology Clinic 24:1–21

Hossman KA (1983). Experimental aspects of stroke. In Vascular Disease of the Central Nervous System, Ross Russell, RW (ed.), pp. 73–100. Edinburgh: Churchill Livingstone.

Hossmann KA (2006). Pathophysiology and therapy of experimental stroke. Cell and Molecular Neurobiology 26:1057–1083

Kaps M, Teschendorf U, Dorndorf W (1992). Haemodynamic studies in early stroke. Journal of Neurology 239:138–142

Lassen NA, Fieschi C, Lenzi GL (1991). Ischaemic penumbra and neuronal death: Comments on the therapeutic window in acute stroke with particular reference to thrombolytic therapy. Cerebrovascular Diseases 1:32–35

Liebeskind DS (2003). Collateral circulation. Stroke 34:2279–2284

Marchal G, Beaudouin V, Rioux P et al. (1996a). Prolonged persistence of substantial volumes of potentially viable brain tissue after stroke. A correlative PET–CT study with voxel-based data analysis. Stroke 27:599–606

Marchal G, Furlan M, Beaudouin V et al. (1996b). Early spontaneous hyperperfusion after stroke. A marker of favourable tissue outcome? Brain 119:409–419

Meyer JS, Obara K, Muramatsu K (1993). Diaschisis. Neurology Research 15:362–366

Nogueira RG, Jadhav AP, Haussen DC et al. (2018) Thrombectomy 6 to 24 hours after stroke with a mismatch between deficit and infarct. New England Journal of Medicine 378:11–21

Rosand J, Eskey C, Chang Y (2002). Dynamic single-section CT demonstrates reduced cerebral blood flow in acute intracerebral hemorrhage. Cerebrovascular Diseases 14:214–220

Siddique MS, Fernandes HM, Wooldridge TD et al. (2002). Reversible ischemia around intracerebral hemorrhage: A single-photon emission computerized tomography study. Journal of Neurosurgery 96:736–741

Symon L, Branston NM, Chikovani O (1979). Ischemic brain edema following middle cerebral artery occlusion in baboons: Relationship between regional cerebral water content and blood flow at 1 to 2 hours. Stroke 10:184–191

Wardlaw JM, Dennis MS, Lindley RI et al. (1993). Does early reperfusion of a cerebral infarct influence cerebral infarct swelling in the acute stage or the final clinical outcome? Cerebrovascular Diseases 3:86–93

Warner DS, Sheng H, Batinic-Haberle I (2004). Oxidants, antioxidants and the ischemic brain. Journal of Experimental Biology 207:3221–3231

Wise RJS, Bernardi S, Frackowiak RSJ et al. (1983). Serial observations on the pathophysiology of acute stroke. The transition from ischaemia to infarction as reflected in regional oxygen extraction. Brain 106:197–222

Zanette EM, Roberti C, Mancini G et al. (1995). Spontaneous middle cerebral artery reperfusion in ischaemic stroke. A follow-up study with transcranial Doppler. Stroke 26:430–433

Zemke D, Smith JL, Reeves MJ et al. (2004). Ischemia and ischemic tolerance in the brain: An overview. Neurotoxicology 25:895–904

Zhang F, Yin W, Chen J (2004). Apoptosis in cerebral ischemia: Executional and regulatory signalling mechanisms. Neurology Research 26:835–845

Zheng Z, Yenari MA (2004). Post-ischemic inflammation: Molecular mechanisms and therapeutic implications. Neurology Research 26:884–892

Causes of Transient Ischemic Attack and Ischemic Stroke

It is important for clinicians to have a thorough understanding of the causes of TIA and ischemic stroke (Table 6.1). Since there is no qualitative difference between TIA and stroke, anything that causes an ischemic stroke may also cause a TIA. The separation of TIA and stroke on the basis of an arbitrary time limit of 24 hours for resolution of symptoms in TIA is useful, not because there is any difference in the underlying causes of TIA and stroke but because the differential diagnosis is not the same for short-lived as for longer focal neurological deficits (Chapters 8 and 9 for the differential diagnosis of TIA and stroke, respectively). Rare causes of TIA and stroke are proportionately more common in young compared with elderly patients, since degenerative arterial disease is unusual in the young. Venous infarction is discussed in Chapter 29.

Approximately 25% of ischemic strokes are caused by identifiable atherothromboembolism from large artery disease, 25% by small vessel disease, 20% by cardioembolism, approximately 5% by rarities, and the remainder are of undetermined etiology (Schulz and Rothwell 2003) (Table 6.2).

Large Vessel Disease and Atherothromboembolism

Atheroma seems to be an almost inevitable accompaniment of aging, at least in developed countries. Atherosclerosis is a multifocal disease affecting large and medium-sized arteries, particularly where there is branching, tortuosity, or confluence of vessels (see Fig. 4.1). Turbulence caused by changes in blood flow direction is thought to contribute to endothelial damage and ultimately to plaque formation. Atheroma begins in childhood as fatty streaks, possibly in response to endothelial injury, and over many years arterial smooth muscle cells proliferate, the intima is invaded by macrophages, fibrosis occurs, and cholesterol is deposited to form fibrolipid plaques (Ross 1999; Goldshmidt-Clermont et al. 2005; Gotto 2005). Individuals with atheroma in one artery usually have widespread vascular disease, making them at high risk of ischemic heart disease, stroke, and claudication (Mitchell and Schwartz 1962; Rothwell 2001), particularly among white males, who often have accompanying hypercholesterolemia. There appear to be important racial differences in the distribution of atheroma, and race is an independent predictor of lesion location. White males tend to develop atheroma in the extracranial cerebral vessels, aorta and coronary arteries, whereas intracranial large vessel disease appears to be relatively more common in black, Hispanic and Asian populations (Feldmann et al. 1990; Leung et al. 1993; Sacco et al. 1995; Wityk et al. 1996; White et al. 2005) and tends to affect younger patients

Table 6.1 Causes of cerebral ischemia

Types	Examples
Arterial wall disorders	Atherothromboembolism
	Intracranial small vessel disease
	Leukoaraiosis
	Dissection (Table 6.4)
	Fibromuscular dysplasia
	Congenital arterial anomalies
	Moyamoya syndrome
	Embolism from arterial aneurysms
	Inflammatory vascular diseases
	Irradiation
Cardioembolism (Table 6.3)	
Hematological disorders (Box 6.1)	
Miscellaneous conditions	Pregnancy/puerperium
	Migraine
	Oral contraceptives and other female sex hormones
	Perioperative
	Recreational drugs
	Cancer
	Chronic meningitis
	Inflammatory bowel disease
	Mitochondrial disease
	Fabry disease
	Homocystinemia
	Hypoglycemia/hypercalcemia
	Fat embolism
	Fibrocartilaginous embolism
	Snake bite
	Epidermal nevus syndrome
	Susac's syndrome
	Cerebral autosomal dominant arteriopathy with subcortical infarcts and leukoencephalopathy (CADASIL)

and those with type 1 diabetes mellitus (Sacco *et al.* 1995). Some but not all sources report that women have more intracranial disease than men.

Pathological, angiographic, and ultrasonic studies show that the most common extracranial sites for atheroma are the aortic arch, the proximal subclavian arteries, the carotid bifurcation (Fig. 6.1), and the vertebral artery origins (Fig. 6.2). Plaques in the subclavian arteries frequently extend into the origin of the vertebral arteries, and similar plaques may occasionally occur at the origin of the innominate arteries. Frequently, the second portion of the vertebral artery as it passes through the transverse foramen is also affected, but the atheroma, which tends to form a ladder-like arrangement opposite cervical discs and osteophytes, does not normally restrict the lumen size significantly.

Table 6.2 Distribution of stroke etiology in four population-based studies

	OXVASC (n = 102)	OCSP (n = 545)	Rochester (n = 454)	Erlangen (n = 531)
Large vessel				
No.	17	77	74	71
% (95% CI)	16.7 (9.4–23.9)	14.1 (11.2–17.1)	16.3 (12.9–19.7)	13.4 (10.5–16.3)
Small vessel				
No.	20	119	72	120
% (95% CI)	19.6 (11.9–27.3)	21.8 (18.4–25.3)	15.9 (12.5–19.2)	22.6 (19.0–26.2)
Cardioembolic				
No.	19	127	132	143
% (95% CI)	18.6 (11.1–26.2)	23.3 (19.8–26.9)	29.1 (24.9–33.3)	26.9 (23.2–30.7)
Other				
No.	3	33	12	9
% (95% CI)	2.9 (0.06–8.4)	6.1 (4.2–8.4)	2.6 (1.4–4.6)	1.7 (0.8–3.2)
Not defined				
No.	43	189	164	188
% (95% CI)	42.2 (32.6–51.7)	34.7 (30.7–38.7)	36.1 (31.7–40.5)	35.4 (31.3–39.5)

Notes: OXVASC, Oxford Vascular Study; OCSP, Oxford Community Stroke Project; CI, confidence interval.
Source: From Schulz and Rothwell (2003).

Intracranial arteries are morphologically different from extracranial arteries in having no external elastic membrane, fewer elastic fibers in the media and adventitia, and a thinner intimal layer. The major sites for atheroma formation in the anterior circulation are the carotid siphon, the proximal middle cerebral artery, and the anterior cerebral artery around the anterior communicating artery origin. In the posterior circulation, the intracranial vertebral arteries are often affected just after they penetrate the dura (Fig. 6.3) and distally near the basilar artery origin. Plaques are also found in the proximal basilar artery and also prior to the origin of the posterior cerebral arteries. The mid-basilar segment may be affected around the origins of the cerebellar arteries (Fig. 6.4). Occlusion of a branch artery at its origin by disease in the parent vessel seems to occur more commonly in the posterior circulation, "basilar branch occlusion", than in the anterior circulation, where occlusion of the small perforating arteries is usually caused by intrinsic small vessel disease.

Atheromatous medium-sized arteries at the base of the brain, particularly the vertebral and basilar arteries, may become affected by dolichoectasia. The arteries are widened, tortuous, and elongated and may be visualized on MRI or, if the walls are calcified, on CT. Dolichoectasia is usually found in elderly patients with hypertension and diabetes, and it may cause stroke through embolization of thrombus or by occlusion of small branch arteries. In younger patients, it should raise the possibility of Fabry disease.

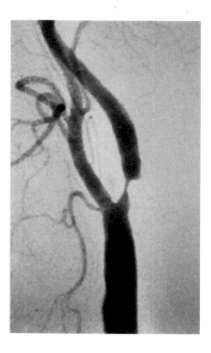

Fig. 6.1 Digitally subtracted arterial angiogram showing a severe stenosis of the internal carotid artery.

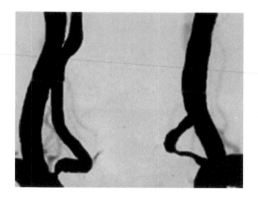

Fig. 6.2 Digitally subtracted arterial angiogram of the origins of both common carotid and vertebral arteries showing bilateral vertebral artery stenosis.

Stroke Mechanisms Related to Large Artery Atherosclerosis

There are four principal mechanisms by which atherosclerotic lesions may cause ischemic stroke.

- Thrombi may form on lesions and cause local occlusion.
- Embolization of plaque debris or thrombus may block a more distal vessel. Emboli are usually the cause of obstruction of the anterior circulation intracranial vessels (Lhermitte *et al.* 1970; Ogata *et al.* 1994), at least in white males in whom intracranial disease is relatively rare. Since emboli follow the prevailing direction of flow in a vessel, most emboli from the internal carotid arteries will travel to the retina or the anterior two-thirds of the ipsilateral cerebral hemisphere. However, in patients with vascular

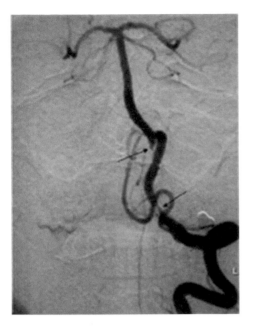

Fig. 6.3 Digitally subtracted arterial angiogram showing occlusion of the distal right vertebral artery (top arrow) and a tight stenosis of the left vertebral artery (lower arrow).

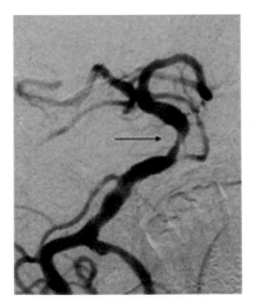

Fig. 6.4 Digitally subtracted arterial angiogram showing stenosis (arrow) of an ecstatic basilar artery.

disease, flow patterns may be abnormal owing to vessel occlusion and collateral flow. Infarction may occur ipsilateral to a chronically occluded internal carotid artery as emboli from the contralateral internal carotid pass via the anterior communicating artery.

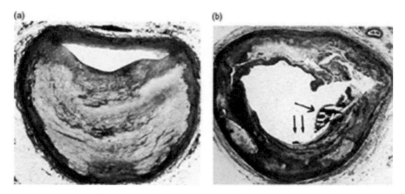

Fig. 6.5 Histological sections showing a quiescent plaque with a thick fibrous cap (a) and a ruptured plaque (b) with adherent thrombus (arrow).

- Small vessel origins may be occluded by growth of plaque in the parent vessel, such as in the basilar artery or proximal middle cerebral artery.
- Severe reduction in the diameter of the vessel lumen caused by plaque growth may lead to hypoperfusion and infarction of distal "borderzone" brain regions where blood supply is poorest.

Approximately 90% of atherothromboembolic strokes in whites are caused by atheroma in the extracranial vessels, whereas intracranial disease appears to be equally important in blacks and Hispanics (Sacco *et al.* 1995; Wityk *et al.* 1996). Atheromatous disease in the ascending aorta and the aortic arch is increasingly recognized as a source of cerebral emboli and an independent risk factor for ischemic stroke in vivo (Amarenco *et al.* 1994; Jones *et al.* 1995; Heinzlef *et al.* 1997; MacLeod *et al.* 2004).

Plaque Activation and Stroke Risk

Atheromatous plaques are typically slow growing or quiescent for long periods but may suddenly develop fissures or ulcers (Fig. 6.5). Activated plaques trigger platelet aggregation, thrombus formation (Viles-Gonzalez *et al.* 2004; Redgrave *et al.* 2006), and embolism. In keeping with the concept of acute intermittent activation of plaques, the likelihood of stroke in patients with cerebral atheromatous disease varies with time, being highest in the few days after a TIA or stroke (Coull *et al.* 2004; Rothwell and Warlow 2005) (Chapter 15). Strokes in large arteries are particularly likely to recur early (Lovett *et al.* 2004). Furthermore, emboli are more often detected with transcranial Doppler sonography if carotid stenosis is recently symptomatic (Dittrich *et al.* 2006; Markus 2006), and the rate of Doppler-detected emboli in the middle cerebral artery tends to decline with time after stroke (Kaposzta *et al.* 1999).

Plaque irregularity or ulceration, which is best visualized on catheter angiography (Fig. 6.6) but can sometimes be seen on contrast-enhanced MR angiography (Fig. 6.7), is independently associated with increased stroke risk. Irregularity of plaque as seen on radiological examination probably represents plaque ulceration and instability with

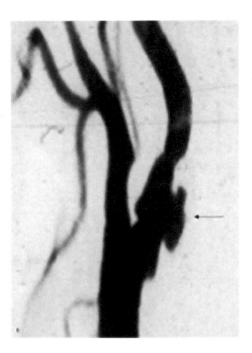

Fig. 6.6 Digitally subtracted arterial angiogram showing an ulcerated plaque at the carotid bifurcation, with contrast seen within the plaque (arrow).

thrombosis, and so the likelihood of complicating embolism (Molloy and Markus 1999; Rothwell *et al.* 2000a; Lovett *et al.* 2004). There is also evidence to suggest that ulcerated carotid plaques are more likely than smooth plaques to be associated with vascular events in other territories, such as the coronary arteries (Rothwell *et al.* 2000b), suggesting that plaque activation is a systemic phenomenon. The trigger for activation is not known, but infective, inflammatory, or genetic mechanisms have been proposed.

Cholesterol Embolization Syndrome

Cholesterol embolization syndrome is a rare disorder that is thought to be caused by rupture of atheromatous plaques particularly in the abdominal aorta, either spontaneously or as a complication of instrumentation of large atheromatous arteries, anticoagulation, or thrombolysis. Cholesterol debris is released and showers of emboli impact in the microcirculation of organs, including the stomach, skin, brain, and spinal cord. Hours or days after instrumentation or surgery, a syndrome very similar to systemic vasculitis or infective endocarditis develops, with malaise, fever, abdominal pain, proteinuria and renal failure, stroke-like episodes, drowsiness, confusion, skin petechiae, splinter hemorrhages, livedo reticularis, cyanosis of fingers and toes, raised erythrocyte sedimentation rate, neutrophil leukocytosis, and eosinophilia. The diagnosis is made by finding cholesterol debris in the microcirculation of biopsy material, usually from the kidney but sometimes from skin or muscle (Cross 1991; Rhodes 1996). The prognosis is poor, with a high mortality rate, and treatment is supportive.

Small Vessel Disease and Leukoaraiosis

Small Vessel Disease

The small penetrating arteries of the brain, less than 0.5 mm in diameter, include the lenticulo-striate branches of the middle cerebral artery, the thalamo-perforating branches of the proximal posterior cerebral artery, and the perforating arteries to the brainstem. Occlusion of one of these small vessels usually causes infarction, albeit in a small area of brain, since there is no significant collateral circulation. Such "lacunar" infarcts make up approximately one-quarter of first ischemic strokes (Bamford *et al.* 1987; Sempere *et al.* 1998; Schulz and Rothwell 2003), but case fatality is low at about 1%. The few pathological data available suggest that these small arteries are much less likely to be occluded by emboli from the heart or from extracranial sites of atherothrombosis compared with the trunk or cortical branches of the middle cerebral artery (Tegeler *et al.* 1991; Boiten *et al.*

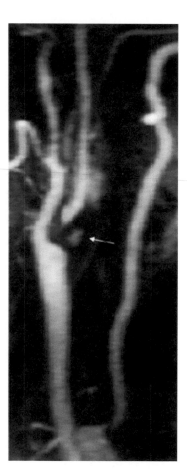

Fig. 6.7 Contrast-enhanced MR carotid angiogram showing a severe stenosis caused by an ulcerated plaque, with contrast seen within the plaque (arrow).

1996; Gan *et al.* 1997). In keeping with the pathological observations, ischemic lacunar strokes are less often associated with middle cerebral artery emboli detected with transcranial Doppler than are large artery strokes (Koennecke *et al.* 1998).

It is thought that the small perforating arteries of the brain are occluded by thrombus complicating a distinct small vessel arteriopathy – "hyaline arteriosclerosis" or "simple small vessel disease" (Lammie *et al.* 1997) – that differs from atheroma. Hyaline arteriosclerosis is an almost universal change in the small arteries and arterioles of the aged brain, particularly in the presence of hypertension or diabetes. The muscle and elastin in the arterial wall are replaced by collagen; there is subintimal hyalinization, the wall thickens, the lumen narrows, and the vessel becomes tortuous. In complex small vessel disease, there is more aggressive disorganization of the small vessel walls, accompanied by foam cell infiltration. Whether simple and complex small vessel diseases are related is unclear.

The current view is that both complex small vessel disease and atheroma at or near the origin of the small perforating vessels arising from the major cerebral arteries cause most of the small deep infarcts responsible for lacunar ischemic strokes, which make up about one-quarter of symptomatic cerebral ischemic events (Bamford *et al.* 1987; Schulz and Rothwell 2003). However, this hypothesis is not universally accepted (Millikan and Futrell 1990) since there is little direct postmortem evidence of occlusion of these vessels leading to lacunar infarcts. Certainly, at least some small infarcts in the brainstem and internal capsule are caused by atheroma at the mouth of the small penetrating vessels spreading from atheroma of the larger parent artery (Fisher and Caplan 1971; Fisher 1979). It is also conceivable that this small vessel arteriopathy can lead to small, deep hemorrhages as well as lacunar infarcts (Labovitz *et al.* 2007); indeed, both types of stroke often coincide (Samuelsson *et al.* 1996; Kwa *et al.* 1998).

Leukoaraiosis

There are a number of alternative terms for leukoaraiosis, including Binswanger's disease, chronic progressive subcortical encephalopathy, subcortical arteriosclerotic encephalopathy, and periventricular leukoencephalopathy. This reflects the confusion between the clinical, radiological, and pathological literature (Munoz 2006). On CT, there is roughly symmetrical but irregular periventricular hypodensity, with or without ventricular dilatation and focal white matter hypodensities. This is better seen as high signal on T_2-weighted MR images (Fig. 6.8). This periventricular radiological appearance is caused by a variety of pathological changes, including demyelination, axonal loss and gliosis, which all are thought to occur as a consequence of diffuse rather than focal ischemia although the exact mechanism remains unclear. Vascular occlusion has not been seen (Caplan 1995; Pantoni and Garcia 1997).

Leuokoaraiosis is frequent in the normal elderly but is more marked in those with hypertension, dementia (Chapter 31), or stroke but not increasing carotid stenosis (Bots *et al.* 1993; Adachi *et al.* 1997; Munoz 2006). It is also common in patients with cerebral amyloid angiopathy (Chapter 7). It is a risk factor for ischemic, particularly lacunar, and hemorrhagic stroke (Inzitari 2003) and is associated with increased bleeding risk with anticoagulants (Gorter 1999). It seems likely that the association between leukoariosis and stroke occurs because hypertension causes both pathological syndromes in the same individual rather than leukoaraiosis itself being the cause of the stroke.

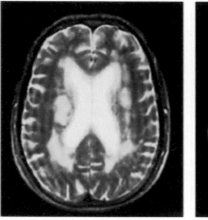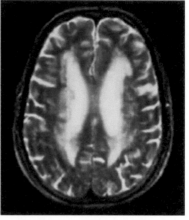

Fig. 6.8 Brain MRI scans showing the typical appearances of advanced periventricular leukoaraiosis.

Cardioembolism

Approximately 20% of ischemic stroke is cardioembolic. There are a large number of potential cardiac sources of embolism (Table 6.3), but it may be difficult to be certain whether an identified putative embolic source is the cause of a stroke. This is especially the case if there are alternative causes such as coexistent large artery disease, or if the stroke is lacunar and unlikely to be caused by cardiac embolism.

Atrial fibrillation is discussed in Chapter 2.

Coronary Artery Disease

Overall, there is approximately a fivefold relative excess risk of stroke in the first few days and weeks after myocardial infarction, but the absolute risk of clinically evident systemic embolism is well under 5% (Dutta *et al.* 2006a). The risk of embolism is higher in anterior infarcts, large infarcts, and the presence of a dyskinetic wall segment. Some post-myocardial infarction strokes may be caused by hypotension and boundary zone infarction, atrial fibrillation with left atrial thrombus, paradoxical embolism, or coronary and aortic instrumentation (see later), while others are primarily hemorrhagic as a consequence of antithrombotic and thrombolytic drugs. Rarely, the same non-atheromatous disorder can cause both ischemic stroke and acute myocardial infarction: giant cell arteritis, aortic arch dissection, or infective endocarditis. The long-term risk of stroke after acute myocardial infarction is approximately 1.5% per annum and 8% in 5 years (Martin *et al.* 1993; Loh *et al.* 1997; Yaghi *et al.* 2015).

Infective Endocarditis

About 30% of patients with infective endocarditis have an ischemic stroke or TIA as a result of embolism of valvular vegetations (Ruttmann *et al.* 2006). Cerebrovascular symptoms usually occur before the infection has been controlled and may be the presenting feature (Hart *et al.* 1990; Salgado 1991). Hemorrhagic transformation of an infarct occurs in 20–40%. Hemorrhagic strokes (intracerebral and subarachnoid) are more commonly

Table 6.3 Causes of cardioembolism

Area affected	Causes
Left atrium	Atrial fibrillation Sinoatrial disease Myxoma Interatrial septal aneurysm
Mitral valve	Infective endocarditis Non-bacterial thrombotic (marantic) endocarditis Rheumatic disease Prosthetic valve Mitral annulus calcification Libman–Sacks endocarditis Papillary fibroelastoma
Aortic valve	Infective endocarditis Non-bacterial thrombotic or marantic endocarditis Rheumatic disease Prosthetic valve Calcification and/or sclerosis Syphilis
Left ventricular mural thrombus	Myocardial infarction Left ventricular aneurysm Cardiomyopathy Myxoma Blunt chest injury Mechanical artificial heart
Paradoxical embolism from the venous system	Atrial septal defect Ventricular septal defect Patent foramen ovale Pulmonary arteriovenous fistula
Congenital cardiac disorders	Particularly with right to left shunt
Cardiac surgery	Catheterization, angioplasty
Others	Primary oxalosis, hydatid cyst

caused by pyogenic vasculitis and vessel wall necrosis than by mycotic aneurysms. These aneurysms can be single or multiple and most often affect the distal branches of the middle cerebral artery (Masuda *et al.* 1992; Krapf *et al.* 1999). They tend to resolve with time, and cerebral angiography to detect unruptured aneurysms with a view to surgery is unnecessary (van der Meulen *et al.* 1992).

Early institution of the correct antibiotic therapy is the most effective way to prevent thromboembolism in infective endocarditis, the risks of which are highest in the first 24–48 hours after diagnosis. Anticoagulation should not be given to patients with native valve or bioprosthetic valve endocarditis because of the risk of intracerebral hemorrhage from mycotic aneurysms and arteritis. Risk of embolism is also reduced with antibiotic therapy. For patients with mechanical valves who are taking long-term anticoagulation at the time of developing infective endocarditis, the correct management is unclear. Other neurological complications of infective endocarditis include meningitis, diffuse encephalopathy, acute mononeuropathy, cerebral abscess, discitis, and headache (Jones and Siekert 1989; Kanter and Hart 1991).

Fever, cardiac murmur, and vegetations are not invariably present in patients with infective endocarditis, and blood cultures are indicated in unexplained stroke particularly if there is raised erythrocyte sedimentation rate, mild anemia, neutrophil leukocytosis, or a history of intravenous drug abuse. The cerebrospinal fluid (CSF) can be normal, but > 100 $\times 10^6$ cells/L polymorphs is said to suggest endocarditis, although similar counts have been described in intracerebral hemorrhage and in hemorrhagic transformation of an infarct but not in ischemic stroke (Powers 1986).

Non-Bacterial Thrombotic or Marantic Endocarditis

Small, friable, and sterile vegetations made of fibrin and platelets can be found on the heart valves of patients with cancer, in those with antiphospholipid antibody syndrome or systemic lupus erythematosus, and possibly in patients with protein C deficiency (Asopa et al. 2007). Thrombotic emboli from such vegetations can be demonstrated using transesophageal echocardiography and are frequently seen in patients with cancer and cerebral ischemia (Dutta et al. 2006b; el-Shami et al. 2007).

Prosthetic Heart Valves

Prosthetic valves, particularly mechanical ones, are associated with thrombosis, embolism, and infective endocarditis. The overall risk of clinically evident embolism is 1–2% per annum in those taking anticoagulants (Vongpatanasin et al. 1996), with mitral valve prostheses being the most prone to thrombosis.

Mitral Leaflet Prolapse

Mitral leaflet prolapse is a common incidental finding. It can be complicated by gross mitral regurgitation, infective endocarditis, atrial fibrillation, and left atrial thrombus and thus embolism to the brain. However, there is no excess risk of first or recurrent stroke in patients with uncomplicated mitral leaflet prolapse (Orencia et al. 1995a, b).

Calcification of the Aortic and Mitral Valves

Calcification, and possibly sclerosis, of the aortic and mitral valves may be a cause of embolism of calcific or complicated thrombotic material. However, these degenerative disorders of heart valves are so common, particularly in the elderly, that it has been very difficult to associate them causally with stroke (Boon et al. 1996).

Paradoxical Embolism, Patent Foramen Ovale, and Atrial Septal Aneurysm

Autopsy examples have established that paradoxical embolism can occur from venous thrombi through the right to the left side of the heart. Emboli may pass through a patent foramen ovale, which is found in approximately one-quarter of healthy people; an atrial septal defect; or a ventriculoseptal defect (Gautier et al. 1991; Jeanrenaud and Kappenberger

1991; Cabanes *et al.* 1993). There is an increased incidence of patent foramen ovale (PFO) in patients with cryptogenic stroke (Mas *et al.* 2001; Lamy *et al.* 2002), but the risk of recurrent stroke in patients with a PFO is low. Although early trials of PFO closure in patients with cryptogenic stroke did not show efficacy over medical treatment alone in their primary intention-to-treat analyses (Furlan *et al.* 2012; Carroll *et al.* 2013; Meier *et al.* 2013), subsequent meta-analysis of these trials demonstrated that closure reduced recurrent stroke risk and had a significant effect on the composite of stroke, TIA, and death (Kent *et al.* 2016).

Recently, the CLOSE trial showed that in carefully selected individuals age < 60 with cryptogenic stroke and with a large PFO (right-to-left shunt > 30 microbubbles) or PFO associated with an atrial septal aneurysm with base of aneurysm 15mm and excursion >10mm, PFO closure with chronic antiplatelet therapy was associated with a significant reduction in risk of stroke recurrence compared with antiplatelet therapy alone (Mas *et al.* 2017). Similarly, the REDUCE trial also showed that in patients age <60 with cryptogenic stroke with a PFO resulting in a right-to-left shunt, PFO closure was associated with a reduced risk of recurrent ischemic stroke (Søndergaard *et al.* 2017). In both trials, however, PFO closure was associated with a small increased risk of subsequent atrial fibrillation (Mas *et al.* 2017; Søndergaard *et al.* 2017). However, although PFO closure may well be beneficial in selected patients with cryptogenic stroke attributable to a PFO, it should be noted that in the REDUCE trial, a large number of patients were lost to follow-up compared with the number of stroke endpoints, rendering the results unreliable. In both the REDUCE and CLOSE trials, there may also be potential bias due to the unblinded referral decisions for endpoint adjudication. Finally, whether PFO closure is superior to anticoagulation in patients with cryptogenic stroke attributable to a PFO remains uncertain.

Atrial septal aneurysm is an echocardiographic finding in some normal people. The combination of atrial septal aneurysm and PFO was thought to carry a higher stroke risk than PFO alone (Mas *et al.* 2001; Lamy *et al.* 2002), with a reported risk of recurrent stroke in such patients as high as 15% (Mas *et al.* 2001), but more recent data from a larger study have cast doubt on this observation (CODICE Study Group 2006). Interestingly, there appears to be an association between PFO and migraine, particularly migraine with aura, and this is particularly strong where there is coexistent atrial septal aneurysm. There are anecdotal reports of improvement in migraine symptoms following PFO closure (Holmes 2004; Diener *et al.* 2005).

Cardiac Myxomas

Cardiac myxomas are rare, are occasionally familial, and arise in any heart chamber, but 75% are found in the left atrium. Tumor material, or complicating thrombus, may embolize, and often there are features of intracardiac obstruction (dyspnea, cardiac failure, syncope) and constitutional upset (malaise, weight loss, fever, rash, arthralgia, myalgia, anemia, raised erythrocyte sedimentation rate, hypergammaglobulinemia) (Ekinci and Donnan 2004). Myxomatous emboli impacted in cerebral arteries may cause aneurysmal dilatation, with subsequent intracerebral or subarachnoid hemorrhage (Sabolek *et al.* 2005).

Dilating Cardiomyopathies

Cardiomyopathies may be complicated by intracardiac thrombus, but associated embolic stroke is rare.

Cardiac Surgery

Cardiac surgery is complicated by stroke or retinal/optic nerve infarction in about 2% of cases, the risk being greater for valve than for coronary artery surgery (Newman *et al.* 2006). Postoperative confusion is much more common, and cognitive deficits may persist for some weeks (Newman *et al.* 2006). Possible mechanisms for postoperative confusion include embolization during or after surgery, hypotension, cholesterol embolization, simultaneous carotid endarterectomy, thrombosis associated with heparin-induced thrombocytopenia, and intracranial hemorrhage caused by anticoagulation or thrombocytopenia.

Sinoatrial Disease

Sinoatrial disease or the sick sinus syndrome is associated with systemic embolism, particularly if there is bradycardia alternating with tachycardia or atrial fibrillation (Bathen *et al.* 1978).

Instrumentation of the Coronary Arteries and Aorta

Instrumental procedures in coronary arteries or the aorta may dislodge valvular or atheromatous debris, causing neurological complications (Ayas and Wijdicks 1995) and cholesterol embolization.

Arterial Dissection and Trauma

Arterial Dissection

Arterial dissection is a common cause of ischemic stroke and TIA in young adults and may also occur in older people. Sometimes there is a predisposing cause (Schievink 2001; Rubinstein *et al.* 2005) (Table 6.4), but often there is no explanation. The artery may become occluded by the wall hematoma itself; thrombosis and embolism may complicate occlusive or non-occlusive dissections, and aneurysmal bulging of the weakened wall may occur (O'Connell *et al.* 1985). Arterial rupture is unusual.

There are a number of characteristic features in the history and examination that point to cervical dissection:

- potential neck injury.
- pain in the neck, side of the head, face, or eye may accompany ipsilateral internal carotid artery dissection; pain at the back of the head and neck, usually unilaterally, may accompany vertebral dissection.
- Horner's syndrome may arise as a result of damage to sympathetic nerves around the internal carotid artery; this occurs in up to 50% of cases.
- a self-audible bruit, which may be described as pulsatile tinnitus, caused by dissection adjacent to the base of the skull occurs in about 30% of cases.
- ipsilateral palsy of a cranial nerve occurs in about 10% of cases, often affecting cranial nerve XII or another lower cranial nerve and rarely cranial nerve III.
- cervical root lesions have been reported in association with vertebral artery dissections from pressure or ischemia.

Table 6.4 Causes of dissection of the extra- and intracranial arteries

Type	Causes
Traumatic	
Penetrating injury	Catheter angiography Jugular vein cannulation Missile wounds Neck/oral injury or surgery
Non-penetrating injury	Blow to the neck Neck injury: fracture, subluxation or dislocation Neck movements: whiplash injury, "head-banging," hairdresser visit, head injury, falls Yoga Chiropractic manipulation Labor Seizures Vomiting Bronchoscopy Atlanto-axial dislocation Occipito-atlantal instability Skull base fracture Cervical rib Fractured clavicle Carotid compression tests Attempted strangulation
Spontaneous	Marfan's syndrome Ehlers–Danlos syndrome Pseudoxanthoma elasticum Inflammatory arterial disease Infective arterial disease, e.g., syphilis Fibromuscular dysplasia Cystic medial necrosis

The presence of cranial neuropathy may result in a misdiagnosis of brainstem stroke. Cranial nerve palsies may result from local pressure from the false internal carotid artery lumen, thromboembolism, or hemodynamic compromise to the blood supply of the nerve. Cranial nerve III receives its blood supply from the ophthalmic artery, branches of the internal carotid, or the posterior cerebral artery and, consequently, may rarely become ischemic after carotid dissection.

The features listed previously may precede the onset of cerebral ischemia by hours or days, and relevant points in the history may, therefore, not be volunteered spontaneously by the patient. Alternatively, diagnostic pointers to dissection may be absent altogether, and then the diagnosis becomes one of exclusion/confirmation on imaging. Secondary aneurysm formation can cause symptoms through local pressure, but it does not appear to increase the risk of thromboembolism.

The incidence of diagnosed internal carotid artery dissection is approximately 1–4 per 100,000 per year. Vertebral dissection is a little less common. The actual incidence

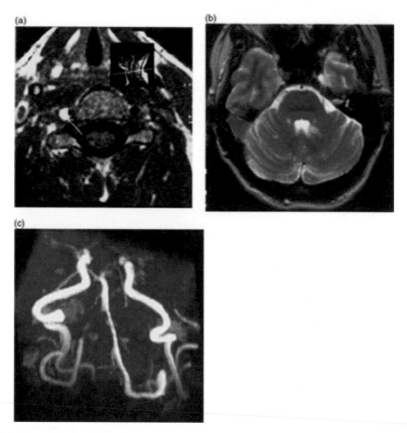

Fig. 6.9 (a) A T_2-weighted MRI scan showing high signal in the wall of the right vertebral artery (arrow) indicating a recent dissection. (b) A T_2-weighted MRI scan showing several areas of cerebellar infarction. (c) An MR angiography showing absence of the right vertebral artery.

of dissections is likely to be considerably higher, but the diagnosis is often missed, particularly in older patients. Usually only one artery is involved, but in about 10%, multiple arteries may be affected simultaneously or in close succession. Recurrence rates are low at approximately 1% per annum except in familial cases of arterial dissection or hereditary connective tissue disorder, where rates are higher (Leys *et al.* 1995).

On angiography, there is usually a long, tapered, narrow, or occluded segment, perhaps with an intimal flap, double lumen, or intraluminal thrombus and sometimes an associated aneurysm. Intracranial arterial occlusion, presumably embolic, may be seen. Carotid dissection can often be strongly suspected on Duplex (Sturzenegger *et al.* 1993, 1995; Flis *et al.* 2007), but the most sensitive and specific imaging evidence of both carotid and vertebral dissection comes from a combination of axial MRI through the lesion, to show the acute hematoma in the arterial wall, with MR angiography (Auer *et al.* 1998; Flis *et al.* 2007) (Fig. 6.9).

Cervical arterial dissection generally has a benign prognosis. The risk of stroke associated with cervical artery dissection is low at ~1.7%, the majority of which occurs within the first 2 weeks after dissection (Morris *et al.* 2017). In patients presenting with an ischemic stroke secondary to cervical artery dissection, the prognosis is similarly good with a risk of recurrent stroke of ~2%, most of which occur within the first 10 days after ischemic stroke (CADISS Trial Investigators 2015). Antiplatelet or anticoagulant drugs are equally effective in preventing stroke (CADISS Trial Investigators 2015).

Intracranial Arterial Dissection

Intracranial dissection is much less common but probably underdiagnosed. It may present with subarachnoid hemorrhage owing to rupture of a pseudo-aneurysm as well as with ischemic stroke and is less often diagnosed during life (Debette *et al.* 2015). Patients who present as a subarachnoid hemorrhage can be considered for surgical or endovascular treatment to prevent rebleeding, while those who present with ischemic symptoms are often treated with antithrombotic agents.

Aortic Arch Dissection

Aortic arch dissection can cause profound hypotension with global, and sometimes boundary zone, cerebral ischemia or focal cerebral ischemia if the dissection spreads up one of the neck arteries. Clues to this diagnosis are anterior chest or interscapular pain, along with diminished, unequal, or absent arterial pulses in the arms or neck and a normal electrocardiogram, unlike acute myocardial infarction, acute aortic regurgitation, and pericardial effusion.

Trauma

Penetrating and non-penetrating neck injuries are more likely to damage the carotid than the better-protected vertebral artery. The vertebral artery appears to be more vulnerable to rotational and hyperextension injuries of the neck, particularly at the level of the atlas and axis. Laceration, dissection, and intimal tears may be complicated by thrombosis and then embolism and, therefore, ischemic stroke at the time of the injury or some days or even weeks after the injury. Later stroke may be a consequence of the formation of a traumatic aneurysm, arteriovenous fistula, or a fistula between the carotid and vertebral arteries (Davis and Zimmerman 1983).

The subclavian artery can be damaged by a fractured clavicle or a cervical rib, with later embolization up the vertebral arteries or even up the right common carotid artery (Prior *et al.* 1979).

Rare Arterial Disorders

There are a large number of rare arterial disorders or anomalies that can cause ischemic stroke (Tables 3.2 and 6.1). The frequency of many of these disorders has probably been underestimated because of under-investigation and lack of radiological imaging of the cerebral vasculature beyond the carotid bifurcation.

Fibromuscular Dysplasia

Fibromuscular dysplasia is a rare segmental disorder with a female preponderance affecting small and medium-sized arteries (Olin *et al.* 2014). There are fibrosis and thickening of the arterial wall alternating with atrophy, giving the typical angiographic appearance of a "string of beads". It is most common in the renal arteries, resulting in hypertension. The mid-cervical portion of the internal carotid artery is the most frequently affected artery to the brain, but the vertebral arteries at the level of the first two cervical vertebrae may also be involved. Intracranial pathology is exceptional (Arunodaya *et al.* 1997). Fibromuscular dysplasia is associated with intracranial saccular aneurysms and arteriovenous malformations and dissection. Since fibromuscular dysplasia of some arteries to the brain is found in up to 1% of routine autopsies, associations with cerebral ischemia or infarction may be coincidental. Occasionally, however, it may be complicated by thrombosis and embolism. The natural history is unknown.

Congenital Arterial Anomalies

Occasionally, the carotid arteries are hypoplastic or absent, and kinking, acute angulation, tortuosity, and looping of the internal carotid artery may be seen on angiograms (Metz *et al.* 1961; Ovchinnikov *et al.* 2007). Such appearances can be caused by atheroma, fibromuscular dysplasia, or congenital abnormality. There is a tendency to regard anomalies in children and young adults as "congenital" and those in the middle aged and elderly as "atherosclerotic".

Congenital Carotid Loops

Carotid loops may be associated with aneurysm formation and rarely with embolism, endothelial damage, and thrombosis; exceptionally there may be focal ischemia on head movement (Sarkari *et al.* 1970; Desai and Toole 1975, Seneviratne *et al.* 2009; Ovchinnikov *et al.* 2007). Rarely, these loops may cause hypoglossal nerve lesions or pulsatile tinnitus.

Some inherited disorders of connective tissue (Table 3.4) can present with or be complicated by arterial dissection or even rupture, intra- and extracranial aneurysm formation, carotico-cavernous fistula, and mitral leaflet prolapse – for example, Ehlers–Danlos syndrome (North *et al.* 1995), pseudoxanthoma elasticum (Lefthériotis *et al.* 2013), and Marfan's syndrome (Wityk *et al.* 2002).

Moyamoya Syndrome

In Japanese, *moyamoya* means "puff of smoke" and describes the characteristic radiological appearance of the fine anastomotic collaterals that develop from the perforating and pial arteries at the base of the brain, the orbital and ethmoidal branches of the external carotid artery, and the leptomeningeal and transdural vessels in response to severe stenosis or occlusion of one or both distal internal carotid arteries (Scott and Smith 2009). The circle of Willis and the proximal cerebral and basilar arteries may also be involved.

Moyamoya is most often encountered in the Japanese and Asians and is much less common in individuals of non-Asian ethnicity (Scott and Smith 2009). In most cases, the cause is unknown. Some cases are familial (Scott and Smith 2009); others appear to be caused by a generalized fibrous disorder of arteries (Aoyagi *et al.* 1996), and a few may result from a congenital hypoplastic anomaly affecting arteries at the base of the brain. Moyamoya is also strongly associated with radiotherapy to the head and neck region (in particular for optic gliomas, craniopharyngiomas, and pituitary tumors), Down syndrome, neurofibromatosis type 1, and sickle cell disease (Scott and Smith 2009). The syndrome may present in infancy with recurrent episodes of cerebral ischemia and infarction, mental retardation, headache, epileptic seizures, and, occasionally, involuntary movements. In adults, subarachnoid or primary intracerebral hemorrhage is also common owing to rupture of collateral vessels. There have also been a few reports of associated intracranial aneurysms (Iwama *et al.* 1997) and also of cerebral arteriovenous malformations.

Embolism from Intra- and Extracranial Arterial Aneurysms

Embolism from thrombus within the cavity of an aneurysm is rare and is difficult to prove in cases where there may be other potential sources of embolization. Intracranial aneurysms more commonly present with rupture and subarachnoid hemorrhage, whereas internal carotid artery aneurysms tend to cause pressure symptoms including a pulsatile and sometimes painful mass in the neck or pharynx, ipsilateral Horner's syndrome, or compression of the lower cranial nerves. Extracranial vertebral artery aneurysms may cause pain in the neck and arm, a mass, spinal cord compression, and upper limb ischemia (Catala *et al.* 1993).

Irradiation

Excessive irradiation of the head and neck can damage intra- and extracranial arteries, both large and small. Within the radiation field, a localized, stenotic, and sometimes apparently atheromatous lesion may become symptomatic months or years later. There can be considerable fibrosis of the arterial wall and even aneurysm formation (O'Connor and Mayberg 2000; Plummer *et al.* 2011). The most common causes of this large artery variant are radiotherapy to the neck following laryngeal carcinoma or nasopharyngeal carcinoma, which leads to disease around the carotid bifurcation, and radiotherapy to pituitary tumors, which leads most commonly to disease in the basilar artery. Optimal medical treatment is uncertain as carotid endarterectomy is affected by the need to operate on scarred tissue planes, while carotid stenting is associated with high restenosis rates. Patients who have had radiotherapy for cerebral tumors more commonly develop a progressive small vessel vasculopathy.

Inflammatory Vascular Disease

There are a number of acute, subacute, and chronic inflammatory "vasculitic" disorders of the arterial or venous wall (Box 6.1). These disorders may be associated with ischemic stroke, intracranial hemorrhage, intracranial venous thrombosis (Chapter 29), or a generalized encephalopathy. Angiographic appearances can be diagnostic, particularly in larger artery vasculitis, but angiography is not particularly sensitive and the abnormalities seen may be nonspecific, and so diagnosis is often made on the basis of the clinical syndrome. Contrast-enhanced high-resolution MRI can be useful in showing contrast uptake in the walls of thickened and inflamed large cerebral arteries.

Giant Cell Arteritis

Giant cell arteritis is the most common vasculitic cause of stroke and is associated particularly with posterior circulation ischemia (Ronthal *et al.* 2003; Muratore *et al.* 2015;

BOX 6.1 Inflammatory Vascular Diseases Causing Stroke	
Giant cell arteritis	Relapsing polychondritis
Systematic lupus erythematosus	Progressive systemic sclerosis
Antiphospholipid antibody syndrome	Sarcoid angiitis Primary vasculitis of the central nervous system
Primary systematic vasculitis	Takayasu's disease
Rheumatoid disease	Buerger's disease
Sjögren's syndrome	Malignant atrophic papulosis
Behçet's disease	Acute posterior multifocal placoid pigment epitheliopathy

Buttgereit *et al.* 2016). Medium and large arteries are affected, especially branches of the external carotid artery, the ophthalmic artery, and the vertebral artery. The patients are elderly, with the diagnosis being rare under age 60 years. Malaise, polymyalgia, and other systemic symptoms are frequently present. The erythrocyte sedimentation rate is usually raised, often to over 100 mm/h in the first hour.

Systemic Lupus Erythematosus

Systemic lupus erythematosus is more likely to cause a subacute or chronic generalized encephalopathy than symptomatic focal ischemia (Jennekens and Kater 2002a, b; Lisnevskaia *et al.* 2014). The underlying vascular pathology, where present, appears to be intimal proliferation rather than a vasculitis. The extracranial arteries are largely unaffected, but embolism from heart valve vegetations is quite common, particularly when there are circulating antiphospholipid antibodies (Mitsias and Levine 1994; Roldan *et al.* 1996). Intracranial venous thrombosis is rare (Vidailhet *et al.* 1990). In some patients with little clinical evidence of systemic lupus erythematosus, there is prominent livedo reticularis, which, when associated with stroke, is referred to as Sneddon's syndrome, in which antiphospholipid antibodies are particularly common (Stockhammer *et al.* 1993; Kalashnikova *et al.* 1994; Boesch *et al.* 2003; Hilton and Footitt 2003).

Antiphospholipid Syndrome

Antiphospholipid syndrome is a constellation of various recurrent clinical events as well as specific immunological features: arterial and venous thrombosis, including recurrent ischemic stroke or TIA and intracranial venous thrombosis; migraine-like episodes; recurrent miscarriage; livedo reticularis; cardiac valvular vegetations; thrombocytopenia; false-positive syphilis serology; and persistently raised circulating IgG anticardiolipin antibodies and/or the circulating lupus anticoagulant, usually detected by prolongation of the activated partial thromboplastin time (Katzav *et al.* 2003; Brey 2005; Sanna *et al.* 2005; Merrill 2007; Ruiz-Irastorza *et al.* 2010). Antiphospholipid antibodies are found in some normal people and in systemic lupus erythematosus; hence, an isolated finding of a raised antibody level in a patient with stroke is of uncertain significance. Antibodies are not uncommonly present after acute stroke but only where they remain on retesting after 6 weeks should the diagnosis of antiphospholipid syndrome be made, particularly if other clinical features are lacking.

Primary Systemic Vasculitis

Primary systemic vasculitis is a group of related disorders including polyarteritis nodosa, granulomatosis with polyangiitis (formerly known as Wegener's granulomatosis), eosinophilic granulomatosis with polyangiitis (formerly known as Churg–Strauss syndrome), and various hypersensitivity vasculitides. Rarely, there is associated cerebrovascular disease, similar to that occurring in systemic lupus erythematosus (Futrell 1995; Savage *et al.* 1997; Ferro 1998). Stroke is usually lacunar (Reichhart *et al.* 2000), and there are often associated hematuria, eosinophilia, and circulating anti-neutrophil cytoplasmic antibodies.

Rheumatoid Disease

Rheumatoid disease is rarely complicated by a systemic vasculitis, which can involve the brain (Genta *et al.* 2006). Occasionally atlanto-axial dislocation causes symptomatic vertebral artery compression (Howell and Molyneux 1988).

Sjögren's Syndrome

Sjögren's syndrome is occasionally complicated by systemic vasculitis, causing focal cerebral ischemia, global encephalopathy, and aseptic meningitis (Hietaharju *et al.* 1993; Bragoni *et al.* 1994; Delalande *et al.* 2004).

Behçet's Disease

Neurological involvement in Behçet's disease may be subclassified into two major forms: a vascular–inflammatory process with focal or multifocal parenchymal involvement and a cerebral venous sinus thrombosis with intracranial hypertension. The vasculitis and meningitis may affect cerebral arteries, particularly in the posterior circulation, to cause ischemic stroke and possibly intracranial hemorrhage (Farah *et al.* 1998; Krespi *et al.* 2001; Siva *et al.* 2004; Borhani Haghighi *et al.* 2005).

Relapsing Polychondritis

Relapsing polychondritis may be complicated by a generalized encephalopathy, stroke-like episodes, and ischemic optic neuropathy as a result of systemic vasculitis (Stewart *et al.* 1988; Hsu *et al.* 2006).

Progressive Systemic Sclerosis

Progressive systemic sclerosis is hardly ever complicated directly by stroke, although a carotid and cerebral vasculopathy has been described (Heron *et al.* 1998; Lucivero *et al.* 2004).

Sarcoid Angiitis

Sarcoid affects the cerebral vessels only rarely, usually causing a generalized encephalo-pathy rather than focal features owing to ischemia or hemorrhage (Hoyle *et al.* 2014; Rosen 2015).

Primary Angiitis of the Central Nervous System

Primary angiitis of the central nervous system (CNS) is a very rare disorder that affects leptomeningeal, cortical, and sometimes spinal cord blood vessels (Birnbaum and Hellmann 2009). It is "isolated" in the sense that it is confined to the CNS. Histologically, it is similar to sarcoid angiitis with granulomatous vasculitic changes. The median age of onset is approximately 50 years, and men are affected twice as often as women. The course is subacute, often leading to death in weeks or months, with progressive headache, mental confusion and impairment, vomiting, stroke-like episodes, and myelopathy. Systemic symptoms are very uncommon. Diagnosis is only really possible from meningeal or cortical biopsy (Birnhaum and Hellmann 2009).

Takayasu's Arteritis

Takayasu's arteritis is a chronic vasculitis, histologically identical to giant cell arteritis but affecting only the aorta and large arteries arising from it; it occurs mainly in young Asian women (Seko 2007). Systemic features are common, including malaise, weight loss, arthralgia, and fever. The neurological complications reflect progressive narrowing and eventual occlusion of the large arteries in the neck: claudication of the jaw muscles, ischemic oculopathy, syncope, seizures, confusion, boundary zone infarction, and, rarely, focal ischemic stroke or TIAs (Hoffmann *et al.* 2000; Hwang *et al.* 2012). In addition, there may be ischemia of the arms and of the kidneys to cause hypertension as well as ischemic necrosis of the lips, nasal septum, and palate. Other causes of a similar aortic arch syndrome include advanced atheroma, giant cell arteritis, syphilis, subintimal fibrosis, arterial dissection, trauma, and coarctation. Treatment is with immunosuppression, which may result in remission (Keser *et al.* 2014). Occasionally surgery in the form of balloon angioplasty, stent graft replacement, or surgical bypass may be useful (Keser *et al.* 2014).

Buerger's Disease

Buerger's disease or "thromboangiitis obliterans" is a rare inflammatory disorder of small and medium-sized arteries and veins, chiefly of the limbs, but very rare cases of TIA or ischemic stroke have been reported. It has a strong male preponderance and mainly affects smokers (Puéchal and Fiessinger 2007).

Malignant Atrophic Papulosis

Malignant atrophic papulosis, or Degos disease, is a very rare syndrome consisting of crops of painless pinkish papules on the trunk and limbs that heal as distinctive circular porcelain-white scars. It may be complicated by ischemic lesions in the gut, brain, spinal cord, and nerve roots owing to endothelial proliferation in small arteries (Sotrel *et al.* 1983; Subbiah *et al.* 1996; Amato *et al.* 2005).

BOX 6.2 Hematological Disorders Causing Ischemic Stroke

Thrombophilia, e.g., antithrombin III deficiency, protein C deficiency, factor V Leiden mutation, protein S deficiency, plasminogen abnormality, or deficiency

Leukemia/lymphoma

Polycythemia

Essential thrombocythemia

Sickle cell disease/trait and other hemoglobinopathies

Iron-deficiency anemia

Paraproteinemias

Paroxysmal nocturnal hemoglobinuria

Thrombotic thrombocytopenic purpura

Disseminated intravascular coagulation

Acute Posterior Multifocal Placoid Pigment Epitheliopathy

Acute posterior multifocal placoid pigment epitheliopathy is a rare and usually benign and self-limiting chorioretinal disorder, with rapidly deteriorating central vision. However, it can be complicated by systemic vasculitis, aseptic meningitis, and stroke (Comu *et al.* 1996; de Vries *et al.* 2006).

Hematological Disorders

A number of hematological disorders may occasionally cause ischemic stroke and TIA (Tatlisumak and Fisher 1996; Arboix and Besses 1997; Markus and Hambley 1998; Matijevic and Wu 2006; Pósfai *et al.* 2014) (Box 6.2).

Thrombophilias

Thrombophilias and other causes of hypercoagulability are rare causes of stroke (Matijevic and Wu 2006). Antithrombin III deficiency, protein C deficiency, activated protein C resistance owing to factor V Leiden mutation, protein S deficiency, and plasminogen abnormality or deficiency can all cause peripheral and intracranial venous thrombosis. Thrombosis is usually recurrent, and there is often a family history. Thrombophilia may cause arterial thrombosis, although the alternative diagnosis of paradoxical embolism should always be considered in patients with these disorders. It should be noted that deficiencies in any one of the factors associated with thrombophilia may be an incidental finding and cannot necessarily be assumed to be the cause of stroke (Hankey *et al.* 2001; Morris *et al.* 2010).

Leukemia and Lymphoma

Leukemia and lymphoma may cause intracranial hemorrhage, particularly in acute myeloid leukemia, most commonly through acute disseminated intravascular coagulation, although other hemostatic defects or CNS infiltration may be responsible (Rogers 2003;

Glass 2006). The hemorrhage is often fulminant, with bleeding usually occurring in the brain or subdural compartment and occasionally in the subarachnoid space. Occasionally, cerebral venous thrombosis or arterial occlusion may occur. **Malignant angioendotheliosis**, an intravascular lymphoma, is a very rare cause of stroke-like episodes and progressive global encephalopathy (Chapin *et al.* 1995; Zuckerman *et al.* 2006; Hundsberger *et al.* 2011).

Polycythemia

Polycythemia is usually defined as a hematocrit above 0.50 in males and 0.47 in females. Polycythemia rubra vera or primary polycythemia, a myeloproliferative disorder, may be complicated by TIAs, ischemic stroke, or intracranial venous thrombosis (Markus and Hambley 1998; Marchioli *et al.* 2005; Spivak 2010; Abdel-Rahman and Murphy 2015). Ischemic complications may occur because the platelet count is raised and platelet activity enhanced or because of increased whole-blood viscosity. Paradoxically, there may also be a hemostatic defect as a result of defective platelet function, resulting in intracranial hemorrhage. Increased stroke risk may also occur with secondary polycythemia caused by chronic hypoxia, smoking, congenital cyanotic heart disease, renal tumor, or cerebellar hemangioblastoma.

Essential Thrombocythemia

Essential thrombocythemia, or idiopathic primary thrombocytosis, is another myeloproliferative disorder in which the platelet count is raised, usually to over $1,000 \times 10^9$ cells/L. Secondary thrombocytosis occurs in malignancy, splenectomy, hyposplenism, surgery, trauma, hemorrhage, iron deficiency, infections, polycythemia rubra vera, myelofibrosis, and the leukemias. There is a tendency for arterial and venous thrombosis and, paradoxically, intracranial hemorrhage because the platelets are hemostatically defective (Arboix *et al.* 1995; Harrison *et al.* 1998; Ogata *et al.* 2005; Pósfai *et al.* 2014).

Sickle Cell Disease and Other Hemoglobinopathies

Sickle cell disease and rarely other hemoglobinopathies may be complicated by ischemic stroke or intracranial hemorrhage (Razvi and Bone 2006; Switzer *et al.* 2006; Talahma *et al.* 2014). Patients are usually children homozygous for the sickle gene, although sometimes a sickle cell crisis, provoked by hypoxia, may occur in an adult heterozygote. Small and large arteries, as well as veins, develop a fibrous vasculopathy and are occluded by thrombi as a result of the abnormally rigid red blood cells and raised whole blood viscosity, thrombocytosis, and impaired fibrinolytic activity.

Iron-Deficiency Anemia

Severe iron-deficiency anemia causes nonspecific neurological symptoms, which are presumably hypoxic in origin, including poor concentration, malaise, giddiness, fatigue, and weakness. Occasionally, TIAs and ischemic strokes seem to be provoked by profound anemia in association with severe extracranial occlusive arterial disease or thrombocytosis (Akins *et al.* 1996; Keung and Owen 2004; Chang *et al.* 2013).

Paraproteinemias

Multiple myeloma and macroglobulinemia cause anemia through defective erythropoiesis and thus produce nonspecific neurological symptoms as described previously. A hemostatic defect caused by reduced platelet number and sometimes associated uremia may cause intracranial hemorrhage. However, most of the "cerebral" features of these patients can be explained by the "hyperviscosity syndrome," which is characterized by headache, ataxia, diplopia, dysarthria, lethargy, drowsiness, poor concentration, visual blurring, and deafness. The same syndrome can be seen in primary polycythemia or leukemia. Arterial or venous cerebral infarction may occur, and at autopsy, the microcirculation is occluded with acidophilic material thought to be precipitates of the abnormal proteins (Davies-Jones 1995). It is exceptional for patients with neurological involvement not to have a raised erythrocyte sedimentation rate.

Paroxysmal Nocturnal Hemoglobinuria

Paroxysmal nocturnal hemoglobinuria is a very rare acquired disorder in which hemopoietic stem cells become particularly sensitive to complement-mediated lysis. Venous and possibly arterial thrombosis occurs in the brain and elsewhere. Patients are nearly always anemic at neurological presentation, and there may be a history of dark urine, evidence of hemolysis, and a low platelet and granulocyte count (Al-Hakim *et al.* 1993; Audebert *et al.* 2005).

Thrombotic Thrombocytopenic Purpura

Thrombotic thrombocytopenic purpura is a rare acute or subacute disease in adults, rather similar to the hemolytic uremic syndrome in children, in which there is systemic malaise, fever, skin purpura, renal failure, hematuria, and proteinuria. Hemorrhagic infarcts caused by platelet microthrombi occur in many organs in the brain. They may cause stroke-like episodes (Matijevic and Wu 2006), although more commonly, there is global encephalopathy. The blood film shows thrombocytopenia, hemolytic anemia, and fragmented red cells. The differential diagnosis includes infective endocarditis, idiopathic thrombocytopenia, heparin-induced thrombocytopenia with thrombosis, systemic lupus erythematosus, non-bacterial thrombotic endocarditis, and disseminated intravascular coagulation.

Disseminated Intravascular Coagulation

Widespread hemorrhagic brain infarcts and intracranial hemorrhages tend to cause an acute or subacute global encephalopathy rather than stroke-like episodes. The diagnosis is confirmed by a low platelet count, low plasma fibrinogen, and raised fibrin degradation products and D-dimer.

Miscellaneous Rare Causes

Other rare causes of cerebral ischemia or infarction include those listed in Table 6.1, some of which are discussed in the following section.

Pregnancy and the Puerperium

Pregnancy is complicated by stroke in approximately 30 per 100,000 deliveries in developed countries, about twice the background rate (Tate and Bushnell 2011).

The risks of stroke are not increased during gestation except for an increased risk in the 2 days prior to birth. During the first 6 weeks and especially the first few days postpartum, there is an increased risk of ischemic stroke and intracerebral hemorrhage.

Causes of stroke particularly relevant to pregnancy include intracranial venous thrombosis, arterial dissection during labor, acute middle cerebral or other large artery occlusion, low-flow infarction and disseminated intravascular coagulation complicating eclampsia, vasoconstriction secondary to drugs, infective endocarditis, peripartum cardiomyopathy, sickle cell crisis and intracranial hemorrhage(s) caused by eclampsia, anticoagulant-use, rupture of a preexisting aneurysm, and vascular malformation (Hender *et al.* 2006). Paradoxical embolism via a PFO may possibly occur as the pregnant woman performs a Valsalva maneuver during labor. Metastases of choriocarcinoma can present with stroke-like episodes and on CT look remarkably like primary intracerebral hemorrhages. Many cases of pregnancy-associated stroke remain cryptogenic, and the risk of recurrent stroke in a future pregnancy is not known.

The diagnostic and therapeutic approaches to stroke are similar during pregnancy and postpartum to those in non-pregnant patients except for consideration of the well-being of the fetus. Although CT or catheter angiography is associated with radiation, the dosage is far lower than the teratogenic dose and hence could be performed in pregnant women with shielding of the abdomen. However, should catheter angiography be performed, fluoroscopy time should be limited. There have been no teratogenic effects of iodinated contrast reported in animal studies, although in pregnant women, there is a slight risk of subsequent treatable fetal hypothyroidism. Similarly, no adverse effects have been reported in pregnant women or their fetuses receiving MRI, and this should be performed if needed regardless of gestational age. MRI contrast agents, however, should be avoided as they cross the placenta, but it remains uncertain whether these are teratogenic (Tate and Bushnell 2011).

In pregnant women with an acute ischemic stroke, case studies have shown that intravenous alteplase is safe with no significant increased risk of intracerebral hemorrhage or poor fetal outcome (del Zotto *et al.* 2010). Intravenous alteplase should therefore be considered in cases of potentially disabling ischemic stroke (Selim and Molina 2013). Endovascular treatment is also considered to be beneficial in suitable cases as it may eliminate the need for thrombolytic agents or allow a reduction in dose. However, ionizing radiation to the fetus should be minimized by an optimal shield.

The safety of aspirin has been debated during the first trimester. However, low-dose (<150 mg) aspirin is safe in the second and third trimester and likely to be safe during pregnancy. Clopidogrel crosses the placenta, and animal studies have failed to demonstrate a risk to the fetus, although there are no adequate well-controlled studies in pregnant women (FDA category B). Intravenous or low-molecular heparin is not associated with teratogenic effects and is compatible with breastfeeding. Warfarin, especially if administered during the first trimester, carries potential serious risks to the fetus including an increased risk of fetal anomalies, prematurity, and low birth weight and hence should be avoided in pregnancy. There are no data on the safety of non-vitamin K antagonist anticoagulants in pregnancy.

Migraine

Migraine is associated with a twofold increased risk of ischemic stroke, in particular cryptogenic stroke, independent of vascular risk factors (Donaghy et al. 2002; Bousser and Welch 2005; Tietjen 2005; Kurth and Diener 2012; Li et al. 2015). Stroke may occur during a migraine attack or remote from it. Cerebral ischemia can induce migrainous symptoms, and migraine aura may resemble TIA, causing diagnostic difficulty (Chapter 8). The term "migrainous stroke" should be reserved for patients who have a history of migraine with aura but have experienced a prolonged typical aura lasting more than 60 minutes with accompanying neuroimaging features of a cerebral infarct in the relevant area. The infarct should not be attributable to another disorder. Migrainous strokes are very rare and account for 0.3–0.5% of all ischemic strokes (Kurth and Diener 2012). Migrainous strokes usually cause a homonymous hemianopia or focal sensory deficit without persisting disability and do not appear to recur very often (Hoekstra-van Dalen et al. 1996).

Sometimes arterial occlusion is demonstrated by angiography in migrainous stroke, and the cause is hypothesized to be in situ thrombosis complicating vasospasm. No provoking factors are known. Other possible causes of stroke in the context of headache must be considered: reversible cerebral vasoconstriction syndrome, carotid dissection, mitochondrial cytopathy, ruptured vascular malformation, antiphospholipid antibody syndrome, and CADASIL (cerebral autosomal dominant arteriopathy with subcortical infarcts and leukoencephalopathy). Migraine auras without headache may be confused with TIA (Chapter 8).

Epidemiological studies suggest the existence of close but complex relationships between estrogens, migraine, and stroke in women before menopause (Donaghy et al. 2002; Bousser 2004). Migraine, particularly without aura, is strongly influenced by estrogens, as illustrated by the frequency of onset at puberty, menstrual migraine, and improvement during pregnancy. The risk of stroke with migraine is further increased by tobacco smoking and oral contraceptive use (Chang et al. 1999; Donaghy et al. 2002). The pathophysiological mechanism underlying these close relationships remains unknown. In practice, given the very low absolute risk of stroke in young women, there is no absolute contraindication to oral contraceptive use in young female migraineurs, but they should be advised strongly not to smoke and to use a form with a low estrogen content or progestogens, particularly if they experience migraine with aura. Elevated blood pressure, an important stroke risk factor, is less common in migraineurs.

Both ischemic stroke and migraine can be consequences of underlying vascular disorders. Hereditary conditions, including CADASIL, MELAS (mitochondrial myopathy, encephalopathy, lactic acidosis, and stroke), and hereditary hemorrhagic telangiectasia, appear to predispose to both migraine and stroke. Acquired antiphospholipid antibodies, while not a cause of migraine per se, may increase the risk of infarction in migraineurs.

Possible mechanisms for migraine-associated stroke include:

- involvement of the vasculature, including vasospasm, arterial dissection, and small vessel arteriopathy.
- hypercoagulability, involving elevated von Willebrand factor or platelet activation.
- elevated risk of cardioembolism through patent foramen ovale or from atrial septal aneurysm.

Triptans and ergotamines, used to treat acute migraine attacks, appear to be safe in low-risk populations but should be avoided in hemiplegic migraine, in basilar migraine, and in patients with prior cerebral or cardiac ischemia.

Cancer

Cancer may cause stroke (Grisold *et al.* 2009) through:

- Cancer-related mechanisms
  - Direct tumor-related
    - Vessel compression or infiltration
    - Cerebral metastases: melanoma, germ cell tumors, choriocarcinoma, lung tumors, hypernephroma
    - Hemorrhage into primary tumors: malignant astrocytoma, oligodendroglioma, medulloblastoma, hemangioblastoma
    - Neoplastic compression or invasion of neck arteries causing ischemic stroke
  - Embolic stroke
    - Tumor embolism
    - Embolism of non-infected heart valve vegetations: non-bacterial thrombotic, or marantic, endocarditis
  - Coagulopathy
    - Hemostatic failure: leukemias with hyperviscosity syndrome or "hypercoagulability"
    - Disseminated intravascular coagulation
    - Intracranial venous thrombosis
- Treatment-related mechanisms
  - Chemotherapy causing coagulopathy
  - Radiation or surgery causing vascular stenosis
  - Infection related: fungi, herpes zoster, bacterial endocarditis

Perioperative Stroke

Incidence of perioperative stroke ranges from 0.08 to 0.7% for general surgical procedures and 0.8 to 3% for peripheral vascular surgeries but can be up to 4–10% for certain head and neck, cardiac, and aortic operations (Selim 2007). It can be caused by hypotension and boundary zone infarction, trauma to and dissection of neck arteries, paradoxical embolism, fat embolism, infective endocarditis, myocardial infarction, atrial fibrillation, or a hemostatic defect caused by antithrombotic drugs or disseminated intravascular coagulation. It is more common in patients aged >70; those with vascular risk factors; those with preexisting vascular, cardiac, or chronic obstructive lung disease; and those with underlying atherosclerosis of the carotid arteries or ascending aorta (Selim 2007). Simultaneous carotid endarterectomy and coronary bypass grafting (Chapter 27) are associated with 10–15% risk of death, stroke, or myocardial infarction, and the risk is higher in those with bilateral as opposed to unilateral carotid disease (Naylor *et al.* 2003a, b).

Recreational Drugs

The use of recreational drugs, including cocaine, amphetamines, and opiates, shows a marked temporal association (often within minutes to an hour) with the onset of both hemorrhagic and ischemic stroke (Neimann *et al.* 2000; O'Connor *et al.* 2005; Westover *et al.* 2007). Possible mechanisms for drug-associated stroke include acute severe elevation of blood pressure, cardiac arrhythmia, cerebral vasospasm, and embolization of foreign material injected with the diluents. Infective endocarditis, particularly associated with *Staphylococcus aureus*, is an important cause of stroke in intravenous drug users. Dilated cardiomyopathy may also occur. Rupture of aneurysms and arteriovenous malformations have been detected in up to half the patients with hemorrhagic stroke caused by cocaine abuse. Cannabis is a potent vasoactive agent and has been associated with ischemic stroke secondary to reversible multifocal intracranial stenosis, a variant of reversible cerebral vasoconstriction syndrome (Wolff *et al.* 2013). Amphetamines can cause a small vessel vasculopathy, leading to intracerebral hemorrhage or infarction (Heye and Hankey 1996). Other sympathomimetic drugs such as ephedrine, phenylpropanolamine, fenfluramine, and phentermine may cause stroke by similar mechanisms, as can ecstasy (3,4-methylenedioxy-*N*-methylamphetamine) (Wen *et al.* 1997).

Chronic Meningitis

Meningitis caused by tuberculous, syphilitic, and fungal infections may involve the arteries at the base of the brain or the perforating arteries and so be complicated by ischemic stroke and intracranial hemorrhage (Lan *et al.* 2001). Very occasionally, acute local infections such as tonsillitis, pharyngitis, or lymphadenitis can cause inflammation and secondary thrombosis in the carotid artery in the neck (Lemierre's syndrome). Otitis media or mastoiditis may cause dural sinus thrombosis. Cerebral arterial and venous thrombosis may result from bacterial meningitis, ophthalmic herpes zoster, chicken pox, leptospirosis, HIV infection, cat scratch disease, neurotrichinosis, and possibly borreliosis.

Inflammatory Bowel Disease

Both ulcerative and Crohn's colitis may occasionally be complicated by intracranial venous thrombosis, arterial occlusion, and intracerebral hemorrhage (Lossos *et al.* 1995; Filimon *et al.* 2015). Mechanisms include thrombocytosis, hyper-coagulability, immobility and paradoxical embolism, vasculitis, and dehydration. The bowel disease is not necessarily severe at the time of the stroke. Celiac disease can also be complicated by a cerebral vasculitis, but this often presents with an encephalopathy rather than a stroke (Mumford *et al.* 1996; Ludvigsson *et al.* 2012).

Mitochondrial Cytopathy

Mitochondrial cytopathy may present with stroke-like episodes often complicated by epilepsy and encephalopathy, a particular example of which is MELAS (Martínez-Fernádez *et al.* 2001; Schapira 2012). Scanning with CT may show hypodensities, particularly in the occipital regions, and calcification of the basal ganglia (Fig. 6.10). In MRI, there are T_2-weighted hyperintensities in the temporo-occipito-parietal regions that do not correspond

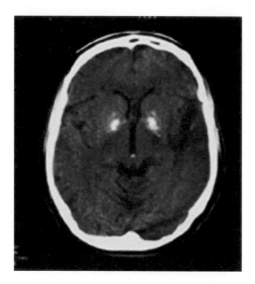

Fig. 6.10 A CT brain scan of a 40-year-old man with mitochondrial cytopathy, showing calcification of the basal ganglia and hypodensity in the left temporal lobe.

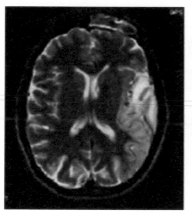 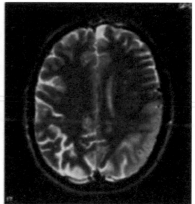

Fig. 6.11 These T$_2$-weighted MRI images of the brain are from a patient with mitochondrial cytopathy and show primarily cortical hyperintensity in the left temporoparietal region not typical of middle cerebral artery branch infarction.

to classical vascular territories (Fig. 6.11) and that may disappear on subsequent scans. Other clinical features often associated with mitochondrial disease include migraine, short stature, sensorineural deafness, diabetes, and learning disability. The blood and CSF lactate are usually raised; most patients have an abnormal muscle biopsy, and diagnosis can often be made by detection of the relevant genetic mutations.

Fabry Disease

Fabry disease is a rare X-linked lysosomal storage disorder that results from a deficiency in or total lack of the enzyme α-galactosidase A due to mutations in the *GLA* gene (Razvi and

Bone 2006; Kolodny *et al.* 2015). About 6% of patients develop strokes (~90% ischemic), mainly due to the progressive accumulation of globotriaosycleramide (GL-3) and other glycosphingolipids in the vascular endothelium (Rolfs *et al.* 2005; Sims *et al.* 2009). Symptoms of Fabry disease usually begin during childhood and include neuropathic pain, gastrointestinal dysfunction, and hypohidrosis. Later on during adulthood, patients may develop renal impairment, cardiovascular dysfunction, and strokes. Treatment is with enzyme replacement therapy with recombinant human α-galactosidase A, which can reduce the plasma and tissue GL-3 accumulation.

Homocystinuria

Homocystinuria is an autosomal recessive inborn error of metabolism that is complicated by cerebral arterial or venous thrombosis (Schimke *et al.* 1965; Visy *et al.* 1991; Rubba *et al.* 1994; Testai and Gorelick 2010). Heterozygotes may have an increased risk of vascular disease.

Hypoglycemia

Hypoglycemic drugs, and rarely an insulinoma, are a well-recognized but uncommon cause of transient focal neurological episodes and patients may be misdiagnosed as TIA (Chapter 8). These episodes tend to occur on waking in the morning or after exercise, and by the time the patient is seen, the blood glucose may well have returned to normal. Persisting focal deficits are unusual (Malouf and Brust 1985; Wallis *et al.* 1985; Service 1995; Shanmugam *et al.* 1997).

Hypercalcemia (Longo and Witherspoon 1980) and **hyponatremia** (Ruby and Burton 1977; Berkovic *et al.* 1984) have been reported to cause TIA-like episodes.

Fat Embolism

Fat embolism, which usually occurs following long bone fracture or surgery, most commonly causes a global encephalopathy, but on occasion there may be focal features, presumably reflecting local ischemia (Jacobson *et al.* 1986; Parizel *et al.* 2001).

Fibrocartilaginous Embolism

Fibrocartilaginous embolism is a rare and curious disorder where fibrocartilaginous emboli, presumably from degenerative intervertebral disc material, are found in various organs, the spinal cord more often than the brain (Freyaldenhoven *et al.* 2001).

Snake Bite

Injection of venom may cause intracranial hemorrhage as a consequence of defibrination and other hemostatic defects and rarely ischemic stroke (Bashir and Jinkins 1985).

Epidermal nevus syndrome, a sporadic neurocutaneous disorder, can be complicated by stroke (Dobyns and Garg 1991).

Susac's Syndrome

Susac's syndrome is a rare triad of branch retinal artery occlusions, sensori-neural hearing loss, and microangiopathy of the brain causing a subacute encephalopathy, almost always in women (García-Carrasco *et al.* 2014).

References

Abdel-Rahman I, Murphy C (2015). Recurrent ischemic stroke unveils polycythemia vera. *BMJ Case Reports* pii:bcr2014207625

Adachi T, Takagi M, Hoshino H *et al.* (1997). Effect of extracranial carotid artery stenosis and other risk factors for stroke on periventricular hyperintensity. *Stroke* 28:2174–2179

Akins PT, Glen S, Nemeth PM *et al.* (1996). Carotid artery thrombus associated with severe iron-deficiency anemia and thrombocytosis. *Stroke* 27:1002–1005

Al-Hakim M, Katirji MB, Osorio I *et al.* (1993). Cerebral venous thrombosis in paroxysmal nocturnal haemoglobinuria: Report of two cases. *Neurology* 43:742–746

Amarenco P (2005). Patent foramen ovale and the risk of stroke: Smoking gun, guilty by association? *Heart* 91:441–443

Amarenco P, Cohen A, Tzourio C *et al.* (1994). Atherosclerotic disease of the aortic arch and the risk of ischemic stroke. *New England Journal of Medicine* 331:1474–1479

Amato C, Ferri R, Elia M *et al.* (2005). Nervous system involvement in Degos disease. *American Journal of Neuroradiology* 26:646–649

Aoyagi M, Fukai N, Yamamoto M *et al.* (1996). Early development of intimal thickening in superficial temporal arteries in patients with Moyamoya disease. *Stroke* 27:1750–1754

Arboix A, Besses C (1997). Cerebrovascular disease as the initial clinical presentation of hematological disorders. *European Neurology* 37:207–211

Arboix A, Besses C, Acin P *et al.* (1995). Ischemic stroke as first manifestation of essential thrombocythemia. Report of six cases. *Stroke* 26:1463–1466

Arunodaya GR, Vani S, Shankar SK *et al.* (1997). Fibromuscular dysplasia with dissection of basilar artery presenting as "locked-in-syndrome." *Neurology* 48:1605–1608

Asopa S, Patel A, Khan OA *et al.* (2007). Non-bacterial thrombotic endocarditis. *European Journal of Cardiothoracic Surgery* 32:696–701

Audebert HJ, Planck J, Eisenburg M *et al.* (2005). Cerebral ischemic infarction in paroxysmal nocturnal haemoglobinuria: Report of 2 cases and updated review of 7 previously published patients. *Journal of Neurology* 252:1379–1386

Auer A, Felber S, Schmidauer C *et al.* (1998). Magnetic resonance angiographic and clinical features of extracranial vertebral artery dissection. *Journal of Neurology, Neurosurgery and Psychiatry* 64:474–481

Ayas N, Wijdicks EFM (1995). Cardiac catheterization complicated by stroke: 14 patients. *Cerebrovascular Diseases* 5:304–307

Bamford J, Sandercock PAG, Jones L *et al.* (1987). The natural history of lacunar infarction: The Oxfordshire Community Stroke Project. *Stroke* 18:545–551

Bashir R, Jinkins J (1985). Cerebral infarction in a young female following snake bite. *Stroke* 16:328–330

Bathen J, Sparr S, Rokseth R (1978). Embolism in sinoatrial disease. *Acta Medica Scandinavica* 203:7–11

Berkovic SF, Bladin PF, Darby DG (1984). Metabolic disorders presenting as stroke. *Medical Journal of Australia* 140:421–424

Birnhaum J, Hellmann DB (2009). Primary angiitis of the central nervous system. *JAMA Neurology* 66:704–709

Boesch SM, Plorer AL, Auer AJ *et al.* (2003). The natural course of Sneddon syndrome: Clinical and magnetic resonance imaging findings in a prospective six year observation study. *Journal of Neurology, Neurosurgery and Psychiatry* 74:542–544

Boiten J, Rothwell PM, Slattery J *et al.* (1996). Ischemic lacunar stroke in the European Carotid Surgery Trial. Risk factors, distribution of carotid stenosis, effect of surgery and type of recurrent stroke. *Cerebrovascular Diseases* 6:281–287

Boon A, Lodder J, Cheriex E *et al.* (1996). Risk of stroke in a cohort of 815 patients with calcification of the aortic valve with or without stenosis. *Stroke* 27:847–851

Borhani Haghighi A, Pourmand R, Nikseresht AR (2005). Neuro–Behçet disease. A review. *Neurologist* 11:80–89

Bots ML, van Swieten JC, Breteler MMB *et al.* (1993). Cerebral white matter lesions and atherosclerosis in the Rotterdam study. *Lancet* 341:1232–1237

Bousser MG (2004). Estrogens, migraine and stroke. *Stroke* 35:2652–2656

Bousser MG, Welch KM (2005). Relation between migraine and stroke. *Lancet Neurology* 4:533–534

Bragoni M, Di Piero V, Priori R *et al.* (1994). Sjögren's syndrome presenting as ischemic stroke. *Stroke* 25:2276–2279

Brey RL (2005). Antiphospholipid antibodies in young adults with stroke. *Journal of Thrombosis and Thombolysis* 20:105–112

Buttgereit F, Dejaco C, Matteson EL *et al.* (2016). Polymyalgia rheumatica and giant cell arteritis – a systematic review. *JAMA* 315:2442–2458

Cabanes L, Mas JL, Cohen A *et al.* (1993). Atrial septal aneurysm and patent foramen ovale as risk factors for cryptogenic stroke in patients less than 55 years of age. A study using transoesophageal echocardiography. *Stroke* 24:1865–1873

CADISS Trial Investigators (2015). Antiplatelet treatment compared with anticoagulation treatment for cervical artery dissection (CADISS): A randomised trial. *Lancet Neurology* 14:361–367

Caplan LR (1995). Binswanger's disease: Revisited. *Neurology* 45:626–633

Carroll JD, Saver JL, Thaler DE *et al.* (2013). Closure of patent foramen ovale versus medical therapy after cryptogenic stroke. *New England Journal of Medicine* 368:1092–1100

Catala M, Rancurel G, Koskas F *et al.* (1993). Ischemic stroke due to spontaneous extracranial vertebral giant aneurysm. *Cerebrovascular Diseases* 3:322–326

Chang YL, Hung SH, Ling W et al. (2013). Association between ischemic stroke and iron-deficiency anemia: A population-based study. *PLos ONE* 8:e82952

Chang CL, Donaghy M, Poulter N *et al.* (1999). Migraine and stroke in young women: Case-control study. *British Medical Journal* 318:13–18

Chapin JE, Davis LE, Kornfeld M *et al.* (1995). Neurologic manifestations of intravascular lymphomatosis. *Acta Neurology Scandinavica* 91:494–499

CODICE Study Group (2006). Recurrent stroke is not associated with massive right-to-left shunt: Preliminary results from the 3-year prospective Spanish Multicentre Centre (CODICE study). *Cerebrovascular Diseases* 21:1

Comu S, Verstraeten T, Rinkoff JS *et al.* (1996). Neurological manifestations of acute posterior multifocal placoid pigment epitheliopathy. *Stroke* 27:996–1001

Coull AJ, Lovett JK, Rothwell PM *et al.* (2004). Population based study of early risk of stroke after transient ischemic attack or minor stroke: Implications for public education and organisation of services. *British Medical Journal* 328:326

Cross SS (1991). How common is cholesterol embolism? *Journal of Clinical Pathology* 44:859–861

Davies-Jones GAB (1995). Neurological manifestations of hematological disorders. In *Neurology and General Medicine*, 2nd edn., Aminoff MJ (ed.), pp. 219–245. New York: Churchill Livingstone.

Davis JM, Zimmerman RA (1983). Injury of the carotid and vertebral arteries. *Neuroradiology* 25:55–69

Debette S, Compter A, Labeyrie MA *et al.* (2015). Epidemiology, pathophysiology, diagnosis, and management of intracranial artery dissection. *Lancet Neurology* 14:640–654

Delalande S, de Seze J, Fauchais AL *et al.* (2004). Neurologic manifestations in primary Sjögren syndrome: A study of 82 patients. *Medicine (Baltimore)* 83:280–291

Del Zotto E, Giossi A, Volonghi I *et al.* (2010). Ischemic stroke during pregnancy and puerperium. *Stroke Research and Treatment* 2011:606780

Desai B, Toole JF (1975). Kinks, coils and carotids: A review. *Stroke* 6:649–653

De Vries JJ, den Dunnen WF, Timmerman EA *et al.* (2006). Acute posterior multifocal placoid pigment epitheliopathy with cerebral vasculitis: A multisystem granulomatous disease. *Archives of Ophthalmology* 124:910–913

Diener HC, Weimar C, Katsarava Z (2005). Patent foramen ovale: Paradoxical connection to migraine and stroke. *Current Opinion in Neurology* 18:299–304

Dittrich R, Ritter MA, Kaps M *et al.* (2006). The use of embolic signal detection in multicenter trials to evaluate antiplatelet efficacy: Signal analysis and quality control mechanisms in the CARESS (Clopidogrel and Aspirin for Reduction of Emboli in Symptomatic carotid Stenosis) trial. *Stroke* 37:1065–1069

Dobyns WB, Garg BP (1991). Vascular abnormalities in epidermal nevus syndrome. *Neurology* 41:276–278

Donaghy M, Chang CL, Poulter N *et al.* (2002). European Collaborators of the World Health Organization Collaborative Study of Cardiovascular Disease and Steroid Hormone Contraception. Duration, frequency, recency, and type of migraine and the risk of ischemic stroke in women of childbearing age. *Journal of Neurology, Neurosurgery and Psychiatry* 73:747–750

Dutta M, Hanna E, Das P *et al.* (2006a). Incidence and prevention of ischemic stroke following myocardial infarction: Review of current literature. *Cerebrovascular Diseases* 22:331–339

Dutta M, Karas MG, Segal AZ *et al.* (2006b). Yield of transoesophageal echocardiography for nonbacterial thrombotic endocarditis and other cardiac sources of embolism in cancer patients with cerebral ischemia. *American Journal of Cardiology* 97:894–898

Ekinci EI, Donnan GA (2004). Neurological manifestations of cardiac myxoma: A review of the literature and report of cases. *Internal Medicine Journal* 34:243–249

el-Shami K, Griffiths E, Streiff M (2007). Nonbacterial thrombotic endocarditis in cancer

patients: pathogenesis, diagnosis, and treatment. *The Oncologist* 12:518–523

Farah S, Al-Shubaili A, Montaser A *et al.* (1998). Behçets syndrome: A report of 41 patients with emphasis on neurological manifestations. *Journal of Neurology, Neurosurgery and Psychiatry* 64:382–384

Feldmann E, Daneault N, Kwan E *et al.* (1990). Chinese–white differences in the distribution of occlusive cerebrovascular disease. *Neurology* 40:1541–1545

Ferro JM (1998). Vasculitis of the central nervous system. *Journal of Neurology* 245:766–776

Filimon AM, Negreanu L, Doca M *et al.* (2015). Cardiovascular involvement in inflammatory bowel disease: Dangerous liaisons. *World Journal of Gastroenterology* 21:9688–9692

Fisher CM (1979). Capsular infarcts: The underlying vascular lesions. *Archives of Neurology and Psychiatry* 36:65–73

Fisher CM, Caplan LR (1971). Basilar artery branch occlusion: A cause of pontine infarction. *Neurology* 21:900–905

Flis CM, Jager HR, Sidhu PS (2007). Carotid and vertebral artery dissections: Clinical aspects imaging features and endovascular treatment. *European Radiology* 17:820–834

Freyaldenhoven TE, Mrak RE, Rock L (2001). Fibrocartilaginous embolization. *Neurology* 56:1354

Furlan AJ, Reisman M, Massaro J *et al.* (2012). Closure or medical therapy for cryptogenic stroke with patent foramen ovale. *New England Journal of Medicine* 366:991–999

Futrell N (1995). Inflammatory vascular disorders: Diagnosis and treatment in ischemic stroke. *Current Opinions in Neurology* 8:55–61

Gan R, Sacco RL, Kargman DE *et al.* (1997). Testing the validity of the lacunar hypothesis: The Northern Manhattan Stroke Study experience. *Neurology* 48:1204–1211

García-Carrasco M, Mendoza-Pinto C, Cervera R (2014). Diagnosis and classification of Susac syndrome. *Autoimmunity Reviews* 13:347–350

Gautier JC, Durr A, Koussa S et al. (1991). Paradoxical cerebral embolism with a patent foramen ovale. A report of 29 patients. *Cerebrovascular Diseases* 1:193–202

Genta MS, Genta RM, Gabay C (2006). Systemic rheumatoid vasculitis: A review. *Seminars in Arthritis and Rheumatism* 36:88–98

Glass J (2006). Neurologic complications of lymphoma and leukemia. *Seminars in Oncology* 33:342–347

Goldschmidt-Clermont PJ, Creager MA, Lorsordo DW et al. (2005). Atherosclerosis 2005: Recent discoveries and novel hypotheses *Circulation* 112:3348–3353

Gorter JW for the Stroke Prevention in Reversible Ischemia Trial (SPIRIT) and the European Atrial Fibrillation Trial (EAFT) Study Groups (1999). Major bleeding during anticoagulation after cerebral ischemia: Patterns and risk factors. *Neurology* 53:1319–1327

Gotto AM Jr., (2005). Evolving concepts of dyslipidaemia, atherosclerosis and cardiovascular disease: The Louis F Bishop Lecture. *Journal of American College of Cardiology* 46:1219–1224

Grisold W, Oberndorfer S, Struhal W (2009). Stroke and cancer: A review. *Acta Neurologica Scandinavica* 119:1–16

Hankey GJ, Eikelboom JW, van Bockxmeer FM et al. (2001). Inherited thrombophilia in ischemic stroke and its pathogenic subtypes. *Stroke* 32:1793–1799

Harrison CN, Linch DC, Machin SJ (1998). Desirability and problems of early diagnosis of essential thrombocythemia. *Lancet* 351:846–847

Hart RG, Foster JW, Lutner MF et al. (1990). Stroke in infective endocarditis. *Stroke* 21:695–700

Heinzlef O, Cohen A, Amarenco P (1997). An update on aortic causes of ischemic stroke. *Current Opinions in Neurology* 10:64–72

Hender J, Harris DG, Bu H et al. (2006). Stroke in pregnancy. *British Journal of Hospital Medicine* 67:129–131

Heron E, Fornes P, Rance A et al. (1998). Brain involvement in scleroderma. Two autopsy cases. *Stroke* 29:719–721

Heye N, Hankey GJ (1996). Amphetamine-associated stroke. *Cerebrovascular Diseases* 6:149–155

Hietaharju A, Jantti V, Korpela M et al. (1993). Nervous system involvement in systemic lupus erythematus, Sjögren syndrome and scleroderma. *Acta Neurology Scandinavica* 88:299–308

Hilton DA, Footitt D (2003). Neuropathological findings in Sneddon's syndrome. *Neurology* 60:1181–1182

Hoekstra-van Dalen RAH, Cillessen JPM, Kappelle LJ et al. (1996). Cerebral infarcts associated with migraine: Clinical features, risk factors and follow up. *Journal of Neurology* 243:511–515

Hoffmann M, Corr P, Robbs J (2000). Cerebrovascular findings in Takayasu disease. *Journal of Neuroimaging* 10:84–90

Holmes DR Jr., (2004). Strokes and holes and headaches: Are they a package deal? *Lancet* 364:1840–1842

Homma S, Sacco RL (2005). Patent foramen ovale and stroke. *Circulation* 112:1063–1072

Howell SJL, Molyneux AJ (1988). Vertebrobasilar insufficiency in rheumatoid atlanto-axial subluxation: A case report with angiographic demonstration of left vertebral artery occlusion. *Journal of Neurology* 235:189–190

Hoyle JD, Jablonski C, Newton HB (2014). Neurosarcoidosis: Clinical review of a disorder with challenging inpatient presentations and diagnostic considerations. *Neurohospitalist* 4:94–101

Hsu KC, Wu YR, Lyu RK et al. (2006). Aseptic meningitis and ischemic stroke in relapsing polychondritis. *Clinical Rheumatology* 25:265–267

Hundsberger T, Cogliatti S, Kleger GR et al. (2011). Intravascular lymphoma mimicking cerebral stroke: Report of two cases. *Case Reports in Neurology* 3:278–283

Hwang J, Kim SJ, Bang OY *et al.* (2012). Ischemic stroke in Takaysu's arteritis: Lesion patterns and possible mechanisms. *Journal of Clinical Neurology* **8**:109–115

Inzitari D (2003). Leukoariaosis: An independent risk factor for stroke? *Stroke* **34**:2067–2071

Iwama T, Hashimoto N, Murai BN *et al.* (1997). Intracranial rebleeding in moyamoya disease. *Journal of Clinical Neuroscience* **4**:169–172

Jacobson DM, Terrence CF, Reinmuth OM (1986). The neurological manifestations of fat embolism. *Neurology* **36**:847–851

Jeanrenaud X, Kappenberger L (1991). Patent foramen ovale and stroke of unknown origin. *Cerebrovascular Diseases* **1**:184–192

Jennekens FG, Kater L (2002a). The central nervous system in systemic lupus erythematous. Part 1. Clinical syndromes: A literature investigation. *Rheumatology (Oxford)* **41**:605–618

Jennekens FG, Kater L (2002b). The central nervous system in systemic lups erythematosus. Part 2. Pathogenic mechanisms of clinical syndromes: a literature investigation. *Rheumatology (Oxford)* **41**:619–630

Jones EF, Kalman JM, Calafiore P *et al.* (1995). Proximal aortic atheroma. An independent risk factor for cerebral ischemia. *Stroke* **26**:218–224

Jones HR, Siekert RG (1989). Neurological manifestations of infective endocarditis: Review of clinical and therapeutic challenges. *Brain* **112**:1295–1315

Kalashnikova LA, Nasonov EL, Stoyanovich LZ *et al.* (1994). Sneddon's syndrome and the primary antiphospholipid syndrome. *Cerebrovascular Diseases* **4**:76–82

Kanter MC, Hart RG (1991). Neurologic complications of infective endocarditis. *Neurology* **41**:1015–1020

Kaposzta Z, Young E, Bath PMW *et al.* (1999). Clinical application of asymptomatic embolic signal detection in acute stroke: A prospective study. *Stroke* **30**:1814–1818

Katzav A, Chapman J, Shoenfeld Y (2003). CNS dysfunction in the antiphospholipid syndrome. *Lupus* **12**:903–907

Kent DM, Ruthazer R, Weimar C *et al.* (2013). An index to identify stroke-related vs. incidental patent foramen ovale in cryptogenic stroke. *Neurology* **81**:619–625

Keser G, Direskeneli H, Aksu K (2014). Management of Takayasu arteritis: A systematic review. *Rheumatology (Oxford)* **53**:793–801

Kent DM, Dahabreh IJ, Ruthazer R *et al.* (2016). Device closure of patent foramen ovale after stroke: Pooled analysis of completed randomized trials. *Journal of American College of Cardiology* **67**:907–917

Keung YK, Owen J (2004). Iron deficiency and thrombosis: Literature review. *Clinical and Applied Thrombolysis and Hemostasis* **10**:387–391

Kizer JR, Devereux RB (2005). Clinical practice. Patent foramen ovale in young adults with unexplained stroke. *New England Journal of Medicine* **353**:2361–2372

Koennecke H, Mast H, Trocio SH *et al.* (1998). Frequency and determinants of microembolic signals on transcranial Doppler in unselected patients with acute carotid territory ischemia. A prospective study. *Cerebrovascular Diseases* **8**:107–112

Kolodny E, Fellgiebel A, Hilz MJ *et al.* (2015). Cerebrovascular involvement in Fabry disease: current status of knowledge. *Stroke* **46**:302–313

Krapf H, Skalej M, Voigt K (1999). Subarachnoid hemorrhage due to septic embolic infarction in infective endocarditis. *Cerebrovascular Diseases* **9**:182–184

Krespi Y, Akman-Demir G, Poyraz M *et al.* (2001). Cerebral vasculitis and ischemic stroke in Behçet's disease: Report of one case and review of the literature. *European Journal of Neurology* **8**:719–722

Kurth T, Diener HC (2012). Migraine and stroke: Perspectives for stroke physicians. *Stroke* **43**:3421–3426

Kwa VIH, Franke CL, Verbeeten B *et al.* (1998). Silent intracerebral microhemorrhages in patients with ischemic stroke for the Amsterdam Vascular Medicine Group. *Annals of Neurology* **44**:372–377

Labovitz DL, Boden-Albala B, Hauser WA *et al.* (2007). Lacunar infarct or deep intracerebral hemorrhage: Who gets which? The Northern Manhattan Study. *Neurology* **68**:606–608

Lammie GA, Brannan F, Slattery J et al. (1997). Nonhypertensive cerebral small-vessel disease. An autopsy study. Stroke 28:2222–2229

Lamy C, Giannesini C, Zuber M et al. (2002). Clinical and imaging findings in cryptogenic stroke patients with and without patent foramen ovale: The PFO–ASA Study (Atrial Septal Aneurysm). Stroke 33:706–711

Lan SH, Chang WN, Lu CH et al. (2001). Cerebral infarction in chronic meningitis: A comparison of tuberculous meningitis and cryptococcal meningitis. Quarterly Journal of Medicine 94:247–253

Lefthériotis G, Omarjee L, Le Saux O et al. (2013). The vascular phenotype in pseudoxanthoma elasticum and related disorders: Contribution of a genetic disease to the understanding of vascular calcification. Frontiers in Genetics 4:4

Leung SY, Ng THK, Yuen ST et al. (1993). Pattern of cerebral atherosclerosis in Hong Kong Chinese: Severity in intracranial and extracranial vessels. Stroke 24:779–786

Leys D, Moulin Th, Stojkovic T et al. (1995). Follow-up of patients with history of cervical artery dissection. Cerebrovascular Diseases 5:43–49

Lhermitte F, Gautier JC, Derouesne C (1970). Nature of occlusions of the middle cerebral artery. Neurology 20:82–88

Li L, Schulz UG, Kuker W et al. (2015). Age-specific association of migraine with cryptogenic TIA and stroke: Population-based study. Neurology 85(17):1444–1451

Lisnevskaia L, Murphy G, Isenberg D (2014). Systemic lupus erythematosus. Lancet 384:1878–1888

Loh E, St John Sutton MS, Wun CC et al. (1997). Ventricular dysfunction and the risk of stroke after myocardial infarction. New England Journal of Medicine 336:251–257

Longo DL, Witherspoon JM (1980). Focal neurologic symptoms in hypercalcemia. Neurology 30:200–201

Lossos A, River Y, Eliakim A, Steiner I (1995). Neurologic aspects of inflammatory bowel disease. Neurology 45:416–421

Lovett JK, Gallagher PJ, Hands LJ et al. (2004). Histological correlates of carotid plaque surface morphology on lumen contrast imaging. Circulation 110:2190–2197

Lucivero V, Mezzapesa DM, Petruzzellis M et al. (2004). Ischemic stroke in progressive system sclerosis. Neurology Science 25:230–233

Ludvigsson JF, West J, Card T et al. (2012). Risk of stroke in 28000 patients with celiac disease: A nationwide cohort study in Sweden. Journal of Stroke and Cerebrovascular Diseases 21:860–867

Macleod MR, Amarenco P, Davis SM et al. (2004). Atheroma of the aortic arch: An important and poorly recognized factor in the aetiology of stroke. Lancet Neurology 3:408–414

Malouf R, Brust JCM (1985). Hypoglycemia: Causes, neurological manifestations and outcome. Annals of Neurology 17:421–430

Marchioli R, Finazzi G, Landolfi R et al. (2015). Vascular and neoplastic risk in a large cohort of patients with polycythemia vera. Journal of Clinical Oncology 23:2224–2232

Markus HS (2006). Can microemboli on transcranial Doppler identify patients at increased stroke risk? Nature Clinical Practice in Cardiovascular Medicine 3:246–247

Markus HS, Hambley H (1998). Neurology and the blood: Hematological abnormalities in ischemic stroke. Journal of Neurology, Neurosurgery and Psychiatry 64:150–159

Martin R, Bogousslavsky J for the Lausanne Stroke Registry Group (1993). Mechanisms of late stroke after myocardial infarct: The Lausanne Stroke Registry. Journal of Neurology, Neurosurgery and Psychiatry 56:760–764

Martínez-Fernádez E, Gil-Peralta A, García-Lozano R et al. (2001). Mitochondrial disease and stroke. Stroke 32:2507–2510

Mas JL (2003). Specifics of patent foramen ovale. Advances in Neurology 92:197–202

Mas JL, Arquizan C, Lamy C et al. (2001). Patent Foramen Ovale and Atrial Septal Aneurysm Study Group. Recurrent cerebrovascular events associated with patent foramen ovale atrial septal aneurysm or both. New England Journal of Medicine 345:1740–1746

Mas JL, Derumeaux G, Guillon B et al. (2017). Patent foramen ovale closure or anticoagulation vs. antiplatelets after stroke. New England Journal of Medicine 377:1011–1021

Masuda J, Yutani C, Waki R et al. (1992). Histopathological analysis of the mechanisms of intracranial haemorrhage complicating infective endocarditis. Stroke 23:843–850

Matijevic N, Wu K (2006). Hypercoagulable states and strokes. Current Atherosclerosis Reports 8:324–329

Meier B, Kalesan B, Mattle HP et al. (2013). Percutaneous closure of patent foramen ovale in cryptogenic stroke. New England Journal of Medicine 368:1083–1091

Merrill JT (2007). Antiphospholipid syndrome: What's new in understanding antiphospholipid antibody-related stroke? Current Rheumatology Reports 8:159–161

Messe SR, Cucchiara B, Luciano J et al. (2005). PFO management: Neurologists vs cardiologists. Neurology 65:172–173

Metz H, Murray-Leslie RM, Bannister RG et al. (1961). Kinking of the internal carotid artery. Lancet i:424–426

Millikan C, Futrell N (1990). The fallacy of the lacune hypothesis. Stroke 21:1251–1257

Mitchell JRA, Schwartz CJ (1962). Relationship between arterial disease in different sites. A study of the aorta and coronary carotid and iliac arteries. British Medical Journal i:1293–1301

Mitsias P, Levine SR (1994). Large cerebral vessel occlusive disease in systemic lupus erythematosus. Neurology 44:385–393

Molloy J, Markus HS (1999). Asymptomatic embolization predicts stroke and TIA risk in patients with carotid artery stenosis. Stroke 30:1440–1443

Morris JG, Singh S, Fisher M (2010). Testing for inherited thrombophilias in arterial stroke: Can it cause more harm than good? Stroke 41:2985–2990

Morris NA, Merkler AE, Gialdini G et al. (2017). Timing of incident stroke risk after cervical artery dissection presenting without ischaemia. Stroke 48:551–555

Mumford CJ, Fletcher NA, Ironside JW et al. (1996). Progressive ataxia, focal seizures and malabsorption syndrome in a 41 year old woman. Journal of Neurology, Neurosurgery and Psychiatry 60:225–230

Munoz DG (2006). Leukoaraiosis and ischemia: Beyond the myth. Stroke 37:1348–1349

Muratore F, Kermani TA, Crowson CS et al. (2015). Large-vessel giant cell arteritis: A cohort study. Rheumatology 54:463–470

Naylor AR, Cuffe RL, Rothwell PM et al. (2003a). A systematic review of outcomes following staged and synchronous carotid endarterectomy and coronary artery bypass. European Journal of Vascular Endovascular Surgery 25:380–389

Naylor R, Cuffe RL, Rothwell PM et al. (2003b). A systematic review of outcome following synchronous carotid endarterectomy and coronary artery bypass: Influence of surgical and patient variables. European Journal of Vascular Endovascular Surgery 26:230–241

Neimann J, Haapaniemi HM, Hillbom M (2000). Neurological complications of drug abuse: Pathophysiological mechanisms. European Journal of Neurology 7:595–606

Newman MF, Matthew JP, Grocott HP et al. (2006). Central nervous system injury associated with cardiac surgery. Lancet 368:694–703

North KN, Whiteman DAH, Pepin MG et al. (1995). Cerebrovascular complications in Ehlers–Danlos syndrome type IV. Annals of Neurology 38:960–964

O'Connell BK, Towfighi J, Brennan RW et al. (1985). Dissecting aneurysms of head and neck. Neurology 35:993–997

O'Connor AD, Rusyniak DE, Bruno A (2005). Cerebrovascular and cardiovascular complications of alcohol and sympathomimetic drug abuse. Medical Clinics of North America 89:1343–1358

O'Connor MM, Mayberg MR (2000). Effects of radiation on cerebral vasculature: A review. Neurosurgery 46:138–149

Ogata J, Masuda J, Yutani C et al. (1994). Mechanisms of cerebral artery thrombosis: A histopathological analysis on eight necropsy cases. Journal of Neurology, Neurosurgery and Psychiatry 57:17–21

Ogata J, Yonemura K, Kimura K et al. (2005). Cerebral infarction associated with essential thrombocythemia: An autopsy case study. Cerebrovascular Diseases 19:201–205

Olin JW, Gornik HL, Bacharach JM *et al.* (2014). Fibromuscular dysplasia: State of the science and critical unanswered questions. A scientific statement from the American Heart Association. *Circulation* 129:1048–1078

Orencia AJ, Petty GW, Khandheria BK *et al.* (1995a). Risk of stroke with mitral valve prolapse in population-based cohort study. *Stroke* 26:7–13

Orencia AJ, Petty GW, Khandheria BK, Fallon WM, Whishant JP (1995b). Mitral valve prolapse and the risk of stroke after initial cerebral ischemia. *Neurology* 45:1083–1086

Ovchinnikov NA, Rao RT, Rao SR (2007). Unilateral congenital elongation of the cervical part of the internal carotid artery with kinking and looping: Two case reports and review of the literature. *Head & Face Medicine* 3:29

Pantoni L, Garcia JH (1997). Pathogenesis of leukoariaosis. A review. *Stroke* 28:652–659

Parizel PM, Demey HE, Veeckmans G *et al.* (2001). Early diagnosis of cerebral fat embolism by diffusion-weighted MRI. *Stroke* 32:2942–2944

Plummer C, Henderson RD, O'Sullivan JD *et al.* (2011). Ischemic stroke and transient ischemic attack after head and neck radiotherapy: A review. *Stroke* 42:2140–2418

Pósfai F., Marton I, Szöke A *et al.* (2014). Stroke in essential thrombocythemia. *Journal of the Neurological Sciences* 336:260–262

Powers WJ (1986). Should lumbar puncture be part of the routine evaluation of patients with cerebral ischemia? *Stroke* 17:332–333

Prior AL, Wilson LA, Gosling RG *et al.* (1979). Retrograde cerebral embolism. *Lancet* ii:1044–1047

Puéchal X and Fiessinger JN (2007). Thromboangiitis obliterans or Buerger's disease: challenges for the rheumatologist. *Rheumatology (Oxford)* 46:192–199

Razvi SS, Bone I (2006). Single gene disorders causing ischemic stroke. *Journal of Neurology* 253:685–700

Redgrave JN, Lovett JK, Gallagher PJ *et al.* (2006). Histological assessment of 526 symptomatic carotid plaques in relation to the nature and timing of ischemic symptoms:

The Oxford Plaque Study. *Circulation* 113:2320–2328

Reichart MD, Bogousslavsky J, Janzer RC (2000). Early lacunar strokes complicating polyarteritis nodosa: Thrombotic microangiopathy. *Neurology* 54:883–889

Rhodes (1996). Cholesterol crystal embolism: An important "new" diagnosis for the general physician. *Lancet* 347:1641

Rogers LR (2003). Cerebrovascular complications in cancer patients. *Neurologic Clinics* 21:167–192

Roldan CA, Shively BK, Crawford MH (1996). An echocardiographic study of valvular heart disease associated with systematic lupus erythematosus. *New England Journal of Medicine* 335:1424–1430

Rolfs A, Bottcher T, Zschiesche M *et al.* (2005). Prevalence of Fabry disease in patients with cryptogenic stroke: A prospective study. *Lancet* 366:1794–1796

Ronthal M, Gonzalez RG, Smith RN *et al.* (2003). Case records of the Massachusetts General Hospital. Weekly clinicopathological exercises. Case 21–2003. A 72 year old man with repetitive strokes in the posterior circulation. *New England Journal of Medicine* 349:170–180

Rosen Y. (2015). Four decades of necrotizing sarcoid granulomatosis. *Archives of Pathology & Laboratory Medicine* 139:252–262

Ross R (1999). Atherosclerosis: An inflammatory disease. *New England Journal of Medicine* 340:115–126

Rothwell PM (2001). The inter-relation between carotid, femoral and coronary artery disease. *European Heart Journal* 22:11–14

Rothwell PM, Warlow CP (2005). Timing of TIAs preceding stroke: Time window for prevention is very short. *Neurology* 64:817–820

Rothwell PM, Gibson R, Warlow CP (2000a). The inter-relation between plaque surface morphology, degree of stenosis and the risk of ischemic stroke in patients with symptomatic carotid stenosis. *Stroke* 31:615–621

Rothwell PM, Villagra R, Gibson R *et al.* (2000b). Evidence of a chronic systemic cause of instability of atherosclerotic plaques. *Lancet* 355:19–24

Rubba P, Mercuri M, Faccenda F *et al.* (1994). Premature carotid atherosclerosis: Does it occur in both familial hypercholesterolemia and homocystinuria? Ultrasound assessment of arterial intima-media thickness and blood flow velocity. *Stroke* **25**:943–950

Rubinstein SM, Peerdeman SM, van Tulder MW *et al.* (2005). A systematic review of the risk factors for cervical artery dissection. *Stroke* **36**:1575–1580

Ruby RJ, Burton JR (1977). Acute reversible hemiparesis and hyponatremia. *Lancet* **i**:1212

Ruiz-Irastorza G, Crowther M, Branch W *et al.* (2010). Antiphospholipid syndrome. *Lancet* **376**:1498–1509

Ruttmann E, Willeit J, Ulmer H *et al.* (2006). Neurological outcome of septic cardioembolic stroke after infective endocarditis. *Stroke* **37**:2094–2099

Sabolek M, Bachus-Banaschak K, Bachus R *et al.* (2005). Multiple cerebral aneurysms as delayed complication of left cardiac myxoma: A case report and review. *Acta Neurology Scandinavica* **111**:345–350

Sacco RL, Kargman DE, Gu Q *et al.* (1995). Race-ethnicity and determinants of intracranial atherosclerotic cerebral infarction. The Northern Manhattan Stroke Study. *Stroke* **26**:14–20

Salgado AV (1991). Central nervous system complications of infective endocarditis. *Stroke* **22**:1461–1463

Samuelsson M, Lindell D, Norrving B (1996). Presumed pathogenetic mechanisms of recurrent stroke after lacunar infarction. *Cerebrovascular Diseases* **6**:128–136

Sanna G, Bertolaccini ML, Hughes GR (2005). Hughes syndrome the antiphospholipid syndrome: A new chapter in neurology. *Annals of the New York Academy of Sciences* **1051**:465–486

Sarkari NBS, Holmes JM, Bickerstaff ER (1970). Neurological manifestations associated with internal carotid loops and kinks in children. *Journal of Neurology, Neurosurgery and Psychiatry* **33**:194–200

Savage COS, Harper L, Adu D (1997). Primary systemic vasculitis. *Lancet* **349**:553–558

Schapira AH (2012). Mitochondrial diseases. *Lancet* **379**:1825–1834

Schievink WI (2001). Spontaneous dissection of the carotid and vertebral arteries. *New England Journal of Medicine* **344**:898–906

Schimke RN, McKusick VA, Huang T *et al.* (1965). Homocystinuria Studies of 20 families with 38 affected members. *Journal of the American Medical Association* **193**:711–719

Schulz UGR, Rothwell PM (2003). Differences in vascular risk factors between aetiological subtypes of ischemic stroke in population-based incidence studies. *Stroke* **34**:2050–2059

Scott RM and Smith ER (2009). Moyamoya disease and moyamoya syndrome. *New England Journal of Medicine* **360**:1226–1237

Seko Y (2007). Giant cell and Takayasu arteritis. *Current Opinions in Rheumatology* **19**:39–43

Selim M (2007). Perioperative stroke. *New England Journal of Medicine* **356**:706–713

Selim MH, Molina CA (2013). The use of tissue plasminogen-activator in pregnancy: A taboo treatment or a time to think out of the box. *Stroke* **44**:868–869

Sempere AP, Duarte J, Cabezas C *et al.* (1998). Aetiopathogenesis of transient ischemic attacks and minor ischemic strokes: A community-based study in Segovia, Spain. *Stroke* **29**:40–45

Seneviratne K, Tam K, Jayatunga A *et al.* (2009). A rare case of a carotid loop anomaly. *BMJ Case Reports* pii:bcr07.2008.0362

Service FJ (1995). Hypoglycemic disorders. *New England Journal of Medicine* **332**:1144–1152

Shanmugam V, Zimnowodzki S, Curtin J *et al.* (1997). Hypoglycemic hemiplegia: Insulinoma masquerading as stroke. *Journal of Stroke and Cerebrovascular Diseases* **6**:368–369

Sims K, Politei J, Banikazemi M *et al.* (2009). Stroke in Fabry disease frequently occurs before diagnosis and in the absence of other clinical events. *Stroke* **40**:788–794

Siva A, Altintas A, Saip S (2004). Behçet's syndrome and the nervous system. *Current Opinions in Neurology* **17**:347–357

Søndergaard L, Kasner SE, Rhodes JF *et al.* (2017). Patent foramen ovale closure or antiplatelet therapy for cryptogenic stroke. *New England Journal of Medicine* **377**:1033–1042

Sotrel A, Lacson AG, Huff KR (1983). Childhood Kohlmeier–Degos disease with atypical skin lesions. *Neurology* **33**:1146–1151

Spivak JL (2010). Narrative review: Thrombocytosis, polycythemia vera, and JAK2 mutations: The phenotypic mimicry of chronic myeloproliferaration. *Annals of Internal Medicine* **152**:300–306

Stewart SS, Ashizawa T, Dudley AW *et al.* (1988). Cerebral vasculitis in relapsing polychondritis. *Neurology* **38**:150–152

Stockhammer G, Felber SR, Zelger B *et al.* (1993). Sneddon's syndrome: Diagnosis by skin biopsy and MRI in 17 patients. *Stroke* **24**:685–690

Sturzenegger M, Mattle HP, Rivoir A *et al.* (1993). Ultrasound findings in spontaneous extracranial vertebral artery dissection. *Stroke* **24**:1910–1921

Sturzenegger M, Mattle HP, Rivoir A *et al.* (1995). Ultrasound findings in carotid artery dissection: Analysis of 43 patients. *Neurology* **45**:691–698

Subbiah P, Wijdicks E, Muenter M *et al.* (1996). Skin lesion with a fatal neurologic outcome (Degos' disease). *Neurology* **46**:636–640

Switzer JA, Hess DC, Nichols FT *et al.* (2006). Pathophysiology and treatment of stroke in sickle-cell disease: Present and future. *Lancet Neurology* **5**:501–512

Talahma M, Strbian D, Sundararajan S (2014). Sickle cell disease and stroke. *Stroke* **45**:e98–e100

Tate J, Bushnell C (2011). Pregnancy and stroke risk in women. *Womens Health (Lond Engl)* **7**:363–374

Tatlisumak T, Fisher M (1996). Hematologic disorders associated with ischemic stroke. *Journal of the Neurological Sciences* **140**:1–11

Tegeler CH, Shi F, Morgan T (1991). Carotid stenosis in lacunar stroke. *Stroke* **22**:1124–1128

Testai FD, Gorelick PB (2010). Inherited metabolic disorders and stroke part 2: Homocystinuria, organic acidurias, and urea cycle disorders. *JAMA Neurology* **67**:148–153

Tietjen GE (2005). The risk of stroke in patients with migraine and implications for migraine management. *CNS Drugs* **19**:683–692

van der Meulen JH, Weststrate W, van Gijn J *et al.* (1992). Is cerebral angiography indicated in infective endocarditis? *Stroke* **23**:1662–1667

Vidailhet M, Piette JC, Wechsler B *et al.* (1990). Cerebral venous thrombosis in systemic lupus erythematosus. *Stroke* **21**:1226–1231

Viles-Gonzalez JF, Fuster V, Badimon JJ (2004). Atherothrombosis: A widespread disease with unpredictable and life-threatening consequences. *European Heart Journal* **25**:1197–1207

Visy JM, Le Coz P, Chadefaux B *et al.* (1991). Homocystinuria due to 5,10-methylenetetrahydrofolate reductase deficiency revealed by stroke in adult siblings. *Neurology* **41**:1313–1315

Vongpatanasin W, Hillis LD, Lange RA (1996). Prosthetic heart valves. *New England Journal of Medicine* **335**:407–416

Wallis WE, Donaldson I, Scott RS *et al.* (1985). Hypoglycemia masquerading as cerebrovascular disease (hypoglycemic hemiplegia). *Annals of Neurology* **18**:510–512

Wen PY, Feske SK, Teoh SK *et al.* (1997). Cerebral haemorrhage in a patient taking fenfluramine and phentermine for obesity. *Neurology* **49**:632–633

Westover AN, McBride S, Haley RW. (2007). Stroke in young adults who abuse amphetamines or cocaine: A population-based study of hospitalized patients. *Archives of General Psychiatry* **64**:495–502

White H, Boden-Albala B, Wang C *et al.* (2005). Ischemic stroke subtype incidence among whites, blacks and Hispanics: The Northern Manhattan Study. *Circulation* **111**:1327–1331

Wityk RJ, Lehman D, Klag M *et al.* (1996). Race and sex differences in the distribution of cerebral atherosclerosis. *Stroke* **27**:1974–1980

Wityk RJ, Zanferrari C, Oppenheimer S (2002). Neurovascular complications of Marfan syndrome: A retrospective, hospital-based study *Stroke* **33**:680–684

Wolff V, Armspach JP, Lauer V *et al.* (2013). Cannabis-related stroke: Myth or reality? *Stroke* **44**:558–563

Yaghi S, Pilot M, Song C *et al.* (2015). Ischemic stroke risk after acute coronary syndrome. *Journal of the American Heart Association* 5: e002590

Zuckerman D, Selim R, Hochberg E (2006). Intravascular lymphoma: The oncologist's "great imitator." *Oncologist* 11:496–502

Causes of Spontaneous Intracranial Hemorrhage

The causes of spontaneous intracerebral hemorrhage are sometimes, but not always, different from those of TIA and ischemic stroke. Spontaneous intracranial hemorrhage may be classified as:

- primary intracerebral hemorrhage: bleeding within the brain substance.
- cerebral microbleeds.
- intraventricular hemorrhage.
- subdural hemorrhage.
- subarachnoid hemorrhage (Chapter 30).

It is often difficult to establish the underlying cause of a spontaneous intracranial hemorrhage. The exact site of origin of bleeding may be unclear: a saccular aneurysm may rupture into the brain as well as into the subarachnoid space, or disruption of a small perforating artery may cause intraventricular hemorrhage as well as a basal ganglia hematoma. Even at autopsy there may be uncertainty because the source of the hemorrhage may have been destroyed. The site of bleeding may give some information as to the likely underlying cause (see later) since the relative frequency of the various pathologies causing intracranial hemorrhage varies by site. However, most parts of the brain may be affected by any of the causes listed in Box 7.1.

Primary Intracerebral Hemorrhage

Primary intracerebral hemorrhage is more common than subarachnoid hemorrhage, and its incidence increases with age (see Fig. 1.1). It is more frequent in Southeast Asian, Japanese, and Chinese populations than in Whites. The most common causes are intracranial small vessel disease, which is associated with hypertension, cerebral amyloid angiopathy (CAA), and intracranial vascular malformations (Qureshi *et al.* 2009). Rarer causes include saccular aneurysms, hemostatic defects (particularly those induced by anticoagulation or therapeutic thrombolysis), antiplatelet drugs, infective endocarditis, cerebral vasculitis, and recreational drug use (Neiman *et al.* 2000; O'Connor *et al.* 2005).

The site of primary intracerebral hemorrhage provides information as to the cause: "hypertensive" hemorrhages (Fig. 7.1a) tend to occur in the basal ganglia, thalamus, and pons, while lobar hemorrhages are more often caused by CAA, vascular malformations, and hemostatic failure (Qureshi *et al.* 2009) (Table 7.1) (Fig. 7.1b and Fig. 7.1c). Multiple hemorrhages suggest certain specific causes:

- cerebral amyloid angiopathy.
- metastatic tumor.
- hemostatic defect.

BOX 7.1 Causes of Spontaneous Intracranial Hemorrhage

Hypertension

Cerebral amyloid angiopathy

Intracranial vascular malformations: arteriovenous, venous, cavernous, telangiectasis

Tumors: melanoma, choriocarcinoma, malignant astrocytoma, oligodendroglioma, medulloblastoma, hemangioblastoma, choroid plexus papilloma, renal cell carcinoma, endometrial carcinoma, bronchogenic carcinoma

Hemostatic failure: hemophilia and other coagulation disorders, anticoagulation therapy, thrombolysis, antiplatelet drugs, disseminated intravascular coagulation, thrombocytopenia, thrombotic thrombocytopenic purpura, polycythemia rubra vera, essential thrombocythemia, paraproteinemias, renal failure, liver failure, snake bite

Aneurysms: saccular, atheromatous, mycotic, myxomatous, dissecting

Inflammatory vascular disease

Hemorrhagic transformation of cerebral infarction, venous more often than arterial

Intracranial venous thrombosis (Chapter 29)

Recreational drugs (Chapter 6)

Infections: infective endocarditis, herpes simplex, leptospirosis, anthrax

Sickle cell disease

Moyamoya syndrome (Chapter 6)

Carotid endarterectomy (Chapter 25)

Intracranial surgery

Alcohol

Wernicke's encephalopathy

Chronic meningitis

- thrombolytic drugs.
- multiple hemorrhagic infarcts (usually embolic from the heart).
- intracranial venous thrombosis.
- inflammatory vascular disease.
- intracranial vascular malformations.
- malignant hypertension.
- eclampsia.
- recreational drug use.

Rarely, primary intracerebral hemorrhage is familial.

The hematoma continues to expand after stroke onset and, in ~30% of patients, causes further neurological deficits (Leira *et al.* 2004; Qureshi *et al.* 2009). Some brainstem hemorrhages evolve subacutely, particularly those caused by a vascular malformation (O'Laoire *et al.* 1982; Howard 1986). Any large hematoma may cause brain shift, transtentorial herniation, brainstem compression, and raised intracranial pressure. Hematomas in the posterior fossa are particularly likely to cause obstructive hydrocephalus. Rupture into the ventricles or onto the surface of the brain is common, causing blood to appear in the subarachnoid space.

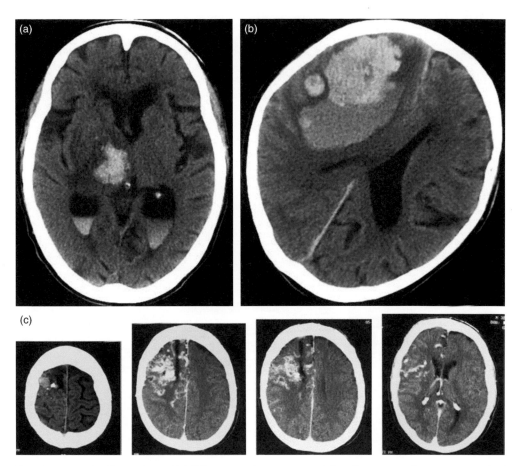

Fig. 7.1 Intracerebral hemorrhage. (a) A CT brain scan showing a typical deep "hypertensive" primary intracerebral hemorrhage at the right thalamus complicated by intraventricular hemorrhage (b) A CT scan showing two lobar primary intracerebral hemorrhages at the right frontal lobe with midline shift, likely due to underlying cerebral amyloid angiopathy (c) These CT brain scans show a right frontal arteriovenous malformation causing hemorrhage.

Cerebral Microbleeds

Cerebral microbleeds are small, perivascular deposits of hemosiderin-laden macrophages that are the result of blood leakage from pathologically fragile small vessels affected by hypertensive or cerebral amyloid angiopathy (Cordonnier *et al.* 2007; Shoamanesh *et al.* 2011; Fisher 2014; van Veluw *et al.* 2016). They can also be secondary to an ischemic insult (Fisher 2014; van Veluw *et al.* 2016). Cerebral microbleeds can be detected using hemosiderin-sensitive sequences on MRI, such as T2* gradient recalled echo (GRE) or susceptibility weighted imaging (SWI), and serve as a neuroimaging biomarker of underlying small vessel disease (Greenberg *et al.* 2009) (Figs. 7.2 and 7.3).

Cerebral microbleeds are seen frequently in patients with primary intracerebral hemorrhage, less commonly in patients with ischemic stroke, and rarely in "healthy controls" (Cordonnier *et al.* 2007; Lovelock *et al.* 2010). Risk factors for cerebral microbleeds include hypertension, increasing age, diabetes, CAA, and, less commonly, cerebral autosomal

Table 7.1 Structural causes of primary intracerebral hemorrhage according to location and patient age, listed according to relative frequency (hematological causes excluded)

Patient age	Anterior hemorrhage		Posterior hemorrhage
	Deep	Lobar	
Younger (< 50 years)	AVM	AVM	AVM
	Cavernous malformations	Cavernous malformations	Hypertension
	Hypertension	Tumor	Tumor
	Tumor		
Older (≥ 50 years)	Hypertension	CAA	Hypertension
	CAA	Hypertension	CAA
	Tumor	Tumor	Tumor

Notes: CAA, cerebral amyloid angiopathy; AVM, arteriovenous malformation.

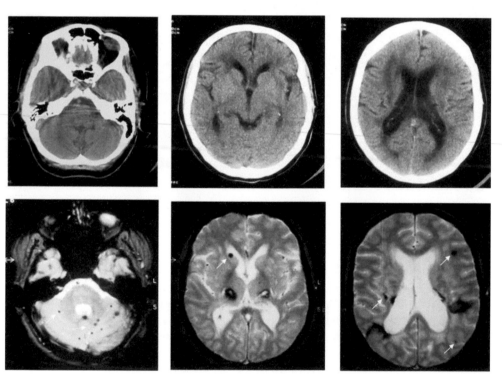

Fig. 7.2 Brain CT scans (top) from a patient with cerebral amyloid angiopathy showing only leukoaraiosis, whereas gradient echo MRI performed on the same day (bottom) shows evidence of several previous intracerebral hemorrhages, multiple microbleeds (arrows), and cortical superficial siderosis.

(a)

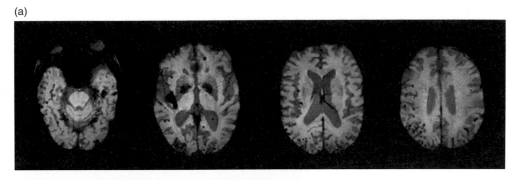

(b)

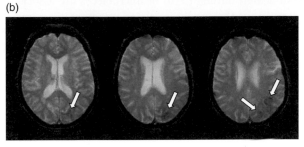

Fig 7.3 Hemosiderin sensitive MRI sequences showing (a) multiple lobar microbleeds and (b) cortical superficial siderosis in patients with cerebral amyloid angiopathy

dominant arteriopathy with silent infarcts and leukoaraiosis (CADASIL) (Cordonnier *et al.* 2007; Lau *et al.* 2017). Prior use of antiplatelet agents or warfarin, particularly in those with a high variability of INR, also appears to be a risk factor of microbleeds (Lovelock *et al.* 2010; Naka *et al.* 2013; Akoudad *et al.* 2014).

The location of microbleeds predicts the underlying type of small vessel disease. Patients with deep (e.g., basal ganglia, thalamus, internal capsule) with or without lobar microbleeds are suggestive of underlying hypertensive angiopathy, while microbleeds that are strictly lobar in location are highly specific for CAA (see following section on CAA) (Kidwell and Wintermark 2008).

In patients with TIA/ischemic stroke, presence of microbleeds is associated with a six-fold increased risk of intracerebral hemorrhage (Wilson *et al.* 2016; Lau *et al.* 2017). The risk of ICH increases steeply with burden of microbleeds, such that in those with ≥ 5 micro-bleeds, risk of ICH is twelvefold compared to those without microbleeds (Wilson *et al.* 2016; Lau *et al.* 2017). In contrast, risk of recurrent ischemic stroke in patients with a high microbleed burden is more modest (2.5-fold increase risk in patients with ≥ 5 microbleeds versus those without) (Wilson *et al.* 2016; Lau *et al.* 2017).

Furthermore, among TIA/ischemic stroke patients with a high burden of microbleeds who are on antiplatelet agents, risk of recurrent stroke appears to be time-dependent, such that within the first year after TIA/ischemic stroke, risk of ischemic stroke and coronary events outweighs the risks of intra- and extracranial bleeds (11.7% versus 3.7%; Lau *et al.* unpublished). However, this ratio appears to change over time, with risk of hemorrhage matching that of ischemic events after 1 year (11.0% versus 10.5%) (Lau *et al.* unpublished).

Withholding antiplatelet drugs during the first year after TIA/ischemic stroke based on microbleed burden may therefore likely be inappropriate. However, the risk of intracerebral hemorrhage is likely to outweigh any benefit thereafter, especially as antiplatelet-associated intracerebral hemorrhage is associated with substantial disability and mortality, and trials of gradual antiplatelet withdrawal in antiplatelet users with a high microbleed burden are justified (Lau *et al.* unpublished).

In ischemic stroke patients with atrial fibrillation on oral anticoagulants, presence of ≥ 5 microbleeds is associated with a pooled annual intracerebral hemorrhage incidence of 2.48% (compared with 0.3% in microbleed-negative patients and 0.81% in microbleed-positive patients) (Charidimou *et al.* 2017). Microbleed presence, especially if ≥ 5, may therefore help with risk stratification and guide anticoagulation decisions (Charidimou *et al.* 2017a). Similarly, ischemic stroke patients with a high burden (>10) of microbleeds are associated with a twelvefold increased risk of intravenous thrombolysis-related symptomatic intracerebral hemorrhage compared with patients with less than 10 microbleeds (Tsivgoulis *et al.* 2016). Benefits and risks of intravenous thrombolysis would therefore need to be carefully balanced in ischemic stroke patients with a known high burden of microbleeds.

Patients with a lobar intracerebral hemorrhage and presence of lobar microbleeds are suggestive of a probable diagnosis of CAA (see Box 7.2 and following section on CAA). Antiplatelet agents and warfarin should be avoided in these situations unless a compelling indication is present.

Primary Intraventricular Hemorrhage

Primary intraventricular hemorrhage is very unusual, except in premature babies. In adults, predisposing causes include hypertension, arterio-venous malformations, Moyamoya disease, lenticulostriate artery aneurysm, arterial dissections, and dural arteriovenous fistulas (Gates *et al.* 1986; Darby *et al.* 1988; Srivastava *et al.* 2014). The clinical features may be indistinguishable from subarachnoid hemorrhage, and it may only be differentiated at autopsy.

Subdural Hemorrhage

Subdural hemorrhage is usually traumatic rather than spontaneous, although the trauma can be very mild or forgotten in elderly patients and alcoholics. Spontaneous causes of subdural hemorrhage include:

- rupture of a vascular malformation in the dura.
- rupture of a peripheral aneurysm, mycotic more likely than saccular.
- a hemostatic defect, particularly therapeutic anticoagulation.
- a superficial cerebral tumor.
- rarely lumbar puncture or spontaneous intracranial hypotension.

Often no cause is found. Acute subdural hemorrhage appears hyperdense on CT brain scan, whereas chronic subdural hematomas appear hypodense (Fig. 7.4). Hematomas of intermediate age, approximately 4 to 6 weeks, are often isodense to gray matter on CT (Fig. 7.4b) and may be overlooked.

Hypertension

Hypertension causes thickening and disruption of the walls of the small arteries that perforate the base of the brain, particularly the lenticulostriate arteries in the region of the

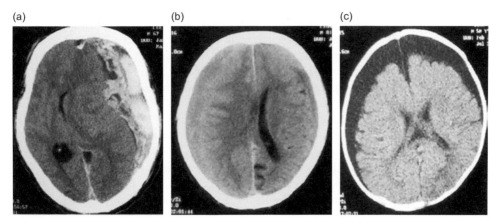

Fig. 7.4 Brain CT scans showing an acute hyperdense left subdural hematoma with mass effect (a), subacute bilateral isodense subdural hematomas (b), and chronic bilateral hypodense subdural hematomas (c).

basal ganglia (Chapter 6). Rupture of these abnormal vessels is thought to cause hypertensive primary intracerebral hemorrhage, although it is almost impossible to prove a cause-and-effect relationship in individuals because the hemorrhage destroys the exact site of the bleeding (Takebayashi and Kaneko 1983). In practice, the clinical diagnosis of "hypertensive" primary intracerebral hemorrhage is based on the lack of any alternative explanation in a patient known to have had hypertension or who clearly has evidence of hypertensive organ damage. Hypertensive intracerebral hemorrhages are often deep-seated (basal ganglia and thalamus most common), and deep (with or without lobar) microbleeds may also be present on MRI scanning, which would be supportive of a hypertension-related hemorrhage. It is also likely that other factors, such as cerebral amyloid angiopathy, may interact with hypertension to cause primary intracerebral hemorrhage in a particular individual.

Cerebral Amyloid Angiopathy

Cerebral amyloid angiopathy (CAA) is an organ-specific form of amyloid-ß protein deposition (Aß40) in small and medium-sized arteries, and less commonly capillaries, of the cerebral cortex and leptomeninges (Attems *et al.* 2011). The majority of cases are sporadic and affect the elderly (Charidimou *et al.* 2012). Hereditary forms of CAA also exist (Chapter 3), and several genetic mutations have been associated with the development of CAA including those affecting the amyloid-ß protein precursor, presenilin, and cystatin C genes (Yamada 2015).

Population-based autopsy studies have shown that CAA is present in 20–40% of elderly without dementia and up to 60% of those with dementia (Charidimou *et al.* 2012). Among patients with Alzheimer's disease, CAA is present in more than 90% of cases – most cases have a mild form of CAA, but severe forms are found in ~25% of cases (Ellis *et al.* 1996; Charidimou *et al.* 2012). Individuals with polymorphisms affecting the apolipoprotein E (apoE) gene, in particular ε2 and ε4, are more likely to develop CAA as well as CAA-related lobar intracerebral hemorrhage (Biffi *et al.* 2011; Verghese *et al.* 2011; Charidimou *et al.* 2012). Those with both ε2 and ε4 alleles are at highest risk of early CAA and intracerebral hemorrhage as ε4 and ε2 works synergistically by promoting amyloid-ß deposition and inducing structural changes in amyloid laden vessels, allowing them to be prone to rupture (Greenberg *et al.* 1998; Walker *et al.* 2000; Charidimou *et al.* 2012).

Individuals with CAA often presents with multiple, recurrent lobar hemorrhages (Charidimou *et al.* 2012). Approximately 15% of patients also present with transient focal neurological episodes (also known as amyloid spells) in the form of recurrent, stereotyped, and short-lasting positive (spreading paresthesias, visual phenomena, or limb jerking) or negative symptoms (sudden-onset limb weakness, dysphasia, or visual loss) (Charidimou *et al.* 2013). Cognitive impairment is also common as a result of vascular amyloid deposition leading to cortical atrophy (Fotiadis *et al.* 2016). Domains in memory, executive function, and processing speed are most frequently affected (Case *et al.* 2016). In a minority of patients with CAA, especially those with apoE ε4/ε4 polymorphisms, amyloid-ß within the vessel wall may trigger an intense inflammatory reaction, and patients may present with neuropsychiatric symptoms, seizures, headache, and focal neurological deficits (Moussaddy *et al.* 2015).

Diagnosis of CAA-related intracerebral hemorrhage is based on the classic and modified Boston criteria (Box 7.2). MRI will frequently show subcortical small vessel disease and demyelination, strictly lobar microbleeds, cortical superficial siderosis, and enlarged centrum semi-ovale perivascular spaces (Esiri *et al.* 2015; Ni *et al.* 2015; Charidimou *et al.* 2017b, c) (Figs. 7.2 and 7.3).

Intracranial Vascular Malformations

Intracranial vascular malformations are uncommon, probably congenital, and sometimes familial (Byrne 2005). Those in the dura, draining into the sinuses rather than cerebral veins, can also be caused by skull fracture, craniotomy, or dural sinus thrombosis. The overall intracranial vascular malformations detection rate is approximately 3 per 100,000 population per annum, and the prevalence is about 20 per 100,000 (Brown *et al.* 1996; Al-Shahi *et al.* 2003).

Arteriovenous Malformations

Arteriovenous malformations present most commonly with signs consistent with a space-occupying lesion or seizures and consist of an abnormal fistulous connection(s) between one or more hypertrophied feeding arteries and dilated draining veins (Clatterbuck *et al.* 2005) (Fig. 7.5). The blood supply is derived from one cerebral artery or, more often, several, sometimes with a contribution from branches of the external carotid artery. Arteriovenous malformations vary from a few millimeters to several centimeters in diameter. Approximately 15% are associated with aneurysms on their feeding arteries. Some grow during life, but a few shrink or even disappear, and some are multiple. These fistulae occur in or on the brain or in the dura of the intracranial sinuses.

Arteriovenous malformations can present at any age with:

- partial or secondarily generalized epileptic seizures.
- hemorrhage, which is more often intracerebral than subarachnoid or subdural.
- a mass lesion.
- TIA-like episodes (Chapter 8)
- a caroticocavernous fistula owing to a dural arteriovenous malformation.
- a self-audible bruit.

BOX 7.2 Classic and Modified Boston Criteria for Diagnosis of CAA-Related Hemorrhage

Definite CAA

Full postmortem examination demonstrating:

- Lobar, cortical, or corticosubcortical hemorrhage
- Severe CAA with vasculopathy
- Absence of other diagnostic lesions

Probable CAA with Supporting Pathology

Clinical data and pathologic tissue (evacuated hematoma or cortical biopsy) demonstrating:

- Lobar, cortical, or corticosubcortical hemorrhage
- Some degree of CAA in the specimen
- Absence of other diagnostic factors

Probable CAA

Clinical data and MRI or CT demonstrating:

- Multiple hemorrhages restricted to lobar, cortical, or corticosubcortical regions (cerebellar hemorrhage allowed) [or single lobar, cortical, or corticosubcortical hemorrhage, and focal[a] or disseminated[b] superficial siderosis]
- Age ≥ 55 years
- Absence of other causes of hemorrhage [or superficial siderosis]

Possible CAA

Clinical data and MRI or CT demonstrating:

- Single lobar, cortical, or corticosubcortical hemorrhage [or focal[a] or disseminated[b] superficial siderosis]
- Age ≥ 55 years
- Absence of other causes of hemorrhage [or superficial siderosis]

Notes: Modified criteria are indicated in brackets.
[a] Siderosis restricted to three or fewer sulci
[b] Siderosis affecting at least four sulci
Sources: From Knudsen *et al.* (2001) and Linn et al. (2010).

- the syndrome of benign intracranial hypertension resulting from increased pressure in cerebral draining veins or sinuses, particularly if a dural arteriovenous malformation is near the transverse/sigmoid sinus and petrous bone.
- high output cardiac failure in neonates and infants.

Headache, although common, is not by itself diagnostically helpful and may well be a coincidence. Rarely, a bruit can be heard over the skull or orbits. A brainstem arteriovenous malformation can present similarly to multiple sclerosis, with fluctuating symptoms and signs of brainstem dysfunction, perhaps caused by recurrent hemorrhage.

A CT scan may show calcification and nonspecific hypo- or hyperdensity, while an enhanced scan is likely to show the dilated vessels of large malformations. Magnetic resonance imaging is more sensitive, showing evidence of old hemorrhage and vascular

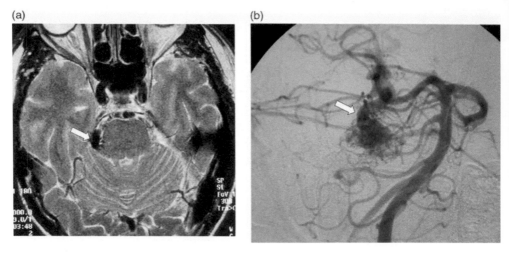

Fig. 7.5 Arteriovenous malformation. A T$_2$-weighted MRI (a) and cerebral angiogram (b) showing a dural arteriovenous malformation (arrows) at the right cerebellopontine angle, causing tinnitus.

flow voids. Angiography is the definitive investigation, but even this may not detect small malformations.

Developmental Venous Anomaly

Developmental venous anomalies (also known as venous angiomas or venous malformations) consist of collections of venous channels and a large draining vein. They are considered as extreme variations of normal transmedullary veins, are present in 2.5–3% of the normal population, and are the most common cerebrovascular malformation. The majority of developmental venous anomalies are asymptomatic and are found incidentally on brain imaging. Symptoms could, however, arise due to mechanical compression of the drainage vein on surrounding structures causing hydrocephalus, tinnitus, brainstem deficits, hemifacial spasm, or trigeminal neuralgia (Pereira *et al.* 2008). Occasionally, in instances where cavernomas or arteriovenous malformations drain directly through a developmental venous anomaly, the chronically increased pressure within the developmental venous anomaly may result in an intracerebral or intraventricular hemorrhage (Pereira *et al.* 2008). Restriction of venous drainage from the developmental venous anomaly may also occur, either by stenosis or thrombosis of the venous anomaly or its drainage vein or by an increased venous pressure secondary to a distant arteriovenous shunt. This may ultimately result in venous congestive edema or venous hemorrhage, presenting with signs and symptoms of raised intracranial pressure, focal neurological deficits, or seizures (Pereira *et al.* 2008).

Neuroimaging may reveal a radially arranged cluster of medullary veins that converge into a large drainage vein, resembling a "Medusa head" or "upside-down umbrella" appearance. These features are usually not present on a non-contrast CT unless the developmental venous anomaly or its drainage vein is very large in size. On contrast-enhanced CT, numerous linear enhancing streaks that converge into a tube-shaped drainage vein may be detected. Similar features may be present on contrast-enhanced T1-weighted image of

MRI, but on T2*GRE or SWI, developmental venous anomalies may appear as linear hypointensities due to the slow flow of deoxygenated blood. The definitive diagnosis is made on the venous phase of a cerebral angiogram.

Developmental venous anomalies do not require treatment unless there are concomitant pathologies such as an arteriovenous malformation.

Cavernous Malformations

Cavernous malformations, or cavernomas, are sharply circumscribed collections of thin-walled sinusoidal vessels lined with a single layer of endothelium without intervening brain parenchyma or identifiable mature vessel wall elements. Cavernomas are occasionally familial, and approximately 15% of individuals with cavernomas have more than one (Labauge et al. 2007; Horne et al. 2016). Most are asymptomatic and picked up incidentally on MRI. They can present with seizures, intracerebral hemorrhage, or a new focal neurological deficit without evidence of hemorrhage on brain imaging (Horne et al. 2016). Cavernomas usually do not show up on non-contrast-enhanced CT scans, as many of them are too small to be detected. They can occasionally appear as hyperdense lesions due to calcifications within the cavernoma but usually without surrounding edema or mass effect. On MRI, cavernomas are often described as a "popcorn ball" in view of the multiple fluid-filled locules of blood of different ages surrounded by a sharply circumscribed hemosiderin rim. They may also appear as multifocal "blooming black dots" on hemosiderin-sensitive sequences of MRI such as T2* GRE or SWI. The angiogram is usually normal.

Meta-analysis of seven cohorts (1,620 patients with cavernomas) revealed that in patients who presented without an intracerebral hemorrhage or focal neurological deficit, the 5-year estimated risk of intracerebral hemorrhage was 3.8% in those with a non-brainstem cavernoma and 8.0% in patients with a brainstem cavernoma (Horne et al. 2016). However, in patients who presented with an intracerebral hemorrhage or focal neurological deficit, the 5-year risk of intracerebral hemorrhage was 18.4% in patients with a non-brainstem cavernoma and 30.8% in those with a brainstem cavernoma (Horne et al. 2016). These risks can therefore be used to inform decisions about whether cavernomas should be treated conservatively, with neurosurgical excision or stereotactic radiosurgery.

Telangiectasias

Telangiectasias are collections of dilated capillaries, most often found in the pons, cerebellum, and spinal cord, that are usually of no clinical significance (Milandre et al. 1987). They may be associated with hereditary hemorrhagic telangiectasia (the Osler–Weber–Rendu syndrome), a rare autosomal dominant monogenetic disorder characterized by multisystem angiodysplastic lesions (mucocutaneous, pulmonary, brain, and gastrointestinal tract being the most common sites). Neurological complications may develop secondary to a pulmonary arteriovenous fistula, which can lead to a right-to-left shunt, resulting in cerebral hypoxia. Such a fistula may also allow for paradoxical emboli to pass through, leading to TIAs, stroke, and cerebral abscesses. Hereditary hemorrhagic telangiectasia is also associated with intracranial arteriovenous malformations, the majority small in size (Govani et al. 2009). If isolated and in the absence of other accompanying vascular malformations, capillary telangiectasias do not require treatment.

Caroticocavernous Fistula

A caroticocavernous fistula is an abnormal connection between the carotid arterial system and the cavernous sinus. It may occur spontaneously, especially in the elderly, or as a result of a ruptured dural arteriovenous malformation, intracavernous internal carotid artery aneurysm, Ehlers–Danlos syndrome, pseudoxanthoma elasticum, or head injury. With a high-flow direct fistulae from the internal carotid artery itself, normal venous return to the cavernous sinus is impeded, resulting in a rapid increase in pressure within the cavernous sinus and engorgement of the draining veins. The onset is dramatic with unilateral pulsating exophthalmos and an orbital bruit, often audible to the patient. In addition, there may be orbital pain, papilledema, dilated conjunctival veins and chemosis, glaucoma, monocular visual loss, and involvement of cranial nerves III, IV, VI, and II and sometimes the second sensory division of the trigeminal nerve. The ophthalmoplegia may also be caused by hypoxia and swelling within the extraocular muscles. Dural fistulae present more insidiously because the blood flow is lower from small meningeal branches of the internal or external carotid arteries in the cavernous sinus. If there is no spontaneous resolution, it may be possible to obliterate the fistula with endovascular treatment (Korkmazer *et al.* 2013).

References

Akoudad S, Darweesh SKL, Leening MJG *et al.* (2014). Use of coumarin anticoagulants and cerebral microbleeds in the general population. *Stroke* 45:3436–3439

Al-Shahi R, Bhattacharya JJ, Currie DG *et al.* (2003). Prospective, population-based detection of intracranial vascular malformations in adults: The Scottish Intracranial Vascular Malformation Study. *Stroke* 34:1163–1169

Attems J, Jellinger K, Thal DR *et al.* (2011). Review: Sporadic cerebral amyloid angiopathy. *Neuropathology and Applied Neurobiology* 37:75–93

Biffi A, Anderson CD, Jagiella JM *et al.* (2011). APOE genotype and extent of bleeding and outcome in lobar intracerebral hemorrhage: A genetic association study. *Lancet Neurology* 10:702–709

Brown RD, Wiebers DO, Torner JC *et al.* (1996). Incidence and prevalence of intracranial vascular malformations in Olmsted, County Minnesota 1965 to 1992. *Neurology* 46:949–952

Byrne JV (2005). Cerebrovascular malformations. *European Radiology* 15:448–452

Case NF, Charlton A, Zwiers A *et al.* (2016). Cerebral amyloid angiopathy is associated with executive dysfunction and mild cognitive impairment. *Stroke* 47:2010–2016

Charidimou A, Gang Q, Werring DJ (2012). Sporadic cerebral amyloid angiopathy revisited: Recent insights into pathophysiology and clinical spectrum. *Journal of Neurology, Neurosurgery and Psychiatry* 83:124–137

Charidimou A, Baron JC, Werring DJ (2013). Transient focal neurological episodes, cerebral amyloid angiopathy, and intracerebral hemorrhage risk: Looking beyond TIAs. *International Journal of Stroke* 8:105–108

Charidimou A, Karayiannis C, Song TJ *et al.* (2017a). Brain microbleeds, anticoagulation, and hemorrhage risk: Meta-analysis in stroke patients with AF. *Neurology* 89:2317–2326

Charidimou A, Boulouis G, Xiong L *et al.* (2017b). Cortical superficial siderosis and first-ever cerebral hemorrhage in cerebral amyloid angiopathy. *Neurology* 88:1–8

Charidimou A, Boulouis G, Pasi M *et al.* (2017c). MRI-visible perivascular spaces in cerebral amyloid angiopathy and hypertensive arteriopathy. *Neurology* 88:1157–1164

Clatterbuck RE, Hsu FP, Spetzler RF (2005). Supratentorial arteriovenous malformations. *Neurosurgery* 57:164–167

Cordonnier C, Al-Shahi Salman R, Wardlaw J (2007). Spontaneous brain microbleeds: Systematic review, subgroup analyses and standards for study design and reporting. *Brain* 130:1988–2003

Darby DG, Donnan GA, Saling MA *et al.* (1988). Primary intraventricular haemorrhage: Clinical and neuropsychological findings in a prospective stroke series. *Neurology* **38**:68–75

Ellis RJ, Olichney JM, Thal LJ *et al.* (1996). Cerebral amyloid angiopathy in the brain of patients with Alzheimer's disease: The CERAD experience, Part XV. *Neurology* **46**:1592–1596

Esiri M, Chance S, Joachim C *et al.* (2015). Cerebral amyloid angiopathy, subcortical white matter disease and dementia: Literature review and study in OPTIMA. *Brain Pathology* **25**:51–62

Fisher M (2014). Cerebral microbleeds: Where are we now? *Neurology* **83**:1304–1305

Fotiadis P, van Rooden S, van der Grond J *et al.* (2016). Cortical atrophy in patients with cerebral amyloid angiopathy: A case-control study. *Lancet Neurology* **15**:811–819

Gates GC, Barnett HJM, Vinters HV *et al.* (1986). Primary intraventricular haemorrhage in adults. *Stroke* **17**:872–877

Govani FS, Shovlin CL (2009). Hereditary hemorrhagic telangiectasia: A clinical and scientific review. *European Journal of Human Genetics* **17**:860–871

Greenberg SM, Vonsattel JP, Segal AZ *et al.* (1998). Association of apolipoprotein E epsilon2 and vasculopathy in cerebral amyloid angiopathy. *Neurology* **50**:961–965

Greenberg SM, Vernooij MW, Cordonnier C *et al.* (2009). Cerebral microbleeds: A guide to detection and interpretation. *Lancet Neurology* **8**:165–174

Horne MA, Flemming KD, Su IC *et al.* (2016). Clinical course of untreated cerebral cavernous malformations: A meta-analysis of individual patient data. *Lancet Neurology* **15**:166–173

Howard RS (1986). Brainstem hematoma due to presumed cryptic telangiectasia. *Journal of Neurology, Neurosurgery and Psychiatry* **49**:1241–1245

Kidwell CS, Wintermark M (2008). Imaging of intracranial hemorrhage. *Lancet Neurology* **7**:256–267

Knudsen KA, Rosand J, Karluk D *et al.* (2001). Clinical diagnosis of cerebral amyloid angiopathy: Validation of the Boston criteria. *Neurology* **56**:537–539

Korkmazer B, Kocak B, Tureci E *et al.* (2013). Endovascular treatment of carotid cavernous sinus fistula: A systematic review. *World Journal of Radiology* **5**:143–155

Labauge P, Denier C, Bergametti F *et al.* (2007). Genetics of cavernous angiomas. *Lancet Neurology* **6**:237–244

Lau KK, Wong YK, Teo KC *et al.* (2017). Long-term prognostic implications of cerebral microbleeds in Chinese with ischemic stroke. *Journal of the American Heart Association* **6**(12)

Lau KK, Lovelock CE, Li L *et al.* (unpublished). Antiplatelet treatment after TIA and ischemic stroke in patients with cerebral microbleeds: Time-course and severity of recurrent stroke in Caucasian and Chinese cohorts

Leira R, Davalos A, Silva Y *et al.* (2004). Early neurologic deterioration in intracerebral hemorrhage: Predictors and associated factors. *Neurology* **63**:461–467

Linn J, Halpin A, Demaerel P *et al.* (2010). Prevalence of superficial siderosis in patients with cerebral amyloid angiopathy. *Neurology* **74**:1346–1350

Lovelock CE, Cordonnier C, Naka H *et al.* (2010). Antithrombotic drug use, cerebral microbleeds, and intracerebral hemorrhage: A systematic review of published and unpublished studies. *Stroke* **41**:1222–1228

Milandre L, Pellissier JF, Boudouresques G *et al.* (1987). Non-hereditary multiple telangiectasias of the central nervous system. *Journal of the Neurological Sciences* **82**:291–304

Moussaddy A, Levy A, Strbian D *et al.* (2015). Inflammatory cerebral amyloid angiopathy, amyloid-β related angiitis, and primary angiitis of the central nervous system – similarities and differences. *Stroke* **46**:e210–213

Naka H, Nomura E, Kitamura J *et al.* (2013). Antiplatelet therapy as a risk factor for microbleeds in intracerebral hemorrhage patients: Analysis using specific antiplatelet agents. *Journal of Stroke and Cerebrovascular Diseases* **22**:834–840

Neimann J, Haapaniemi HM, Hillbom M (2000). Neurological complications of drug abuse: Pathophysiological mechanisms. *European Journal of Neurology* **7**:595–606

Ni J, Auriel E, Martinez-Ramirez S *et al.* (2015). Cortical localization of microbleeds in cerebral amyloid angiopathy: An ultra high-field 7T MRI study. *Journal of Alzheimer's Disease.* **43**:1325–1330

O'Connor AD, Rusyniak DE, Bruno A (2005). Cerebrovascular and cardiovascular complications of alcohol and sympathomimetic drug abuse. *Medical Clinics of North America* **89**:1343–1358

O'Laoire SA, Crockard A, Thomas DGT *et al.* (1982). Brain-stem hematoma. A report of six surgically treated cases. *Journal of Neurosurgery* **56**:222–227

Pereira VM, Geibprasert S, Krings T *et al.* (2008). Pathomechanisms of symptomatic developmental venous anomalies. *Stroke* **39**:3201–3215

Qureshi AI, Mendelow AD, Hanley DF (2009). Intracerebral hemorrhage. *Lancet* **373**:1632–1644

Shoamanesh A, Kwok CS, Benavente O. (2011). Cerebral microbleeds: Histopathological correlation of neuroimaging. *Cerebrovascular diseases* **32**:528–534

Srivastava T, Sannegowda RB, Satija V *et al.* (2014). Primary intraventricular hemorrhage: Clinical features, risk factors, etiology, and yield of diagnostic cerebral angiography. *Neurology India* **62**:144–148

Takebayashi S, Kaneko M (1983). Electron microscopic studies of ruptured arteries in hypertensive intracerebral haemorrhage. *Stroke* **14**:28–36

Tsivgoulis G, Zand R, Katsanos AH *et al.* (2016). Risk of symptomatic intracerebral hemorrhage after intravenous thrombolysis in patients with acute ischemic stroke and high cerebral microbleed burden: A meta-analysis. *JAMA Neurology* **73**:675–683

van Veluw SJ, Biessels GJ, Klijn CJM *et al.* (2016). Heterogeneous histopathology of cortical microbleeds in cerebral amyloid angiopathy. *Neurology* **86**:867–871

Verghese PB, Castellano JM, Holtzman DM (2011). Apolipoprotein E in Alzheimer's disease and other neurological disorders. *Lancet Neurology* **10**:241–252

Walker LC, Pahnke J, Madauss M *et al.* (2000). Apolipoprotein E4 promotes the early deposition of Abeta42 and then Abeta 40 in the elderly. *Acta Neuropathologica* **100**:36–42

Wilson D, Charidimou A, Ambler G *et al.* (2016). Recurrent stroke risk and cerebral microbleed burden in ischemic stroke and TIA: A meta-analysis. *Neurology* **87**:1–10

Yamada M (2015). Cerebral amyloid angiopathy: Emerging concepts. *Journal of Stroke* **17**:17–30

8 Clinical Features and Differential Diagnosis of a Transient Ischemic Attack

The causes of TIAs are the same as the causes of stroke, with the caveat that the vast majority of TIAs appear to be caused by ischemia rather than hemorrhage (Chapter 9). The differential diagnosis of TIA differs from that of stroke owing to the transient nature of the symptoms (Box 8.1). A careful history and examination is important since this may provide clues to the underlying cause of the TIA (Chapter 6) or may indicate a non-vascular cause for the focal symptoms. Identification of the underlying affected vascular territory from the clinical features of the TIA is important for targeting further investigation and secondary preventive treatments. Localization of the site of ischemia may be aided by brain imaging, which is also used to exclude structural lesions causing "transient focal neurological attacks," and to differentiate between hemorrhage and ischemia (Chapter 10).

Symptoms and Ischemic Territory

Symptoms are of sudden onset and are "focal", indicating a disturbance in a particular area of brain or in one eye (Flemming *et al.* 2004; Sherman 2004). Motor symptoms are the most common: weakness, clumsiness or heaviness usually on just one side of the body (Table 8.1). Unilateral sensory symptoms are described as numbness, tingling, or deadness. Speech may be dysphasic, dysarthric, or both. Transient monocular blindness (amaurosis fugax) affects the upper or lower half of vision or all the vision of one eye and is often described like a "blind or shutter" coming down from above or up from below. However, transient monocular ischemia can also cause partial visual loss, such as blurring or dimming.

BOX 8.1 Causes of Transient Focal Neurological Attacks

Transient ischemic attack

Migraine with aura

Partial epileptic seizures

Structural intracranial lesions: tumor, chronic subdural hematoma, vascular malformation, giant aneurysm

Cerebral amyloid angiopathy

Multiple sclerosis

Labyrinthine disorders: Meniere's disease or benign paroxysmal positional vertigo

Peripheral nerve or root lesion

Metabolic: hypo- or hyperglycemia, hypercalcemia, hyponatremia

Psychological

Table 8.1 Clinical features and vascular distribution of transient ischemic attacks

Symptoms	Vascular distribution		Frequency (%)
	Carotid	Vertebrobasilar	
Unilateral weakness, heaviness, or clumsiness	+	+	50
Unilateral sensory symptoms	+	+	35
Dysarthria[a]	+	+	23
Transient monocular blindness	+	−	18
Dysphasia	+	(+)	18
Unsteadiness/ataxia[a]	(+)	+	12
Bilateral simultaneous blindness	−	+	7
Vertigo[a]	−	+	5
Homonymous hemianopia	(+)	+	5
Diplopia	−	+	5
Bilateral motor loss	−	+	4
Dysphagia[a]	(+)	+	1
Crossed sensory and motor loss	−	+	1

[a] In general, if these symptoms are isolated, it is best not to diagnose definite transient ischemic attack.

Transient monocular blindness must be distinguished from transient homonymous hemi-anopia, although this can be difficult even when the patient is a very good historian.

Simultaneous bilateral transient motor or sensory loss is almost always caused by brainstem ischemia. Sudden simultaneous bilateral blindness in elderly patients usually indicates bilateral occipital ischemia. Vertigo, diplopia, dysphagia, unsteadiness, tinnitus, amnesia, drop attacks, and dysarthria may be caused by posterior circulation or more global cerebral ischemia, or by non-vascular causes such as motor neuron disease or myesthenia in the case of dysarthria. If these symptoms occur in isolation, the diagnosis of TIA should only be considered after exclusion of other possibilities (Gomez *et al.* 1996; Bos *et al.* 2007). Global symptoms such as a reduced level of consciousness are almost never caused by a TIA. They can only be accepted as resulting from a TIA if there are additional focal symptoms that are unlikely to be epileptic or syncopal.

If more than one body part is involved, the symptoms usually start simultaneously in all parts, persist for a while, and then gradually wear off over a few minutes, particularly in the case of transient monocular blindness, or an hour or so. If a patient still has symptoms more than an hour after the onset, the chances are that complete recovery will take more than 24 hours. A mild headache accompanying the neurological symptoms is quite common, usually ipsilateral to the affected carotid territory but most common in posterior circulation TIAs. If cerebral symptoms last less than a minute, particularly if they are "sensory," the diagnosis of TIA is difficult to sustain. In contrast, symptoms of retinal ischemia may be very short-lived.

The symptoms of a TIA enable categorization of attacks by arterial territory affected: carotid in approximately 80% or vertebrobasilar in 20%. This has important implications for further investigation and secondary prevention. Such categorization may be straightforward where there are definite cortical symptoms such as dysphasia or brainstem symptoms such as diplopia. However, because the motor and sensory pathways are supplied by both vascular systems at different points in their course, it is not always possible to distinguish which territory is involved (Table 8.1). One study found that the agreement between the clinical diagnosis of vascular territory in patients with TIA or minor stroke made by three neurologists compared with the near "gold standard" of lesion location on diffusion-weighted MRI was only moderate, with the kappa statistics varying from 0.48 to 0.54 for each neurologist (Flossmann et al. 2006). Interobserver agreement on territory ranged from 0.46 to 0.60, and only the presence of visual symptoms improved the accuracy of vascular territory diagnosis (Flossmann et al. 2006). Ischemia in the territory of supply of the deep perforating arteries may be suspected if the patient has a transient lacunar syndrome and no positive evidence of cortical involvement such as dysphasia.

Mechanisms of Ischemia

Most TIAs are probably caused by arterial occlusion (Bogousslavsky et al. 1986) (Chapter 6). Less commonly, they may be secondary to low-flow distal to a severely stenosed or occluded artery in the neck following a fall in blood pressure, as after antihypertensive medication or vasodilators, after standing or sitting up quickly, after a heavy meal or a hot bath, on exercise, or during cardiac arrhythmia (Caplan and Sergay 1976; Ruff et al. 1981; Russell and Page 1983; Kamata et al. 1994). Such low-flow TIAs may be atypical: symptoms may take some minutes to develop; there may be irregular shaking or dystonic posturing of the arm or leg contralateral to the cerebral ischemia; or there may be monocular or binocular visual blurring, dimming, fragmentation, or bleaching, often just in bright light (Hess et al. 1991; Schulz and Rothwell 2002). Symptoms of focal brainstem ischemia caused by intermittent obstruction of a vertebral artery by cervical osteophytes are rare, presumably because collateral blood flow to the brainstem is usually sufficient.

"Subclavian steal" is caused by retrograde flow in the vertebral artery. It is a common angiographic or ultrasound finding when there is stenosis or occlusion of the subclavian artery proximal to the vertebral artery origin, particularly on the left, or of the innominate artery. When the ipsilateral arm is exercised, the increased blood flow to meet the metabolic demand may be enough to "steal" more blood down the vertebral artery, away from the brainstem into the axillary artery. If there is poor collateral blood flow to the brainstem, then symptoms may occur, but this is very rare. The subclavian disease is almost always severe enough to be detectable by unequal radial pulses and blood pressures, and often there is a supraclavicular bruit (Cho et al. 2007).

Signs

Owing to their brief duration, patients are rarely examined during a TIA at a time when focal neurological signs might indicate the site of the lesion, although this now occurs more frequently with the advent of acute stroke services and thrombolysis. However, non-neurological signs, including carotid bruits, retinal emboli, cardiac dysrhythmia, and signs of peripheral vascular disease, may help to elucidate the cause of the attacks (Chapter 9).

BOX 8.2 Causes of Transient Monocular Blindness (Amaurosis Fugax)	
Transient ischemic attack	Intraorbital tumor
Glaucoma	Caroticocavernous fistula
Uhthoff's phenomenon in retrobulbar neuritis	Retinal migraine
Raised intracranial pressure with papilloedema	Intracranial dural malformation
Retinal hemorrhage	Paraneoplastic retinopathy
Retinal venous thrombosis	Reversible diabetic cataract
Retinal detachment	Uveitis–glaucoma–hyphema syndrome
Macular degeneration	

Differential Diagnosis and Mimics of Transient Ischemic Attacks

Transient ischemic attacks are but one cause of "transient focal neurological attacks" (Box 8.1) and "transient monocular blindness" (Box 8.2). There is no test to confirm a TIA, and the gold standard method of diagnosis remains a thorough clinical assessment as soon as possible after the event by an experienced stroke physician, although the advent of new imaging techniques, particularly diffusion-weighted MRI (Chapter 10), has allowed the diagnosis to be made or excluded with more certainty in some patients. A diagnosis of TIA is supported by a sudden onset and definite focal symptoms in the history and evidence of vascular disease on examination (Hand *et al.* 2006).

Some conditions and syndromes are particularly frequently misdiagnosed as TIA (Table 8.2), but features in the history are often helpful in distinguishing TIA and minor stroke from mimics (Table 8.3).

Migraine with Aura

Migraine is not a major diagnostic problem if the aura is associated with a headache with or without nausea and vomiting or if a known migraineur develops a typical aura without headache. However, occasionally migraine auras start in middle or old age, and if there is no headache, they can be confused with TIAs. The time course of the symptoms is the key to distinguishing between TIA and migraine aura: migrainous auras start slowly, spread and intensify over several minutes, and usually fade in 20–30 minutes (Dennis and Warlow 1992). The symptoms tend to begin in one domain, particularly vision, fade and move on to another, such as language, and tend to be positive involving flashing lights or tingling rather than the negative symptoms typical of a TIA such as weakness, visual loss, or numbness. However, it is important to note that a progressive or stuttering pattern of symptom onset, positive visual phenomena, and headache are also compatible with vertebrobasilar TIA.

Epilepsy

Epilepsy is not a diagnostic problem unless the seizures are partial. Partial sensory seizures tend to cause positive symptoms such as tingling. Symptoms often "march" across a hand or foot and up the limb in around a minute and may eventually be accompanied by focal motor seizures or secondary generalization. Sudden speech arrest seems to be more often epileptic,

Table 8.2 Numbers of patients referred to dedicated "TIA clinics" in whom a non-neurovascular diagnosis was eventually made in Oxford Vascular Study (OXVASC; 2002–2004) and the Oxford Community Stroke Project (OCSP; 1981–1986)

Diagnosis	OXVASC (n = 112)	Diagnosis	OCSP (n = 317)
Migraine	25	Migraine	52
Anxiety	14	Syncope	48
Seizure	9	"Possible TIA"	46
Peripheral neuropathy	8	"Funny turn"	45
Arrhythmia	6	Isolated vertigo	33
Labyrinthine	6	Epilepsy	29
Postural hypotension	6	Transient global amnesia	17
Transient global amnesia	6	Lone bilateral blindness	14
Syncope	5	Isolated diplopia	4
Tumor or metastases	4	Drop attack	3
Cervical spine disease	3	Meningioma	2
Dementia	2	Miscellaneous	24
Myasthenia gravis	1		
Multiple sclerosis	1		
Parkinson's disease	1		
Miscellaneous	15		

Note: TIA, transient ischemic attack.
Source: From Martin et al. (1989).

and not necessarily arising from the dominant hemisphere, than caused by ischemia, which is more likely to cause dysphasic speech (Cascino et al. 1991). Transient inhibitory seizures may mimic the focal motor weakness of TIA but are most unusual (Kaplan 1993). Todd's paresis is a focal neurological deficit that can follow up to 10% of seizures, most commonly grand mal seizures, and typically causes a unilateral motor weakness but can also cause diplopia or speech disturbance. The cause of Todd's paresis is unknown, but "exhaustion" of the primary motor cortex or inactivation of motor fibers by NMDA receptors has been postulated. Like a TIA, Todd's paresis can last for several hours, and differentiation can be difficult but depends mainly on establishing the presence of seizure activity at onset (Gallmetzer et al. 2004).

Intracranial Structural Lesions

Occasionally, but importantly, intracranial structural lesions such as subdural hematoma (see Fig. 7.4), tumor (Fig. 8.1), or cerebral amyloid angiopathy (CAA) (Figs 7.2 and 7.3) may cause TIA-like symptoms, although such lesions may sometimes be incidental.

Table 8.3 Features of a patient's history that are less typical of a transient ischemic attack and alternative (non-neurovascular) diagnosis suggested

Symptom	Description	Non-neurovascular diagnosis suggested	Notes
Timing	Recurrent/ stereotypical episodes	Anxiety related	Especially hemisensory loss
Onset	Stuttering	Tumor	Over hours/days
	Progressive	Migraine	Over minutes
		Cerebral amyloid angiopathy	Over minutes
	Ill defined	Delirium	
Symptoms	Prodrome	Aura	Migraine, seizure
	Non-focal	Syncope	Loss of consciousness
		Delirium	Reduced attention
		Labyrinthine dysfunction	Balance disturbance
	Positive	Seizure	Motor symptom
		Migraine	Visual spectra
		Cerebral amyloid angiopathy	Motor, sensory and/or visual
	Negative	Cerebral amyloid angiopathy	Limb-weakness, dysphasia or visual loss
	Additional symptoms	Migraine	Headache
		Labyrinthine dysfunction	Hearing loss/tinnitus
Course	Fluctuating	Tumor	
		Delirium	
Recall	Absent	Transient global amnesia	
		Seizure	Generalized seizure
	Patchy	Delirium	

Compression of an intracranial artery is perhaps an explanation for those patients with a space-occupying lesion, while focal seizures misdiagnosed as TIAs are another possibility. Intracerebral tumors can suddenly expand in size as a result of in situ hemorrhage (Fig. 8.1b), edema, or both, and these are further causes of symptoms coming on suddenly in an otherwise "chronic" condition. Intracranial vascular malformations might cause local steal of blood, thereby causing a TIA, or perhaps cause focal epileptic attacks that mimic TIAs. CAA is due to amyloid-β deposition in the wall of cortical and leptomeningeal arterioles and may result in transient focal neurological episodes in approximately 15% of patients (Charidimou *et al.* 2013). These transient focal neurological episodes are often recurrent, stereotyped, and short-lasting (usually subsiding within minutes). They may be in the form of positive and negative symptoms.

Although intracranial structural lesions can cause focal neurological deficits, these are almost never the sole clinical feature. Cerebral imaging with MRI is, therefore, important to exclude space-occupying lesions in patients with stuttering, deficits of gradual onset, more prolonged histories, or additional features such as headache or

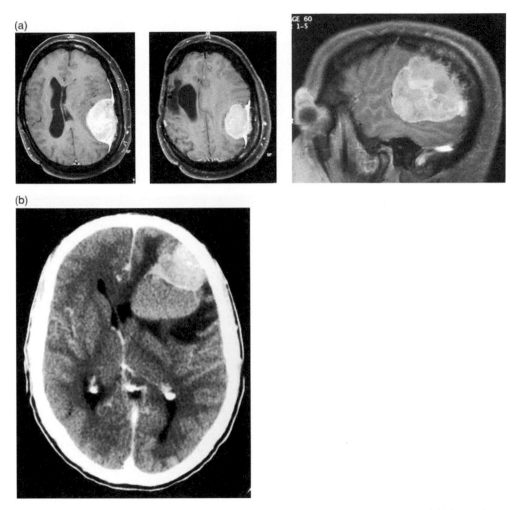

Fig. 8.1 Examples of tumors that may cause symptoms mimicking TIA: (a) meningioma, and (b) hemorrhagic melanoma metastasis

nausea. A hemosiderin-sensitive sequence on MRI such as T2*-gradient echo (GRE) or susceptibility weighted imaging (SWI) may also need to be incorporated to detect lobar microbleeds and/or cortical superficial siderosis in CAA (Figs 7.2 and 7.3). Imaging with non-contrast CT lacks sensitivity for space-occupying lesions and is not recommended (Chapter 10).

Transient Global Amnesia

Transient global amnesia is a characteristic but uncommon clinical syndrome, usually occurring in the middle aged or elderly (Hodges and Warlow 1990a, b; Quinette *et al.* 2006). The onset is sudden, with severe anterograde amnesia usually accompanied by retrograde amnesia. The attack lasts several hours, after which the patient recovers the ability to lay down new memories and recall old ones but never has recollection of the period of the attack itself. During the attack, the patient is fully conscious, has no loss of personal identity, looks normal if not a little subdued and bewildered, and has no other symptoms apart perhaps from some headache and nausea. The patient can perform normal everyday activities, even driving, but typically asks the same question repetitively because of the anterograde amnesia. A witness account is required to differentiate such attacks from hysterical fugues, alcoholic amnesic states, or complex partial seizures. Emotional upset, Valsalva maneuvers, defecation, sexual intercourse, and other physical exertions, often outdoor activities on a cold day, may be precipitants (Quinette *et al.* 2006). In most cases, the prognosis is excellent and attacks do not usually recur.

The etiology of transient global amnesia is unclear. Various mechanisms have been proposed, including temporary metabolic abnormality in the medial temporal lobes, venous hypertension, and ischemia (Bettermann 2006; Menendez-Gonzalez and Rivera 2006; Roach 2006). Sometimes a diagnosis of epilepsy, usually of complex partial type, becomes apparent subsequently. This is particularly likely if the transient global amnesia had been short-lived, for less than an hour, had occurred on wakening, and had recurred early (Zeman *et al.* 1998). Neuroimaging has confirmed that medial temporal lobe changes accompany transient global amnesia (Sander and Sander 2005). The presence of abnormality on diffusion-weighted MRI (Sander and Sander 2005; Sedlaczek *et al.* 2004) has led to the proposal that transient global amnesia may be an ischemic phenomenon. However, such changes are not diagnostic of ischemia and can occur following seizures.

Vestibular Dysfunction

The acute onset of vertigo is a common complaint and presents a diagnostic challenge, especially in elderly patients with preexisting risk factors for vascular disease. An essential part of the evaluation should be the distinction between "true vertigo," put simply the false illusion of movement, and other less-specific symptoms of "unsteadiness" or "light-headedness." The differential diagnosis of "true vertigo" is traditionally divided into peripheral causes, including benign paroxysmal positional vertigo, vestibular neuritis, and Meniere's disease; and central causes, one of which is TIA or stroke affecting the brainstem. Generally, peripheral causes of vertigo are more common than central causes, and one study found stroke or TIA to be the cause of only 3.2% of presentations with "dizziness symptoms" to an emergency department (Kerber *et al.* 2006).

Important features in the history that help in the differential diagnosis and indicate an alternative cause to TIA or stroke include the recurrent stereotypical episodes, presence of provoking factors (head movement), presence of features of middle ear disease (tinnitus, hearing loss), and absence of other focal neurological symptoms of sudden onset that might be attributable to the brainstem (visual or speech disturbance, weakness, or numbness). Features on examination that are thought to identify a central cause of vertigo include nystagmus that is not suppressed by visual fixation, a normal head thrust test, and other features of posterior circulation ischemia, including dysphagia, dysarthria, limb or facial weakness, gaze palsies, or upgoing plantar responses. Despite these clinical indicators, the differential diagnosis is challenging and is sometimes only made when imaging is suggestive of focal ischemia (Schwartz *et al.* 2007).

Delirium or Toxic Confusional State

Delirium, toxic confusional state, metabolic encephalopathy, and acute confusional state are terms that are used interchangeably and often loosely to describe a syndrome of acutely disordered cognition, sometimes associated with reduced level of consciousness and abnormal attention (see Table 31.3). The syndrome is very common, especially in the elderly and in patients with dementia, and presentations vary widely both in the speed of onset and severity (Siddiqi *et al.* 2006). The differential diagnosis is broad and includes almost any medical condition, but the commonest causes are sepsis, adverse drug reaction, and metabolic derangement (Francis *et al.* 1990).

Delirium can be mistaken for a TIA if mild, when the predominant feature is interpreted as language disorder as opposed to confusion and when important clinical details are unclear such as when a witness account is unavailable, the patient has cognitive impairment, or there is a long delay between the event and assessment. Reliable differentiation between TIA and delirium is important because each carries a potentially poor prognosis, though for very different reasons, and the treatments are dissimilar (Siddiqi *et al.* 2006). Features suggestive of delirium as opposed to TIA include the presence of a causative factor such as urinary tract sepsis, an inability of the patient to remember the event clearly, fluctuating disturbance in attention and consciousness, and the absence of a clearly sudden onset of symptoms.

Syncope and Presyncope

Syncope is the abrupt loss of consciousness associated with the loss of postural tone, usually followed by a rapid and complete recovery. Presyncope is a premonitory sensation of syncope. The differential diagnosis of syncope is very broad and is divided into cardiovascular causes (most commonly tachy- or bradyarrhythmias) and non-cardiovascular causes (most commonly vasovagal syncope, orthostatic hypotension, and carotid sinus hypersensitivity). Although the time course of syncope is consistent with TIA, the lack of focal neurological disturbance is definitely not, and the diagnosis should, therefore, only be made with considerable caution. Diagnostic confusion can sometimes be caused by a TIA of the brainstem, causing transient quadriparesis presenting with a sudden loss of postural tone, but loss of consciousness is not a feature. Less infrequently, embolus to the tip of the basilar artery can present with sudden-onset coma, but this is virtually never a transient, self-limiting condition, and other signs of brainstem dysfunction are always present and obvious, so this should not cause difficulties in diagnosis (Voetsch *et al.* 2004).

Other Neurological Disorders

Occasionally, non-structural neurological disorders such as motor neuron disease, multiple sclerosis (Rolak and Fleming 2007), or myasthenia gravis may present with transient symptoms of sudden onset. Although these conditions usually follow a progressive course, the initial clinical course can occasionally be rapid and may resemble a TIA or minor stroke. Both motor neuron disease and myasthenia gravis occur more commonly in the elderly and can present with isolated dysarthria or dysphagia, and unless the diagnosis is made initially, subsequent deterioration can often be put down to "recurrent stroke" (Libman *et al.* 2002; Kleiner-Fisman and Kott 1998).

Cryptogenic Drop Attacks

Drop attacks affect middle-aged and elderly women, almost only when walking rather than just standing or sitting (Stevens and Matthews 1973). Without warning, the patient falls to the ground. There is no loss of consciousness or leg weakness. The attacks may recur but then disappear as mysteriously as they came. There is usually no known cause, although carotid sinus syncope and orthostatic hypotension are possibilities (Dey *et al.* 1996). There appear to be no serious prognostic implications. Sudden weakness of both legs can occur in brainstem ischemia and, rarely, if both anterior cerebral arteries are supplied from the same stenosed internal carotid artery. Bilateral motor, sensory, or visual impairments can also be caused by bihemispheric boundary zone ischemia distal to severe carotid disease (Sloan and Haley 1990). Finally, spinal cord "TIAs" do occur but are even rarer than spinal cord infarction (Cheshire *et al.* 1996). Cataplexy is almost invariably precipitated by excitement or emotion, seldom causes the patient to fall over, and usually presents fairly early in life.

Psychogenic Attacks

Psychogenic attacks are usually situational, for instance occurring in open spaces. Suggestive features include age less than 50 years, lack of vascular risk factors, symptoms affecting the non-dominant side (Rothwell 1994), hyperventilation, other medically unexplained symptoms, or non-organic motor or sensory signs.

Isolated Transient Focal Neurological Disturbance of Uncertain Significance

In a significant proportion of patients referred to a neurovascular service with suspected TIA or minor stroke, no clear diagnosis of either a cerebrovascular event or a mimic can be reached, even after thorough clinical assessment and investigation. In our experience, these are often presentations with isolated focal neurological disturbance with sudden onset and gradual recovery, over seconds to minutes. Several distinct syndromes can be recognized, for instance isolated and transient vertigo with no other features to suggest a central or peripheral cause, isolated slurred speech, or isolated hemisensory loss (Paul *et al.* 2013). A history of these transient isolated symptoms that do not satisfy traditional definitions of TIA are present in up to 16% of patients with a definite vertebrobasilar ischemic stroke but are much less common in patients with a definite carotid territory ischemic stroke (1.6%) (Paul *et al.* 2013).

References

Bettermann K (2006). Transient global amnesia: The continuing quest for a source. *Archives of Neurology* 63:1336–1338

Bogousslavsky J, Hachinski VC, Boughner DR et al. (1986). Clinical predictors of cardiac and arterial lesions in carotid ischaemic attacks. *Archives of Neurology* 43:229–233

Bos MJ, van Rijn MJ, Witteman JC et al. (2007). Incidence and prognosis of transient neurological attacks. *Journal of the American Medical Association.* 298:2877–2885

Caplan LR, Sergay S (1976). Positional cerebral ischaemia. *Journal of Neurology, Neurosurgery and Psychiatry* 39:385–391

Cascino GD, Westmoreland BF, Swanson TH et al. (1991). Seizure-associated speech arrest in elderly patients. *Mayo Clinic Proceedings* 66:254–258

Charidimou A, Baron JC, Werring DJ (2013). Transient focal neurological episodes, cerebral amyloid angiopathy, and intracerebral hemorrhage risk: Looking beyond TIAs. *International Journal of Stroke* 8:105–108

Cheshire WP, Santos CC, Massey EW *et al.* (1996). Spinal cord infarction: Aetiology and outcome. *Neurology* 47:321–330

Cho HJ, Song SK, Lee DW *et al.* (2007). Carotid-subclavian steal phenomenon. *Neurology* 68:702

Dennis M, Warlow CP (1992). Migraine aura without headache: transient Ischaemic attack or not? *Journal of Neurology, Neurosurgery and Psychiatry* 55:437–440

Dey AB, Stout NR, Kenny RA (1996). Cardiovascular syncope is the commonest cause of drop attacks in the older patient. *European Journal of Cardiac Pacing and Electrophysiology* 6:84–88

Flemming KD, Brown RD Jr., Petty GW *et al.* (2004). Evaluation and management of transient ischaemic attack and minor cerebral infarction. *Mayo Clinic Proceedings* 79:1071–1086

Flossmann E, Redgrave JN, Schulz UG *et al.* (2006). Reliability of clinical diagnosis of the symptomatic vascular territory in patients with recent TIA or minor stroke. *Cerebrovascular Diseases* 21(Suppl 4):18

Francis J, Martin D, Kapoor WN (1990). A prospective study of delirium in hospitalized elderly. *Journal of the American Medical Association* 263:1097

Gallmetzer P, Leutmezer F, Serles W *et al.* (2004). Postictal paresis in focal epilepsies – incidence, duration, and causes: A video-EEG monitoring study. *Neurology* 62:2160–2164

Gomez CR, Cruz-Flores S, Malkoff MD *et al.* (1996). Isolated vertigo as a manifestation of vertebrobasilar ischaemia. *Neurology* 47:94–97

Hand PJ, Kwan J, Lindley RI *et al.* (2006). Distinguishing between stroke and mimic at the bedside: the brain attack study. *Stroke* 37:769–775

Hess DC, Nichols FT, Sethi KD *et al.* (1991). Transient cerebral ischaemia masquerading as paroxysmal dyskinesia. *Cerebrovascular Diseases* 1:54–57

Hodges JR, Warlow CP (1990a). Syndromes of transient amnesia: Towards a classification. A study of 153 cases. *Journal of Neurology, Neurosurgery and Psychiatry* 53:834–843

Hodges JR, Warlow CP (1990b). The aetiology of transient global amnesia. A case–control study of 114 cases with prospective follow-up. *Brain* 113:639–657

Kamata T, Yokata T, Furukawa T *et al.* (1994). Cerebral ischaemic attack caused by postprandial hypotension. *Stroke* 25:511–513

Kaplan PW (1993). Focal seizures resembling transient ischaemic attacks due to subclinical ischaemia. *Cerebrovascular Diseases* 3:241–243

Kerber KA, Brown DL, Lisabeth LD *et al.* (2006). Stroke among patients with dizziness, vertigo, and imbalance in the emergency department: A population-based study. *Stroke* 37:2484–2487

Kleiner-Fisman G, Kott HS (1998). Myasthenia gravis mimicking stroke in elderly patients. *Mayo Clinic Proceedings.* 73:1077–1078

Libman R, Benson R, Einberg K (2002). Myasthenia mimicking vertebrobasilar stroke. *Journal of Neurology* 249:1512–1514

Martin MS, Bamford JM, Sandercock PA (1989). Incidence of transient ischemic attacks in Oxfordshire. *Stroke* 20: 333–339

Menendez Gonzalez M, Rivera MM (2006). Transient global amnesia: Increasing evidence of a venous etiology. *Archives of Neurology* 63:1334–1336

Paul NL, Simoni M, Rothwell PM (2013). Transient isolated brainstem symptoms preceding posterior circulation stroke: A population-based study. *Lancet Neurology* 12:65–71

Quinette P, Guillery-Girard B, Dayan J et al. (2006). What does transient global amnesia really mean? Review of the literature and thorough study of 142 cases. *Brain* 129:1640–1658

Roach ES (2006). Transient global amnesia: Look at mechanisms not causes. *Archives of Neurology* 63:1338–1339

Rolak LA, Fleming JO (2007). The differential diagnosis of multiple sclerosis. *Neurologist* 13:57–72

Russell RW, Page NGR (1983). Critical perfusion of brain and retina. *Brain* 106:419–434

Rothwell PM (1994). Investigation of unilateral sensory or motor symptoms: Frequency of neurological pathology depends on side of symptoms. *Journal of Neurology, Neurosurgery and Psychiatry* 57:1401–1402

Ruff RL, Talman WT, Petito F (1981). Transient ischaemic attacks associated with hypotension in hypertensive patients with carotid artery stenosis. *Stroke* 12:353–355

Sander K, Sander D (2005). New insights into transient global amnesia: Recent imaging and clinical findings. *Lancet Neurology* 4:437–444

Schulz UG, Rothwell PM (2002). Transient ischaemic attacks mimicking focal motor seizures. *Postgraduate Medicine Journal* 78:246–247

Schwartz NE, Venkat C, Albers GW (2007). Transient isolated vertigo secondary to an acute stroke of the cerebellar nodulus. *Archives of Neurology* 64:897

Sedlaczek O, Hirsch JG, Grips E *et al.* (2004). Detection of delayed focal MR changes in the lateral hippocampus in transient global amnesia. *Neurology* 62:2165–2170

Sherman DG (2004). Reconsideration of TIA diagnostic criteria. *Neurology* **62**:S20–S21

Siddiqi N, House AO, Holmes JD (2006). Occurrence and outcome of delirium in medical in-patients: A systematic literature review. *Age Ageing* 35:350–364

Sloan MA, Haley EC (1990). The syndrome of bilateral hemispheric border zone ischaemia. *Stroke* 21:1668–1673

Stevens DL, Matthews WB (1973). Cryptogenic drop attacks: An affliction of women. *British Medical Journal* i: 439–442

Voetsch B, DeWitt LD, Pessin MS *et al.* (2004). Basilar artery occlusive disease in the New England Medical Center Posterior Circulation Registry. *Archives of Neurology* 61:496–504

Zeman AZJ, Boniface SJ, Hodges JR (1998). Transient epileptic amnesia: A description of the clinical and neuropsychological features in 10 cases and a review of the literature. *Journal of Neurology, Neurosurgery and Psychiatry* 64:435–443

The Clinical Features and Differential Diagnosis of Acute Stroke

The diagnosis of stroke is often fairly straightforward. However, clinicians should be aware of the conditions that can mimic stroke since diagnostic errors will have important consequences. In common with TIA, determining the site of the cerebrovascular lesion is important since this narrows down the likely underlying etiology and enables appropriate targeting of investigations (Chapters 10–13). There may be important clues from the history and examination suggesting the underlying cause of the stroke or that there may be a non-vascular cause for the patient's symptoms and signs. Establishing the underlying cause of the stroke enables specific treatment and secondary prevention (see later).

Diagnosis of Stroke

The diagnosis of stroke is relatively straightforward if there is focal brain dysfunction of sudden onset or that was first present on waking. There may be some progression over the first few minutes or hours, particularly in posterior circulation stroke (Brandt *et al.* 2000). Usually the deficit stabilizes by 12–24 hours, and if the patient survives, recovery starts within a few days in most cases. Various scoring systems or similar strategies have been developed as aids in diagnosing stroke (Nor *et al.* 2005; Hand *et al.* 2006), but these are not infallible, and clinicians should always consider the potential differential diagnoses (Box 9.1).

BOX 9.1 Differential Diagnosis of Acute Stroke

Intracranial tumor, e.g., glioma, meningioma

Subdural hematoma

Epileptic seizure

Metabolic/toxic encephalopathy: hypoglycemia, hepatic failure, alcohol intoxication

Cerebral abscess

Viral encephalitis

Hypertensive encephalopathy

Multiple sclerosis

Head injury

Peripheral nerve lesion

Psychogenic (somatization, hysteria)

Creutzfeldt–Jakob disease

Cervical cord pathology, e.g., spontaneous spinal epidural hematoma

---

If the history is consistent with stroke, there is only a 5% chance of a CT or MR brain scan showing an intracranial mass lesion rather than the expected changes consistent with stroke (Sandercock *et al.* 1985). If the history is consistent with TIA, the likelihood of findings on neuroimaging suggestive of an alternative diagnosis is even lower (Chapter 10). This risk is higher when the speed of onset is uncertain. Features indicative of an **intracranial tumor** (see Fig. 8.1) include recent headaches, seizures, papilledema, a worsening deficit over days or weeks, and the presence of a primary tumor elsewhere. Chronic **subdural hematoma** (see Fig. 7.4) is suggested by prior head injury, more drowsiness, confusion and headache out of proportion to the severity of the neurological deficit, a fluctuating course, use of anticoagulants, or chronic alcohol abuse. Other diagnoses are usually obvious: **multiple sclerosis** occurs at a younger age; **peripheral nerve or root lesion** is accompanied by clinical signs and or pain; **postseizure hemiparesis** is suggested by the history; **metabolic encephalopathy** by global rather than focal neurological features; **somatization and hysteria** by young age and inconsistent signs; **encephalitis** by fever, clinical symptoms, and signs and a diffusely abnormal EEG; and **intracranial abscess** by fever and a predisposing cause such as sinusitis or a congenital heart lesion (Norris and Hachinski 1982). Very occasionally, more unusual conditions such as Wilson's disease (Pendlebury *et al.* 2004), Creutzfelt–Jacob disease, and spontaneous spinal epidural hematomas (Matsumoto *et al.* 2012) may present with stroke-like symptoms.

Occasionally, head injury causing intracerebral hemorrhage can be missed, while hemorrhagic stroke may cause a fall and subsequent head injury; consequently the sequence of events may be unclear (Berlit *et al.* 1991). Ischemic stroke following head injury may be caused by neck artery dissection (Chapter 6). Residual signs from an old stroke may become more pronounced with intercurrent illness or after a seizure.

Determining the Site of the Lesion

Determining the location of the stroke provides useful prognostic information and helps to establish the underlying cause for the stroke, since the various clinical syndromes (described later) have differing probabilities of being caused by large or small vessel disease or cardioembolism.

Strokes can be divided into four main clinical syndromes on the basis of symptoms and clinical signs (Bamford *et al.* 1991; Mead *et al.* 1999):

- total anterior circulation syndrome.
- partial anterior circulation syndrome.
- lacunar syndrome.
- posterior circulation syndrome.

These categories provide information on early prognosis, residual disability, and risk of recurrence.

Stroke localization using clinical data is not infallible: in about a quarter of cases where a recent lesion is visible on brain imaging, it is not in the expected place (Mead *et al.* 1999). For example, although most pure motor strokes are caused by a lacunar infarct as a result of small vessel disease, in a few cases the CT or MR scan shows striatocapsular infarction caused by middle cerebral artery occlusion with good cortical collaterals (Fig. 9.1). Therefore, patients may need to be reclassified on the basis of the brain imaging results.

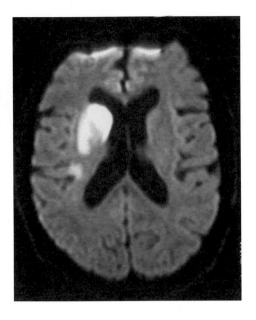

Fig. 9.1 Diffusion-weighted MRI showing a striatocapsular infarct.

Total Anterior Circulation Syndrome

A large hematoma in one cerebral hemisphere or an infarct affecting a large proportion of the middle cerebral artery territory causes a characteristic clinical syndrome:

- contralateral hemiparesis, with or without a sensory deficit and involving the whole of at least two of the three body areas: the face, upper limb, or lower limb.
- a homonymous visual field defect.
- a cortical deficit consisting of dysphasia, neglect, or visuospatial problems.

Cognitive or visual field defects may have to be assumed in drowsy patients. Deviation of the eyes toward the affected hemisphere is common but recovers in a few days. A large hematoma may cause midline shift, transtentorial herniation, and coma within 24 hours (Fig. 9.2). By contrast, these changes take 2 or 3 days to evolve with large infarcts as cerebral edema develops.

Total anterior circulation infarcts are usually the result of acute occlusion of the internal carotid artery or embolic occlusion of the proximal middle cerebral artery from a cardiac or proximal arterial source (Caplan 1993; Lindgren *et al.* 1994; Wardlaw *et al.* 1996, Georgiadis *et al.* 2004) (see Fig. 5.1). Sometimes the cortex is relatively spared owing to good pial collaterals or rapid recanalization of the occluded artery, and infarction is largely subcortical in the distribution of several lenticulostriate arteries. This may be seen as a characteristic area of "striatocapsular infarction" on brain imaging (Fig. 9.1). This clinical syndrome is not as severe as a total anterior circulation syndrome, having less cognitive deficit and often being without homonymous hemianopia (Nicolai *et al.* 1996).

Partial Anterior Circulation Syndrome

A lobar hemorrhage, or a cortical infarct, causes a more restricted clinical syndrome (Bassetti *et al.* 1993; Aerden *et al.* 2004):

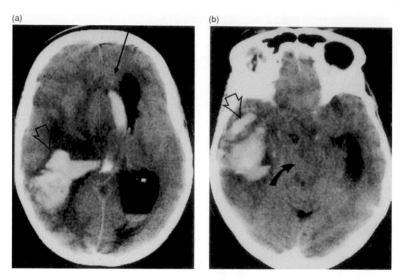

Fig. 9.2 Large intracerebral hematoma with mass effect.

- any two of the following three components of a total anterior circulation syndrome: hemiparesis or hemiplegia contralateral to hemispheric lesion, homonymous visual field defect, and cortical deficit (dysphasia, neglect, or visuospatial problems); or
- motor/sensory deficit restricted to one body area or part of one body area; or
- isolated cortical deficit such as dysphasia.

It may be difficult to distinguish between some partial anterior circulation syndromes and a "lacunar" stroke.

Partial anterior circulation infarcts (Fig. 9.3) are caused by occlusion of a branch of the middle cerebral artery or rarely the trunk of the anterior cerebral artery. They are usually a consequence of embolism from the heart or proximal atherothrombosis as in total anterior circulation infarcts. Investigation should be prompt because of the high risk of recurrence. Anterior cerebral artery infarcts cause contralateral weakness predominantly of the lower limb, sometimes with cortical sensory loss, and aphasia if in the dominant hemisphere. Left and rarely right anterior cerebral artery infarcts can cause a curious dyspraxia of the left upper limb owing to infarction of the corpus callosum disconnecting the right motor centers from the left language centers (Kazui et al. 1992). Bilateral leg and even additional bilateral arm weakness has been described when both anterior cerebral arteries are supplied from one stenosed internal carotid artery or if both anterior cerebral arteries are occluded by embolism, so mimicking a brainstem or spinal cord syndrome (Borggreve et al. 1994).

Some anterior circulation syndromes, usually classified as partial anterior circulation syndromes, are caused by boundary zone infarcts. The rare anterior choroidal artery distribution infarcts, which can be defined only by the CT or MRI pattern, are probably caused by large artery atherosclerosis or cardio-embolism, and they can lead to a partial anterior circulation syndrome or lacunar syndrome (Leys et al. 1994).

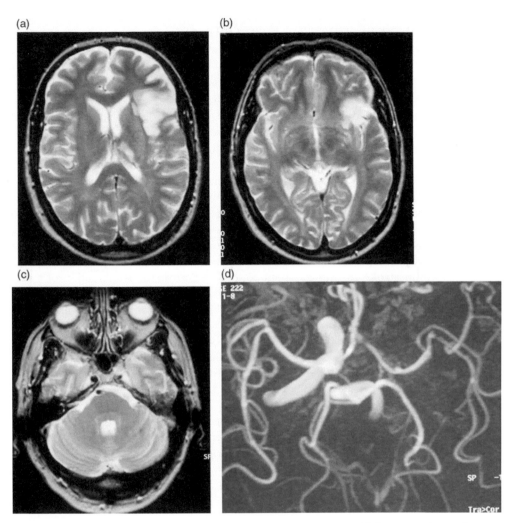

Fig. 9.3 Axial T_2-weighted MRI scans (a–c) and a magnetic resonance angiogram (d) showing a right partial anterior circulation infarct secondary to right carotid occlusion.

Lacunar Syndrome

Lacunar syndromes are defined clinically. They are highly predictive of small, deep lesions affecting the motor and/or sensory pathways in the corona radiata, internal capsule, thalamus, cerebral peduncle, or pons. Although a few patients have a partial anterior circulation infarct (Bamford *et al.* 1987; Anzalone and Landi 1989; Arboix *et al.* 2007), the great majority have small infarcts, which are sometimes visible on CT, more often on MRI. These are caused by presumed occlusion of a small perforating artery affected by intracranial small vessel disease (see Fig. 10.3). There is no visual field defect, no new cortical defect, no impairment of consciousness, and nothing to suggest a brainstem syndrome, for instance diplopia or crossed motor and sensory deficits.

The four main lacunar syndromes are:

- pure motor deficit: involving two or three of the areas face, arm, and leg.
- pure sensory deficit: involving two or three of the areas face, arm, and leg.
- sensorimotor deficit.
- ataxic hemiparesis (hemiparesis with ipsilateral cerebellar ataxia).

Pure motor stroke constitutes about 50% of lacunar stroke cases. It consists of a unilateral motor deficit involving two or three areas – the face, upper arm, and/or leg – including the whole of each area that is affected. There are often sensory symptoms but no sensory signs. The lesion occurs at locations where the motor pathways are closely packed together and separate from other pathways: usually in the internal capsule or pons, sometimes in the corona radiata or cerebral peduncle, and rarely in the medullary pyramid. There may be a flurry of immediately preceding TIAs, the so-called capsular warning syndrome (Paul *et al.* 2012).

Pure sensory stroke constitutes about 5% of cases. It has the same distribution as pure motor stroke, but the symptoms are of sensory loss, with or without sensory signs affecting all modalities equally, or sparing proprioception. The lesion is usually in the thalamus (see Fig. 10.3) but can be in the brainstem.

Sensorimotor stroke constitutes about 35% of cases. It is the combination of a pure motor stroke with sensory signs in the affected body parts. The lesion is usually in the thalamus or internal capsule, but it can be in the corona radiata or pons. A similar clinical picture can be caused by cortical infarcts, leading to misclassification (Blecic *et al.* 1993).

Ataxic hemiparesis constitutes about 10% of cases. It is the combination of cortico-spinal and ipsilateral cerebellar-like dysfunction affecting the arm and/or leg. It includes a syndrome in which there is little more than dysarthria and one clumsy hand. The lesion is usually in the pons, internal capsule, or cerebral peduncle. Dysarthria, with or without upper motor neuron facial weakness, may also be a lacunar syndrome with similar lesion localization as ataxic hemiparesis, but there are other localizing possibilities as well.

Small deep infarcts in the subcortical white matter of the corona radiata may result from small vessel disease affecting the long medullary perforating arteries extending down from cortical branches of the middle cerebral artery or from embolism. Such centrum semiovale infarcts present either as a lacunar syndrome or, occasionally, as a partial anterior circulation syndrome with "cortical" features (Read *et al.* 1998; Lammie and Wardlaw 1999). They are not, however, easy to classify or to distinguish from border zone infarcts deeper in the white matter lying between the arterial territories of the deep perforators from the first part of the middle cerebral artery and the superficial medullary perforators.

Various other lacunar syndromes have been described with rather poor clinical–pathological–anatomical correlation; for example, chorea or hemiballismus usually appears to be caused by a lesion in the contralateral subthalamic nucleus or elsewhere in the basal ganglia and tends to get better (Ghika and Bogousslavsky 2001).

Posterior Circulation Syndrome

Brainstem, cerebellar, thalamic, or occipital lobe signs normally indicate infarction in the distribution of the vertebrobasilar circulation or a localized hemorrhage.

The posterior circulation syndrome consists of any one of the following:

- motor and/or sensory deficit and cranial nerve palsy.
- bilateral motor and/or sensory deficit.
- deficit of conjugate eye movement.

- cerebellar deficit.
- isolated hemianopia or cortical blindness.

A combination of brainstem and occipital lobe signs is highly suggestive of infarction caused by thromboembolism within the basilar and posterior cerebral artery territories. Occasionally, proximal posterior cerebral artery occlusion causes extensive temporal, thalamic, and perhaps midbrain infarction. This results in contralateral hemiparesis and sensory loss and a marked cognitive deficit such as aphasia as well as the expected homonymous hemianopia. This syndrome may be confused with occlusion of the middle cerebral artery or one of its branches (Argentino *et al.* 1996). This is the so-called "walking total anterior circulation syndrome" because although it fulfills the definition of a total anterior circulation syndrome, the motor loss is occasionally mild. Cerebellar hematomas have fairly characteristic clinical features except in the case of massive hemorrhage, which is clinically indistinguishable from a brainstem stroke, and very small hemorrhages, which may simulate a peripheral disorder of the vestibular system (Jensen and St. Louis 2005).

The causes of infarction in the vertebrobasilar territory are heterogeneous. Often they are difficult to establish since vertebral angiography is seldom carried out, although noninvasive arterial imaging is increasingly helpful. Some lacunar syndromes result from small brainstem or thalamic infarcts following small vessel occlusion: intracranial small vessel disease or atheroma at the mouth of small perforating arteries. However, both small and large infarcts can be caused by embolism from the heart by atherothrombosis, affecting the vertebral and basilar arteries; thrombotic occlusion complicating atheroma of the basilar artery or its major branches; or low flow distal to vertebral and other arterial occlusions.

Although a large number of posterior circulation syndromes have been described, there is no clear association with a unique pattern of arterial occlusion or with prognosis. Syndromes include the "top of the basilar" syndrome (Caplan 1980), various other midbrain syndromes (Bogousslavsky *et al.* 1994), the locked-in syndrome (Patterson and Grabois 1986), pontine syndromes (Bassetti *et al.* 1996), lateral medullary syndromes (Kim *et al.* 1998), and medial medullary syndromes (Bassetti *et al.* 1997). Recognition of these is more an exercise in clinical–anatomical correlation rather than being very useful for clinical management. Because thalamic and cerebellar strokes can cause diagnostic confusion and the latter may require surgical treatment, they are given separate consideration later.

Thalamic Stroke

Small thalamic lesions may cause a pure sensory stroke or sensorimotor stroke, sometimes with ataxia in the same limbs (Schmahmann 2003). However, other deficits may occur in isolation or in combination depending on which thalamic nuclei are involved. These include paralysis of upward gaze, small pupils, apathy, depressed consciousness, hypersomnolence, disorientation, visual hallucinations, aphasia and impairment of verbal memory attributable to the left thalamus, and visuospatial dysfunction attributable to the right thalamus. Occlusion of a single small branch of the proximal posterior cerebral artery (artery of Percheron) in individuals with this anatomical variant can cause bilateral paramedian thalamic infarction with severe retrograde and anterograde amnesia.

Thalamic stroke should be considered when there is a sudden onset of behavioral disturbance. The diagnosis is often missed since patients are thought to have primary psychiatric disorders, especially when neurological dysfunction is lacking. Distinct behavioral patterns can be delineated on the basis of the four main arterial thalamic territories (Schmahmann 2003; Carrera and Bogousslavsky 2006):

- the anterior pattern consists mainly of perseverations, apathy, and amnesia.
- paramedian infarction causes disinhibition and personality change, amnesia, and, in the case of extensive lesions, thalamic "dementia."
- in inferolateral lesions, executive dysfunction may develop but is often overlooked, although it may occasionally lead to severe long-term disability.
- posterior lesions are known to cause cognitive dysfunction, including neglect and aphasia, but no specific behavioral syndrome has been reported.

Cerebellar Strokes

Cerebellar strokes can be mild, with sudden vertigo, nausea, imbalance, and horizontal nystagmus, which soon recover. They are frequently misdiagnosed as labyrinthitis. More extensive infarction or hemorrhage causes additional ipsilateral limb and truncal ataxia as well as dysarthria. Very severe strokes cause occipital headache, vomiting, and depressed consciousness, making it difficult to detect limb or truncal ataxia. There are often additional brainstem signs such as ipsilateral facial weakness and sensory loss, a gaze palsy to the side of the lesion, ipsilateral deafness and tinnitus, and bilateral extensor plantar responses. These occur because of pressure from a large edematous infarct or hematoma or because an occluded artery supplying the cerebellum may also supply parts of the brainstem. Mass effect can obstruct flow of cerebrospinal fluid from the fourth ventricle, causing acute or subacute hydrocephalus. The consequent coma and meningism may be mistaken for subarachnoid hemorrhage. A CT scan will reveal a hematoma, but the signs of an infarct are more subtle, with disappearance or shift of the fourth ventricle owing to mass effect before the low density of the lesion itself appears. Magnetic resonance is more sensitive in infarction and provides detail of any additional brainstem involvement. It should be noted that initial mild symptoms may be misleading and patients may deteriorate rapidly. Accordingly, urgent brain imaging is mandatory in suspected cerebellar stroke, irrespective of apparent clinical severity.

Patients who become acutely or subacutely comatosed have a very poor prognosis. However, if there is little evidence of primary brainstem infarction, drainage of any hydrocephalus and/or decompression of the posterior fossa may sometimes be followed by relatively good-quality survival.

Boundary Zone Infarcts

Boundary zone infarcts occur in the border zones *between* arterial territories:

- anterior boundary zone: between the superficial territories of the middle cerebral artery and anterior cerebral artery in the frontoparasagittal region.
- posterior boundary zone: between the superficial territories of the middle cerebral artery and posterior cerebral artery in the parieto-occipital region.
- subcortical boundary zone: between the superficial medullary penetrators and deep lenticulostriate territories of the middle cerebral artery in the paraventricular white matter of the corona radiation.

There is evidence that both low flow and microembolism may be important in causing boundary zone infarction (Momjian-Mayor and Baron 2005). The evidence strongly favors a hemodynamic mechanism for internal boundary zone infarction, especially in the centrum semiovale. However, the relationship between cortical boundary zone infarction and hemodynamic compromise appears more complicated, and artery-to-artery embolism may play an important role. Based on the high prevalence of microembolic signals documented by ultrasound in symptomatic carotid disease, embolism and hypoperfusion may play a synergistic role, with small emboli lodging in distal field arterioles being more likely to result in cortical microinfarcts when chronic hypoperfusion prevails. Future studies combining imaging of brain perfusion, diffusion-weighted imaging, and ultrasound detection of microembolic signals should help to resolve these issues.

Low flow may occur secondary to systemic hypotension, as during cardiac arrest. This results in bilateral infarcts, usually in the posterior boundary zones, and causes cortical blindness, visual disorientation and agnosia, and amnesia. Alternatively, a relatively small fall in systemic blood pressure in the presence of internal carotid occlusion or stenosis may cause unilateral boundary zone infarction, usually in the anterior and subcortical regions. This causes contralateral weakness of the leg more than the arm, with sparing of the face, some impaired sensation in the same areas, and aphasia if the dominant hemisphere is affected. Unilateral posterior boundary zone infarcts are less common and cause contralateral hemianopia and cortical sensory loss, along with aphasia if the dominant hemisphere is affected.

Miscellaneous Clinical Features

Cranial Nerves

Unilateral supratentorial stroke lesions can cause contralateral weakness of the bulbar muscles, with unilateral weakness of the palate, tongue, and forehead musculature, resembling a lower motor-neuron rather than upper motor-neuron facial palsy. Because all these muscles have a strong *bilateral* upper motor-neuron innervation, this weakness tends to disappear quite quickly in most cases. The bulbar muscle weakness may be enough to cause significant dysphagia; therefore, dysphagia is not a symptom exclusively confined to brainstem strokes. Dysarthria is common in supratentorial strokes, usually in proportion to any facial weakness, and is a defining feature of the clumsy hand–dysarthria syndrome, but it can be isolated with no localizing value (Ichikawa and Kageyama 1991). Any weakness of the sternomastoid muscle is ipsilateral to a supratentorial lesion, so there is difficulty turning the head away from the side of the lesion. Lower cranial nerve lesions ipsilateral to a supratentorial infarct suggest dissection of the internal carotid artery. Lesions of cranial nerves III, IV, and VI have rarely been described ipsilateral to internal carotid artery occlusion or dissection, presumably caused by ischemia of the nerve trunks.

Headache

Headache is not uncommon around the time of stroke onset. It is more often severe in primary intracerebral hemorrhage than ischemic stroke and more often severe with posterior than anterior circulation strokes. If the headache is localized at all, it tends to be over the site of the lesion. Headache is more common in cortical and posterior circulation than lacunar infarcts (Kumral *et al.* 1995). Severe unilateral neck, orbital, or scalp pain suggests internal carotid artery dissection, particularly if there is an ipsilateral Horner's syndrome. Severe occipital headache can occur with vertebral artery dissection. Headache is also a particular feature of venous infarcts. Unusual headache in the days before stroke would suggest giant cell arteritis or perhaps a mass lesion rather than a stroke.

Movement Disorders

Acute hemiparkinsonism contralateral to a basal ganglia stroke is rare. Contralateral chorea, hemiballismus, and sometimes tremor or dystonia are more common (D'Olhaberriague *et al.* 1995; Scott and Jankovic 1996; Giroud *et al.* 1997). Dystonia often develops gradually in a hemiplegic limb some weeks after the stroke, particularly in children and young adults. Rather nondescript "limb-shaking" has been described in patients with "low flow" TIA and can occur in stroke, particularly in brainstem infarction.

Determining the Cause of the Stroke: Pathophysiological Mechanism

The four main classifications described previously (Bamford *et al.* 1991; Mead *et al.* 1999) are clinical and can be determined at the bedside and following the results of brain imaging. Further classification is possible in ischemic stroke by etiology, and this is most commonly done according to the TOAST (Trial of ORG 10172 in Acute Stroke Treatment) criteria.

TOAST Classification

The TOAST system attempts to classify ischemic strokes according to the major causative pathophysiological mechanisms. It assigns ischemic strokes to five subtypes based upon clinical features and the results of investigations including brain and vascular imaging, cardiac tests, and laboratory tests for a prothrombotic state (Adams *et al.* 1993). It was originally developed in a clinical trial of heparin (Trial of ORG 10172) but has been used extensively in both research and clinical practice and has been modified only slightly since its first description in 1993 (Adams *et al.* 1993; Ay *et al.* 2005).

The five TOAST subtypes of ischemic stroke are:

- large artery atherosclerosis.
- cardioembolism.
- small vessel occlusion.
- stroke of other determined etiology.
- stroke of undetermined etiology.

Large artery atherosclerosis is confirmed by the presence of brain or vascular imaging findings of either significant stenosis (> 50%) or occlusion of a major brain artery or branch cortical artery, presumably through atherosclerosis. Cortical, cerebellar, brainstem, or large subcortical lesions on CT or MRI are supportive of the diagnosis, as are symptoms or signs of large artery disease elsewhere.

For cardioembolic stroke, the most frequent sources of cardioembolism (Chapter 6) are:

- atrial fibrillation.
- a mechanical prosthetic valve.
- mitral stenosis.
- left atrial or left ventricular thrombus.
- recent myocardial infarction.
- dilated cardiomyopathy.

- infective endocarditis.

The small vessel occlusion category corresponds to the lacunar syndrome described by Bamford *et al.* (1991) and is supported by normal brain imaging or a relevant subcortical or brainstem infarct measuring < 1.5 cm.

"Other determined etiologies" include non-atherosclerotic vasculopathies, hypercoagulable states, and hematological disorders.

Stroke of undetermined etiology includes those in which evaluation has been inadequate, adequate evaluation has not revealed a cause ("cryptogenic stroke"), and those in which two or more potential causes have been identified (for instance a patient who has atrial fibrillation and an ipsilateral carotid stenosis of 60% or a patient with a traditional lacunar syndrome and an ipsilateral carotid stenosis of 60%).

Some overlap exists between the clinical classification (Bamford *et al.* 1991) and the etiological TOAST classification. In a large hospital-based series of patients with ischemic stroke, total and partial anterior circulation infarcts were most likely to be caused by large artery atherosclerosis, cardioembolism or both (Wardlaw *et al.* 1999).

Determining the Cause of the Stroke: Clues from the History

In the vast majority of strokes, there is the sudden onset of focal symptoms without any other features. However, it is important to take a detailed history since occasionally there may be a more gradual onset of symptoms, thus widening the differential diagnosis, or there may be points in the history suggesting an underlying cause for the stroke or an indication that the presentation is of a condition mimicking stroke (Table 9.1).

Gradual Onset

Gradual onset of stroke over hours or days, rather than seconds or minutes, is unusual and is much more likely to occur in ischemic than in hemorrhagic stroke. If the onset is gradual and not likely to be caused by low flow or migraine (Chapter 8), then a structural intracranial lesion must be excluded. In younger patients, multiple sclerosis should also be considered. However, focal neurological deficits that develop over hours or up to 2 days in elderly patients are still most likely to have a vascular cause since vascular disease is so common in older patients.

Precipitating Factors

The activity being undertaken at stroke onset and the time of onset may both be important. Anything to suggest a fall in cerebral perfusion or blood pressure may be relevant, as is pregnancy and any operative procedure. Activities affecting head position or head and neck trauma (see Chapter 6) may indicate dissection. Recurrent attacks first thing in the morning or during exercise suggest hypoglycemia (may be the presenting feature of insulinoma or related to drugs such as pentamidine as well as diabetes). Onset during a Valsalva maneuver such as lifting suggests a low-flow ischemic stroke or paradoxical embolism (Chapter 6).

Headache

Headache at around the onset of ischemic stroke or TIA occurs in about 25% of patients, is usually mild, and, if localized at all, tends to be related to the position of the brain or eye

Table 9.1 Important clues from the history that may suggest the cause of an ischemic stroke or that the diagnosis of cerebrovascular disease should be reconsidered

Type	Features
Gradual onset	Low cerebral blood flow without acute occlusion (Chapter 6) Migraine (Chapter 8) Structural intracranial lesion (Chapters 8 and 9) Multiple sclerosis
Precipitating factors	Suspected systemic hypotension or low cerebral perfusion pressure (standing up or sitting up quickly, heavy meal, hot weather, hot bath, warming the face, exercise, coughing, hyperventilation, chest pain or palpitations, starting or changing blood pressure–lowering drugs) Pregnancy/puerperium Surgery Head turning Hypoglycemia Valsalva maneuver (paradoxical embolism, or low flow)
Recent headache	Carotid/vertebral dissection (Chapter 6) Migrainous stroke/transient ischemic attack (Chapter 8) Intracranial venous thrombosis (Chapter 29) Giant cell arteritis (or other inflammatory vascular disorders) (Chapter 6) Structural intracranial lesion (Chapters 8 and 9)
Epileptic seizures	Intracranial venous thrombosis (Chapter 29) Mitochondrial diseases (Chapter 6) Non-vascular intracranial lesion (Chapters 8 and 9)
Malaise	Inflammatory arterial disorders (Chapter 6) Infective endocarditis (Chapter 6) Cardiac myxoma (Chapter 6) Cancer (Chapter 6) Thrombotic thrombocytopenic purpura (Chapter 6) Sarcoidosis (Chapter 6)
Chest pain	Myocardial infarction Aortic dissection Paradoxical embolism (Chapter 6)
Non-stroke vascular disease or vascular risk factors	Ischemic heart disease (Chapter 2) Claudication (Chapter 2) Hypertension (Chapter 2) Smoking (Chapter 2)
Drugs	Oral contraceptives (Chapter 2) Estrogens in men (Chapter 2) Blood pressure-lowering/vasodilators (Chapter 6) Hypoglycemic drugs (Chapter 6) Cocaine, ecstasy (Chapter 6) Amphetamines (Chapter 6) Ephedrine (Chapter 6)

Table 9.1 (cont.)

Type	Features
	Phenylpropanolamine (Chapter 6)
	Atypical antipsychotic drugs
Injury	Chronic subdural hematoma (Chapter 7)
	Vertebral/carotid artery dissection (Chapter 6)
	Fat embolism (Chapter 6)
Self-audible bruits	Internal carotid artery stenosis (distal)
	Dural arteriovenous fistula (Chapter 7)
	Glomus tumor
	Caroticocavernous fistula (Chapter 7)
	Raised intracranial pressure
	Intracranial venous thrombosis (Chapter 29)
Past medical history	Inflammatory bowel disease (Chapter 6)
	Celiac disease (Chapter 6)
	Homocystinuria (Chapter 6)
	Cancer (Chapter 6)
	Irradiation of the head or neck (Chapter 6)
	Recurrent deep venous thrombosis
	Recurrent miscarriages
	Recent surgery/long-distance travel
Family history	
(Table 3.2)	

lesion. It is more common with ischemia in the vertebrobasilar than carotid distribution and is less common with lacunar ischemia. Severe pain unilaterally in the head, face, neck, or eye at around or before the time of stroke onset is highly suggestive of carotid dissection, while vertebral dissection tends to cause unilateral or sometimes bilateral occipital pain (Chapter 6). Migrainous stroke may be accompanied by headache (Chapters 6 and 8), and patients with cerebral autosomal dominant arteriopathy with subcortical infarcts and leukoencephalopathy (CADASIL) usually have a history of migraine. In the context of the differential diagnosis of TIAs, migraine should be fairly obvious, unless there is no headache (Chapter 8). It is important to note that vertebrobasilar ischemia may cause similar symptoms to migraine with headache, with gradual onset of focal neurological symptoms and visual disturbances.

Although intracranial venous thrombosis usually causes either a benign intracranial hypertension syndrome or a subacute encephalopathy, sometimes the onset is focal. The diagnosis may be suggested by headache, which occurs in the majority of patients (around 75%) (Chapter 29). Stroke (or TIA) in the context of a headache occurring for days or weeks previously must raise the possibility of giant cell arteritis and other inflammatory vascular disorders (Chapter 6). Pain in the jaw muscles with chewing, which resolves with rest, strongly suggests claudication, caused more frequently by giant cell arteritis than atherothrombosis of the external carotid artery.

Epileptic Seizures

Epileptic seizures, partial or generalized, within hours of stroke onset are unusual in adults (5%) and should lead to a reconsideration of non-stroke brain pathologies, particularly since contrast enhancement of a tumor on CT can be misinterpreted as an infarct. The risk of seizure is higher with hemorrhagic than ischemic strokes and if the lesion is large and involves the cerebral cortex (Arboix *et al.* 2003). Seizures are common in venous infarction (up to 40%) and mitochondrial cytopathy. Partial motor seizures can be confused with limb-shaking TIAs (Chapter 8), but the former are more clonic and the jerking spreads in a typical Jacksonian way from one body part to another and the latter are supposed never to involve the face. Rarely, transient focal ischemia seems to cause partial epileptic seizures, but proving a causal relationship is seldom possible (Kaplan 1993). Interestingly, onset of idiopathic seizures late in life is a powerful independent predictor of subsequent stroke (Cleary *et al.* 2004) and of dementia after stroke (Cordonnier *et al.* 2007). Seizures preceded by malaise, headache, and fever suggest encephalitis.

Malaise

Stroke in the context of preceding malaise for up to some months suggests an inflammatory arterial disorder, particularly giant cell arteritis, infective endocarditis, cardiac myxoma, cancer, thrombotic thrombocytopenic purpura, or even sarcoidosis (Chapter 6).

Chest Pain

Chest pain may be indicative of a recent myocardial infarction complicated with stroke, aortic dissection (particularly if the pain is also interscapular), or pulmonary embolism and raises the possibility of paradoxical embolism.

Vascular Risk Factors

Vascular risk factors (Chapter 2) and diseases should be sought. It is unusual for an ischemic stroke or TIA to occur in someone with no vascular risk factors, unless they are very old or are young with some unusual cause of stroke (Chapter 6). A history of heart disease may be relevant, and cardiac symptoms should be specifically inquired about.

Drugs

Drugs may be relevant: oral contraceptives in women, estrogens in men, hypotensive agents, hypoglycemic agents, and recreational drugs.

Injury

Any injury in the days and weeks before ischemic stroke or TIA onset is important and may not be spontaneously volunteered by the patient particularly where this occurred some time previously. A head or neck injury might have caused a chronic subdural hematoma (highly unlikely if more than 3 months previously) or carotid or vertebral dissection (Chapter 6).

Self-Audible Bruits

Pulsatile self-audible bruits are rare. They can be differentiated from tinnitus because they are in time with the pulse. They may be audible to the examiner on auscultation of the neck, eye, or cranium and may indicate:

- distal internal carotid artery stenosis (dissection or, rarely, atherothrombosis).
- dural arteriovenous fistula near the petrous temporal bone.
- glomus tumor.
- caroticocavernous fistula.
- intracranial venous thrombosis.
- symptomatic and idiopathic intracranial hypertension.
- loop in the internal carotid artery.

Past Medical History

Recurrent deep venous thrombosis suggests thrombophilia, particularly if there is a family history, or antiphospholipid syndrome, the latter being suggested by the accompanying feature of recurrent miscarriages. Any reason for a recent deep vein thrombosis (e.g., a long-haul flight or surgery) should raise the question of paradoxical embolism. Past medical history of a condition predisposing to stroke (Chapters 2, 3, and 6) may be present.

Previous Strokes and/or Transient Ischemic Attacks

Previous strokes and/or TIAs in different vascular territories are more likely with a proximal embolic source in the heart or arch of the aorta than with a single arterial lesion. Attacks going back months or more make certain causes such as infective endocarditis and arterial dissection unlikely.

Family History

There are several rare familial conditions that may be complicated by ischemic stroke and TIAs (Table 3.4). However, family history of stroke is only a modest risk factor for sporadic ischemic stroke (Flossmann and Rothwell 2004), and a family history of stroke is associated with little or no increased risk of future stroke (Flossmann and Rothwell 2005, 2006) (Chapter 3).

Determining the Cause of Stroke: Clues from the Examination

Similar to a detailed history, careful clinical examination of the patient with suspected stroke may provide clues to the underlying cause of the stroke (Table 9.1).

Neurological Examination

Neurological examination is primarily to localize the brain lesion, but there may also be clues as to the cause of the stroke: a Horner's syndrome ipsilateral to a carotid distribution infarct suggests dissection of the internal carotid artery or sometimes acute atherothrombotic carotid occlusion. Lower cranial nerve lesions ipsilateral to a hemispheric cerebral infarct can also occur in carotid dissection.

Total anterior circulation syndromes or brainstem strokes often cause some drowsiness, but in smaller lesions, consciousness is normal. Therefore, if consciousness is impaired and yet the focal deficit is mild, it is important to:

- reconsider the differential diagnosis (particularly chronic subdural hematoma).
- consider the diffuse encephalopathic disorders that have focal features and that may masquerade as stroke, for example cerebral vasculitis, non-bacterial thrombotic endocarditis, intracranial venous thrombosis, mitochondrial cytopathy, thrombotic thrombocytopenic purpura, familial hemiplegic migraine, and Hashimoto's encephalitis.
- be aware that comorbidity, such as pneumonia, sedative drugs, infection, and hypoglycemia, may exacerbate the neurological deficit.

Eyes

The eyes may provide general clues to the cause of a stroke (e.g., diabetic or hypertensive retinopathy) or may reveal papilledema, which would make the diagnosis of ischemic stroke or even intracerebral hemorrhage most unlikely. There may be evidence of retinal emboli, which are often asymptomatic. Roth spots in the retina are very suggestive of infective endocarditis. Dislocated lenses should suggest Marfan's syndrome or homocystinuria. Angioid streaks in the retina suggest pseudoxanthoma elasticum, and in hyperviscosity syndromes there is a characteristic retinopathy.

Dilated episcleral vessels are a clue to abnormal anastamoses between branches of the external carotid artery and orbital branches of the internal carotid artery, distal to severe internal carotid artery disease. With extreme ischemia, ischemic oculopathy may develop, with impaired visual acuity, eye pain, rubeosis of the iris (dilated blood vessels), fixed dilated pupil, "low-pressure" glaucoma, cataract, and corneal edema.

Arterial Pulses

Both radial pulses should be examined simultaneously since inequality in timing or volume suggests subclavian or innominate stenosis or occlusion and, importantly, aortic dissection.

Tenderness of the branches of the external carotid artery (occipital, facial, superficial temporal) points toward giant cell arteritis. Tenderness of the common carotid artery in the neck can occur in acute carotid occlusion but is more likely to be a sign of dissection or arteritis. Absence of several neck and arm pulses in a young person may occur in Takayasu's arteritis (Chapter 6). Delayed or absent leg pulses suggest coarctation of the aorta or, much more commonly, peripheral vascular disease. Other causes of widespread disease of the aortic arch are atheroma, giant cell arteritis, syphilis, subintimal fibrosis, arterial dissection, and trauma. The prevalence of abdominal aortic aneurysms in patients with stroke and TIA is high with one study showing up to 11% of men aged 59 years or older with TIA /stroke having subclinical abdominal aortic aneurysms on ultrasound screening (van Lindert et al. 2009).

Cervical Bruits

A localized bruit over the carotid bifurcation (under the jaw) is predictive of some degree of carotid stenosis, but very tight stenosis or occlusion may not cause a bruit at all. Bruits may be asymptomatic, particularly in women, probably owing to sex differences in carotid bifurcation anatomy (Schulz and Rothwell 2001) and less likely to be associated with carotid stenosis.

Cardiac Examination

Thorough cardiac examination should look for possible cardiac source of embolism, including atrial fibrillation, mitral stenosis, and prosthetic heart valves. Left ventricular hypertrophy suggests hypertension or aortic stenosis, and a displaced apex from a dilated left ventricle indicates underlying cardiac or valvular pathology.

Fever

Fever is unusual in the first few hours after stroke onset, and endocarditis or other infections, inflammatory vascular disorders, or cardiac myxoma should be considered. Later fever is quite common and usually reflects a complication of the stroke (Chapter 16).

Other Indications

Clues as to the cause of a stroke may be obtained from examination of the skin and nails (Table 9.2).

Table 9.2 Clues to the cause of ischemic stroke/transient ischemic attack from examination of the skin and nails

Feature	Possible cause
Finger clubbing	Right-to-left intracardiac shunt Cancer (Chapter 6) Pulmonary arteriovenous malformation (Chapter 6) Infective endocarditis (Chapter 6) Inflammatory bowel disease (Chapter 6)
Splinter hemorrhages	Infective endocarditis (Chapter 6) Cholesterol embolization syndrome (Chapter 6) Vasculitis (Chapter 6)
Scleroderma	Systemic sclerosis (Chapter 6)
Livedo reticularis	Sneddon's syndrome (Chapter 6) Systemic lupus erythematosus (Chapter 6) Polyarteritis nodosa (Chapter 6) Cholesterol embolization syndrome (Chapter 6)
Lax skin	Ehlers–Danlos syndrome (Chapter 3) Pseudoxanthoma elasticum (Chapter 3)
Skin color	Anemia (Chapter 6) Polycythemia (Chapter 6) Cyanosis (right-to-left intracardiac shunt, pulmonary arteriovenous malformation) (Chapter 6)
Porcelain-white papules/scars	Kohlmeier–Degos disease (Chapter 6)
Skin scars	Ehlers–Danlos syndrome (Chapter 3)

Table 9.2 (cont.)

Feature	Possible cause
Petechiae/purpura/bruising	Thrombotic thrombocytopenic purpura (Chapter 6) Fat embolism (Chapter 6) Cholesterol embolization syndrome (Chapter 6) Ehlers–Danlos syndrome (Chapter 3)
Orogenital ulceration	Behçet's disease (Chapter 6)
Rash	Fabry's disease (Chapter 6) Systemic lupus erythematosus (Chapter 6) Tuberous sclerosis (Chapter 6)
Epidermal nevi	Epidermal nevus syndrome
Café-au-lait patches	Neurofibromatosis
Thrombosed superficial veins, needle marks	Intravenous drug use (Chapter 6)

References

Adams HP Jr., Bendixen BH, Kappelle LJ et al. (1993). Classification of subtype of acute ischemic stroke. Definitions for use in a multicenter clinical trial. TOAST. Trial of Org 10172 in Acute Stroke Treatment. *Stroke* **24**:35–41

Aerden L, Luijckx GJ, Ricci S et al. (2004). Validation of the Oxfordshire Community Stroke Project syndrome diagnosis derived from a standard symptom list in acute stroke. *Journal of Neurology Science* **220**:55–58

Anzalone N, Landi G (1989). Non ischaemic causes of lacunar syndromes: Prevalence and clinical findings. *Journal of Neurology, Neurosurgery and Psychiatry* **52**:1188–1190

Arboix, A, Comes, E, Garcia-Eroles et al. (2003). Prognostic value of very early seizures for in-hospital mortality in atherothrombotic infarction. *European Neurology* **50**:78–84

Arboix A, Garcia-Eroles L, Massons J et al. (2007). Haemorrhagic pure motor stroke. *European Journal of Neurology* **14**:219–223

Argentino C, De Michele M, Fiorelli M et al. (1996). Posterior circulation infarcts simulating anterior circulation stroke: Perspective of the acute phase. *Stroke* **27**:1306–1309

Ay H, Furie KL, Singhal A et al. (2005). An evidence-based causative classification system for acute ischemic stroke. *Annals of Neurology* **58**:688–697

Bamford J, Sandercock PAG, Jones L et al. (1987). The natural history of lacunar infarction: The Oxfordshire Community Stroke Project. *Stroke* **18**:545–551

Bamford J, Sandercock P, Dennis M et al. (1991). Classification and natural history of clinically identifiable subtypes of cerebral infarction. *Lancet* **337**:1521–1526

Bassetti C, Bogousslavsky J, Regli F (1993). Sensory syndromes in parietal stroke. *Neurology* **43**:1942–1949

Bassetti C, Bogousslavsky J, Barth A, Regli F (1996). Isolated infarcts of the pons. *Neurology* **46**:165–175

Bassetti C, Bogousslavsky J, Mattle H et al. (1997). Medial medullary stroke: Report of seven patients and review of the literature. *Neurology* **48**:882–890

Berlit P, Rakicky J, Tornow K (1991). Differential diagnosis of spontaneous and traumatic intracranial haemorrhage. *Journal of Neurology, Neurosurgery and Psychiatry* **54**:1118

Blecic SA, Bogousslavsky J, van Melle et al. (1993). Isolated sensorimotor stroke: A re-evaluation of clinical topographic and aetiological patterns. *Cerebrovascular Diseases* **3**:357–363

Bogousslavsky J, Maeder P, Regli F *et al.* (1994). Pure midbrain infarction: Clinical syndromes MRI and aetiologic patterns. *Neurology* 44:2032–2040

Borggreve F, de Deyn PP, Marien P *et al.* (1994). Bilateral infarction in the anterior cerebral artery vascular territory due to an unusual anomaly of the circle of Willis. *Stroke* 25:1279–1281

Brandt T, Steinke W, Thie A *et al.* (2000). Posterior cerebral artery territory infarcts: Clinical features, infarct topography, causes and outcome. Multicenter results and a review of the literature. *Cerebrovascular Diseases* 10:170–182

Caplan LR (1980). "Top of the basilar" syndrome. *Neurology* 30:72–79

Caplan LR (1993). Brain embolism revisited. *Neurology* 43:1281–1287

Carrera E, Bogousslavsky J (2006). The thalamus and behaviour: Effects of anatomically distinct strokes. *Neurology* 66:1817–1823

Cleary P, Shorvon S, Tallis R. (2004). Late-onset seizures as a predictor of subsequent stroke. *Lancet* 363:1184–1186

Cordonnier C, Hénon H, Derambure P *et al.* (2007). Early epileptic seizures after stroke are associated with increased risk of new-onset dementia. *Journal of Neurology, Neurosurgery and Psychiatry* 78:514–516

D'Olhaberriague L, Arboix A, Marti-Vilalta JL *et al.* (1995). Movement disorders in ischaemic stroke: Clinical study of 22 patients. *European Journal of Neurology* 2:553–557

Flossman E, Rothwell PM (2004). Systematic review of methods and results of studies of the genetic epidemiology of ischaemic stroke. *Stroke* 35:212–227

Flossmann E, Rothwell, PM (2005). Family history of stroke in patients with TIA in relation to hypertension and other intermediate phenotypes. *Stroke* 36:830–835

Flossmann E, Rothwell PM (2006). Family history of stroke does not predict risk of stroke after transient ischemic attack. *Stroke* 37:544–546

Georgiadis D, Oehler J, Schwarz S *et al.* (2004). Does acute occlusion of the carotid T invariably have a poor outcome? *Neurology* 63:22–26

Ghika J, Bogousslavsky J (2001). Abnormal movements. In *Stroke Syndromes* Bogousslavsky J, Caplan L (eds.), pp. 162–181. Cambridge, UK: Cambridge University Press

Giroud M, Lemesle M, Madinier G *et al.* (1997). Unilateral lenticular infarcts: Radiological and clinical syndromes, aetiology and prognosis. *Journal of Neurology, Neurosurgery and Psychiatry* 63:611–615

Hand PJ, Kwan J, Lindley RI *et al.* (2006). Distinguishing between stroke and mimic at the bedside: The brain attack study. *Stroke* 37:769–775

Ichikawa K, Kageyama Y (1991). Clinical anatomic study of pure dysarthria. *Stroke* 22:809–812

Jensen MB, St. Louis EK (2005). Management of acute cerebellar stroke. *Archives of Neurology* 62:537–544

Kaplan PW (1993). Focal seizures resembling transient ischaemic attacks due to subclinical ischaemia. *Cerebrovascular Diseases* 3:241–243

Kazui S, Sawada T, Naritomi H *et al.* (1992). Left unilateral ideomotor apraxia in ischaemic stroke within the territory of the anterior cerebral artery. *Cerebrovascular Diseases* 2:35–39

Kim JS, Lee JH, Choi CG (1998). Patterns of lateral medullary infarction. Vascular lesion: Magnetic resonance imaging correlation of 34 cases. *Stroke* 29:645–652

Kumral E, Bogousslavsky J, van Melle G *et al.* (1995). Headache at stroke onset: The Lausanne Stroke Registry. *Journal of Neurology, Neurosurgery and Psychiatry* 58:490–492

Lammie GA, Wardlaw JM (1999). Small centrum ovale infarcts: A pathological study. *Cerebrovascular Diseases* 9:82–90

Leys D, Mounier-Vehier F, Lavenu I *et al.* (1994). Anterior choroidal artery territory infarcts: Study of presumed mechanisms. *Stroke* 25:837–842

Lindgren A, Roijer A, Norrving B *et al.* (1994). Carotid artery and heart disease in subtypes of cerebral infarction. *Stroke* 25:2356–2362

Matsumoto H, Miki T, Miyaji Y *et al.* (2012). Spontaneous spinal epidural hematoma with hemiparesis mimicking acute cerebral infarction: Two case reports. *The Journal of Spinal Cord Medicine* **35**:262–266

Mead GE, Lewis SC, Wardlaw JM *et al.* (1999). Should CT appearance of lacunar stroke influence patient management? *Journal of Neurology, Neurosurgery and Psychiatry* **67**:682–684

Momjian-Mayor I, Baron JC (2005). The pathophysiology of watershed infarction in internal carotid artery disease: Review of cerebral perfusion studies. *Stroke* **36**:567–577

Nicolai A, Lazzarino LG, Biasutti E (1996). Large striatocapsular infarcts: Clinical features and risk factors. *Journal of Neurology* **243**:44–50

Nor AM, Davis J, Sen B *et al.* (2005). The Recognition of Stroke in the Emergency Room (ROSIER) scale: Development and validation of a stroke recognition instrument. *Lancet Neurology* **4**:727–734

Norris JW, Hachinski VC (1982). Misdiagnosis of stroke. *Lancet* **i**:328–331

Patterson JR, Grabois M (1986). Locked-in syndrome: A review of 139 cases. *Stroke* **17**:758–764

Paul NL, Simoni M, Chandratheva A *et al.* (2012). Population-based study of capsular warning syndrome and prognosis after early recurrent TIA. *Neurology* **79**:1356–1362

Pendlebury ST, Rothwell PM, Dalton A, Burton EA (2004). Strokelike presentation of Wilson's disease with homozygosity for a novel T766 R mutation. *Neurology* **63**:1982–1983

Read SJ, Pettigrew L, Schimmel L *et al.* (1998). White matter medullary infarcts: Acute subcortical infarction in the centrum ovale. *Cerebrovascular Diseases* **8**:289–295

Sandercock PAG, Molyneux A, Warlow C (1985). Value of computed tomography in patients with stroke: Oxfordshire Community Stroke Project. *British Medical Journal* **290**:193–197

Schmahmann JD (2003). Vascular syndromes of the thalamus. *Stroke* **34**:2264–2278

Schulz UG, Rothwell PM (2001). Major variation in carotid bifurcation anatomy: A possible risk factor for plaque development? *Stroke* **32**: 2522–2529

Scott BL, Jankovic J (1996). Delayed-onset progressive movement disorders after static brain lesions. *Neurology* **46**:68–74

van Lindert NH, Bienfait HP, Gratama JW *et al.* (2009). Screening for aneurysm of the abdominal aorta: Prevalence in patients with stroke or TIA. *European Journal of Neurology* **16**:602–607

Wardlaw JM, Merrick MV, Ferrington CM *et al.* (1996). Comparison of a simple isotope method of predicting likely middle cerebral artery occlusion with transcranial Doppler ultrasound in acute ischaemic stroke. *Cerebrovascular Diseases* **6**:32–39

Wardlaw JM, Lewsi SC, Dennis MS *et al.* (1999). Is it reasonable to assume a particular embolic source from the type of stroke? *Cerebrovascular Diseases* **9**(Suppl 1):14

Chapter 10

Brain Imaging in Transient Ischemic Attack and Minor Stroke

The main modalities for imaging the brain parenchyma are CT and MRI, and these are increasingly used to assess the cerebral vasculature in TIA and stroke. They differ in a number of technical aspects (Table 10.1). At present there is little consensus on optimal imaging strategies after TIA or minor stroke or indeed if imaging is required at all in some cases. The role of imaging differs from that in major stroke for a number of reasons. First, in patients with TIA or minor stroke, the likelihood of alternative, non-neurovascular diagnoses is higher than in patients with major stroke, and so imaging is important in identifying mimics. Second, minor stroke is less likely to be caused by hemorrhage than major stroke, and the risk is lower still in TIA, although it is not negligible (Gunatilake 1998; Werring *et al.* 2005; Kumar *et al.* 2016). Third, although there is little or no neurological deficit, the risk of recurrent and possibly severe ischemic events is high, and imaging has a role in identifying high-risk patients. In TIA and minor stroke, brain imaging is required to:

- exclude stroke mimics.
- differentiate between ischemic and hemorrhagic events.
- determine etiology, for example, carotid stenosis or cardioembolic source with lesions in multiple vascular territories.
- identify patients at high risk of early recurrent stroke in order to target suitable treatment.

The sensitivity and specificity of different imaging modalities vary with the pretest probability, the nature of the lesion in question, and the delay from event to imaging, while the availability of and expertise in imaging techniques will vary from center to center. When making decisions about imaging after TIA and minor stroke, the choice of imaging will depend on all these factors as well as patient safety, tolerability, and contraindications (Table 10.2).

The Identification of Non-Neurovascular Diagnoses

The most important mimics to identify with brain imaging after suspected TIA or minor stroke are subdural hematomas and brain tumors (see Figs. 7.4 and 8.1). The likelihood of these diagnoses will depend on the clinical setting. For example, high rates of non-vascular pathology have been reported in early studies conducted in specialist units before CT was widely available, where patients referred for imaging were highly selected (Weisberg and Nice 1977; Weisberg 1986). In cohorts of patients with suspected TIA who were referred directly for scanning by primary care physicians, prior to expert review by a stroke physician, rates of alternative diagnoses were also high, probably reflecting a high rate of pre-

Table 10.1 Technical aspects of imaging using computed tomography (CT) and magnetic resonance imaging (MRI)

Modality	Usage
CT	An X-ray tube rotates helically around the subject while an array of detectors opposite the tube measures the residual radiation that has passed through the body according to the density of local tissues to X-rays. Cross-sectional images are constructed using mathematical algorithms.
MRI	The subject is exposed to a strong external magnetic field, causing nuclei containing an odd number of neutrons or protons to align themselves within the field. When a pulse of radiofrequency energy of a particular frequency is applied, the protons are perturbed initially and then realign, producing a radiofrequency signal that is proportional to the surrounding "magnetic micro-environment". Radiofrequency signals are detected and processed to form an image; it provides better contrast between soft tissues than CT.
T_1-weighted	Sequence that demonstrates anatomy. Fluid (e.g., cerebrospinal fluid) has a low signal and appears black, while tissues with high fat content (e.g., subcutaneous tissues) has a high signal and appears bright. In the cerebral hemisphere, gray matter has a lower signal (appears gray) than white matter (appears white).
T_2-weighted	Sequence that demonstrates pathology. Fluid (e.g., cerebrospinal fluid) has a high signal and appears bright. Gray matter has an intermediate or slightly high signal, while white matter has a low signal.
Fluid attenuation inversion recovery (FLAIR)	Good to pick up cerebral edema and subarachnoid blood (appears bright in subarachnoid spaces). Can be T1 or T2 FLAIR. However, generally T_2 is used. The normally high signal of cerebrospinal fluid seen on T_2 is suppressed to a low signal and appears black.
T2*-gradient echo (GRE) or susceptibility weighted imaging (SWI)	Most sensitive to hemoglobin degradation products and detects hemorrhage, including microbleeds and cortical superficial siderosis
Diffusion weighted	Detects abnormalities caused by ischemia in the hyper-acute phase
Perfusion (CT or MR)	Quantifies the amount of contrast (exogenous or endogenous) reaching the brain tissue

imaging misdiagnosis (Lemesle *et al.* 1998). Low rates have been reported in retrospective case series, but these studies are likely not to have included patients in whom the initial diagnosis was changed in light of brain imaging results (Rolak *et al.* 1990; Douglas *et al.* 2003). Secondary prevention trials of aspirin in TIA and minor stroke have also reported very low numbers of patients subsequently shown to have non-vascular pathologies after randomization into the trials, but these studies did not report the number of patients with suspected TIAs who were scanned and excluded before randomization because a non-

Table 10.2 Advantages and disadvantages of computed tomography (CT) and magnetic resonance imaging (MRI) in minor stroke and transient ischemic attack

Modality	Advantages	Disadvantages
CT	Low cost and wide availability	Low sensitivity for small acute ischemic lesions
	Superior detection of hemorrhage in the early phase[a]	Low sensitivity for posterior fossa lesions Low sensitivity for mimics, especially early tumor Lacks spatial resolution to detect microbleeds and enlarged perivascular spaces Radiation exposure Intravenous contrast nephrotoxic and potentially allergenic
MRI	Superior sensitivity for small ischemic lesions, posterior fossa lesions, and stroke mimics	Patient tolerability and contraindications (e.g., non-MRI compatible pacemaker implants, recent surgery with metallic implant, claustrophobia)
	Superior spatial resolution to detect microbleeds and enlarged perivascular spaces	Risk of systemic nephrogenic fibrosis in patients with moderate-severe renal impairment receiving intravenous gadolinium contrast
	Provides prognostic information Superior detection of hemorrhage in the subacute and chronic phase[a]	

[a] Although pretest probability of hemorrhage is low in patients with a high clinical suspicion of transient ischemic attack or minor stroke.

vascular cause was identified (Dutch TIA Study Group 1993; UK TIA Study Group 1993). Finally, many studies have described relatively young cohorts, but the prevalence of non-vascular pathologies is likely to increase with age. Therefore, it is difficult to be either reassured by low rates of non-vascular pathology in cohorts diagnosed with TIA or convinced of the need for routine neuroimaging by high rates.

Brain Imaging after Transient Ischemic Attack and Minor Stroke: The Oxford Vascular Study (OXVASC)

The Oxford Vascular Study (OXVASC) is a population-based study in which all patients with suspected TIA or stroke are ascertained prospectively and reviewed by an experienced stroke physician who determines the probability of a vascular diagnosis before brain imaging. Events are described as definite, when the diagnosis is clearly neurovascular in origin, or possible, when an alternative explanation for the event could be found but a minor stroke or TIA could not be completely excluded on clinical grounds. This study has the

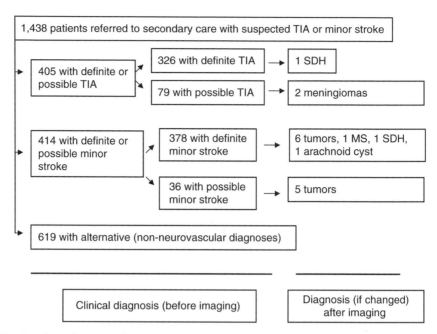

Fig. 10.1 Numbers of patients referred to the Oxford Vascular Study (OXVASC) between 2002 and 2007 with suspected transient ischemic attack (TIA) or minor stroke showing clinical diagnosis (before imaging) and revised diagnosis following brain imaging. SDH, subdural hematoma; MS, multiple sclerosis.

advantages that all patients are studied irrespective of whether they are referred to the clinic or hospital, pre-imaging diagnoses are reliably recorded and imaging is near complete.

During 2002–2007, 1,438 patients were referred either to the hospital or to the study clinic with a suspected TIA or minor stroke (defined on assessment as a score of ≤ 3 on the National Institutes of Health Stroke Scale [NIHSS]) (Wityk *et al.* 1994) (Fig. 10.1). Of these, a pre-scan diagnosis of definite or possible TIA was made in 405 patients (46% male, mean age 74 years) and definite or possible minor stroke in 414 patients (54% male, mean age 76 years). Overall, 97% underwent brain imaging for definite or possible events (699 CT, 93 MRI).

Of 326 patients with a clinical diagnosis of definite TIA, only one patient (0.3%; confidence interval [CI], 95% 0.1–1.7) was subsequently found to have symptomatic non-vascular pathology, a small subdural hematoma. Of 79 patients with a clinical diagnosis of possible TIA, two patients (2.5%; 95% CI, 0.7–8.8) were subsequently diagnosed with symptomatic non-vascular pathology, a meningioma in both cases.

Of 378 patients with a clinical diagnosis of definite minor stroke, there were nine (2.4%; 95% CI, 1.3–4.5) with non-vascular pathology (six intracranial tumors, one demyelination, one arachnoid cyst, one subdural hematoma). Possible minor stroke was diagnosed in thirty-six, and non-vascular pathology was identified in five (13.9%; 95% CI, 6.1–28.7), all of whom had intracranial tumors.

Importantly, of the eleven patients in total with intracranial tumors, five were not identified on initial non-contrast CT, and the correct diagnosis was made only after the patient deteriorated and repeat neuroimaging was performed. The yield of CT imaging for non-vascular pathology in patients with definite TIA or minor stroke is, therefore, low, and it is only slightly higher in possible events where additional clinical features such as seizure at the time of ictus or prominent confusion cast doubt on the pre-imaging diagnosis. Imaging with CT, therefore, does not add significantly to bedside assessment by an expert clinician, and MRI is recommended as first-line brain imaging in recent guidelines (Jauch *et al.* 2013; National Institute for Health and Clinical Excellence 2017). From 2010 onward, cerebral MRI and MR angiography of the intra- and extracranial vessels has since become the first-line imaging methods for all patients presenting to OXVASC with a TIA or minor stroke.

The Identification of Infarction and Hemorrhage

The rapid and accurate identification of intracerebral hemorrhage with brain imaging in patients with TIA or minor stroke is essential to direct timely, safe, and effective secondary prevention. For example, the misdiagnosis of a cerebral hemorrhage as an infarct may lead to a patient erroneously receiving antithrombotic or anticoagulant medication, with consequent increased risk of further hemorrhage, while a delay to rapid initiation of secondary preventive medication while imaging is awaited may expose a patient with an infarct to an unacceptably high risk of further ischemia. These scenarios are particularly relevant as the initiation of aspirin before brain imaging is recommended in some guidelines (National Institute for Health and Clinical Excellence 2017).

As mentioned previously, the sensitivity and specificity of different imaging modalities for infarction versus hemorrhage vary with pretest probability and delay from event to imaging. Acute primary intracerebral hemorrhage is seen on CT scanning as an area of well-defined hyperdensity. Soon, a surrounding area of low density appears that is attributable to edema, clot retraction, and infarction of the surrounding brain. The hemoglobin in the hematoma itself is broken down to oxyhemoglobin through deoxyhemoglobin and methemoglobin prior to red cell lysis and breakdown into ferritin and hemosiderin, causing the initial area of hyperdensity to become isodense and then hypodense, at which stage it becomes indistinguishable from an infarct (Fig. 11.1). When the volume of hemorrhage is small, as in minor stroke, the rate of change of imaging abnormalities is faster, and so the sensitivity of CT for hemorrhage diminishes more quickly with time (Fig. 10.2) (Dennis *et al.* 1987). In cases when there is a delay from event to imaging, MRI becomes more sensitive for the detection of hemorrhage than CT, although the exact timing of this process is not clear and will vary with size of hemorrhage. Decisions about choice of imaging modality should be made according to these factors and local availability and expertise.

Rates of Hemorrhage in Transient Ischemic Attack and Minor Stroke

The risk associated with a policy of "blind" treatment prior to imaging depends on the frequency of intracranial hemorrhage among patients with TIA or minor stroke. However, few published studies have reported this frequency.

One prospective study of consecutive patients (both inpatients and outpatients) presenting to a single center with mild stroke after a delay of more than 4 days reported imaging findings after both CT and MRI scanning were performed (Wardlaw *et al.* 2003). Among 228 patients scanned after a median delay of 20 days, primary intracerebral hemorrhage was identified by CT in two patients (0.9%; 95% CI, 0.1–3.1) and MRI in eight (3.5%; 95% CI, 1.5–6.8). Both hemorrhages identified by CT were identified on MRI. The study concluded with the recommendation that MRI was the modality of choice in patients with minor

Day 1   Day 3

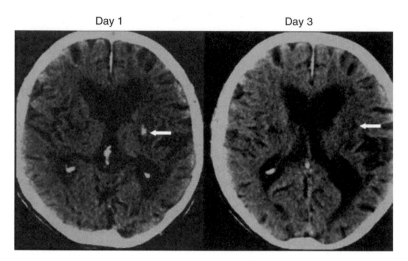

Fig. 10.2 These CT brain scans show a small hemorrhage in the left basal ganglia/internal capsule (arrow) visible as a hyperintense area on day 1 that has become hypodense by day 3.

stroke where there is a delay to imaging, owing to the unacceptable rate of misdiagnosis with CT. More recently, in a study composed of 3,207 patients with intracerebral hemorrhage, seventeen (0.53%) presented with rapidly resolving deficits resembling TIAs (Kumar *et al.* 2016). These results reinforce the importance of prompt brain imaging, even among patients with rapidly resolving stroke-like symptoms.

In the OXVASC cohort (2002–2007) of patients with probable or definite TIA or minor stroke, 699 were imaged with CT. Rates of infarction and hemorrhage detected with CT are listed in Table 10.3.

Among 334 patients with definite or possible minor stroke in OXVASC in whom hemorrhage could be detected reliably by either CT performed within 10 days or MRI (regardless of delay), primary hemorrhage was detected in seventeen (5.1%; 95% CI, 3. 2–8.0) and hemorrhagic transformation of an infarct in four (1.2%; 95% CI, 0.5–3.0).

Similar rates of primary intracerebral hemorrhage were reported in an unpublished study of consecutive patients with minor stroke attending a neurovascular clinic in Buckinghamshire, UK, who were all imaged with MRI on the day of attendance. Of 280 patients (59% male, mean age 72 years), primary intracerebral hemorrhage was detected in 15 (5.4%; 95% CI, 3.3–8.7) and hemorrhagic transformation in six (2.1%; 95% CI, 1. 0–4.6). The median delay to assessment and scanning was 15 days (interquartile range, 10–23).

In the OXVASC and Buckinghamshire neurovascular clinic cohorts of minor stroke patients, the clinical factors identified as being predictive of hemorrhage were blood pressure on initial assessment ≥ 180/110 mmHg, vomiting and confusion at onset, and premorbid anticoagulation. Headache was only very weakly predictive, and age was not predictive at all. In settings where access to MRI is limited and delays from event to presentation and imaging do occur, these factors might be used to identify patients with a high pretest probability of hemorrhage and in whom MRI imaging will have a higher positive yield.

Table 10.3 Rates of infarction, primary hemorrhage, or hemorrhagic infarction on CT scan among subjects with probable or definite transient ischemic attack or minor stroke in the Oxford Vascular Study (OXVASC)

Event	Appropriate infarction (%; 95% CI)	Primary hemorrhage or hemorrhagic infarction (%; 95% CI)
Transient ischemic attack		
Definite	10.1 (7.0–14.3)	0
Possible	3.0 (0.8–10.40)	0
Minor stroke		
Definite	40.4 (35.3–45.7)	5.9 (3.9–8.9)
Possible	19.2 (8.5–379)	3.9 (0.7–18.9)

Note: CI, confidence interval.

Microbleeds and Transient Ischemic Attack and Minor Stroke

Echo-planar gradient-echo T_2-weighted imaging (GRE) or susceptibility weighted imaging (SWI) MRI, which exploits the paramagnetic effects of deoxyhemoglobin, has a high sensitivity for detecting primary intracerebral hemorrhage. Studies comparing CT and GRE MRI for detection of hemorrhage in acute stroke show that GRE MRI is as good as or better than CT, particularly for small or chronic bleeds (Schellinger *et al.* 1999, 2007; Fiebach *et al.* 2004; Kidwell *et al.* 2004; Chalela *et al.* 2007). Use of GRE or SWI MRI has led to the increasing detection of apparently spontaneous cerebral microbleeds, which are small, round, homogeneous foci of low signal intensity (see Figs. 7.2 and 7.3). They were first described in the mid-1990s (Chan *et al.* 1996; Greenberg *et al.* 1996; Offenbacher *et al.* 1996) and have led to considerable research interest, although their pathological and clinical significance is still unclear (Chapter 7).

The few pathological data available indicate that cerebral microbleeds identified on MRI correspond to clusters of perivascular hemosiderin-laden macrophages, as a result of blood leakage from pathologically fragile small vessels affected by hypertensive or cerebral amyloid angiopathy (Fazekas *et al.* 1999; Cordonnier *et al.* 2007; Shoamanesh *et al.* 2011; Fisher 2014; van Veluw *et al.* 2016). They can also be secondary to an ischemic insult (Fisher 2014; van Veluw *et al.* 2016). Patients with hypertensive angiopathy tend to have "deep-seated" microbleeds located in the basal ganglia, thalamus, brainstem, and cerebellum (Fazekas *et al.* 1999), while cerebral microbleeds in patients with cerebral amyloid angiopathy tends to be of lobar distribution (Knudsen *et al.* 2001).

In a rigorous systematic review, microbleeds were found to be infrequent in "healthy adults", with a prevalence of 5.0% (95% CI, 3.9–6.2) pooled across four studies of 1,411 individuals, and more common in patients with ischemic stroke, with a prevalence of 33.5% (95% CI, 30.7–36.4) pooled across sixteen studies of 1,075 individuals. It should be noted that individual studies of ischemic stroke reported prevalences ranging from 12% to 71% (Cordonnier *et al.* 2007). In a cohort of 129 consecutive patients attending a neurovascular clinic, microbleeds were detected in 1/43 (2%) with TIA and 20/86 (23%) with stroke, although patients with TIA who had suffered a previous stroke were excluded (Werring *et al.* 2005). Given that the cohort was recruited from an outpatient setting, it is likely that the stroke patients included had suffered non-disabling strokes, although specific data on severity were not described. Data from OXVASC during 2004–2014 showed that microbleeds were detected in 63/572 (11%) of patients with TIA and 94/508 (18.7%) in patients with ischemic stroke.

Unpublished data from OXVASC demonstrated that among patients with TIA/ischemic stroke, microbleed burden is independently associated with a history of hypertension and renal impairment. Microbleeds are also strongly associated with other neuroimaging markers of small vessel disease such as white matter disease and enlarged basal-ganglia perivascular spaces. In TIA/ischemic stroke patients, presence of microbleeds is associated with a six-fold increased risk of intracerebral hemorrhage (Wilson *et al.* 2016; Lau *et al.* 2017). The risk of ICH increases steeply with burden of microbleeds, such that in those with ≥ 5 microbleeds, risk of ICH is twelvefold compared to those without microbleeds. In contrast, risk of recurrent ischemic stroke in patients with a high microbleed burden is more modest (2.5-fold increase in risk in patients with ≥ 5 microbleeds versus those without) (Wilson *et al.* 2016; Lau *et al.* 2017). The implications of use of antiplatelet agents, anticoagulants, and thrombolysis in TIA/ischemic stroke patients with microbleeds are discussed in Chapter 7.

Imaging: Diagnosis and Prognostication

Previous studies have demonstrated the usefulness of MRI in patients with suspected TIA, particularly diffusion-weighted imaging (DWI) (Figs. 10.3–10.9) (Schulz *et al.* 2003; Schulz *et al.* 2004). This modality relies on changes in the Brownian motion of water molecules to generate contrast. During early ischemia, there is decreased water proton movement caused by cytotoxic edema as water moves from the less-restricted extracellular environment into the more-restricted intracellular environment. Reduced proton diffusion leads to a bright,

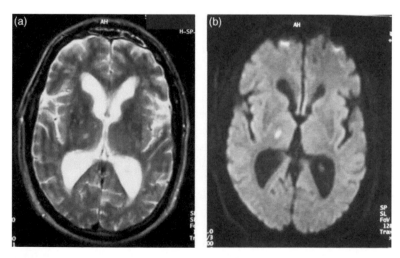

Fig. 10.3 Images with T$_2$-weighted (a) and diffusion-weighted (b) MRI in a 70-year-old man who presented with a history of sudden-onset numbness and tingling in the left face, arm and leg. On examination there was sensory loss over the left hand but nothing else. The diffusion-weighted images confirm a thalamic infarct consistent with the clinical diagnosis of pure sensory stroke.

high-signal DWI lesion. The degree of water proton restriction can be quantitatively measured using maps of the apparent diffusion coefficient (ADC). In contrast to DWI, ADC maps depict reduced diffusion as a dark, low signal (Figs. 10.4, 10.7, and 10.9). The value of the ADC changes with time after stroke onset, being reduced for the first few days after which it rises (pseudonormalization) to become hyperintense in the chronic phase when there is vasogenic edema and cellular necrosis (Table 10.4). This allows DWI to distinguish between acute and chronic infarction, unlike conventional MRI (Schaefer et $al.$ 2005), although it should be noted that the DWI-detectable lesion persists for at least a week since it detects prolonged T_2 signal "T_2 shine-through", so correct interpretation of DWI including identifying acute recurrence of ischemia requires consideration of the ADC map. Subacute lesions may also enhance on post-contrast T_1-weighted sequences (Figs. 10.6, 10.7, and 10.9) (Table 10.4).

Approximately 50% of patients with TIA have a focal abnormality on DWI if scanned within 24 hours; of these 25% do not have a lesion correlate on T_2-weighted MRI (Kidwell et $al.$ 1999; Ay et $al.$ 2002). Presence of DWI abnormalities is associated with some clinical characteristics of the presenting event. For example, in a systematic review of all studies reporting DWI findings and clinical characteristics of presenting TIA, symptom duration over 1 hour, dysarthria, dysphasia, and weakness were all significantly associated with abnormalities on DWI, as were atrial fibrillation and carotid stenosis > 50%, while hypertension, diabetes, and patient age were not (Redgrave et $al.$ 2007). Use of DWI alters the attending physician's opinion regarding vascular localization, anatomical localization, and probable TIA/minor stroke mechanism in a significant number of patients (Figs. 10.3–10.9) (Albers et $al.$ 2000; Schulz et $al.$ 2004; Gass et $al.$ 2004).

Approximately 25% of patients with TIA have cerebral infarction with transient signs in which DWI positivity corresponds to cytotoxic edema; this progresses to permanent parenchymal injury and increased tissue water content visible as a lesion on T_2-weighted MRI. Approximately 20% of patients have early DWI abnormality but no evidence of later T_2-weighted abnormality. This suggests reversibility of the initial DWI abnormality if blood flow is restored early enough to prevent permanent parenchymal injury, as seen in patients with stroke in whom the DWI-detected lesion may regress with reperfusion. In patients with negative DWI, a very brief period of ischemia may have been sufficient to disrupt neuronal activity but insufficient to cause cytotoxic edema.

Many patients with TIA or minor stroke delay seeking medical attention. Often there is a further delay before they are seen by specialist stroke services. In these patients, a clear history may be more difficult to obtain; clinical signs may have resolved, and it may be difficult to make a definite diagnosis of a cerebral ischemic event or to be certain of the vascular territory or territories involved. Studies suggest that DWI is also of use in diagnosis and management of patients presenting later with TIA or minor stroke symptoms (Schulz et $al.$ 2003, 2004) (Fig. 10.3). Clinically appropriate ischemic lesions are detected by DWI in a high proportion of patients with minor stroke when they are scanned 2 weeks or more after their event (Schulz et $al.$ 2004). Interobserver agreement for identifying recent ischemic lesions in this patient group is much higher for DWI than for T_2-weighted scans, and DWI provides useful information over and above T_2-weighted imaging in approximately a third of patients, most commonly by increasing diagnostic certainty and by indicating the vascular territory involved (Figs. 10.3–10.9). The presence of lesions seen with DWI decreases with time since symptom onset, and increases with NIHSS and age, and

Table. 10.4 Dating a cerebral infarction based on MRI findings

	Hyperacute (0–6 hours)	Hyperacute (6–24 hours)	Acute (24 hours–1 week)	Subacute (1–3 weeks)	Chronic (> 3 weeks)
DWI	High signal intensity			High signal intensity for 10–14 days, then iso or hypointense. Hyperintense if T_2 shine-through	Variable signal intensity. May be isointense, hyperintense if T_2 shine-through or hypointense in the presence of cystic encephalomalacia
ADC	Low signal intensity			Low signal intensity up to around 10 days. May pseudonormalize at days 10–15 then high signal intensity	High signal intensity
FLAIR	Variable signal intensity	High signal intensity			Low signal intensity if gliosis or cystic encephalomalacia
T_2	Isointense. Loss of flow void in patients with large artery occlusion may be seen.	Variable, usually high signal intensity after 8 hours	High signal intensity		
T_1	Isointense	Low signal intensity after 16 hours	Low signal intensity, but may have areas of hyperintensity (usually resolving by 3 months) in the cortical necrosis is present		

| Contrast-enhanced T$_1$ | Arterial enhancement may occur. Parenchymal cortical enhancement may occur after 2–4 hours in incomplete infarction | Arterial and meningeal enhancement may occur. Parenchymal enhancement may occur after 5–7 days in complete infarction. | Parenchymal enhancement may occur for up to 8 weeks in patients with complete infarction. |

Note: DWI, diffusion-weighted imaging; ADC, apparent diffusion coefficient; FLAIR, fluid attenuation inversion recovery
Source: Allen et al. (2012).

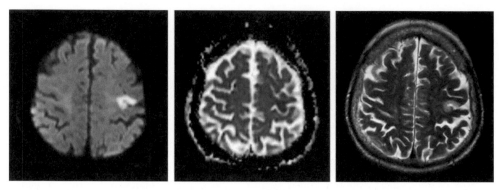

Fig. 10.4 These diffusion-weighted (DWI) (left), apparent diffusion coefficient (ADC) (middle), and T_2-weighted (right) scans were taken 36 hours after an 84-year-old woman presented with a sudden onset of right hand weakness. She was newly diagnosed to have atrial fibrillation. DWI confirms a small area of hyperintensity involving the left precentral area with corresponding hypointensity in the ADC map. There is also hyperintensity in the T_2-weighted sequences.

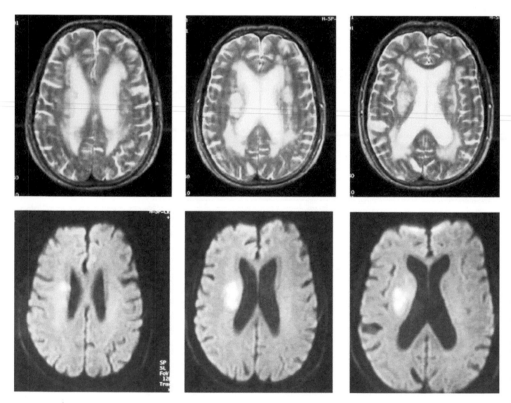

Fig. 10.5 These T_2-weighted (top) and diffusion-weighted (bottom) MRI scans were taken of an 80-year-old woman who had developed dysarthria and left-sided weakness 2 weeks previously. The T_2-weighted images show extensive leukoaraiosis, making it impossible to be certain which is the acute lesion. This, however, is clearly shown in the diffusion-weighted images.

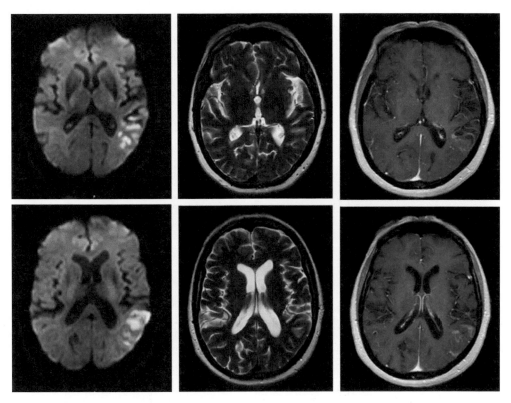

Fig. 10.6 These diffusion-weighted (DWI) (left panel), T_2-weighted (middle panel), and T_1-contrast enhanced (right panel) scans were taken 1 week after a 70-year-old woman presented with sudden onset of isolated expressive dysphasia. She was newly diagnosed to have atrial fibrillation. DWI demonstrates an acute infarct affecting the left posterior temporal lobe with a mild degree of corresponding hyperintensity on T_2-weighted imaging. There is intraparenchymal contrast enhancement, suggesting the subacute nature of the infarct.

is positively associated with stroke rather than TIA, motor deficit, and dysarthria (Schulz *et al.* 2004).

Preliminary studies using DWI suggest that the presence, absence and pattern of DWI-detectable lesions in patients with TIA and minor stroke provide prognostic information (Chapter 14) (Wen *et al.* 2004; Purroy *et al.* 2004; Bang *et al.* 2005; Coutts *et al.* 2005; Sylaja *et al.* 2007).

References

Albers GW, Lansberg MG, Norbash AM *et al.* (2000). Yield of diffusion-weighted MRI for detection of potentially relevant findings in stroke patients. *Neurology* **54**:1562–1567

Allen LM, Hasso AN, Handwerker J *et al.* (2012). Sequence-specific MR imaging findings that are useful in dating ischemic stroke. *Radiographics* **32**:1285–1297

Ay H, Oliveira-Filho J, Buonanno FS *et al.* (2002). "Footprints" of transient ischemic attacks: A diffusion-weighted MRI study. *Cerebrovascular Digest* **14**:177–186

Bang OY, Lee PH, Heo KG *et al.* (2005). Specific DWI lesion patterns predict prognosis after acute ischaemic stroke within the MCA territory. *Journal of Neurology, Neurosurgery and Psychiatry* **76**:1222–1228

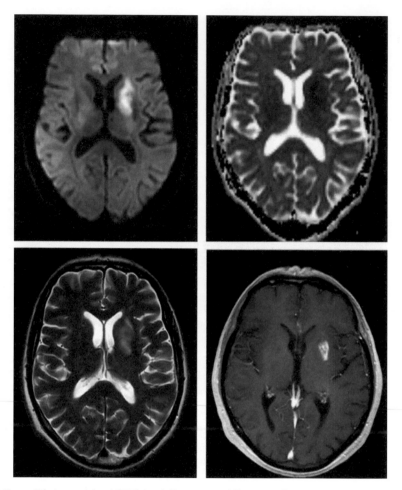

Fig. 10.7 These diffusion-weighted (DWI) (top left), apparent diffusion coefficient (ADC) (top right), T_2-weighted (bottom left), and T_1-contrast enhanced (bottom right) scans were taken 1 week after a 77-year old man presented with a sudden onset of isolated expressive dysphasia. DWI and ADC confirmed presence of an ischemic lesion with restricted diffusion affecting the left anterior basal ganglia. The lesion was also hyperintense on T_2 and contrast-enhancing on T_1 scans, suggesting the subacute nature of the infarct.

Chalela JA, Kidwell CS, Nentwich L *et al.* (2007). Magnetic resonance imaging and computed tomography in emergency assessment of patients with suspected acute stroke: A prospective study. *Lancet* **369**:293–298

Chan S, Kartha K, Yoon SS *et al.* (1996). Multifocal hypointense cerebral lesions on gradient-echo MR are associated with chronic hypertension. *American Journal of Neuroradiology* **17**:1821–1827

Cordonnier C, Al-Shahi Salman R, Wardlaw J (2007). Spontaneous brain microbleeds: Systematic review, subgroup analyses and standards for study design and reporting. *Brain* **130**:1988–2003

Coutts SB, Simon JE, Eliasziw M *et al.* (2005). Triaging transient ischemic attack and minor stroke patients using acute magnetic resonance imaging. *Annals of Neurology* **57**:848–854

Dennis MS, Bamford JM, Molyneux AJ *et al.* (1987). Rapid resolution of signs of primary intracerebral hemorrhage in computed

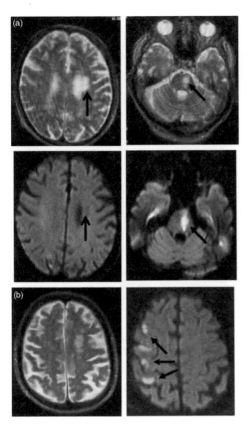

Fig. 10.8 Distinguishing the region of circulation affected (a) Anterior circulation or posterior circulation event? A patient presented with right arm weakness that developed 8 days previous and a history of a previous stroke with a right hemiparesis. The T_2-weighted MRI (upper images) shows two possibly relevant lesions (left corona radiata and left pons, arrows). The diffusion-weighted images (lower images) show that the pontine lesion is recent (arrow). (b) Lacunar or cortical event? A patient presented with a 12-day history of left hemiparesis involving face, arm, and leg. The T_2-weighted MRI (left) shows widespread "small vessel disease" throughout both hemispheres, but diffusion-weighted MRI (right) shows acute right hemispheric cortical infarcts (arrows).

tomograms of the brain. *British Medical Journal* **295**:379–381

Douglas VC, Johnston CM, Elkins J *et al.* (2003). Head computed tomography findings predict short-term stroke risk after transient ischemic attack. *Stroke* **34**:2894–2898

Dutch TIA Trial Study Group (1993). Predictors of major vascular events in patients with a transient ischemic attack or nondisabling stroke. *Stroke* **24**:527–531

Fazekas F, Kleinert R, Roob G *et al.* (1999). Histopathologic analysis of foci of signal loss on gradient-echo T_2-weighted MR images in patients with spontaneous intracerebral hemorrhage: Evidence of microangiopathy-related microbleeds. *American Journal of Neuroradiology* **20**:637–642

Fiebach JB, Schellinger PD, Gass A *et al.* (2004). Stroke magnetic resonance imaging is accurate in hyperacute intracerebral hemorrhage:

A multicenter study on the validity of stroke imaging. *Stroke* **35**:502–506

Fisher M (2014). Cerebral microbleeds: Where are we now? *Neurology* **83**:1304–1305

Gass A, Ay H, Szabo K *et al.* (2004). Diffusion-weighted MRI for the "small stuff": The details of acute cerebral ischaemia. *Lancet Neurology* **3**:39–45

Greenberg SM, Finklestein SP, Schaefer PW (1996). Petechial hemorrhages accompanying lobar hemorrhage: Detection by gradient-echo MRI. *Neurology* **46**:1751–1754

Gunatilake SB (1998). Rapid resolution of symptoms and signs of intracerebral hemorrhage: Case reports. *British Medical Journal* **316**:1495–1496

Kidwell CS, Alger JR, Di Salle F *et al.* (1999). Diffusion MRI in patients with transient ischemic attacks. *Stroke* **30**:1174–1180

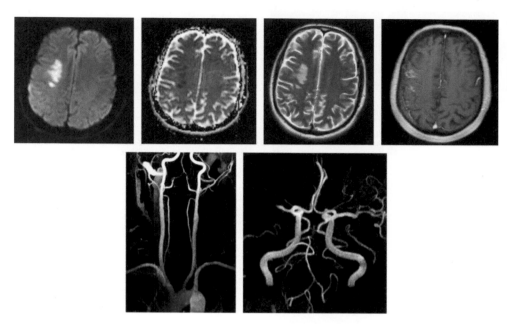

Fig. 10.9 These diffusion-weighted (DWI) (upper panel, far left), apparent diffusion coefficient (ADC) (upper panel, second left), T_2-weighted (upper panel, third left), and T_1-contrast enhanced (upper panel, far right) scans were taken 9 days after a 56-year-old man from Pakistan presented with sudden onset of dysarthria, and left face and hand weakness. DWI and ADC confirmed an ischemic lesion with restricted diffusion affecting the right hemispheric deep white matter. The lesion was also hyperintense on T_2 and contrast-enhancing on T_1 scans indicating the subacute nature of the infarct. Contrast-enhanced MR angiogram demonstrated presence of an occluded M1 branch of the right middle cerebral artery (lower panel, right), but otherwise no significant extracranial atherosclerosis (lower panel, left).

Kidwell CS, Chalela JA, Saver JL *et al.* (2004). Comparison of MRI and CT for detection of acute intracerebral hemorrhage. *JAMA* **292**:1823–1830

Knudsen KA, Rosand J, Karluk D *et al.* (2001). Clinical diagnosis of cerebral amyloid angiopathy: Validation of the Boston Criteria. *Neurology* **56**:537–539

Kumar S, Selim M, Marchina S *et al.* (2016). Transient neurological symptoms in patients with intracerebral hemorrhage. *JAMA Neurology* **73**:316–320

Jauch EC, Saver JL, Adams HP Jr *et al.* (2013). Guidelines for the early management of patients with acute ischemic stroke: A guideline for healthcare professionals from the American Heart Association/ American Stroke Association. *Stroke* **44**:870–947

Lau KK, Wong YK, Teo KC *et al.* (2017). Long-term prognostic implications of cerebral microbleeds in Chinese with ischemic stroke. *Journal of the American Heart Association* **6**(12)

Lemesle M, Madinier G, Menassa M *et al.* (1998). Incidence of transient ischemic attacks in Dijon, France. A 5-year community-based study. *Neuroepidemiology* **17**:74–79

National Institute for Health and Clinical Excellence (2017). *Stroke and Transient Ischemic Attack in Over 16s: Diagnosis and Initial Management*. London: NICE

Offenbacher H, Fazekas F, Schmidt R *et al.* (1996). MR of cerebral abnormalities concomitant with primary intracerebral hematomas. *American Journal of Neuroradiology* **17**:573–578

Purroy F, Montaner J, Rovira A *et al.* (2004). Higher risk of further vascular events among transient ischaemic attack patients with diffusion-weighted imaging acute lesions. *Stroke* 35:2313–2319

Redgrave JN, Coutts SB, Schulz UG *et al.* (2007). Systematic review of associations between the presence of acute ischemic lesions on diffusion-weighted imaging and clinical predictors of early stroke risk after transient ischemic attack. *Stroke* 38:1482–1488

Rolak LA, Gilmer W, Strittmatter WJ (1990). Low yield in the diagnostic evaluation of transient ischemic attacks. *Neurology* 40:747–748

Schaefer PW, Copen WA, Lev MH *et al.* (2005). Diffusion-weighted imaging in acute stroke. *Neuroimaging Clinics of North American* 15:503–530

Schellinger PD, Jansen O, Fiebach JB *et al.* (1999). A standardized MRI stroke protocol: Comparison with CT in hyperacute intracerebral hemorrhage. *Stroke* 30:765–768

Schellinger PD, Thomalla G, Fiehler J *et al.* (2007). MRI-based and CT-based thrombolytic therapy in acute stroke within and beyond established time windows: An analysis of 1210 patients. *Stroke* 38:2640–2645

Schulz UGR, Briley D, Meagher T *et al.* (2003). Abnormalities on diffusion weighted magnetic resonance imaging performed several weeks after a minor stroke or transient ischaemic attack. *Journal of Neurology, Neurosurgery and Psychiatry* 74:734–738

Schulz UG, Flossman E, Rothwell PM (2004). Heritability of ischemic stroke in relation to age, vascular risk factors and subtypes of incident stroke in population-based studies. *Stroke* 35:819–824

Shoamanesh A, Kwok CS, Benavente O (2011). Cerebral microbleeds: Histopathological correlation of neuroimaging. *Cerebrovascular diseases* 32:528–534

Sylaja PN, Coutts SB, Subramaniam S *et al.* (2007). Acute ischemic lesions of varying ages

predict risk of ischemic events in stroke/TIA patients. *Neurology* 68:415–419

UK TIA Study Group (1993). Intracranial tumours that mimic transient cerebral ischaemia: Lessons from a large multicentre trial. *Journal of Neurology, Neurosurgery and Psychiatry* 56:563–566

van Veluw SJ, Biessels GJ, Klijn CJM *et al.* (2016). Heterogeneous histopathology of cortical microbleeds in cerebral amyloid angiopathy. *Neurology* 86:867–871

Wardlaw JM, Keir SL, Dennis MS (2003). The impact of delays in computed tomography of the brain on the accuracy of diagnosis and subsequent management in patients with minor stroke. *Journal of Neurology, Neurosurgery and Psychiatry* 74:77–81

Weisberg LA (1986). Computerized tomographic abnormalities in patients with hemispheric transient ischemic attacks. *South Medical Journal* 79:804–807

Weisberg LA, Nice CN (1977). Intracranial tumors simulating the presentation of cerebrovascular syndromes. Early detection with cerebral computed tomography (CCT). *American Journal of Medicine* 63:517–524

Wen HM, Lam WW, Rainer T *et al.* (2004). Multiple acute cerebral infarcts on diffusion-weighted imaging and risk of recurrent stroke. *Neurology* 63:1317–1319

Werring DJ, Coward LJ, Losseff NA *et al.* (2005). Cerebral microbleeds are common in ischemic stroke but rare in TIA. *Neurology* 65:1914–1918

Wilson D, Charidimou A, Ambler G *et al.* (2016). Recurrent stroke risk and cerebral microbleed burden in ischemic stroke and TIA: A meta-analysis. *Neurology* 87:1–10

Wityk RJ, Pessin MS, Kaplan RF *et al.* (1994). Serial assessment of acute stroke using the NIH Stroke Scale. *Stroke* 25:362–365

Brain Imaging in Major Acute Stroke

In patients with major stroke, investigations are required to:

- differentiate between infarction and hemorrhage.
- exclude stroke mimics.
- inform treatment decisions: identify vascular occlusion or stenosis and identify areas of completed and threatened infarction.
- provide prognostic information.

Brain imaging is required to distinguish between primary intracerebral hemorrhage and cerebral infarction since this distinction cannot be made reliably on clinical criteria alone (Hawkins *et al.* 1995). Developments in brain imaging, in particular MRI sequences (e.g., diffusion-weighted imaging and perfusion), and also CT techniques (e.g., perfusion), have enabled visualization of the pathophysiological processes involved in brain infarction. These techniques are particularly useful to select patients suitable for endovascular therapy beyond the 6-hour time window and may in the future enable targeting of treatments such as neuroprotection (Chapter 21).

At present in most centers in most countries, CT remains the imaging modality used routinely to distinguish between hemorrhage and infarction in acute stroke: it is better tolerated, easier to perform in sick patients, and more widely available than MRI. Further, the various randomized trials of thrombolysis in ischemic stroke used CT criteria to guide treatment decisions and showed thrombolysis to be effective if given within 3–4.5 hours of stroke (Chapter 21). Consequently, CT is felt to be sufficient to select patients for thrombolysis within 3–4.5 hours of stroke onset by most centers. Although conventional T_1- and T_2-weighted MR sequences have a low sensitivity acutely for intracranial hemorrhage, sequences such as $T2^*$ gradient echo (GRE) and susceptibility-weighted imaging (SWI) have greater sensitivity for hemorrhage than CT. Consequently, some centers advocate the use of multi-modal MRI as the imaging modality of choice in acute stroke (Chalela *et al.* 2007) particularly beyond the 3-hour time window, although the use of perfusion CT to image cerebral blood flow is also becoming more common (Table 11.1).

Computed Tomography and Conventional Magnetic Resonance Imaging

Hemorrhage

Hemorrhage is seen as a hyperdense region by CT, often in the form of a space-occupying mass (Fig. 9.2). The sensitivity of CT for parenchymal hemorrhage is almost 100%, but small parenchymal hemorrhage or subarachnoid hemorrhage may be missed (Schriger *et al.*

Table 11.1 Advantages and disadvantages of computed tomography (CT) and magnetic resonance imaging (MRI) in major stroke

Modality	Advantages	Disadvantages
CT	Low cost and wide availability Safe for medically unstable patients High sensitivity for hemorrhage in the acute phase	Radiation exposure Poor image resolution for posterior structures Iodinated contrast required if CT angiogram is to be performed (relatively contraindicated in patients with renal impairment or allergic to iodinated contrast)
	Rapid acquisition of images CT angiogram can be performed quickly in the same setting to exclude a large artery occlusion or intracranial aneurysm	
MRI	High sensitivity for stroke mimics High sensitivity for ischemia (with DWI) and cerebral perfusion	Patient tolerability and contraindications Low sensitivity for cerebral hemorrhage, unless incorporation of sequences that are sensitive for blood products such as GRE or SWI
	High resolution for imaging of vasculature	Slower image acquisition Gadolinium contrast required if MR angiogram is to be performed (contraindicated in patients with severe renal impairment due to risk of nephrogenic systemic fibrosis)

Notes: DWI, diffusion-weighted imaging; GRE, gradient echo; SWI, susceptibility-weighted imaging.

1998). With increasing passage of time after the onset of the hemorrhage, CT becomes progressively less good at distinguishing between hemorrhage and infarction as the initial hyperdensity becomes iso- and then hypodense (Fig. 11.1). Consequently, MRI is better than CT for diagnosing hemorrhage more than a week after onset, particularly in defining possible underlying pathology.

There is usually not a large amount of edema early after intracerebral hemorrhage, and the finding of edema should prompt a search for an underlying tumor or venous obstruction. Hemorrhages related to coagulopathies, anticoagulants or to cerebral amyloid angiopathy are often inhomogeneous with fluid levels. Recently, it has been shown that the combination of subarachnoid hemorrhage, lobar intracerebral hemorrhage with finger-like projections and *APOE* E4 possession is highly suggestive of cerebral amyloid angiopathy-associated intracerebral hemorrhage, although this model still requires external validation (Rodrigues *et al.* 2018). The location and number of hemorrhages may provide clues as to the underlying cause and hence guide further investigation and treatment (see Chapter 7).

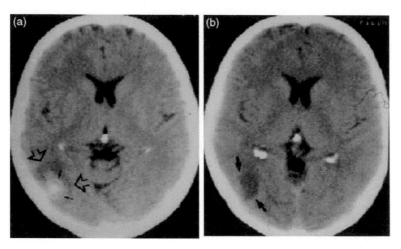

Fig. 11.1 These CT brain scans show an acute right cortical hemorrhage on the day of the stroke (a, open arrow), which has become hypodense on repeat scanning 7 days later (b, black arrow).

As stated previously, conventional MRI is not the modality of choice for distinguishing between hemorrhage and infarction in acute stroke. The appearance of primary intracerebral hemorrhage on conventional MRI sequences at different time periods following stroke onset is complex since the T_1 and T_2 relaxation rates vary with the concentration of breakdown products of hemoglobin (Table 11.2). As the hematoma ages, it is converted from oxyhemoglobin to deoxyhemoglobin and then to methemoglobin prior to red cell lysis and breakdown into ferritin and hemosiderin. Acute hematoma is characterized by central hypointensity on T_2-weighted and isointensity on T_1-weighted MRI. Methemoglobin formation leads to shortening of T_1 relaxation and to central hyperintensity on T_1-weighted images, with hyperintensity on T_2-weighted images. Days and weeks after onset of bleeding, a hypo-intense border zone caused by the paramagnetic rim of methemoglobin demarcates the border zone of the hematoma. The complexity and subtlety of these changes have resulted in a strong preference by clinicians and radiologists for CT over conventional MRI in the acute evaluation of intracerebral hemorrhage.

Ischemic Changes

Knowledge of the nature and time course of ischemic changes on CT and conventional MRI is necessary as an aid to diagnosis, infarct localization, and selection of patients for acute stroke therapy. While hemorrhage is visible almost immediately on CT, ischemia takes longer to manifest, although changes have been reported as early as 22 minutes in one study (von Kummer *et al.* 2001). Consistent with its end-artery vascular system, the striatocapsular area exhibits irreversible damage very early in patients with middle cerebral artery stem occlusion, whereas the cortical areas usually fall within the penumbra. The earliest signs of ischemia are of brain tissue swelling, as shown by effacement of cortical sulci, asymmetry of the sylvian fissures, and ventricular distortion (Fig. 11.2) (Kucinski *et al.* 2002). Occasionally the segment of the artery occluded by the thrombus, particularly in the case of the main trunk of the middle cerebral artery, may appear hyperdense, although interobserver agreement on such signs is only moderate (Fig. 11.3) (von Kummer *et al.* 1996;

Table 11.2 Appearance of intracerebral hemorrhage on computed tomography (CT) and magnetic resonance imaging (MRI) at different time periods

Stage	Time (range)	Blood product	CT	T$_1$-weighted MRI	T$_2$-weighted MRI
Hyperacute	< 24 hours	Oxyhemoglobin	Hyperdense	Isointense	High signal intensity
Acute	1–3 days	Deoxyhemoglobin	Hyperdense	Isointense	Low signal intensity
Early subacute	3–7 days	Intracellular methemoglobin	Isodense	High signal intensity	Low signal intensity
Late subacute	1 week to months	Extracelluar methemoglobin	Hypodense	High signal intensity	High signal intensity
Chronic	Months	Hemosiderin	Hypodense	Low signal intensity	Low signal intensity

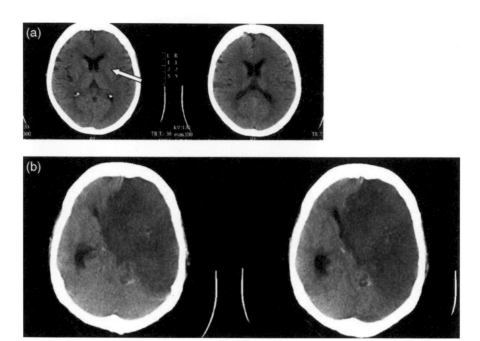

Fig. 11.2 Early ischemic change on CT (a) showing very subtle loss of gray-white matter differentiation in the internal capsule/basal ganglia (arrow) in a patient with a massive infarction in the left middle cerebral artery territory. This is seen clearly on CT scan 3 days after stroke onset (b).

Grotta *et al.* 1999). Early brain swelling is followed by the development of parenchymal hypodensity, corresponding to cytotoxic edema, and is seen on CT as loss of the normal gray-white matter differentiation in the cortex, insular ribbon, or basal ganglia (Fig. 11.4).

The early ischemic changes on CT are subtle, and the CT may appear normal if performed in the first few hours. The sensitivity of CT within 5 hours of ischemic stroke was reported as 58% in one early study (Horowitz *et al.* 1991) although a higher rate of 68% has been reported within 2 hours (von Kummer *et al.* 1994) and even higher of 75% within 3 hours with middle cerebral artery infarction (Barber *et al.* 2000). The interobserver reliability and reproducibility of CT in the estimation of the degree of ischemic change are modest (von Kummer *et al.* 1996, 1997; Grotta *et al.* 1999; Schriger *et al.* 1998), although use of a systematic CT review system, the Alberta Stroke Program Early CT Score (ASPECTS), by trained observers has better interrater reliability (Coutts *et al.* 2004). Sensitivity is less for small infarcts and infarcts in the posterior fossa, and a significant minority of clinically definite strokes are not associated with an appropriate lesion on CT even after 2 or 3 days. "Re-windowing" the CT images to ~35:35 may increase the differentiation between gray and white matter and may facilitate detection of early signs of ischemia such as loss of gray-white differentiation.

One to 2 days after stroke onset, the infarcted area appears as an ill-defined hypodense area as vasogenic edema becomes predominant. Within 2 or 3 days, the attenuation values become lower, the ischemic area is better demarcated, and there may be evidence of mass effect (Figs. 5.1 and 11.5). Later, there may be ipsilateral ventricular dilatation owing to loss of brain substance. Hemorrhagic transformation usually occurs a few days after stroke onset

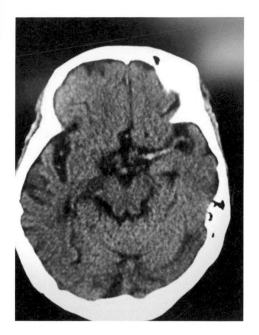

Fig. 11.3 Hyperdense left middle cerebral artery sign.

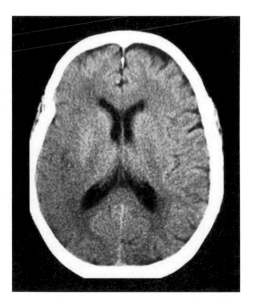

Fig. 11.4 Patient with a right middle cerebral artery territory infarction. A number of early radiological signs of ischemia are present including: sulcal effacement, asymmetry of the sylvian fissures, and loss of the normal gray-white matter differentiation in the cortex, insular ribbon, and, to a lesser extent, the basal ganglia.

in large infarcts, but it may develop within hours and result in appearances very similar to primary intracerebral hemorrhage (Fig. 16.1) (Bogousslavsky 1991).

The site of any hypodensity relates to the underlying arterial distribution, allowing for differences between individuals in arterial anatomy. A small proportion of patients with first-ever strokes have focal hypodensities on CT in areas inconsistent with the

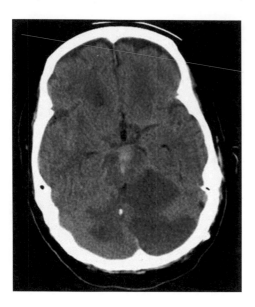

Fig. 11.5 Later ischemic changes in a patient with bilateral cerebellar infarcts due to cardioembolism. Mass effect is also present with compression of the forth ventricle.

presenting symptoms. Others have widespread diffuse periventricular hypodensity, making any new infarcts difficult to delineate (Chodosh *et al.* 1988). Further, despite the temporal sequence of ischemic changes on CT, it is often difficult to determine the age of an infarct from the CT appearance. Diffusion-weighted MR imaging overcomes these limitations (Figs. 10.3–10.9).

In summary, one of the main roles of CT in acute stroke is to exclude hemorrhage. In patients with acute ischemic stroke who may be eligible for intravenous thrombolysis or endovascular therapy, CT angiography also has an important role in determining whether an underlying large artery occlusion is present as well as assessing the status of collateral blood flow (see Chapters 12 and 21). However, owing to the limitations in visualization of ischemia, especially in the early stages, CT cannot be used to stratify participants reliably according to infarct location or size in trials of acute stroke therapy, although it is currently used to exclude major completed infarction prior to early thrombolysis.

The earliest ischemic change on conventional MRI, immediately detectable, is loss of the normal flow void in the affected artery, the MRI equivalent of the hyperdense artery sign on CT, and arterial enhancement if contrast has been used (Mohr *et al.* 1995; Allen *et al.* 2012) (see Table 10.4). Subsequent changes are swelling on T_1-weighted images caused by cytotoxic edema, which is present in up to half of patients within 6 hours; hyperintensity on T_2-weighted images from vasogenic edema, present within 8 hours; and T_1-weighted signal change, within 16 hours (Yuh *et al.* 1991). Consequently, the sensitivity of conventional MRI is low in the first few hours following the onset of stroke symptoms, with values similar to CT (Mohr *et al.* 1995; Mullins *et al.* 2002). In subacute ischemic stroke, conventional MRI has higher sensitivity than CT owing to its better spatial resolution and lack of posterior fossa artifact (Simmons *et al.* 1986; Bryan *et al.* 1991), but conventional MRI may still be normal in clinically definite stroke.

Conventional MRI is poor at distinguishing acute from chronic infarction. This is a particular problem in patients with multiple infarcts and in the elderly, in whom multiple

T_2-weighted abnormalities in the corona radiata, basal ganglia, and brainstem are common and in whom neurological symptoms may develop with intercurrent illness on a background of previous stroke. This, together with the poor sensitivity in the acute stroke period, means that, as for CT, conventional MRI is often unable to stratify patients according to infarct presence, ischemic stroke subtype, size, or location prior to therapy or randomization in acute stroke trials. Both MRI and MR venography will help where there is a possibility of venous rather than arterial infarction.

Gradient-Echo, Susceptibility-Weighted Imaging and Primary Intracerebral Imaging Hemorrhage

There are limitations to the information on cerebrovascular pathophysiology in vivo that can be provided by CT and conventional MRI. Specifically, these include lack of sensitivity for acute ischemic stroke, difficulty in determining infarct age, lack of demonstration of the ischemic penumbra, and low sensitivity and specificity for primary intracerebral hemorrhage in the case of MRI.

Advances in MRI sequences have now led to the routine use of gradient-echo (GRE) or susceptibility-weighted imaging (SWI) to detect hemorrhage, including microbleeds and cortical superficial siderosis (see Chapters 7 and 10). This would avoid the need to perform two imaging modalities in acute stroke, CT followed by MRI, in patients in whom further characterization of pathophysiology is necessary, for instance to determine selection for thrombolysis.

Diffusion-Weighted Imaging

Diffusion-weighted imaging (DWI) has a high sensitivity for acute ischemic stroke, at approximately 90–95% (Makin *et al.* 2015; Edlow *et al.* 2017), although other conditions such as abscesses, intracerebral lymphomas, and acute disseminated encephalomyelitis may also result in lesions detected by DWI (see Chapter 10). DWI is abnormal within minutes of stroke onset (Hjort *et al.* 2005a). Interobserver agreement is also better for DWI than with conventional MRI (Lutsep *et al.* 1997; Lansberg *et al.* 2000). However, there appears to be a lower sensitivity for DWI in posterior circulation acute stroke, and patients with neurological deficits consistent with posterior circulation ischemia have five times the odds of having a negative DWI scan compared with patients with anterior circulation ischemia (Edlow *et al.* 2017).

The fact that DWI distinguishes between acute and chronic infarction and has high sensitivity in acute stroke makes it a valuable tool in the diagnosis and management of patients with acute stroke. It has been reported to show localization in a different vascular territory from that initially suspected on the basis of clinical features and conventional MRI in 18% of patients (Albers *et al.* 2000; Schulz *et al.* 2004). It can confirm that a new ischemic cerebrovascular event has occurred in a confused elderly patient with previous strokes or in patients with nonspecific symptoms such as confusion or dizziness. The presence of bilateral multiple acute infarcts as shown on DWI may suggest cardioembolism, prompting further cardiac investigation, whereas one acute infarct with several old infarcts might be more suggestive of a thromboembolic event. Multiple recent infarcts in the anterior circulation of the same hemisphere suggest critical carotid stenosis (Gass *et al.* 2004), dissection, or proximal middle cerebral artery stenosis (Lee *et al.* 2005) and warrant urgent imaging of the anterior circulation vessels with referral for surgery where appropriate. Demonstration of posterior circulation infarction may prompt further assessment of the vertebrobasilar vessels.

Diffusion and Perfusion Imaging on Magnetic Resonance and the Ischemic Penumbra

There is a need to identify those patients with a small infarct but a large ischemic penumbra, in whom the risk–benefit ratio of thrombolysis and endovascular therapy is likely to be favorable, and to exclude from treatment patients at high risk of hemorrhagic transformation or with small lacunar infarcts. Qualitative information on the ischemic penumbra can be obtained using DWI in combination with MR perfusion-weighted imaging (Kidwell and Hsia 2006; Muir *et al.* 2006).

Perfusion-weighted imaging measures the relative blood flow rate through the brain and can be achieved using an injected contrast agent such as gadolinium (e.g., dynamic susceptibility contrast-enhanced or dynamic contrast-enhanced MR perfusion) or endogenous techniques such as arterial spin labeling (ASL), which utilizes magnetically labeled blood as an endogenous tracer (Zaharchuk *et al.* 2014). The latter has the advantage of being noninvasive and could be used for multiple repeat investigations. However, compared with contrast-enhanced MR perfusion, ASL is less well studied, has a lower signal-to-noise ratio (which limits its temporal and spatial resolution), and requires a much longer scan time (8–10 minutes at 1.5-T MRI or 4–5 minutes at 3-T MRI), therefore increasing the susceptibility to motion artifacts (Essig *et al.* 2013). Hence, although ASL holds much promise, its widespread clinical use is limited at present.

In contrast to lesion volumes seen with DWI, those with perfusion-weighted imaging are typically largest acutely and resolve over time. Consistent with earlier positron emission tomography studies, perfusion changes precede the development of DWI-detected lesions. In the absence of reperfusion, lesions detected by DWI progressively extend over 24 hours into the area of reduced perfusion-weighted imaging. Severity of perfusion deficit has therefore been proposed as a surrogate marker for subsequent infarction (Thijs *et al.* 2001; Shih *et al.* 2003).

Two patterns of DWI and perfusion-weighted imaging abnormalities have been observed in acute ischemic stroke:

* perfusion-weighted imaging shows less damage than DWI: the volume of abnormal perfusion is less than that of the hyperintense DWI signal.
* perfusion-weighted imaging shows more damage than DWI: the volume of abnormal perfusion is greater than the volume of hyperintense DWI change.

When perfusion-weighted imaging shows a larger abnormality than DWI, at least half of patients show an increase in DWI-detectable lesion volume over the 3–11 days after stroke onset (Sorensen *et al.* 1996; Baird *et al.* 1997; Barber *et al.* 1998; van Everdingen *et al.* 1998; Beaulieu *et al.* 1999; Karonen *et al.* 1999). Lesion growth is amplified by hyperglycemia, high hematocrit, old age, and hypoxia (Baird *et al.* 2003; Allport *et al.* 2005; Ay *et al.* 2005; Singhal *et al.* 2005). When perfusion-weighted imaging shows less abnormality than does DWI initially, no significant lesion growth occurs (Barber *et al.* 1998). Consequently, it has been proposed that when there is "perfusion–diffusion mismatch," that is, where there is reduced perfusion but not yet DWI signal change, this tissue area represents the ischemic penumbra

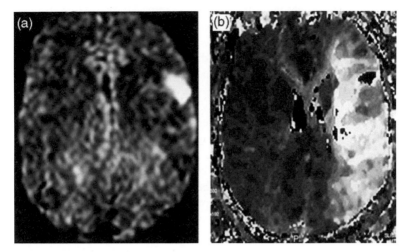

Fig. 11.6 A patient with acute ischemic stroke where MRI shows a perfusion–diffusion mismatch with a relatively small area of high signal on diffusion-weighted imaging (a) but a large area of reduced perfusion on perfusion-weighted imaging (b).

and thus tissue that may be salvaged if perfusion can be restored quickly enough (Fig. 11.6). Indeed, recent randomized-controlled trials such as DAWN (DWI or CTP Assessment with Clinical Mismatch in the Triage of Wake-Up and Late Presenting Strokes Undergoing Neurointervention with Trevo) (Nogueira *et al.* 2018) and DEFUSE 3 (Endovascular Therapy Following Imaging Evaluation for Ischemic Stroke) (Albers *et al.* 2018) were able to demonstrate that in carefully selected patients with acute ischemic stroke due to anterior circulation large vessel occlusion and with presentation 6 to 24 hours from symptom onset, presence of significant perfusion-diffusion mismatch on MRI is useful in selecting patients who may benefit from mechanical thrombectomy (Powers *et al.* 2018).

Perfusion Computed Tomography

CT perfusion studies can also be used to examine cerebral blood flow (Wintermark and Bogousslavsky 2003) using existing CT technology. Cerebral blood flow measurement using CT can be achieved using existing CT-based technology; it is easier to perform in sick patients than MRI and is not contraindicated in those with pacemakers, ferromagnetic implants, mechanical heart valves, and those with claustrophobia. The CT perfusion technique uses exogenous contrast and enables calculation of cerebral blood flow (CBF), cerebral blood volume (CBV), and mean transit time (MTT). CBF is equivalent to CBV divided by MTT where CBF represents the volume of blood flowing through a given volume of brain matter during a specified time period, CBV being the volume of blood flowing within a given volume of brain matter and MTT representing the average time for blood to transit through the given volume of brain matter.

One of the main aims of CT perfusion studies is to identify whether there is any penumbra that may be potentially salvageable by revascularization strategies. In infarcted tissue, there is a matched reduction in both CBF and CBV, while the CBF is reduced but with CBV maintained in the ischemic penumbra. However, quantification of CBF is problematic, and most studies use ratios comparing values with homologous areas of the contralateral hemisphere, which itself may show a reduced CBF in acute stroke, for example in diaschisis. In addition, current technology allows only limited brain coverage, which means that large areas of ischemia are imaged inadequately and small ones may be missed altogether. Lesions in the posterior fossa are difficult to image and CT perfusion studies also lack sensitivity in patients who have an inadequate CBF, for example, in patients with cardiac failure, arrhythmia, or underlying severe intra- or extracranial atherosclerosis. Currently, there is also significant variability and lack of standardization in how software packages acquire and process raw data. Nevertheless, there is evidence in acute stroke that perfusion CT values correlate with angiographic findings and can predict infarction and clinical outcome (Nabavi et al. 2002; Meuli 2004; Parsons et al. 2005; Wintermark et al. 2007). In the recent DAWN (Nogueira et al. 2018) and DEFUSE 3 (Albers et al. 2018) trials, CT perfusion studies have been shown to be valuable in selecting acute ischemic stroke patients, presenting 6 to 24 hours from symptom onset, who may benefit from mechanical thrombectomy (Powers et al. 2018) (see following discussion).

Radiological Selection of Patients for Thrombolysis and Endovascular Therapy

Radiological investigation to exclude hemorrhage is essential in selecting patients for thrombolysis and endovascular therapy. It may also help to identify patients with large completed infarcts, a small ischemic penumbra, or TIA, in whom revascularization therapy would not be beneficial. The majority of centers currently rely on CT rather than MRI as the first-line investigation in stroke.

There is currently insufficient evidence to suggest a threshold of acute hypoattenuation severity or extent on CT that affects treatment response to alteplase (Powers et al. 2018). Nevertheless, current international stroke guidelines do not recommend administrating intravenous alteplase to patients whose CT brain shows extensive regions of clear hypoattentuation (Powers et al. 2018). Severe hypoattenuation represents irreversible injury and these patients have a poor prognosis despite intravenous alteplase. Similarly, a pooled analysis of previous randomized controlled trials did not show any significant interaction between baseline CT leukoaraiosis and the effect of intravenous alteplase (Charidimou et al. 2016). Initial small studies investigating cerebral microbleeds and the risk of hemorrhagic transformation after thrombolysis showed an uncertain relationship (Derex et al. 2005; Koennecke 2006; Cordonnier et al. 2007), but more recent data do show an increased thrombolysis risk (Tsivgoulis et al. 2016) (Chapter 21). Intravenous alteplase may still be reasonable in patients with <10 cerebral microbleeds, but in those with >10 cerebral microbleeds, the benefits of intravenous alteplase are uncertain, but may still be administered if the perceived benefits significantly outweigh the increased risk of intracerebral hemorrhage (Powers et al. 2018). Presence of a large lesion on DWI (Singer et al. 2007) or high permeability (Bang et al. 2007) is also associated with hemorrhage.

The theory that the ischemic penumbra represents salvageable tissue has led to the proposal that thrombolysis and endovascular therapy is likely to be most effective in those patients with diffusion–perfusion mismatch. Despite the fact that the area of diffusion–perfusion mismatch does not precisely delineate the penumbra, it appears reasonably robust in representing tissue at risk of infarction. Use of recombinant tissue plasminogen activator is associated with early resolution of perfusion-weighted imaging lesions in less than 36 hours, reduced DWI lesion growth, smaller final stroke volumes, and better clinical outcome on follow-up (Hjort *et al.* 2005b). It has been suggested that diffusion–perfusion mismatch might be mirrored by a clinical–diffusion mismatch, but current data suggest that this is not the case (Lansberg *et al.* 2007; Messe *et al.* 2007).

In patients with matched images by DWI and perfusion-weighted imaging, it is unclear whether reperfusion will be of benefit since it is uncertain whether the area detected by DWI still contains a significant penumbra. In these cases, MR angiographic findings and the clinical picture should be taken into account. A severe neurological deficit and middle cerebral artery occlusion predict a malignant middle cerebral artery infarction. A DWI lesion with normal or increased perfusion indicates spontaneous recanalization and is inappropriate for thrombolysis or endovascular treatment.

In acute ischemic stroke patients that meet criteria for mechanical thrombectomy (see Chapter 21), current international stroke guidelines recommend noninvasive intracranial vascular studies, for example CT angiography during the initial imaging evaluation (Powers *et al.* 2018). However, these tests should not delay intravenous alteplase if clinically indicated. In carefully selected patients with acute ischemic stroke presenting within 6 to 24 hours of symptom onset time, who have demonstrable anterior circulation large artery occlusion, CT perfusion or MRI-DWI and perfusion studies is recommended to aid patient selection for mechanical thrombectomy (Powers *et al.* 2018). Routine use of MRI to exclude cerebral microbleeds before intravenous alteplase is not recommended, nor is the use of perfusion studies to select patients who present beyond the currently accepted time window for administration of intravenous alteplase. Perfusion studies are also not required for selection of patients for suitability of mechanical thrombectomy if they present within 6 hours of symptom onset (Powers *et al.* 2018).

References

Albers GW, Lansberg MG, Norbash AM *et al.* (2000). Yield of diffusion-weighted MRI for detection of potentially relevant findings in stroke patients. *Neurology* 54:1562–1567

Albers GW, Marks MP, Kemp S *et al.* (2018). Thrombectomy for stroke at 6 to 16 hours with selection by perfusion imaging. *New England Journal of Medicine* 378:708–718

Allen LM, Hasso AN, Handwerker J *et al.* (2012). Sequence-specific MR imaging findings that are useful in dating ischemic stroke. *Radiographics* 32:1285–1297

Allport LE, Parsons MW, Butcher KS *et al.* (2005). Elevated hematocrit is associated with reduced reperfusion and tissue survival in acute stroke. *Neurology* 65:1382–1387

Ay H, Koroshetz WJ, Vangel M *et al.* (2005). Conversion of ischemic brain tissue into infarction increases with age. *Stroke* 36:2632–2636

Baird AE, Benfield A, Schlaug G *et al.* (1997). Enlargement of human cerebral ischemic lesion volumes measured by diffusion-weighted magnetic resonance imaging. *Annals of Neurology* 41:581–589

Baird TA, Parsons MW, Phanh T *et al.* (2003). Persistent poststroke hyperglycemia is independently associated with infarct expansion and worse clinical outcome. *Stroke* 34:2208–2214

Bang OY, Buck BH, Saver JL *et al.* (2007). Prediction of hemorrhagic transformation after recanalization therapy using T_2^*-permeability magnetic resonance imaging. *Annals of Neurology* 62:170–176

Barber PA, Darby DG, Desmond PM *et al.* (1998). Prediction of stroke outcome with echoplanar perfusion-and diffusion-weighted MRI. *Neurology* 51:418–426

Barber PA, Demchuk AM, Zhang J *et al.* (2000). Validity and reliability of a quantitative computed tomography score in predicting outcome of hyperacute stroke before thrombolytic therapy. ASPECTS Study Group. Alberta Stroke Programme Early CT Score. *Lancet* **355**:1670–1674

Beaulieu C, de Crespigny A, Tong DC *et al.* (1999). Longitudinal magnetic resonance imaging study of perfusion and diffusion in stroke: Evolution of lesion volume and correlation with clinical outcome. *Annals in Neurology* **46**:568–578

Bogousslavsky J (1991). Topographic patterns of cerebral infarcts: Correlation with aetiology. *Cerebrovascular Diseases* **1**:61–68

Bryan RN, Levy LM, Whitlow WD *et al.* (1991). Diagnosis of acute cerebral infarction: Comparison of CT and MR imaging. *American Journal of Neuroradiology* **12**:611–620

Campbell BC, Mitchell MJ, Kleinig TJ *et al.* (2015). Endovascular therapy for ischemic stroke with perfusion-imaging selection. *New England Journal of Medicine* **372**:1009–1018

Chalela JA, Kidwell CS, Nentwich LM *et al.* (2007). Magnetic resonance imaging and computed tomography in emergency assessment of patients with suspected acute stroke: A prospective comparison. *Lancet* **369**:293–298

Charidimou A, Pasi M, Fiorelli M *et al.* (2016). Leukoaraiosis, cerebral hemorrhage, and outcome after intravenous thrombolysis for acute ischemic stroke: A meta-analysis. *Stroke* **47**:2364–2372

Chodosh EH, Foulkes MA, Kase CS *et al.* (1988). Silent stroke in the NINCDS stroke data bank. *Neurology* **38**:1674–1679

Cordonnier C, Al-Shahi Salman R, Wardlaw J (2007). Spontaneous brain microbleeds: Systematic review subgroup analyses and standards for study design and reporting. *Brain* **130**:1988–2003

Coutts SB, Demchuk AM, Barber PA *et al.* (2004). Interobserver variation of ASPECTS in real time. *Stroke* **35**:103–105

Derex L, Hermier M, Adeleine P *et al.* (2005). Clinical and imaging predictors of intracerebral hemorrhage in stroke patients treated with intravenous tissue lasminogen activator. *Journal of Neurology, Neurosurgery and Psychiatry* **76**:70–75

Edlow BL, Hurwitz S, Edlow JA (2017). Diagnosis of DWI-negative acute ischaemic stroke. *Neurology* **89**:256–262

Essig M, Shiroishi MS, Nguyen TB *et al.* (2013). Perfusion MRI: The five most frequently asked technical questions. *American Journal of Roentgenology* **200**:24–34

Gass A, Ay H, Szabo K *et al.* (2004). Diffusion-weighted MRI for the "small stuff": The details of acute cerebral ischemia. *Lancet Neurology* **3**:39–45

Goyal M, Menon BK, van Zwam WH *et al.* (2016). Endovascular thrombectomy after large-vessel ischemic stroke: A meta-analysis of individual patient data from five randomized trials. *Lancet* **387**:1723–1731

Grotta JC, Chiu D, Lu M *et al.* (1999). Agreement and variability in the interpretation of early CT changes in stroke patients qualifying for intravenous rtPA therapy. *Stroke* **30**:1528–1533

Hand PJ, Wardlaw JM, Rivers CS *et al.* (2006). MR diffusion-weighted imaging and outcome prediction after ischemic stroke. *Neurology* **66**:1159–1163

Hawkins GC, Bonita R, Broad JB *et al.* (1995). Inadequacy of clinical scoring systems to differentiate stroke subtypes in population-based studies. *Stroke* **26**:1338–1342

Hjort N, Christensen S, Solling C *et al.* (2005a). Ischemic injury detected by diffusion imaging 11 minutes after stroke. *Annals of Neurology* **58**:462–465

Hjort N, Butcher K, Davis SM *et al.* (2005b). Magnetic resonance imaging criteria for thrombolysis in acute cerebral infarct. *Stroke* **36**:388–397

Horowitz SH, Zito JL, Donnarumma R *et al.* (1991). Computed tomographic–angiographic findings within the first five hours of cerebral infarction. *Stroke* **22**:1245–1253

IST-3 Collaborative Group (2015). Association between brain imaging signs, early and late outcomes, and response to intravenous alteplase after acute ischemic stroke in the third International Stroke Trial (IST-3): Secondary analysis of a randomized controlled trial. *Lancet Neurology* **14**:485–496

Karonen JO, Vanninen RL, Liu Y *et al.* (1999). Combined diffusion and perfusion MRI with correlation to single-photon emission CT in acute ischemic stroke. Ischemic penumbra predicts infarct growth. *Stroke* **30**:1583–1590

Kidwell CS, Hsia AW (2006). Imaging of the brain and cerebral vasculature in patients with suspected stroke: Advantages and disadvantages of CT and MRI. *Current Neurology and Neuroscience Reports* **6**:9–16

Koennecke HC (2006). Cerebral microbleeds on MRI: Prevalence associations and potential clinical implications. *Neurology* **66**:165–171

Kucinski T, Vaterlein O, Glauche V *et al.* (2002). Correlation of apparent diffusion coefficient and computed tomography density in acute ischemic stroke. *Stroke* **33**:1786–1791

Lansberg MG, Norbash AM, Marks MP *et al.* (2000). Advantages of adding diffusion-weighted magnetic resonance imaging to conventional magnetic resonance imaging for evaluating acute stroke. *Archives of Neurology* **57**:1311–1316

Lansberg MG, Thijs VN, Hamilton S for the DEFUSE Investigators (2007). Evaluation of the clinical–diffusion and perfusion–diffusion mismatch models in DEFUSE. *Stroke* **38**:1826–1830

Lee DK, Kim JS, Kwon SU *et al.* (2005). Lesion patterns and stroke mechanism in atherosclerotic middle cerebral artery disease: Early diffusion-weighted imaging study. *Stroke* **36**:2583–2588

Lutsep HL, Albers GW, DeCrespigny A *et al.* (1997). Clinical utility of diffusion-weighted magnetic resonance imaging in the assessment of ischemic stroke. *Annals of Neurology* **41**:574–580

Makin SDJ, Doubal FN, Dennis MS *et al.* (2015). Clinically confirmed stroke with negative diffusion-weighted imaging magnetic resonance imaging. *Stroke* **46**:3142–3148

Messe SR, Kasner SE, Chalela JA *et al.* (2007). CT–NIHSS mismatch does not correlate with MRI diffusion–perfusion mismatch. *Stroke* **38**:2079–2084

Meuli RA (2004). Imaging viable brain tissue with CT scan during acute stroke. *Cerebrovascular Disease* **17**:28–34

Mohr JP, Biller J, Hilal SK *et al.* (1995). Magnetic resonance versus computed tomographic imaging in acute stroke. *Stroke* **26**:807–812

Muir KW, Buchan A, von Kummer R *et al.* (2006). Imaging of acute stroke. *Lancet Neurology* **5**:755–768

Mullins ME, Schaefer PW, Sorensen AG *et al.* (2002). CT and conventional and diffusion-weighted MR imaging in acute stroke: Study in 691 patients at presentation to the emergency department. *Radiology* **224**:353–360

Nabavi DG, Kloska SP, Nam EM *et al.* (2002). MOSAIC: Multimodal stroke assessment using computed tomography: Novel diagnostic approach for the prediction of infarction size and clinical outcome. *Stroke* **33**:2819–2826

Nogueira RG, Jadhav AP, Haussen DC *et al.* (2018). Thrombectomy 6 to 24 hours after stroke with a mismatch between deficit and infarct. *New England Journal of Medicine* **378**:11- 21

Parsons MW, Pepper EM, Chan V *et al.* (2005). Perfusion computed tomography: Prediction of final infarct extent and stroke outcome. *Annals of Neurology* **58**:672–679

Powers WJ, Rabinstein AA, Ackerson T *et al.* (2018). 2018 Guidelines for the early management of patients with acute ischemic stroke: A guideline for healthcare professionals from the American Heart Association/American Stroke Association. *Stroke* **49**:e46–e110

Rodrigues MA, Samarasekera N, Lerpiniere C *et al.* (2018). The Edinburgh CT and genetic diagnostic criteria for lobar intracerebral hemorrhage associated with cerebral amyloid angiopathy: Model development and diagnostic test accuracy study. *Lancet Neurology* **17**:232–240

Schriger DL, Kalafut M, Starkman S *et al.* (1998). Cranial computed tomography interpretation in acute stroke: Physician accuracy in determining eligibility for thrombolytic therapy. *JAMA* **279**:1293–1297

Schulz UG, Flossman E, Rothwell PM (2004). Heritability of ischemic stroke in relation to age, vascular risk factors and subtypes of incident stroke in population-based studies. *Stroke* **35**:819–824

Shih LC, Saver JL, Alger JR *et al.* (2003). Perfusion-weighted magnetic resonance imaging thresholds identifying core, irreversibly infarcted tissue. *Stroke* 34:1425–1430

Simmons Z, Biller J, Adams HP, Jr. *et al.* (1986). Cerebellar infarction: Comparison of computed tomography and magnetic resonance imaging. *Annals of Neurology* 19:291–293

Singer OC, Humpich MC, Fiehler J for the MR Stroke Study Group Investigators (2007). Risk for symptomatic intracerebral hemorrhage after thrombolysis assessed by diffusion-weighted magnetic resonance imaging. *Annals of Neurology* 63:52–60

Singhal AB, Benner T, Roccatagliata L *et al.* (2005). A pilot study of normobaric oxygen therapy in acute ischemic stroke. *Stroke* 36:797–802

Sorensen AG, Buonanno FS, Gonzalez RG *et al.* (1996). Hyperacute stroke: Evaluation with combined multisection diffusion-weighted and haemodynamically weighted echo-planar MR imaging. *Radiology* 199:391–401

Thijs VN, Afami A, Neumann-Haefelin T *et al.* (2001). Relationship between severity of MR perfusion deficit and DWI lesion evolution. *Neurology* 57:1205–1211

Tsivgoulis G, Zand R, Katsanos AH *et al.* (2016). Risk of symptomatic intracerebral hemorrhage after intravenous thrombolysis in patients with acute ischemic stroke and high cerebral microbleed burden: A meta-analysis. *JAMA Neurology* 73:675–683

van Everdingen KJ, van der Grond J, Kappelle LJ *et al.* (1998). Diffusion-weighted magnetic resonance imaging in acute stroke. *Stroke* 29:1783–1790

von Kummer R, Meyding-Lamade U, Forsting M *et al.* (1994). Sensitivity and prognostic value of early CT in occlusion of the middle cerebral artery trunk. *American Journal of Neuroradiology* 15:9–15

von Kummer R, Holle R, Gizyska U *et al.* (1996). Interobserver agreement in assessing early CT signs of middle cerebral artery infarction. *American Journal of Neuroradiology* 17:1743–1748

Wintermark M, Bogousslavsky J (2003). Imaging of acute ischemic brain injury: The return of computed tomography. *Current Opinions in Neurology* 16:59–63

Wintermark M, Meuli R, Browaeys P *et al.* (2007). Comparison of CT perfusion and angiography and MRI in selecting stroke patients for acute treatment. *Neurology* 68:694–697

Yuh WT, Crain MR, Loes DJ *et al.* (1991). MR imaging of cerebral ischemia: Findings in the first 24 hours. *American Journal of Neuroradiology* 12:621–629

Zaharchuk G (2014). Arterial spin labeled perfusion imaging in acute ischemic stroke. *Stroke* 45:1202–1207

Chapter 12

Vascular Imaging in Transient Ischemic Attack and Stroke

The main clinical indications for imaging the cerebral circulation are TIA (e.g., to identify arterial stenosis), acute ischemic stroke (e.g., to identify vessel occlusion), intracerebral hemorrhage (e.g., to identify an underlying vascular malformation), and possible arterial dissection, fibromuscular dysplasia or other arteriopathies, cerebral aneurysm, intracranial venous thrombosis, or cerebral vasculitis.

In contrast to pharmaceutical products, diagnostic and imaging technologies are not subject to stringent regulatory control, and no standards are set for validation. As a result, the evidence base on important issues such as diagnostic sensitivity and specificity is often poor. For example, although several hundred studies of carotid imaging have been published over the past few decades, most are undermined by poor design, inadequate sample size, and inappropriate analysis and presentation of data (Rothwell *et al.* 2000a).

Catheter Angiography

Cerebral angiography, introduced by Moniz in Portugal in the 1930s, was the first method to display the cerebral circulation during life (Chapter 25). Originally it required the intracarotid injection of material that was opaque to X-rays. Over the years, the technology has improved, with less toxic contrast material, femoral artery catheterization, digital imaging, and catheters that can be controlled and introduced into vessels as small as the cortical branches of the middle cerebral artery.

Before the introduction of axial imaging of the brain in the early 1970s, first by computed tomography (CT) and then by magnetic resonance imaging (MRI), catheter angiography was used to identify intracranial mass lesions, hydrocephalus, and other structural abnormalities. Nowadays, with the increased use of CT angiography, MR angiography, and ultrasound imaging, catheter angiography is more or less confined to TIA/ischemic stroke patients in whom endovascular treatment is considered (e.g., prior to mechanical thrombectomy in patients with acute ischemic stroke due to large artery occlusion or for confirmation of symptomatic cases of severely stenotic intra- or extracranial arteries prior to angioplasty or stenting) and patients with intracranial hemorrhage where there remains a high suspicion of an underlying vascular abnormality (e.g., small cerebral aneurysm or intracranial vascular malformation) in whom noninvasive methods are nondiagnostic. The reasons for this diminishing role are that although catheter angiography remains the "gold standard" technique in many situations, it is inconvenient, invasive, uncomfortable, and costly and it requires hospital admission and carries a risk (Table 12.1). For example, a systematic review of prospective studies of the risks of catheter angiography in patients with cerebrovascular disease reported a 0.1% risk of death and

Table 12.1 Complications of catheter angiography

	Complication
Related to the catheter placement	TIA, stroke, or death as a result of dislodgement of atheromatous plaque by the catheter tip; dissection of the arterial wall; thrombus formation on the catheter tip; air embolism
Related to arterial puncture and cannulation	Hematoma
	Aneurysm Nerve injury Exacerbation of peripheral vascular disease distal to puncture site
Related to intravenous contrast	Allergic reaction
	Cardiac failure owing to the volume of injected contrast Renal toxicity

Note: TIA, transient ischemic attack.
Source: From Gerraty *et al.* (1996).

a 1.0% risk of permanent neurological sequelae (Hankey and Warlow 1990), although more recent studies have reported lower risks (Johnston *et al.* 2001).

Compared with cut-film selective intra-arterial catheter angiography recorded directly onto X-ray film, intra-arterial digital subtraction angiography (DSA) (Fig. 12.1) is quicker; the images are easier to manipulate and store, and contrast resolution is better, although spatial resolution is less. However, there is no evidence that less contrast is used or that it is much safer (Warnock *et al.* 1993). Even for imaging only as far as the carotid bifurcation, neither intravenous DSA nor arch aortography is a satisfactory alternative to selective intra-arterial angiography (Pelz *et al.* 1985; Rothwell *et al.* 1998; Cuffe and Rothwell 2006).

Even with selective catheter angiography, there can be difficulty in distinguishing occlusion from extreme internal carotid artery stenosis, and then late views are needed to see contrast eventually passing up into the head. Moreover, because of the localized and nonconcentric nature of atherosclerotic plaques, biplanar, and preferably triplanar (Jeans *et al.* 1986; Cuffe and Rothwell 2006), views of the carotid bifurcation are required to measure the degree of carotid stenosis accurately: that is, to visualize the residual lumen without overlap of other vessels, to measure at the narrowest point, and to compare with a suitable denominator to derive the percentage diameter stenosis.

Catheter angiography can also provide information about ulceration of carotid plaque and complicating luminal thrombosis, albeit with only moderate interobserver agreement (Streifler *et al.* 1994; Rothwell *et al.* 1998). However, angiographic irregularity and ulceration predict a higher risk of stroke than if the plaque is smooth, given the same degree of stenosis (Eliasziw *et al.* 1994; Rothwell *et al.* 2000b), and there is good correlation between catheter angiographic plaque morphology and histology when the latter is rigorously

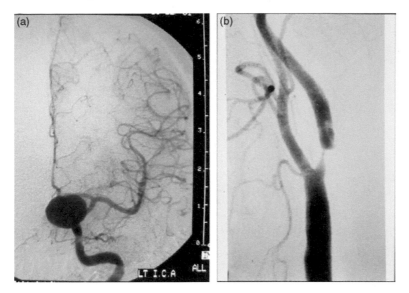

Fig. 12.1 Digitally subtracted arterial angiograms showing a large distal internal carotid artery aneurysm (a) and a severe stenosis of the proximal internal carotid artery (b).

evaluated (Lovett *et al.* 2004). Luminal thrombus is relatively unusual but is thought to be associated with a high risk of stroke (Martin *et al.* 1992).

With the advances in MRI, CT, and MR angiography, underlying structural vascular causes of intracerebral hemorrhage are increasingly being detected without the need of catheter angiography (discussed later). MRI can even be more sensitive than catheter angiography in detecting certain vascular malformations such as cavernomas. However, catheter angiography still has a role in revealing small vascular malformations or aneurysms in patients whom the cause of intracerebral hemorrhage cannot be identified via CT or MR angiography, and the suspicion of an underlying structural vascular cause remains high (Zhu *et al.* 1997; Wilson *et al.* 2015).

In the past, catheter angiography was the standard imaging modality to confirm or exclude carotid or vertebral artery dissection (Fig. 12.2) because ultrasound was neither specific nor sensitive enough. However, there is now a widespread consensus that cross-sectional MRI, to show thrombus within the widened arterial wall, combined with MR angiography is the safest and best option.

Catheter Angiography versus Noninvasive Imaging

Although noninvasive methods of imaging continue to improve, catheter angiography remains the gold standard against which other vessel imaging methods must be compared, and it is also the underpinning method for the interventional neuroradio-logical treatment of arterial stenoses, aneurysms, and vascular malformations. However, the clinician is often faced with the question as to whether to base decision making on noninvasive imaging alone or whether to proceed to catheter angiography. For example, multi-slice CT angiography is widely used in the screening for cerebral aneurysms because of its speed, tolerability, safety, and potential for three-dimensional

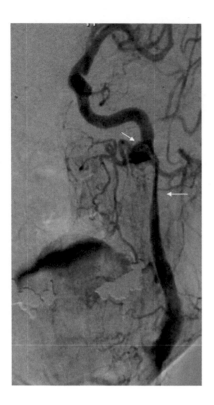

Fig. 12.2 Digitally subtracted arterial angiogram showing a distal internal carotid artery dissection (tapering lumen; lower arrow) and a complicating aneurysm (upper arrow).

reconstructions. The sensitivity of CT angiography compared with conventional angiography for aneurysms ≥ 10 mm is 100%, but the sensitivity decreases with aneurysm size (5 to < 10 mm: 98.4%; 3 to < 5 mm: 94% and < 3 mm: 91.3%) (Lu *et al.* 2012). The sensitivity for detecting ruptured aneurysms with CT angiography, with conventional angiography as the gold standard, is approximately 95% (Villablanca *et al.* 2002; Chappell *et al.* 2003; Wintermark *et al.* 2003). MR angiography has similar resolution to CT angiography but is less easy to use in sick patients. Four-vessel catheter angiography may still, therefore, be required when noninvasive imaging is negative.

A similar trade-off between diagnostic accuracy and risk is necessary when imaging the carotid bifurcation in patients with TIA or ischemic stroke. Performing intra-arterial catheter angiography in everyone is clearly unacceptable because of the risks and cost. Fewer than 20% of patients will have an operable carotid stenosis, even if only those with "cortical" rather than "lacunar" events are selected (Hankey and Warlow 1991; Hankey *et al.* 1991; Mead *et al.* 1999). Confining angiography to patients with a carotid bifurcation bruit will miss some patients with severe stenosis and still subject too many with mild or moderate stenosis to the risks. Nor will a combination of a cervical bruit with various clinical features do much better (Mead *et al.* 1999).

Therefore, noninvasive imaging is required at least as an initial screening tool. In many centers, decisions about endarterectomy are now based solely on noninvasive imaging.

However, because benefit from endarterectomy is highly dependent on the degree of symptomatic carotid stenosis as measured on catheter angiography, misclassification of stenosis with noninvasive methods will lead to some patients being operated on unnecessarily and others being denied appropriate surgery. A meta-analysis of studies of noninvasive carotid imaging published prior to 1995 concluded that noninvasive methods could not substitute for catheter angiography as the sole pre-endarterectomy imaging because of the frequency with which the degree of stenosis was misclassified (Blakeley *et al.* 1995). More recent studies have confirmed this (Johnston and Goldstein 2001; Norris *et al.* 2003; Norris and Halliday 2004; Chappell *et al.* 2006). For example, in a comparison of catheter angiography with Doppler ultrasound in 569 consecutive patients in "accredited" laboratories with experienced radiologists, 28% of decisions about endarterectomy based on Doppler ultrasound alone were inappropriate (Johnston and Goldstein 2001). However, the combination of Doppler ultrasound with another noninvasive method of imaging, such as MR angiography, reduced inappropriate decisions in comparison with catheter angiography to less than 10% in patients for whom the results of Doppler ultrasound and MR angiography were concordant (Johnston and Goldstein 2001). Similar approaches based on two different methods of noninvasive imaging have been shown by other groups to be effective in routine clinical practice (Johnston *et al.* 2002; Barth *et al.* 2006). Catheter angiography is still required in the patients in whom Doppler ultrasound and MR angiography do not produce concordant results. Catheter angiography is also required for confirmation of lesion severity in patients with suspected symptomatic severe vertebrobasilar or intracranial stenosis in whom angioplasty or stenting is being contemplated.

Duplex Sonography

Duplex sonography combines real-time ultrasound imaging to display the arterial anatomy with pulsed Doppler flow analysis at any point of interest in the vessel lumen. Its accuracy is enhanced and it is technically easier to carry out if the Doppler signals are color-coded to show the direction of blood flow and its velocity (Fig. 12.3). Power Doppler and intravenous echocontrast may also help (Droste *et al.* 1999; Gaitini and Soudack 2005; Wardlaw and Lewis 2005). The degree of carotid luminal stenosis is calculated not only from the real-time ultrasound image, which can be inaccurate when the lesion is echolucent or calcification scatters the ultrasound beam, but also from the blood flow velocities derived from the Doppler signal. If color Doppler is not available but only grayscale duplex, it is usually helpful to insonate the supraorbital artery first with a simple continuous-wave Doppler probe because *inward* flow of blood strongly suggests severe internal carotid artery stenosis or occlusion, although not necessarily at the origin.

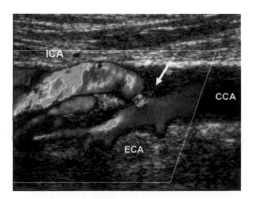

Fig. 12.3 A color-flow Doppler ultrasound of the carotid bifurcation showing a plaque (arrow) at the origin of the internal carotid artery (ICA) and the resulting stenosis. ECA, external carotid artery; CCA, common carotid artery.

BOX 12.1 Difficulties Encountered with Carotid Duplex Sonography

- Operator dependent, so requires training, skill, and experience to ensure accuracy of and consistency in measurement of stenosis
- Plaque or peri-arterial calcification causes difficulty in interpretation
- Lack of reliability in distinguishing very severe stenosis (> 90%) from occlusion and resultant uncertainty in decision making about surgery
- Only moderate-to-good sensitivity and specificity for severe internal carotid artery stenosis (70–99%)
- Variability between machines in accuracy of measurement of carotid stenosis
- Little information provided about proximal or distal arterial anatomy (although this is sometimes not relevant to the surgeon nor affected by disease)

Although duplex sonography is noninvasive and widely available, there are some difficulties that any ultrasound service must deal with (Box 12.1). Nonetheless, with stringent quality control and ideally with confirmation of stenosis by an independent observer, duplex sonography is now the most common way that carotid stenosis severe enough to warrant surgery is diagnosed (Chappell *et al.* 2006).

There are no standard and commonly used definitions for the ultrasound appearance of plaques (soft, hard, calcified, etc.) and there is also considerable variation in reporting between and even within the same observers at different times (Arnold *et al.* 1999). Therefore, although unstable and ulcerated plaques are more likely to be symptomatic than stable plaques with fibrous caps, the ultrasound inaccuracy compromises any study of the relationship between plaque characteristics on duplex sonography and the risk of later stroke, and so the selection for carotid surgery (Gronholdt 1999). In asymptomatic stenosis, there is some evidence that a hypoechoic plaque predicts an increased risk of stroke (Polak *et al.* 1998), but this was not confirmed in the Asymptomatic Carotid Surgery Trial (Halliday *et al.* 2004). Until it becomes possible to translate carotid plaque irregularity as seen on catheter angiography, which does add to the risk of stroke over and above the degree of stenosis, into what is seen on duplex sonography, it will remain difficult to use anything other than stenosis to predict stroke risk if only duplex is being used.

Despite these limitations, duplex sonography is a remarkably quick and simple investigation in experienced hands, and it is neither unpleasant nor risky. Very rarely, the pressure of the Doppler probe on the carotid bifurcation can dislodge thrombus or cause enough carotid sinus stimulation to lead to bradycardia or hypotension (Rosario *et al.* 1987; Friedman 1990). The same conceivably applies to the various arterial compression maneuvers that may be carried out during transcranial Doppler, and any such compression should be avoided in patients who may have carotid bifurcation disease.

Computed Tomography Angiography

Computed tomography is now a widely used method for imaging the cerebral circulation as well as the carotid and vertebral arteries (Brink *et al.* 1997; Josephson *et al.* 2004; Bartlett *et al.* 2006; Khan *et al.* 2007). CT angiography is very quick (takes less than 1 minute) and

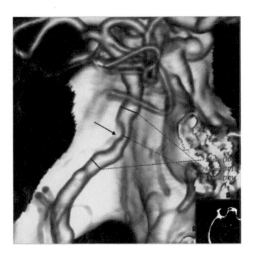

Fig. 12.4 A CT angiogram three-dimensional reconstruction showing a stenosis (arrow) of the distal vertebral artery.

easy to perform, is widely available, and is not contraindicated in those with pacemakers, ferromagnetic implants, mechanical heart valves, or claustrophobia. It can thus be performed in very sick patients in whom MRI may be difficult. However, it does require ≈100 ml of iodinated contrast to outline the arterial lumen and hence may be contraindicated in patients with known severe renal impairment or severe allergies to iodinated contrast. Nevertheless, the incidence of significant contrast-induced renal impairment in acute stroke patients undergoing urgent CT scanning with contrast is low (Krol *et al.* 2007; Hopyan *et al.* 2008) and it is reasonable to proceed with an urgent CT angiogram before obtaining a serum creatinine concentration in patients without a history of renal impairment if clinically indicated (Powers *et al.* 2018). Patients undergoing CT angiography will be subjected to X-ray exposure; the images obtained depend on the proficiency of the operator in their selection, and it tends to underestimate vessel stenosis. Nevertheless, it does provide multiple viewing angles, three-dimensional reconstruction (Fig. 12.4), and imaging of calcium deposits separately from the vessel lumen outlined by the contrast (Heiken *et al.* 1993; Leclerc *et al.* 1995; Nandalur *et al.* 2006).

Compared with DSA, CT angiography is highly sensitive in detecting intracranial (97.1%), carotid (96–100%), and vertebral artery atherosclerosis (~100%) (Josephson *et al.* 2004; Khan *et al.* 2007; Nguyen-Huynh *et al.* 2008) as well as in detecting intracranial aneurysms (aneurysm size < 3 mm: 91.3%, 3 to < 5 mm: 94.0%; 5 to < 10 mm: 98.4% and ≥ 10 mm: 100%) (Lu *et al.* 2012). Importantly, CT angiography provides a rapid and convenient means of identifying patients with acute ischemic stroke due to large artery occlusion. It can be performed right after the brain parenchyma is scanned and hence can quickly identify potential candidates that would qualify for endovascular treatment (Powers *et al.* 2015) (see Chapter 21). Recently, the "clot-burden score" was developed, which aims to quantify the extent of intracranial thrombosis visualized on CT angiography (Tan *et al.* 2009). This score is composed of 10 points in total, and points are subtracted if presence of occlusion or nonocclusive clots are noted at certain locations (2 points deducted if presence of clot noted within the supraclinoid internal carotid artery, proximal or distal M1 of middle cerebral artery; 1 point deducted if presence of clot noted within the infraclinoid internal carotid artery, anterior cerebral artery, or M2 segment of middle cerebral artery). A clot burden score of 0 therefore indicates complete multi-segmental vessel occlusion. Lower scores have been shown to predict larger infarcts, a higher risk of hemorrhagic transformation, lower recanalization rates with intravenous thrombolysis, and an overall poor outcome (Puetz *et al.* 2008).

CT angiography in patients with acute ischemic stroke also allows collateral blood flow (e.g., leptomeningeal arteries), an important determinant of the rate that penumbral tissue evolves into an irreversible infarct, to be imaged (Campbell *et al.* 2013). Collateral blood flow differs from individual to individual and is dependent on variations in vascular anatomy, presence of underlying atherosclerosis, clot location, and burden. There are currently a number of scoring systems, such as the regional leptomeningeal collateral score and collateral score (Menon *et al.* 2011; Fanou *et al.* 2015). Both scores have been shown to independently predict infarct volume, risk of hemorrhagic transformation, and poor outcome in patients with acute ischemic stroke due to a large artery occlusion (Menon *et al.* 2011; Fanou *et al.* 2015). However, the optimal scoring method remains uncertain.

Recently, multiphase CT angiography, performed during three different phases (peak arterial, peak venous, and late venous) after contrast injection, has been shown to be superior to single-phase CT angiography by providing a more comprehensive picture of the underlying collateral blood flow (Menon *et al.* 2015). Furthermore, CT angiogram source images could be re-windowed to look for early ischemic changes in the brain parenchyma. The Alberta Stroke Program Early CT score (ASPECTS) could also be calculated based on these CT angiogram-derived source images, and it has been shown that these images are superior to those obtained from non-contrast CT in predicting final infarct volumes of strokes affecting both the anterior and posterior circulations (Coutts *et al.* 2004; Schramm *et al.* 2004; Camargo *et al.* 2007; Puetz *et al.* 2011).

Magnetic Resonance Angiography

MR angiography is noninvasive and safe if done without contrast ("time of flight" imaging) (Fig. 12.5). Contrast-enhanced imaging provides improved resolution and reduces problems with flow voids at points of stenosis, and it is necessary for detecting cerebral aneurysms or determining the severity of carotid stenosis. However, even with contrast, MR angiography is unlikely to be accurate enough in estimating carotid stenosis, at least at the present stage of development (Graves 1997; Chappell *et al.* 2006; DeMarco *et al.* 2006). The pictures are not always adequate to allow measurement of the carotid stenosis (movement and swallowing artifacts are particular problems); the severity of the stenosis tends to be overestimated; there may be a flow gap distal to a stenosis of as little as 60%, making precise stenosis measurement impossible even in the posterior part of the carotid bulb, in both cases probably because of loss of laminar flow and increased residence times of the blood; irregularity/ulceration are not well seen; and severe stenosis can be confused with occlusion (Siewert *et al.* 1995; Levi *et al.* 1996; Fox *et al.* 2005). However, image quality and reproducibility of measurement of stenosis are significantly improved with contrast-enhanced MR angiography (DeMarco *et al.* 2006; Mitra *et al.* 2006). So far, there have not been enough methodologically sound comparisons of MR angiography with catheter angiography (U-King-Im *et al.* 2005; Chappell *et al.* 2006). The comparative studies that have been carried out have frequently been overtaken by changes in MR technology. For example, in the recent years, high-resolution MRI of the carotid and intracranial artery

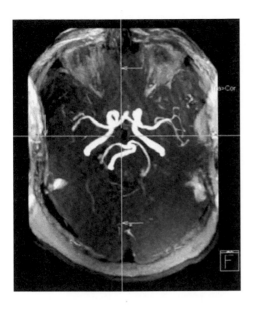

Fig. 12.5 A "time of flight" MR angiogram of the circle of Willis in a patient with no posterior communicating arteries.

plaques has gained popularity (Watanabe and Nagayama 2010; Ryu *et al.* 2014). This technique aims to characterize the overall condition of the plaque (e.g., nature of fibrous cap, size of necrotic core, whether any intra-plaque hemorrhage is present, extent of inflammatory activity within the plaque) as well as the underlying vessel wall. Although these techniques have potential as a means of further risk stratifying patients beyond severity of atherosclerosis (e.g., by identifying suitable patients for endarterectomy or intracranial artery stenting), these techniques are currently not widely available in routine clinical practice.

Imaging the Posterior Circulation

Vertebrobasilar TIAs were thought for many years to be associated with a lower risk of stroke than carotid territory TIAs, but recent work has shown that the risk of stroke is at least as high (Flossmann and Rothwell 2003; Flossmann *et al.* 2006). There is, therefore, an increasing interest in angioplasty and stenting of atherothrombotic stenoses of the vertebral or proximal basilar arteries (see Chapter 26). Angiography with MR or CT is the most useful noninvasive method of imaging the posterior circulation (Fig. 12.6), although catheter angiography is often still necessary to confirm or exclude significant stenosis.

Although asymptomatic **subclavian steal** is quite common (reversed vertebral artery flow detected by ultrasound or vertebral angiography), *symptomatic* subclavian steal is rare, presumably because collateral blood flow to the brainstem is enough to compensate for the reversed vertebral artery blood flow distal to ipsilateral subclavian stenosis or occlusion. The clinical syndrome is quite easily recognized by unequal blood pressures between the two arms, a supraclavicular bruit, and vertebrobasilar TIAs, which may or may not be brought on by exercise of the arm ipsilateral to the subclavian stenosis or occlusion, so increasing blood flow down the vertebral artery from the brainstem to the arm muscles (Bornstein and Norris 1986; Hennerici *et al.* 1988). It is only this type of symptomatic patient who may

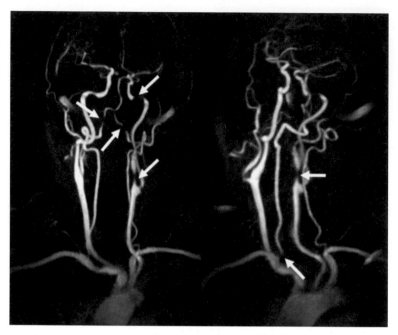

Fig. 12.6 Contrast-enhanced magnetic resonance angiography revealing multiple severe stenotic lesions affecting both vertebral arteries (right V1 and V4 segments, left V4 segment) and the left internal carotid artery (proximal and distal).

require surgery and, therefore, who has to accept the risk of any preceding angiography. **Innominate artery steal** is even rarer, with retrograde vertebral artery flow distal to innominate rather than subclavian artery occlusion (Kempczinski and Hermann 1979; Grosveld *et al.* 1988).

Transcranial Doppler Sonography

Transcranial Doppler sonography provides information on the velocity of blood flow, and its direction in relation to the ultrasound probe, in the major intracranial arteries at the base of the brain and so whether they are occluded or stenosed. It is noninvasive, safe, repeatable, and not too difficult to perform accurately; can be performed at the bedside; and is not expensive. However, the patient has to keep reasonably still; the examination can take as long as an hour; the skull is impervious to ultrasound in 5–10% of individuals, more with increasing age and in females but less if intravenous echocontrast is used; exact vessel identification may be difficult, but color-flow real-time imaging makes this easier; spatial resolution is poor; diagnostic criteria vary; and the technique is not always accurate in comparison with cerebral catheter angiography (Baumgartner *et al.* 1997; Baumgartner 1999; Gerriets *et al.* 1999; Markus 1999).

Despite the fact that transcranial Doppler sonography, like positron emission tomography, has increased our knowledge of the cerebral circulation in health and disease and even though it is inexpensive and quite widely available and repeatable on demand (unlike positron emission tomography), it still has rather a minor role in *routine* clinical management.

Possible indications for transcranial Doppler ultrasound in routine clinical practice (Babikian *et al.* 1997; Molloy and Markus 1999; Alexandrov *et al.* 2004; Kim *et al.* 2005; Dittrich *et al.* 2006; Markus 2006) include:

- operative monitoring during carotid endarterectomy.
- diagnosis of patent foramen ovale and other right-to-left shunts.
- identification of patients with carotid stenosis at high risk of stroke.
- display of intracranial arterial occlusion and stenosis.
- assessment of cerebrovascular reactivity.
- acceleration of clot lysis during or after thrombolysis for acute ischemic stroke.

Detection of emboli as high-intensity transient signals on the sonogram, so-called microembolic signals, might be of clinical relevance in certain situations. The vast majority of such signals appear to be from asymptomatic emboli, but their detection may help in distinguishing cardiac and aortic arch emboli from carotid emboli because with the first two, emboli should be detected in several arterial distributions; whereas with the last, in only the one arterial distribution distal to the supposed embolic source (Markus *et al.* 1994; Sliwka *et al.* 1997; Markus 2006). However, the frequency of microembolic signals can be so frustratingly low and variable, and so their detection requires prolonged monitoring and automation (Markus 1999, 2006; Dittrich *et al.* 2006). Consequently, their detection is currently used mainly as a research tool, most usefully perhaps as a surrogate outcome in trials of secondary prevention of stroke (Dittrich *et al.* 2006; Markus 2006).

Transcranial Doppler sonography can also be used to assess cerebrovascular reactivity as indicated by the capacity for intracranial vasodilatation in response to acetazolamide, carbon dioxide inhalation, or breath holding, although these three methods do not always produce concordant results (Bishop *et al.* 1986; Markus and Harrison 1992; Dahl *et al.* 1995; Derdeyn *et al.* 2005). However, there is still debate about exactly how to standardize this test, and it is not widely used in routine clinical practice. Impaired reactivity may have some prognostic significance for identifying individual patients at particularly high risk of stroke from among those with carotid stenosis and internal carotid artery occlusion, although the numbers studied have been small and the situation is not yet clear-cut (Derdeyn *et al.* 1999, 2005; Vernieri *et al.* 2001). With time and presumably increasing collateralization, any impairment of reactivity can return to normal (Kleiser and Widder 1992; Widder *et al.* 1994; Gur *et al.* 1996; Vernieri *et al.* 1999).

References

Alexandrov AV, Molina CA, Grotta JC *et al.* (2004). Ultrasound-enhanced systemic thrombolysis for acute ischemic stroke. *New England Journal of Medicine* **351**:2170–2178

Arnold JA, Modaresi KB, Thomas N *et al.* (1999). Carotid plaque characterization by duplex scanning: Observer error may undermine current clinical trials. *Stroke* **30**:61–65

Babikian VL, Wijman CAC, Hyde C *et al.* (1997). Cerebral microembolism and early recurrent cerebral or retinal ischemic events. *Stroke* **28**:1314–1318

Bartlett ES, Symons SP, Fox AJ (2006). Correlation of carotid stenosis diameter and cross-sectional areas with CT angiography. *American Journal of Neuroradiology* **27**:638–642

Barth A, Arnold M, Mattle HPC *et al.* (2006). Contrast-enhanced 3-D MRA in decision making for carotid endarterectomy: A 6-year experience. *Cerebrovascular Diseases* **21**:393–400

Baumgartner RW (1999). Transcranial color-coded duplex sonography. *Journal of Neurology* **246**:637–647

Baumgartner RW, Mattle HP, Aaslid RC *et al.* (1997). Transcranial colour-coded duplex sonography in arterial cerebrovascular disease. *Cerebrovascular Diseases* **7**:57–63

Bishop CCR, Powell S, Insall MC *et al.* (1986). Effect of internal carotid artery occlusion on middle cerebral artery blood flow at rest and in response to hypercapnia. *Lancet* **i**:710–712

Blakeley DD, Oddone EZ, Hasselblad VC *et al.* (1995). Non-invasive carotid artery testing: A meta-analytic review. *Annals of Internal Medicine* **122**:360–367

Bornstein NM, Norris JW (1986). Subclavian steal: A harmless haemodynamic phenomenon? *Lancet* **ii**:303–305

Brink JA, McFarland EG, Heiken JP (1997). Helical/spiral computed body tomography. *Clinical Radiology* **52**:489–503

Camargo EC, Furie KL, Singhal AB *et al.* (2007). Acute brain infarct: Detection and delineation with CT angiographic source images versus nonenhanced CT scans. *Radiology* **244**:541–548

Campbell BC, Christensen S, Tress BM *et al.* (2013). Failure of collateral blood flow is associated with infarct growth in ischemic stroke. *Journal of Cerebral Blood Flow and Metabolism* **33**:1168–1172

Campbell BC, Mitchell MJ, Kleinig TJ *et al.* (2015). Endovascular therapy for ischemic stroke with perfusion-imaging selection. *New England Journal of Medicine* **372**:1009–1018

Chappell ET, Moure FC, Good MC (2003). Comparison of computed tomographic angiography with digital subtraction angiography in the diagnosis of cerebral aneurysms: A meta-analysis. *Neurosurgery* **52**:624–631

Chappell F, Wardlaw J, Best JKK *et al.* (2006). Non-invasive imaging compared with intra-arterial angiography in the diagnosis of symptomatic carotid stenosis: A meta-analysis. *Lancet* **376**:1503–1512

Coutts SB, Lev MH, Eliasziw M *et al.* (2004). ASPECTS on CTA source images versus unenhanced CT: Added value in predicting final infarct extent and clinical outcome. *Stroke* **35**:2472–2476

Cuffe R, Rothwell PM (2006). Effect of non-optimal imaging on the relationship between the measured degree of symptomatic carotid stenosis and risk of ischemic stroke. *Stroke* **37**:1785–1791

Dahl A, Russell D, Rootwelt KC *et al.* (1995). Cerebral vasoreactivity assessed with transcranial Doppler and regional cerebral blood flow measurements: Dose serum concentration and time course of the response to acetazolamide. *Stroke* **26**:2302–2306

DeMarco JK, Huston J III, Nash AK (2006). Extracranial carotid MR imaging at 3T. *Magnetic Resonance Imaging Clinics of North America* **14**:109–1021

Derdeyn CP, Grubb RL, Powers WJ (1999). Cerebral haemodynamic impairment: Methods of measurements and association with stroke risk. *Neurology* **53**:251–259

Derdeyn CP, Grubb RL Jr., Powers WJ (2005). Indications for cerebral revascularization for patients with atherosclerotic carotid occlusion. *Skull Base* **15**:7–14

Dittrich R, Ritter MA, Kaps MC *et al.* (2006). The use of embolic signal detection in multicenter trials to evaluate antiplatelet efficacy: Signal analysis and quality control mechanisms in the CARESS (Clopidogrel and Aspirin for Reduction of Emboli in Symptomatic carotid Stenosis) trial. *Stroke* **37**:1065–1069

Droste DW, Jurgens R, Nabavi DGC *et al.* (1999). Echocontrast-enhanced ultrasound of extracranial internal carotid artery high-grade stenosis and occlusion. *Stroke* **30**:2302–2306

Eliasziw M, Streifler JY, Fox AJC for the North American Symptomatic Carotid Endarterectomy Trial (1994). Significance of plaque ulceration in symptomatic patients with high-grade carotid stenosis. *Stroke* **25**:304–308

Fanou EM, Knight J, Aviv RI *et al.* (2015). Effect of collaterals on clinical presentation, baseline imaging, complications, and outcome in acute stroke. *American Journal of Neuroradiology* **36**:2285–2291

Flossmann E, Rothwell PM (2003). Prognosis of verterobrobasilar transient ischemic attack and minor ischemic stroke. *Brain* **126**:1940–1954

Flossmann E, Redgrave JN, Schulz UGC et al. (2006). Reliability of clinical diagnosis of the symptomatic vascular territory in patients with recent TIA or minor stroke. *Cerebrovascular Diseases* **21**(Suppl 4):18

Fox AJ, Eliasziw M, Rothwell PMC et al. (2005). Identification prognosis and management of patients with carotid artery near occlusion. *American Journal of Neuroradiology* **26**:2086–2094

Friedman SG (1990). Transient ischemic attacks resulting from carotid duplex imaging. *Surgery* **107**:153–155

Gaitini D, Soudack M (2005). Diagnosing carotid stenosis by Doppler sonography: State of the art. *Journal of Ultrasound Medicine* **24**:1127–1136

Gerraty RP, Bowser DN, Infeld BC et al. (1996). Microemboli during carotid angiography: Association with stroke risk factors or subsequent magnetic resonance imaging changes? *Stroke* **27**:1543–1547

Gerriets T, Seidel G, Fiss IC et al. (1999). Contrast-enhanced transcranial colour-coded duplex sonography: Efficiency and validity. *Neurology* **52**:1133–1137

Graves MJ (1997). Magnetic resonance angiography. *British Journal of Radiology* **70**:6–28

Gronholdt MLM (1999). Ultrasound and lipoproteins as predictors of lipid-rich rupture-prone plaques in the carotid artery. *Arteriosclerosis Thrombosis and Vascular Biology* **19**:2–13

Grosveld WJ, Lawson JA, Eikelboom BCC et al. (1988). Clinical and haemodynamic significance of innominate artery lesions evaluated by ultrasonography and digital angiography. *Stroke* **19**:958–962

Gur AY, Bova I, Bornstein NM (1996). Is impaired cerebral vasomotor reactivity a predictive factor of stroke in asymptomatic patients? *Stroke* **27**:2188–2190

Halliday A, Mansfield A, Marro JC for the MRC Asymptomatic Carotid Surgery Trial (ACST) Collaborative Group (2004). Prevention of disabling and fatal strokes by successful carotid endarterectomy in patients without recent neurological symptoms: Randomised controlled trial. *Lancet* **363**:1491–1502

Hand PJ, Wardlaw JM, Rivers CS et al. (2006). MR diffusion-weighted imaging and outcome prediction after ischemic stroke. *Neurology* **66**:1159–1163

Hankey GJ, Warlow CP (1990). Symptomatic carotid ischemic events: Safest and most cost effective way of selecting patients for angiography before carotid endarterectomy. *British Medical Journal* **300**:1485–1491

Hankey GJ, Warlow CP (1991). Lacunar transient ischemic attacks: A clinically useful concept? *Lancet* **337**:335–338

Hankey GJ, Slattery JM, Warlow CP (1991). The prognosis of hospital-referred transient ischemic attacks. *Journal of Neurology, Neurosurgery and Psychiatry* **54**:793–802

Heiken JP, Brink JA, Vannier MW (1993). Spiral (helical) CT. *Radiology* **189**:647–656

Hennerici M, Klemm C, Rautenberg W (1988). The subclavian steal phenomenon: A common vascular disorder with rare neurologic deficits. *Neurology* **38**:669–673

Hopyan JJ, Gladstone DJ, Mallia G et al. (2008). Renal safety of CT angiography and perfusion imaging in the emergency evaluation of acute stroke. *American Journal of Neuroradiology* **29**:1826–1830

Jeans WD, Mackenzie S, Baird RN (1986). Angiography in transient cerebral ischemia using three views of the carotid bifurcation. *British Journal of Radiology* **59**:135–142

Johnston DC, Goldstein LB (2001). Clinical carotid endarterectomy decision making: Noninvasive vascular imaging versus angiography. *Neurology* **56**:1009–1015

Johnston DC, Chapman KM, Goldstein LB (2001). Low rate of complications of cerebral angiography in routine clinical practice. *Neurology* **57**:2012–2014

Johnston DC, Eastwood JD, Nguyen TC et al. (2002). Contrast-enhanced magnetic resonance angiography of carotid arteries: Utility in routine clinical practice. *Stroke* **33**:2834–2838

Josephson SA, Bryant SO, Mak HK et al. (2004). Evaluation of carotid stenosis using CT angiography in the initial evaluation of stroke and TIA. *Neurology* **63**:457–460

Kempczinski R, Hermann G (1979). The innominate steal syndrome. *Journal of Cardiovascular Surgery* 20:481–486

Khan S, Cloud GC, Kerry S *et al.* (2007). Imaging of vertebral artery stenosis: A systematic review. *Journal of Neurology, Neurosurgery and Psychiatry* 78:1218–1225

Kim YS, Garami Z, Mikulik RC for the CLOTBUST Collaborators (2005). Early recanalization rates and clinical outcomes in patients with tandem internal carotid artery/middle cerebral artery occlusion and isolated middle cerebral artery occlusion. *Stroke* 36:869–871

Kleiser B, Widder B (1992). Course of carotid artery occlusions with impaired cerebrovascular reactivity. *Stroke* 23:171–174

Krol AL, Dzialowski I, Roy J *et al.* (2008). Incidence of radiocontrast nephropathy in patients undergoing acute stroke computed tomography angiography. *Stroke* 38:2364–2366

Leclerc X, Godefroy O, Pruvo JPC *et al.* (1995). Computed tomographic angiography for the evaluation of carotid artery stenosis. *Stroke* 26:1577–1581

Levi CR, Mitchell A, Fitt GC *et al.* (1996). The accuracy of magnetic resonance angiography in the assessment of extracranial carotid artery occlusive disease. *Cerebrovascular Diseases* 6:231–236

Lovett JK, Gallagher PJ, Hands LJC *et al.* (2004). Histological correlates of carotid plaque surface morphology on lumen contrast imaging. *Circulation* 110:2190–2197

Lu L, Zhang LJ, Poon CS *et al.* (2012). Digital subtraction CT angiography for detection of intracranial aneurysms: Comparison with three-dimensional digital subtraction angiography. *Radiology* 262:605–612

Markus HS (1999). Transcranial Doppler ultrasound. *Journal of Neurology, Neurosurgery and Psychiatry* 67:135–137

Markus HS (2006). Can microemboli on transcranial Doppler identify patients at increased stroke risk? *Nature Clinical Practice in Cardiovascular Medicine* 3:246–247

Markus HS, Harrison MJG (1992). Estimation of cerebrovascular reactivity using transcranial Doppler, including the use of breath-holding as the vasodilatory stimulus. *Stroke* 23:668–673

Markus HS, Droste DW, Brown MM (1994). Detection of asymptomatic cerebral embolic signals with Doppler ultrasound. *Lancet* 343:1011–1012

Martin R, Bogousslavsky J, Miklossy J *et al.* (1992). Floating thrombus in the innominate artery as a cause of cerebral infarction in young adults. *Cerebrovascular Diseases* 2:177–181

Mead GE, Wardlaw JM, Lewis SCC *et al.* (1999). Can simple clinical features be used to identify patients with severe carotid stenosis on Doppler ultrasound? *Journal of Neurology, Neurosurgery and Psychiatry* 66:16–19

Menon BK, Smith EE, Modi J et al. (2011). Regional leptomeningeal score on CT angiography predicts clinical and imaging outcomes in patients with acute anterior circulation occlusions. *American Journal of Neuroradiology* 32:1640–1645

Menon BK, d'Esterre CD, Qazi EM *et al.* (2015). Multiphase CT angiography: A new tool for the imaging triage of patients with acute ischemic stroke. *Radiology* 275:510–520

Meuli RA (2004). Imaging viable brain tissue with CT scan during acute stroke. *Cerebrovascular Diseases* 17:28–34

Mitra D, Connolly D, Jenkins SC *et al.* (2006). Comparison of image quality, diagnostic confidence and interobserver variability in contrast enhanced MR angiography and 2D time of flight angiography, in evaluation of carotid stenosis. *British Journal of Radiology* 79:201–207

Molloy J, Markus HS (1999). Asymptomatic embolization predicts stroke and TIA risk in patients with carotid artery stenosis. *Stroke* 30:1440–1443

Nabavi DG, Kloska SP, Nam EM *et al.* (2002). MOSAIC: Multimodal stroke assessment using computed tomography: Novel diagnostic approach for the prediction of infarction size and clinical outcome. *Stroke* 33:2819–2826

Nandalur KR, Baskurt E, Hagspiel KDC *et al.* (2006). Carotid artery calcification on CT may independently predict stroke risk. *American Journal of Radiology* 186:547–552

Nguyen-Huynh MN, Wintermark M, English J et al. (2008). How accurate is CT angiography in evaluating intracranial atherosclerotic disease? *Stroke* **39**:1184–1188

Norris JW, Halliday A (2004). Is ultrasound sufficient for vascular imaging prior to carotid endarterectomy? *Stroke* **35**:370–371

Norris JW, Morriello F, Rowed DW et al. (2003). Vascular imaging before carotid endarterectomy. *Stroke* **34**:e16

Parsons MW, Pepper EM, Chan V et al. (2005). Perfusion computed tomography: Prediction of final infarct extent and stroke outcome. *Annals of Neurology* **58**:672–679

Pelz DM, Fox AJ, Vinuela F (1985). Digital subtraction angiography: Current clinical applications. *Stroke* **16**:528–536

Polak JF, Shemanski L, O'Leary DH for the Cardiovascular Health Study (1998). Hypoechoic plaque at US of the carotid artery: An independent risk factor for incident stroke in adults aged 65 years or older. *Radiology* **208**:649–654

Puetz V, Dzialowski I, Hill MD et al. (2008). Intracranial thrombus extent predicts clinical outcome, final infarct size and hemorrhagic transformation in ischemic stroke: The clot burden score. *International Journal of Stroke* **3**:230–236

Puetz V, Khomenko A, Hill MD et al. (2011). Extent of hypoattenuation on CT angiography source images in basilar artery occlusion: Prognostic value in the Basilar Artery International Cooperation Study. *Stroke* **42**:3454–3459

Rosario JA, Hachinski VA, Lee DH et al. (1987). Adverse reactions to duplex scanning. *Lancet* **ii**:1023

Rothwell PM, Gibson RJ, Villagra RC et al. (1998). The effect of angiographic technique and image quality on the reproducibility of measurement of carotid stenosis and assessment of plaque surface morphology. *Clinical Radiology* **53**:439–443

Rothwell PM, Pendlebury ST, Wardlaw J et al. (2000a). Critical appraisal of the design and reporting of studies of the imaging and measurement of carotid stenosis. *Stroke* **31**:1444–1450

Rothwell PM, Gibson R, Warlow CP on behalf of the European Carotid Surgery Trialists' Collaborative Group (2000b). Interrelation between plaque surface morphology and degree of stenosis on carotid angiograms and the risk of ischemic stroke in patients with symptomatic carotid stenosis. *Stroke* **31**:615–621

Ryu CW, Kwak HS, Jahng GH et al. (2014). High-resolution MRI of intracranial atherosclerotic disease. *Neurointervention* **9**:9–20

Schramm P, Schellinger PD, Klotz E et al. (2004). Comparison of perfusion computed tomography and computed tomography angiography source images with perfusion-weighted imaging and diffusion-weighted imaging in patients with acute stroke of less than 6 hours' duration. *Stroke* **35**:1652–1658

Siewert B, Patel MR, Warach S (1995). Magnetic resonance angiography. *Neurologist* **1**:167–184

Sliwka U, Lingnau A, Stohlmann WD et al. (1997). Prevalence and time course of microembolic signals in patients with acute stroke: A prospective study. *Stroke* **28**:358–363

Streifler JY, Eliaziw M, Fox AJ, for the North American Symptomatic Carotid Endarterectomy Trial (1994). Angiographic detection of carotid plaque ulceration: Comparison with surgical observations in a multicentre study. *Stroke* **25**:1130–1132

Tan IY, Demchuk AM, Hopyan J et al. (2009). CT angiography clot burden score and collateral score: Correlation with clinical and radiologic outcomes in acute middle cerebral artery infarct. *American Journal of Neuroradiology* **30**:525–531

U-King-Im JM, Hollingworth W, Trivedi RAC et al. (2005). Cost-effectiveness of diagnostic strategies prior to carotid endarterectomy. *Annals of Neurology* **58**:506–515

Vernieri F, Pasqualetti P, Passarelli FC et al. (1999). Outcome of carotid artery occlusion is predicted by cerebrovascular reactivity. *Stroke* **30**:593–598

Vernieri F, Pasqualetti P, Matteis MC et al. (2001). Effect of collateral blood flow and cerebral vasomotor reactivity on the outcome of carotid artery occlusion. *Stroke* **32**:1552–1558

Villablanca JP, Hooshi P, Martin N *et al.* (2002). Three-dimensional helical computerized tomography angiography in the diagnosis characterization and management of middle cerebral artery aneurysms: Comparison with conventional angiography and intraoperative findings. *Journal of Neurosurgery* **97**:1322–1332

Wardlaw JM, Lewis S (2005). Carotid stenosis measurement on colour Doppler ultrasound: Agreement of ECST NASCET and CCA methods applied to ultrasound with intra-arterial angiographic stenosis measurement. *European Journal of Radiology* **56**:205–211

Warnock NG, Gandhi MR, Bergvall UC *et al.* (1993). Complications of intra-arterial digital subtraction angiography in patients investigated for cerebral vascular disease. *British Journal of Radiology* **66**:855–858

Watanabe Y, Nagayama M (2010). MR plaque imaging of the carotid artery. *Neuroradiology* **52**:253–274

Widder B, Kleiser B, Krapf H (1994). Course of cerebrovascular reactivity in patients with carotid artery occlusions. *Stroke* **25**:1963–1967

Wilson D, Adams ME, Robertson F *et al.* (2015). Investigating intracerebral hemorrhage. *British Medical Journal* **350**:h2484

Wintermark M, Uske A, Chalaron M *et al.* (2003). Multislice computerized tomography angiography in the evaluation of intracranial aneurysms: A comparison with intraarterial digital subtraction angiography. *Journal of Neurosurgery* **98**:828–836

Wintermark M, Bogousslavsky J (2003). Imaging of acute ischemic brain injury: The return of computed tomography. *Current Opinions in Neurology* **16**:59–63

Wintermark M, Meuli R, Browaeys P *et al.* (2007). Comparison of CT perfusion and angiography and MRI in selecting stroke patients for acute treatment. *Neurology* **68**:694–697

Zhu XL, Chan MSY, Poon WS (1997). Spontaneous intracranial hemorrhage: Which patients need diagnostic cerebral angiography? A prospective study of 206 cases and review of the literature. *Stroke* **28**:1406–1409

Chapter 13

Non-Radiological Investigations for Transient Ischemic Attack and Stroke

The clinical syndrome – total anterior circulation stroke, partial anterior circulation stroke, lacunar infarction, or posterior circulation stroke – gives an indication as to the site and size of the lesion, which, together with brain imaging findings, often gives clues as to the likely underlying cause, for example large vessel disease versus small vessel disease (Chapters 6 and 9). Although brain imaging is of paramount importance in TIA and stroke (Chapters 10–12), non-radiological investigations may help to identify the cause of the cerebrovascular event, eliminate stroke and TIA mimics, and enable appropriate secondary preventive therapy. Investigations are likely to be more extensive in patients without evidence of vascular disease or embolism from the heart, in whom there may be a rare underlying cause for the stroke.

First-Line Investigations

In general, all patients with a TIA or stroke should have basic blood and urine tests at presentation (Table 13.1). Patients with hemorrhagic stroke should have a clotting screen, particularly if they are already taking anticoagulation medication. The likelihood of finding a relevant abnormality may be low for some tests, such as full blood count and erythrocyte sedimentation rate, but such straightforward tests may reveal a serious treatable disorder, such as giant cell arteritis. Many patients are hypercholesterolemic, although immediately after stroke, but probably not TIA, there is a transient fall in plasma cholesterol, which will lead to underestimation of the usual level (Mendez *et al.* 1987; Woo *et al.* 1990).

Second-Line Investigations

Second-line investigations (Table 13.2) must be targeted appropriately since the likelihood of a relevant result depends on the selection of patients and further investigation will incur more cost. There are numerous rare causes of stroke (Chapter 6) for which highly specialized tests may be required.

Routine lumbar puncture is not indicated after stroke and may be dangerous in the presence of a large intracerebral hematoma or edematous infarct causing brain shift. Examination of the cerebrospinal fluid may be necessary in diagnostic uncertainty where there is a possibility of encephalitis or multiple sclerosis or if the stroke is thought to have been caused by infective endocarditis or by chronic meningitis in syphilis or tuberculosis. The cerebrospinal fluid after stroke is usually acellular, but there may be up to 100×10^6 cells/L. Levels above this suggest septic emboli to the brain (Powers 1986). A lumbar puncture may also be required in patients with suspected subarachnoid hemorrhage who present beyond 6 hours of symptom onset (Chapter 30).

Routine electroencephalography is not indicated in stroke but may be helpful where there is a possibility of encephalitis, generalized encephalopathy, or focal seizure activity.

Table 13.1 Baseline non-imaging tests for transient ischemic attack and stroke

Investigation	Disorders detected
Full blood count	Anemia Polycythemia Leukemia Thrombocythemia/thrombocytopenia
Erythrocyte sedimentation rate/C-reactive protein	Vasculitis Infective endocarditis Hyperviscosity Myxoma
Electrolytes	Hyponatremia Hypokalemia
Urea and creatinine	Renal impairment
Plasma glucose	Diabetes Hypoglycemia
Plasma lipids	Hyperlipidemia
Urine analysis	Diabetes Renal disease Vasculitis

Table 13.2 Second-line investigations for selected transient ischemic attack or stroke patients

Investigation	Comments
Blood	
Liver function	Fever, malaise, raised ESR, suspected malignancy, temporal arteritis
Calcium	Recurrent focal neurological symptoms are occasionally caused by hypercalcemia
Thyroid function tests	Atrial fibrillation
Body red cell mass	Raised hematocrit
Activated partial thromboplastin time, anticardiolipin antibody,[a] antinuclear and other autoantibodies	Young (< 50 years) and no other cause found; past history or family history of venous thrombosis, especially if unusual site (cerebral, mesenteric, hepatic veins); recurrent miscarriage; thrombocytopenia; cardiac valve vegetations; livedo reticularis; raised ESR; malaise; positive syphilis serology
Serum proteins, serum protein electrophoresis, plasma viscosity	Myeloma
Hemoglobin electrophoresis	Hemoglobinopathies, e.g., sickle cell anemia

Table 13.2 (cont.)

Investigation	Comments
Protein C and S, antithrombin III, activated protein C resistance, thrombin time[b]	Thrombophilia: personal or family history of thrombosis (usually venous, particularly in unusual sites such as hepatic vein) at unusually young age
Blood cultures	Infective endocarditis: fever, cardiac murmur, hematuria, deranged liver function, raised ESR, malaise
HIV serology	Unexplained stroke in the young, drug addiction, homosexuality, blood product transfusion, lymphadenopathy, pneumonia, cytomegalovirus retinitis
Lipoprotein fractionation	Elevated cholesterol or strong family history, hyperlipoproteinemia
Serum homocysteine	Marfanoid habitus, high myopia, dislocated lenses, osteoporosis, mental retardation
Leukocyte α-galactosidase A	Corneal opacities, cutaneous angiokeratomas, paresthesias and pain, renal failure
Blood/cerebrospinal fluid lactate	MELAS/mitochondrial cytopathy: young patient, basal ganglia calcification, epilepsy, parieto-occipital ischemia
Syphilis serology	Young patient, high risk of sexually transmitted disease
Cardiac enzymes	History or ECG evidence of recent electrocardiographic myocardial infarction
Drug screen	Cocaine/amphetamine/ecstasy: young patient, no other obvious cause
Urine	
Amino acids	Marfanoid habitus, high myopia, dislocated lenses, osteoporosis, mental retardation
Drug screen	Young patient, no other obvious cause, cocaine/ amphetamine, etc.
Others	
Electroencephalography	Doubt about diagnosis of TIA or stroke: ?epilepsy
Temporal artery biopsy	Age > 60 years, jaw claudication, headache, polymyalgia, malaise, anemia, raised ESR[a]

Notes: ESR, erythrocyte sedimentation rate; MELAS, mitochondrial encephalopathy, lactic acidosis, and stroke-like episodes; TIA, transient ischemic attack; ECG, electrocardiogram.
[a] Repeat to ensure persistently raised.
[b] Transient falls occur after stroke so any low level must be repeated and family members investigated.

It should be noted that there may be transient focal weakness after a seizure – "Todd's paresis" (Chapter 8).

Temporal artery biopsy may be required in patients with suspected temporal arteritis (Chapter 6).

Cardiac Investigations

Given the high prevalence of cardiovascular disease in patients with cerebrovascular disease (about one-third have angina or have had a myocardial infarction) (Chapter 6), there is a strong likelihood of electrocardiography (ECG) abnormalities in patients presenting with TIA and stroke. The ECG may show evidence of coronary artery disease, previous or current myocardial infarction, or disorders of rhythm, such as atrial fibrillation (AF). It should be noted that stroke can itself cause ECG changes in approximately 15–20% of patients, ranging from left-axis deviation to a variety of repolarization abnormalities including QT prolongation, septal U waves, and ST segment changes (Chapter 20). The insular cortex is a crucial center for control of autonomic function and may be a possible cortical site for generation of some of these ECG changes in patients with stroke affecting the insula. Patients with left insular stroke may result in sympathetic overactivity, tachyarrhythmias, and ventricular fibrillation, while strokes involving the right insula may result in parasympathetic overactivity, bradyarrhythmias, and asystole (Sörös *et al.* 2012). Such changes may contribute to the excess cardiac mortality in stroke patients.

Many patients will require cardiac investigations beyond ECG (Table 13.3), although the likelihood of finding a significant cardiac abnormality on routine transthoracic

Table 13.3 Cardiac investigations in stroke

Investigation	Comments
ECG	Left ventricular hypertrophy Arrhythmia Conduction block Myocardial infarction
Chest X-ray	Hypertension, finger clubbing, cardiac murmur or abnormal ECG, ill patient
Echocardiography (transthoracic)	Valvular heart disease, left ventricular dyskinesias, left ventricular thrombus
Echocardiography (transesophageal)	Patent foramen ovale, atrial septal aneurysm, left atrial spontaneous echo contrast, left atrial thrombus, mitral and aortic valve vegetations
External cardiac monitoring (24-hour Holter monitoring, extended Holter monitoring, patch monitors, etc.)	AF detection in cryptogenic stroke Monitoring for 24 hours–30 days AF detection yield 2.5–16%
Insertable cardiac monitors*	AF detection in cryptogenic stroke Monitoring for 6 months to > 1 year AF detection yield 9–34%

Notes: *Not generally used in routine practice
ECG, electrocardiography; TIA, transient ischemic attack; AF, atrial fibrillation.

Table 13.4 Pooled prevalence of various cardiac abnormalities on transthoracic echocardiography in patients with ischemic stroke without prior known cardiac disease

Abnormality	Pooled prevalence (%)	
	< 45 years	> 45 years
Myxoma	0.7	0.1
Vegetations	1	1
Mitral stenosis	2	2
Left atrial thrombus	0.5	0.3
Left ventricular thrombus/ cardiomyopathy	3	10

Source: From Beattie *et al.* (1998).

Table 13.5 Comparison of transthoracic and transesophageal echocardiography for detecting potential cardiac sources of embolism

Transthoracic preferred	Transesophageal preferred
Left ventricular thrombus	Left atrial thrombus
Left ventricular dyskinesis	Left atrial appendage thrombus
Mitral stenosis	Spontaneous echo contrast
Mitral annulus calcification	Intracardiac tumors
Aortic stenosis	Atrial septal defect[a]
	Atrial septal aneurysm
	Patent foramen ovale[a]
	Mitral and aortic valve vegetations
	Prosthetic heart valve malfunction
	Aortic arch atherothrombosis/dissection
	Mitral valve prolapse

[a] A less-invasive alternative is to inject air bubbles or other echo contrast material intravenously. If there is a patent foramen ovale, they can be detected by transcranial Doppler sonography of the middle cerebral artery, particularly with a provocative Valsalva maneuver. There is considerable variation in the methods used to detect patent foramen ovale and this influences the diagnostic sensitivity and specificity. It is also uncertain what size of shunt is "clinically relevant," and some bubbles may pass to the brain through pulmonary rather than cardiac shunts (Droste *et al.* 1999, 2002; Schwarze *et al.* 1999).

echocardiography in patients without prior known cardiac abnormality or a normal cardiovascular examination is low (Table 13.4) (Beattie *et al.* 1998; Douen *et al.* 2007). Patients with a suspected cardiac source of embolism should certainly have a transthoracic echocardiography and/or transesophageal examination (Table 13.5). Specific echocardiographic techniques may be required where there is the possibility of a patent foramen ovale (Table 13.5; Chapter 6). In patients with cryptogenic TIA or ischemic stroke, prolonged rhythm recording using an external cardiac monitor for 5–30 days is recommended to exclude paroxysmal AF (Table 13.3) (Kernan *et al.* 2014; Albers *et al.* 2016). However, the question of how much AF detected on these monitors should trigger anticoagulation use remains, although current authorities recommend anticoagulation if 2 or more minutes of AF is detected (Albers *et al.* 2016).

References

Albers GW, Berstein RA, Brachmann J *et al.* (2016). Heart rhythm monitoring strategies for cryptogenic stroke: 2015 diagnostics and monitoring stroke focus group report. *Journal of the American Heart Association* 5:e002944

Beattie JR, Cohen DJ, Manning WJ, Douglas PS (1998). Role of routine transthoracic echocardiography in evaluation and management of stroke. *Journal of Internal Medicine* 243:281–291

Douen A, Pageau N, Medic S (2007). Usefulness of cardiovascular investigations in stroke management. *Stroke* 38:1956–1958

Droste DW, Kriete JU, Stypmann J *et al.* (1999). Contrast transcranial Doppler ultrasound in the detection of right-to-left shunts: Comparison of different procedures and different procedures and different contrast agents. *Stroke* 30:1827–1832

Droste DW, Lakemeier S, Wichter T *et al.* (2002). Optimizing the technique of contrast transcranial Doppler ultrasound in the detection of right-to-left shunts. *Stroke* 33: 2211–2216

Kernan WN, Ovbiagele B, Black HR *et al.* (2014). Guidelines for the prevention of stroke in patients with stroke and transient ischemic attack: A guideline for healthcare professionals from the American Heart Association/American Stroke Association. *Stroke* 45:2160–2236

Mendez I, Hachinski V, Wolfe B (1987). Serum lipids after stroke. *Neurology* 37:507–511

Powers WJ (1986). Should lumbar puncture be part of the routine evaluation of patients with cerebral ischemia? *Stroke* 17:332–333

Schwarze JJ, Sander D, Kukla C *et al.* (1999). Methodological parameters influence the detection of right-to-left shunts by contrast transcranial Doppler ultrasonography. *Stroke* 30:1234–1239

Sörös P, Hachinski V (2012). Cardiovascular and neurological causes of sudden death after ischaemic stroke. *Lancet Neurology* 11:179–188

Woo J, Lam CWK, Kay R *et al.* (1990). Acute and long term changes in serum lipids after acute stroke. *Stroke* 21:1407–1411

Methods of Determining Prognosis

Why Study Prognosis?

Once a diagnosis has been made, the issue of prognosis is as important to patients as treatment. There are many examples in neurology of the usefulness of simple prognostic studies of groups of patients, such as the demonstrations of the relatively benign long-term outcome after transient global amnesia (Hodges and Warlow 1990a, b), after cryptogenic drop-attacks in middle-aged women (Stevens and Matthews 1973) and the more recent data on the risks of major congenital malformations when taking various antiepileptic drugs in pregnancy (Morrow *et al.* 2006). Prognostic studies not only provide patients with useful information on the average risk of a poor outcome but also provide data that can be used to inform decisions for individuals about treatment by allowing an estimation of the likely absolute risk reduction (ARR) of a poor outcome with treatment, derived from the relative risk reduction provided by clinical trials. The ARR indicates what the chance of benefit from treatment is (e.g., an ARR of 25% – from 50% to 25% – tells us that four patients has to be treated for one to avoid a poor outcome or, put in another way, there is a 1 in 4 chance of benefit for the individual treated patient). In contrast, a relative risk reduction gives no information about the likelihood of benefit. For example, the relative reductions in the risk of stroke in the Swedish Trial in Old Patients with Hypertension (STOP-hypertension) (Dahlof *et al.* 1991) and MRC (Medical Research Council Working Party 1985) trials of blood pressure lowering in primary prevention were virtually identical (47% versus 45%). However, there was a twelvefold difference in the ARR and hence the probability of benefit for individual patients. All other things being equal, 166 of the young hypertensives in the MRC trial would have to be treated for 5 years to prevent one stroke, compared with 14 of the elderly hypertensives in STOP-hypertension. Therefore, without an understanding of prognosis (i.e., absolute risk of a poor outcome), the likelihood that a treatment is worth having is impossible to judge (unless of course it is to relieve a symptom such as pain).

Why Predict an Individual's Prognosis?

Patients and their doctors are understandably keen to go further than simply defining average or overall prognosis. They want to understand how a combination of factors might determine prognosis for the individual concerned: "How do *my* particular characteristics influence the likely outcome, doctor?"

Where possible, treatments should always be targeted at those individuals who are likely to benefit and be avoided in those with little chance of benefit or in whom the risks of complications are too great compared with the expected benefit. A targeted approach based on risk is most useful for treatments with modest benefits (e.g., lipid lowering in primary prevention of vascular disease), for costly treatments with moderate overall benefits (e.g., beta-interferon in multiple sclerosis), if the availability of treatment is limited (e.g., organ transplantation), in developing countries with limited healthcare budgets, and, most importantly, for treatments that although of overall benefit are associated with a significant risk of harm (such as carotid endarterectomy or anticoagulation).

However, without formal risk models, clinicians are often inaccurate in assessment of risk in their patients (Grover *et al.* 1995). Moreover, the absolute risk of a poor outcome for patients with multiple specific characteristics cannot simply be derived arithmetically from data on the effect of each individual characteristic such as age or severity of illness: that is, one cannot simply multiply risk ratios for these characteristics together as if they were independent. Even if one could, it would still be rather complicated. In a patient with symptomatic carotid stenosis, for example, what would the risk of stroke without endarterectomy be in a 78-year-old (high risk) female (lower risk) with 80% stenosis who presented within 2 days (high risk) of an ocular ischemic event (low risk) and was found to have an ulcerated carotid plaque (high risk)?

Models that combine prognostic variables to predict risk are, therefore, essential if we want reliable prognostication at the individual level.

What Is a Prognostic Model?

A prognostic model is the mathematical combination of two or more patient or disease characteristics to predict outcome. Confusingly, prognostic models are also termed prognostic indexes, risk scores, probability models, risk stratification schemes, or clinical prediction rules (Reilly and Evans 2006). To be useful, they must be shown to predict clinically relevant outcomes reliably. They must, therefore, be derived from a representative cohort in which outcome has been measured accurately. Next, they must be validated, not just in the data from which they were derived (internal validation) but also on data from independent cohorts (external validation) (Wyatt and Altman 1995; Justice *et al.* 1999; Altman and Royston 2000). Lastly, a model must be simple to use and have clinical credibility; otherwise, it is unlikely to be taken up in routine clinical practice (Table 14.1).

A model for prediction of stroke on medical treatment in patients with recently symptomatic carotid stenosis is shown in Table 14.2 (Rothwell *et al.* 2005). The numeric weights for each variable are coefficients from a fitted regression model (Lewis 2007), and the model can be simplified to produce a simple risk score. Examples of other models are also given showing prediction of stroke in patients with non-valvular atrial fibrillation (the CHADS2 scheme; Box 14.1; Gage *et al.* 2004; Hart 2007), prediction of recurrence after a single seizure or in early epilepsy (Kim *et al.* 2006 Box 14.2) and the prediction of outcome in the Guillain–Barré syndrome (van Koningsveld *et al.* 2007; Box 14.3). Further examples of prognostic models are given elsewhere in the book, including the ABCD tool (Chapter 15).

The best evidence of the impact of using prognostic models comes from stratification of the results of randomized trials by predicted baseline risk, and the usefulness of this approach in targeting treatment has been demonstrated particularly well in patients with vascular disease. Predictable qualitative heterogeneity of relative treatment effect (i.e., benefit in some patients and harm in others) in relation to baseline risk has been demonstrated for anticoagulation therapy in primary prevention of stroke in patients with non-valvular atrial fibrillation (Laupacis *et al.* 1994), carotid endarterectomy for symptomatic

Table 14.1 Prerequisites for the clinical credibility of a prognostic model

	Prerequisites
Use of relevant data	All clinically relevant patient data should have been tested for inclusion in the model. Many models are developed in retrospective studies using those variables that happen to have been collected already for other reasons. Thus, potentially valuable variables may be omitted if data for them are unavailable.
Simplicity of data collection	It should be simple for doctors to obtain all of the patient data required in the model reliably and without expending undue resources in time to generate the prediction and so guide decisions. Data should be obtainable with high reliability, particularly in those patients for which the model's prediction are most likely to be needed.
Avoidance of arbitrary thresholds	Model builders should avoid arbitrary thresholds for continuous variables because categorization discards potentially useful information.
Derivation	The statistical modeling method must be correctly applied. Black box models, such as artificial neural networks, are less suitable for clinical applications.
Simplicity of use	It should be simple and intuitive for doctors to calculate the model's prediction for a patient. The model's structure should be apparent, and its predictions should make sense to the doctors who will rely on it. This will increase the likelihood of uptake of a model in routine practice.

Sources: From Wyatt and Altman (1995) and Altman and Royston (2000).

stenosis (Rothwell *et al.* 2005), coronary artery bypass grafting (Yusuf *et al.* 1994), and anti-arrhythmic drugs following myocardial infarction (Boissel *et al.* 1993). Clinically important heterogeneity has also been demonstrated for blood pressure lowering (Li *et al.* 1998), aspirin (Sanmuganathan *et al.* 2001), lipid lowering in primary prevention of vascular disease (West of Scotland Coronary Prevention Group 1996), and many other areas of medicine and surgery (Pagliaro *et al.* 1992; International Study of Unruptured Intracranial Aneurysms Investigators 1998).

How to Measure Prognosis

In order to develop a prognostic model, prognosis itself must first be measured reliably, although there is limited consensus on the ideal methodology required to achieve this. As there is little evidence to support the importance of features of study method that might affect the reliability of findings, particularly the avoidance of bias, researchers have tended to devise their own criteria or to ignore the issue altogether. As a result, many prognostic studies have been found to be of poor quality in both TIA and stroke (Kernan *et al.* 1991) and other fields of medicine (Altman 2001; Hayden *et al.* 2006). Despite the lack of accepted criteria, both theoretical considerations and common sense point toward the importance of various aspects of study method that would be

Table 14.2 A Cox model for the 5-year risk of ipsilateral ischemic stroke in patients with recently symptomatic carotid stenosis on medical treatment[a]

	Model			Scoring system		
Risk factor	Hazard ratio (95% CI)	p value		Risk factor	Score	Example
Stenosis (per 10%)	1.18 (1.10–1.25)	< 0.0001		Stenosis (%)		
				50–59	2.4	2.4
				60–69	2.8	
				70–79	3.3	
				80–89	3.9	
				90–99	4.6	
Near occlusion	0.49 (0.19–1.24)	0.1309		Near occlusion	0.5	No
Male sex	1.19 (0.81–1.75)	0.3687		Male sex	1.2	No
Age (per 10 years)	1.12 (0.89–1.39)	0.3343		Age (years)		
				31–40	1.1	
				41–50	1.2	
				51–60	1.3	
				61–70	1.5	1.5
				71–80	1.6	
				81–90	1.8	
Time since last event (per 7 days)	0.96 (0.93–0.99)	0.0039		Time since last event (days)		
				0–13	8.7	8.7
				14–28	8.0	
				29–89	6.3	
				90–365	2.3	
Presenting event		0.0067		Presenting event		
Ocular	1.000			Ocular	1.0	
Single TIA	1.41 (0.75–2.66)			Single TIA	1.4	
Multiple TIAs	2.05 (1.16–3.60)			Multiple TIAs	2.0	
Minor stroke	1.82 (0.99–3.34)			Minor stroke	1.8	
Major stroke	2.54 (1.48–4.35)			Major stroke	2.5	2.5
Diabetes	1.35 (0.86–2.11)	0.1881		Diabetes	1.4	1.4
Previous MI	1.57 (1.01–2.45)	0.0471		Previous MI	1.6	No
PVD	1.18 (0.78–1.77)	0.4368		PVD	1.2	No

Table 14.2 (cont.)

	Model			Scoring system		
Risk factor	Hazard ratio (95% CI)	p value	Risk factor	Score	Example
Treated hypertension	1.24 (0.88–1.75)	0.2137	Treated hypertension	1.2	1.2
Irregular/ ulcerated plaque	2.03 (1.31–3.14)	0.0015	Irregular/ plaque ulcerated	2.0	2.0
Total risk score					263
Predicted 5-year risk of stroke (derived using a nomogram)					37%

Notes: CI, confidence interval; MI, myocardial infarction; PVD, peripheral vascular disease; TIA, transient ischemic attack.
[a] Hazard ratios derived from the model are used for the scoring system. The score for the 5-year risk of stroke is the product of the individual scores for each of the risk factors present. The score is converted into a risk with a graph.
Source: Rothwell *et al.* (2005).

required for the reliable measurement of prognosis (Sackett and Whelan 1980; Kernan *et al.* 1991; Altman 2001) (Table 14.3).

In the case of TIA and stroke, the diagnostic criteria used and by whom the diagnosis was made must be adequately described, especially because the definition of TIA has changed over time (Chapter 1) and diagnostic sensitivity may vary between individuals and groups of clinicians, for example between neurologists and emergency department physicians. Methods of ascertainment of cases from the study population should be described, as should all demographic and clinical characteristics of the cohort; where relevant, this includes the methods of measurement themselves. Adequate description of the derivation cohort allows an assessment of how representative it is of the population in which the prognostic tool is intended for use. Only patients at a similar point in the course of the condition should be included, a point that has previously been taken to be the time of diagnosis, referral to secondary care or initiation of treatment. However, ideally, this point should be as early as possible into the condition ("inception cohort"), and this is the reason that some studies of the prognosis of TIA that ascertained patients some weeks or months after the initial event underestimated the immediate risk of stroke (Rothwell 2003). Intensity and setting of treatment should be described as both of these factors will have an impact on prognosis (Giles and Rothwell 2007). Methods of follow-up must be appropriately sensitive to identify outcomes and criteria for such outcomes, and methods of adjudication must be fully described.

Although, in general, prospective cohort studies of well-defined groups of patients are superior, retrospective studies may have the advantage of longer follow-up, which might be necessary for a clinically relevant prognosis or simply in order to have a sufficient number of outcome events to construct a reasonably precise prediction model. However, retrospective studies often have vague inclusion criteria, selection biases, incomplete baseline data, variable use of diagnostic tests, nonstandard methods of measurement, and inconsistent treatment (Laupacis *et al.* 1997).

BOX 14.1 Prediction of Stroke in Patients with Non-Valvular Atrial Fibrillation

Why Predict Risk?

The absolute risk of stroke varies twenty fold among patients with non-valvular atrial fibrillation, depending on age and associated vascular diseases. Estimating an individual's stroke risk is, therefore, essential when considering potentially hazardous anticoagulation therapy. More than 10 similar stroke risk models for patients with atrial fibrillation have been published, but the CHADS2 scheme was one of the most widely used.

What Is the Score?

The CHADS2 scheme awards 1 point each for **c**ongestive heart failure, **h**ypertension, **a**ge ≥ 75 years, and **d**iabetes mellitus and 2 points for prior **s**troke or TIA.

Does It Work?

The CHADS2 score has been validated in many groups of patients, three of which are shown in the following table (Gage *et al.* 2004; Hart 2007). In each of the validation studies, those with CHADS2 scores of 0 or 1 had stroke rates of ≤ 3% per year, whereas those with higher scores had progressively increasing risks. The lower risks in the outpatient cohort very likely reflect the small numbers of patients with previous TIA or stroke compared with the other groups.

	Hospital discharge cohort	Outpatient cohort	Aspirin-treated clinical trial participants
No.	1733	5089	2580
Prior stroke no. [%]	433 (25)	204 (4)	568 (22)
Overall annual stroke rate	4.4	2.0	4.2
CHADS2 score (95% CI)	Stroke + TIA rate (%/year)	Stroke + systemic embolism rate (%/year)	Stroke rate (%/year)
0	1.9 (1.2–3.0)	0.5 (0.3–0.8)	0.8 (0.4–1.7)
1	2.8 (2.0–3.8)	1.5 (1.2–1.9)	2.2 (1.6–3.1)
2	4.0 (3.1–5.1)	2.5 (2.0–3.2)	4.5 (3.5–5.9)
3	5.9 (4.6–7.3)	5.3 (4.2–6.7)	8.6 (6.8–11.0)
4	8.5 (6.3–11)	6.0 (3.9–9.3)	10.9 (7.8–15.2)
5–6	> 12	6.9 (3.4–13.8)	> 12

Note: CI, confidence interval.

What Are Its Potential Deficiencies?

For patients with prior stroke/TIA who have no other risk factors, a CHADS2 score of 2 yields an estimated stroke risk of 2.5–4.5% per year, which is probably too low. All patients with atrial fibrillation and prior stroke or TIA, recent or remote, should be considered high risk. The stroke risk associated with a CHADS2 score of 2 is very different according to primary versus secondary prevention. The use of a CHAD score (i.e., dropping "S2") for primary prevention or a CHADS3 score for secondary prevention appears to fit available data better. If echocardiographic data are available, the Stroke Prevention in Atrial Fibrillation (SPAF) III risk stratification scheme has also been validated in several, albeit smaller, groups of patients (Stroke Prevention in Atrial Fibrillation Investigators 1995). Furthermore, the CHADS2 score has been criticized that even patients categorized as "low-risk" by a CHADS2 score of 0 are not necessarily at a low risk of stroke. The CHA_2DS_2-VASc score (see Chapter 24 Box 24.2) was subsequently developed and validated in numerous populations of different settings and has been shown to be superior to the CHADS2 score in identifying patients truly at low risk of an atrial fibrillation–related thromboembolic event.

Sources: From Gage *et al.* (2004); Hart (2007); Lip *et al.* (2010); Friberg *et al.* (2012).

BOX 14.2 Prediction of Recurrence after a Single Seizure and in Early Epilepsy

Why Predict Risk?

Outcome after a first seizure varies, with approximately 65% of newly diagnosed people rapidly entering remission after starting treatment and approximately 25% developing drug-resistant epilepsy. Treatment for most patients is with antiepileptic drugs, which carry risks of acute idiosyncratic reactions, dose-related and chronic toxic effects, and teratogenicity. The benefits of treatment will outweigh the risks for most patients, but for those who have had only a single seizure, the risk–benefit ratio is more finely balanced.

What Is the Score?

A prognostic model was developed based on individual patient data from the Multicentre Trial for Early Epilepsy and Single Seizures (MESS) to enable identification of patients at low, medium, or high risk of seizure recurrence (Kim *et al.* 2007). A 60:40 split-sample approach was used in which the model was developed on a subsample (885 patients) of the full dataset and validated on the remainder of the sample (535 patients). The significant predictors of future seizures, on which the score was based, were number of seizures of all types at presentation (one scored 0, two or three scored 1, and four or more scored 2 points), presence of a neurological disorder or learning disability (1 point), and an abnormal electro-encephalogram (1 point).

Does It Work?

Patients with a single seizure and no other high-risk characteristics (i.e., 0 points) were classified as low risk; those with two or three seizures, a neurological disorder, or an abnormal EEG (1 point) were classified as medium risk; and those with ≥ 2 points were classified as high risk. In trial patients randomized to delayed treatment, the probabilities of a recurrent seizure were 19%, 35%, and 59%, respectively, at 1 year, and 30%, 56%, and 73%, respectively, at 5 years. The score was also used to stratify the analysis of the effect of antiepileptic treatment in the trial (patients had been randomized to immediate treatment or delayed treatment if required). There was no benefit to immediate treatment in patients at low risk of seizure recurrence, but there were potentially worthwhile benefits in those at medium and high risk.

What Are Its Potential Deficiencies?

The split sample approach is not an independent validation, and so further validations are required, preferably in non-trial groups of patients.

Source: From Kim *et al.* (2006).

BOX 14.3 Prediction of Outcome in Guillain–Barré Syndrome

Why Predict Risk?

Guillain–Barré syndrome (GBS) is characterized by rapidly progressive weakness, which is usually followed by slow clinical recovery, but outcome is variable, with some patients remaining bedridden or wheelchair bound. Previous studies showed that preceding infection, age, rapid progression, disability at nadir, and electrophysiological characteristics were associated with long-term prognosis, but a readily applicable and validated model was required to predict outcome.

What Is the Score?

The Erasmus GBS Outcome Score (EGOS) was derived and validated on patients in the acute phase of GBS who were unable to walk independently (van Koningsveld et al. 2007). The derivation set included 388 patients from randomized controlled trials, and the outcome was inability to walk independently at 6 months. A simple score was developed from the coefficients in a regression model: age, preceding diarrhea, and GBS disability score at 2 weeks after entry. Scores range from 1 to 7, with three categories for age (≤ 40, 41–60, and > 60 years scoring 0, 0.5, and 1, respectively), 1 point for recent diarrhea, and 1–5 points for disability score at 2 weeks.

Does It Work?

The score was validated in a set of 374 patients from another randomized trial. Predictions of the inability to walk independently at 6 months ranged from 1% for a score of 1 to 83% for patients with a score of 7. Predictions agreed well with observed outcome frequencies (i.e., good calibration) and showed very good discriminative ability (C statistic = 0.85).

Score	Derivation set ($n = 388$)	Validation set ($n = 374$)	Combined set ($n = 762$)
1–3	1/107 (1%)	0/86 (0%)	1/193 (0.5%)
3.5–4.5	7/116 (6%)	9/110 (8%)	16/226 (7%)
5	20/81 (25%)	23/80 (29%)	43/161 (27%)
5.5–7	43/84 (51%)	51/98 (22%)	94/182 (53%)
Total	71/388 (18%)	83/374 (22%)	154/762 (20%)

What Are Its Potential Deficiencies?

The EGOS was derived and validated on patients from randomized controlled trials, who may have been unrepresentative. The score was also derived and validated on patients with moderately severe GBS (unable to walk independently) and might work less well in milder cases – but then the prognosis for full recovery is known to be good in mild cases, and so a score is not necessary in these instances. There are also geographical differences in the type of GBS and its outcome. The EGOS was derived and validated on European populations, and so further validations in other areas would be helpful. It has not yet been validated by independent researchers. Furthermore, the EGOS was designed to be applied at 2 weeks after hospital admission. This may limit the use of the score for testing new treatment strategies, which should be administered as soon as possible. A modified version of EGOS was subsequently developed that similarly predicts 6-month functional outcome but could be used at hospital admission and at day 7 of admission.

Sources: From van Koningsveld *et al.* (2007); Walgaard *et al.* (2011).

Table 14.3 Table of quality criteria for study method for reliable measurement of prognosis

Study feature	Qualities sought
Sample of patients	Methods of patient selection from study population described
	Inclusion and exclusion criteria defined
	Diagnostic criteria defined
	Clinical and demographic characteristics fully described
	Representative
	Assembled at common (usually early) point in course of disease
	Complete (all eligible patients included)
Follow-up of patients	Sufficiently long, thorough and sensitive to outcomes of interest
	Loss to follow-up provided
Outcome	Objective, unbiased and fully defined (e.g., assessment blinded to prognostic information)
	Appropriate
	Known for all or high proportion of patients
Prognostic variable	Fully defined
	Details of measurement available (methods if relevant)
	Available for all or high proportion of patients
Analysis	Continuous predictor variable analyzed appropriately
	Statistical adjustment for all important prognostic factors
Treatment subsequent to inclusion in cohort	Fully described
	Treatment standardized or randomized

Source: From Altman and Royston (2000).

Developing a Prognostic Model

The purpose of a prognostic model is usually to predict the risk of an event. Although the outcome is, therefore, binary (i.e., yes or no), the predictions are almost always intermediate probabilities rather than 0% (will definitely not happen) or 100% (definitely will happen). A model should, therefore, successfully distinguish between high- and low-risk *groups*, but the ability to predict an *individual's* outcome is almost always limited (Henderson and Keiding 2005). Nevertheless, even relatively modest risk stratification can be clinically useful. For example, given a 5% operative risk of stroke and death for endarterectomy for patients with asymptomatic carotid stenosis and an average 5-year risk of stroke on medical treatment of about 10%, simply separating patients into a group with a mere 5% 5-year unoperated risk and a group with a more worrying 20% 5-year risk would substantially improve the targeting of treatment (avoid for the former, recommend for the latter perhaps).

The quality of the data is also important. Measurements should ideally have been made with reliable and reasonably standard methods, preferably without categorization (i.e., they should be recorded as continuous variables as opposed to ad hoc categories, which might limit their predictive value). In multicenter trials or cohorts, it is particularly important to have consistent methods of measurements and similar definitions of variables across centers (e.g., are the centers all using the same definitions of hypertension?). As complete a set of data as possible is also essential for the development of reliable prognostic models. Even when each variable is reasonably complete, many patients will have missing data for at least one variable, often the majority of patients (Clark and Altman 2003). Excluding such cases, as standard statistical packages would automatically do, reduces statistical power and may also introduce bias. The alternative to exclusion of patients with missing data is to impute the missing values (Vach 1997; Schafer and Graham 2002). Although imputation requires certain assumptions about why data are missing, it is often preferable to risk selection bias by using only cases with complete data (Schafer and Graham 2002; Burton and Altman 2004).

Prognostic models are usually derived using logistic regression (for predicting binary outcomes) or Cox regression (for time-to event data). The sample size required depends on the number of outcomes and *not* the number of patients (Feinstein 1996; Schmoor *et al.* 2000). Cohorts with few events per prognostic variable studied are likely to produce unreliable results. It is generally recommended that there should be at least 10 to 20 outcome events per prognostic variable studied (i.e., *not* 10 to 20 per variable eventually included in the model), although reliable models have been derived on smaller numbers (Harrell *et al.* 1984; Feinstein 1996). However, with a small derivation cohort, there will always be a risk of selecting unimportant variables and missing important ones by chance.

Before performing multivariable analysis, many researchers try to reduce the number of candidate variables by means of univariate analyses, eliminating those variables that are not significant univariate predictors (often with a cutoff of $p < 0.1$). However, this step is not strictly necessary, and it may introduce bias (Sun *et al.* 1996; Babyak 2004). It makes more sense to reduce the number of candidate variables using clinical criteria, such as by eliminating variables that are difficult to measure in routine practice (e.g., emboli on transcranial Doppler) or a variable that is likely to be closely correlated with another (e.g., systolic and diastolic blood pressure).

The initial selection of variables can be further reduced automatically using a selection algorithm (often backward elimination or forward selection). Such an automated procedure sounds as though it should produce the optimal choice of predictive variables, but it is often necessary in practice to use clinical knowledge to override the statistical process, either to ensure inclusion of a variable that is known from previous studies to be highly predictive or to eliminate variables that might lead to overfitting (i.e., overestimation of the predictive value of the model by inclusion of variables that appear to be predictive in the derivation cohort, probably by chance, but are unlikely to be predictive in other cohorts).

It is also important to look for potential interactions between the predictive value of particular variables (i.e., the predictive value of one variable may depend on the presence or absence of another), especially if there is some a priori clinical or biological reason to suspect an interaction. For example, the predictive value of cholesterol level is likely to fall with age in a model predicting the risk of vascular events (total cholesterol is highly predictive of myocardial infarction in patients in their 40s and 50s, of less value in 60s and early 70s, and of little value in the 80s). Such interactions can be taken into account in the model by including an interaction term, which will increase the predictive power of the model, assuming that the interaction is generalizable to future patients.

Studies developing models should be reported in adequate detail. Several reviews of papers presenting prognostic models have found common deficiencies in methodology and reporting, including a lack of information on the method for selecting the variables in the model and on the coding of variables and a tendency to have too few events per variable in the derivation cohort (Concato *et al.* 1993; Coste *et al.* 1995; Laupacis *et al.* 1997; Counsell and Dennis 2001; Hackett and Anderson 2005; Jacob *et al.* 2005). Authors must report the model in enough detail so that someone else can use it in the clinic and can validate it with their own data. The main issues in assessing studies reporting prognostic models are internal validity, external validity, statistical validity, evaluation of the model, and practicality of the model (Counsell and Dennis 2001; Jacob *et al.* 2005).

How to Derive a Simple Risk Score

Ideally, in order for risk scores to be useful in clinical practice, they should be simple enough to be calculated without the need for a calculator or computer and to be memorized and so should be based only on a small number of variables (Table 14.3). In practice, a few variables with strong predictive effects usually account for most of the prognostic power, with the remaining weaker variables contributing relatively little. However, a large number of candidate variables are often available for initial consideration, and so a balance is required between fitting the current data as well as possible and developing a model that will be generalizable *and* will actually be used in day-to-day practice. On the one hand, models that are "overfitted" to the derivation cohort often perform badly when independently validated (Harrell *et al.* 1984; Babyak 2004). This is because they generally contain some variables that were only marginally statistically significant predictors in the derivation cohort, often through chance, or they overestimated the predictive value of genuinely predictive variables, both of which will result in a model that "overpredicts".

On the other hand, a potential problem with simple risk scores is that they may not use the full information from the prognostic variables (Christensen 1987; Royston *et al.* 2006). If continuous predictors such as age are dichotomized (e.g., old versus young), power is usually reduced (Altman and Royston 2000). Furthermore, if the dichotomy is data derived at the point where "it looks best," it may also compromise the generalizability of the score. However, although some loss of prognostic power is almost inevitable, simple scores often perform almost as well as more complex models. One reason for this is that a simple score based on a small number of highly predictive variables is much less likely to be overfitted than a complex score with additional weakly predictive variables and interaction terms.

Assuming that there are no complex interaction terms in a multivariable model, it is relatively easy to convert a model to a simple score. The numeric weights allocated to each variable in the model (i.e., the coefficients from the fitted regression model) provide the basis of the score. Simply using the same numeric weights and adding them up to produce a simple score will actually result in the same ranking of patients as the more complex mathematical model. The only thing that is lost is the exact predicted risk. However, the exact predicted risk can be obtained from a simple graph of score versus risk.

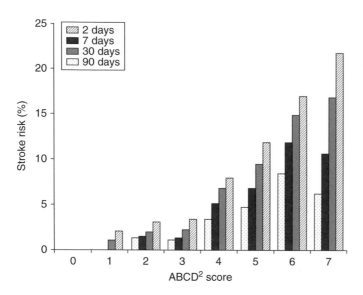

Fig. 14.1 Short-term stroke risk stratified by ABCD^2 score in six cohort studies combined ($n =$ 4,799 patients). Stroke risks are shown at 2, 7, 30, and 90 days (Johnston *et al.* 2007).

Validation of a Prognostic Model or Score

A prognostic model or score must always be independently validated. Simply because a model seems to include appropriately modeled powerful predictors does not mean that it will necessarily validate well because associations might just occur by chance and predictors may not be as powerful as they appear.

External validation of a model means determining whether it performs well in groups of patients other than those on whom it was derived: that is, how it is likely to do in real clinical practice. These other groups almost certainly will differ in case mix, referral patterns, treatment protocols, methods of measurement of variables, and definition of outcomes. Nevertheless, if a prognostic model includes powerful predictive variables, appropriately modeled, it should validate reasonably well in other groups of patients. For example, Fig. 14.1 shows the validation of the ABCD^2 score on pooled individual patient data from six independent groups of patients with TIA (Johnston *et al.* 2007) (Chapter 15).

The two main aims of a validation are to calibrate the model (i.e., to compare observed and predicted event rates for groups of patients) and to assess its discrimination (i.e., how well it distinguishes between patients who do or do not have an outcome event) (Harrell *et al.* 1996; Mackillop and Quirt 1997; Altman and Royston 2000).

Calibration is assessed by comparing the observed with the predicted proportions of events in groups defined by the risk prediction or score.

Discrimination can be summarized by various single statistics, such as the area under the receiver operating characteristic curve (or the equivalent C statistic), R^2 measures, or the d statistic, although all of these measures have limitations (Royston and Sauerbrei 2004; Altman and Royston 2007; Lewis 2007).

In reality, the best measure of the performance of a model is whether the risk stratification that it provides is likely to be useful in routine clinical practice. A relatively poorly predictive model can be useful when, for example, the overall risks of treatment versus no treatment are finely balanced, whereas a very powerfully predictive model may be unhelpful if a very high or low probability of a poor outcome is needed to affect clinical management. For example, use of a model predicting risk of death in a patient with prolonged refractory septic shock would only be helpful in the decision to withdraw active treatment if it could reliably predict probabilities of death of 95% or higher.

Internal validation of a model uses the same dataset as was used for derivation and will, therefore, almost inevitably overestimate its discriminatory power – sadly, this rather lazy approach is all too common, and external validation of the model is often not attempted. Better, in the absence of a new group of patients, is to use new data from the same source as the derivation sample. Several approaches are possible and will give useful information about predictive power (although *not* about generalizability):

- split the dataset into two parts before the modeling begins: the model is derived on the first portion of the data (the "training" set), and its ability to predict outcome is evaluated on the second portion (the "test" set).
- a bootstrapping approach, i.e., leave-one-out cross-validation.
- split the data in a non-random way, such as by time period or source of referral.
- prospective validation on subsequent patients from the same center(s).

These types of partially independent validation are of course tempting, and they do allow refinement of models and scores (Verweij and van Houwelingen 1993; Schumacher *et al.* 1997; Babyak 2004), but they are not a sufficient validation. Clearly, with each of the approaches listed previously, there will be many similarities between the derivation and validation sets of patients and between the clinical and laboratory techniques used in evaluating them. Indeed, this lack of true independence of the validation group of patients probably explains, in part, the fact that researchers tend to confirm the validity of their own models more often than do independent researchers (Altman and Royston 2000, 2007). The likely generalizability and so usefulness of a model can usually only be shown convincingly in a completely independent group of patients.

Even when a model has been independently validated and performs well, it must still be shown that it is useful in clinical practice. For helping treatment decisions in individual patients, usefulness is generally best tested by stratifying patients in a randomized controlled trial by estimated baseline risk of a poor outcome. Fig. 14.2 shows an external validation in an independent trial of the model detailed in Table 14.2 for the 5-year risk of stroke on medical treatment in patients with recently symptomatic carotid stenosis (Rothwell *et al.* 2005). Predicted medical risk is plotted against observed risk of stroke or death in patients randomized to medical or surgical treatment. Given that surgical treatment is associated with an additional 1–2% stroke risk per year over and above the operative risk, it is clear that surgery should probably only be considered in patients in the top two quintiles of predicted risk on medical treatment. Surgery will be harmful or of no benefit in the lower-risk individuals. This type of stratification of trial data using an independently derived model is usually essential to convince clinicians that the risk modeling approach is clinically useful. It is important to recognize, however, that even if the model has been validated previously in several non-trial groups of patients, it may perform differently in a trial because of the tendency to recruit relatively low-risk individuals. The distribution of risks in patients who are considered for treatment in routine clinical practice may be closer to that in the non-trial observational groups of patients used for derivation and validation of the model.

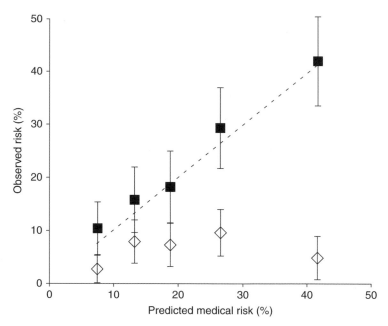

Fig. 14.2 An external validation of the model detailed in Table 14.2 for the 5-year risk of stroke on medical treatment in an independent randomized trial of endarterectomy versus medical treatment for symptomatic carotid stenosis (Rothwell *et al.* 2005). Predicted risk of stroke on medical treatment is plotted against the observed risk of stroke in patients randomized to medical treatment in the trial (squares) and against the observed operative risk of stroke and death in patients randomized to surgical treatment (diamonds). Groups are quintiles of predicted risk.

Reilly and Evans (2006) have defined five levels of evidence to assess the usefulness of a clinical prediction model (Box 14.4).

Another important issue is the need for updating of predictive models and scores if new predictors are discovered, requiring the addition of new variables to the model, or if new treatments reduce the risk of a poor outcome in general, requiring recalibration of the model. In general, minor recalibration of the prognostic index from the original model would be preferable to complete reconstruction (van Houwelingen and Thorogood 1995).

Reporting of Studies Developing, Validating, or Updating a Prediction Model

Previous reviews have noted that the quality of reporting prediction models in medicine is generally poor (Mallet *et al.* 2010; Collins *et al.* 2011, 2013). Recently, the Transparent Reporting of a multivariable prediction model for Individual Prognosis Or Diagnosis (TRIPOD) Initiative was established and developed a set of recommendations – "The TRIPOD Statement" (Collins *et al.* 2015). These recommendations are in the form of a checklist of 22 items that aims to improve the transparent reporting of studies developing, validating or updating a prediction model, be it for diagnostic or prognostic purposes.

BOX 14.4 Five Levels of Evidence Suggested by Reilly and Evans (2006) to Assess the Usefulness of a Clinical Prediction Rule

1. Derivation of the prediction rule
2. Narrow validation of the prediction rule (i.e., prospective evaluation in one setting)
3. Broad validation of the prediction rule (i.e., prospective evaluation in varied settings with a wide spectrum of patients and physicians)
4. Narrow impact analysis of the prediction rule used as a decision rule (i.e., prospective demonstration in one setting that the use of the prediction rule improves clinical decision making)
5. Broad impact analysis of the prediction rule used as a decision rule (i.e., prospective demonstration in varied settings that use of the prediction rule improves clinical decision making in a wide spectrum of patients)

References

Altman DG (2001). Systematic reviews of evaluations of prognostic variables. *British Medical Journal* **323**:224–228

Altman DG, Royston P (2000). What do we mean by validating a prognostic model? *Statistics in Medicine* **19**:453–473

Altman DG, Royston P (2007). Evaluating the performance of prognostic models. In *Treating Individuals: From Randomized Trials to Personalised Medicine*, Rothwell PM (ed.), pp. 213–30. London: Elsevier

Babyak MA (2004). What you see may not be what you get: A brief, nontechnical introduction to overfitting in regression-type models. *Psychosomatic Medicine* **66**:411–421

Boissel JP, Collet JP, Lievre M *et al.* (1993). An effect model for the assessment of drug benefit: Example of antiarrhythmic drugs in postmyocardial infarction patients. *Journal of Cardiovascular Pharmacology* **22**:356–363

Burton A, Altman DG (2004). Missing covariate data within cancer prognostic studies: A review of current reporting and proposed guidelines. *British Journal of Cancer* **91**:4–8

Christensen E (1987). Multivariate survival analysis using Cox's regression model. *Hepatology* **7**:1346–1358

Clark TG, Altman DG (2003). Developing a prognostic model in the presence of missing data: An ovarian cancer case study. *Journal of Clinical Epidemiology* **56**:28–37

Collins GS, Mallett S, Omar O *et al.* (2011). Developing risk prediction models for type 2 diabetes: A systematic review of methodology and reporting. *BMC Medicine* **9**:103

Collins GS, Omar O, Shanyinde M *et al.* (2013). A systematic review finds prediction models for chronic kidney disease were poorly reported and often developed using inappropriate methods. *Journal of Clinical Epidemiology* **66**:268–277

Collins GS, Reitsma JB, Altman DG *et al.* (2015). Transparent Reporting of a multivariable prediction model for Individual Prognosis or Diagnosis (TRIPOD): The TRIPOD statement. *Annals of Internal Medicine* **162**:600

Concato J, Feinstein AR, Holford TR (1993). The risk of determining risk with multivariable models. *Annals of Internal Medicine* **118**:201–210

Coste J, Fermanian J, Venot A (1995). Methodological and statistical problems in the construction of composite measurement scales: A survey of six medical and epidemiological journals. *Statistics in Medicine* **14**:331–345

Counsell C, Dennis M (2001). Systematic review of prognostic models in patients with acute stroke. *Cerebrovascular Diseases* **12**:159–170

Dahlof B, Lindholm LH, Hansson L *et al.* (1991). Morbidity and mortality in the Swedish trial in old patients with hypertension (STOP-hypertension). *Lancet* **338**:1281–1285

Feinstein AR (1996). *Multivariable Analysis: An Introduction*. New Haven, CT: Yale University Press

Friberg L, Rosenqvist M, Lip GY (2012). Evaluation of risk stratification schemes for ischemic stroke and bleeding in 182678 patients with atrial fibrillation: The Swedish Atrial

Fibrillation cohort study. *European Heart Journal* 33:1500–1510

Gage BF, van Walraven C, Pearce LA *et al.* (2004). Selecting patients with atrial fibrillation for anticoagulation. Stroke risk stratification in patients taking aspirin. *Circulation* 110:2287–2292

Giles MF, Rothwell PM (2007). Risk of stroke early after transient ischaemic attack: A systematic review and meta-analysis. *Lancet Neurology* 6:1063–1072

Grover SA, Lowensteyn I, Esrey KL *et al.* (1995). Do doctors accurately assess coronary risk in their patients? Preliminary results of the coronary health assessment study. *British Medical Journal* 310:975–978

Hackett ML, Anderson CS (2005). Predictors of depression after stroke: A systematic review of observational studies. *Stroke* 36:2296–2301

Harrell FE Jr., Lee KL, Califf RM *et al.* (1984). Regression modelling strategies for improved prognostic prediction. *Statistics in Medicine* 3:143–152

Harrell FE Jr., Lee KL, Mark DB (1996). Multivariable prognostic models: Issues in developing models, evaluating assumptions and adequacy, and measuring and reducing errors. *Statistics in Medicine* 15:361–387

Hart RG (2007). Antithrombotic therapy to prevent stroke in patients with atrial fibrillation. In *Treating Individuals: From Randomized Trials to Personalised Medicine*, Rothwell PM (ed.) pp. 265–278. London: Elsevier

Hayden JA, Côté P, Bombardier C (2006). Evaluation of the quality of prognosis studies in systematic reviews. *Annals of Internal Medicine* 144:427–437

Henderson R, Keiding N (2005). Individual survival time prediction using statistical models. *Journal of Medical Ethics* 31:703–706

Hodges JR, Warlow CP (1990a). Syndromes of transient amnesia: Towards a classification. A study of 153 cases. *Journal of Neurology, Neurosurgery Psychiatry* 53:834–843

Hodges JR, Warlow CP (1990b). The aetiology of transient global amnesia. A case–control study of 114 cases with prospective follow-up. *Brain* 113:639–657

International Study of Unruptured Intracranial Aneurysms Investigators (1998). Unruptured intracranial aneurysms: Risks of rupture and risks of surgical intervention. *New England Journal of Medicine* 1998 339:1725–1733

Jacob M, Lewsey JD, Sharpin C *et al.* (2005). Systematic review and validation of prognostic models in liver transplantation. *Liver Transplantation* 11:814–825

Johnston SC, Rothwell PM, Nguyen-Huynh MN *et al.* (2007). Validation and refinement of scores to predict very early stroke risk after transient ischaemic attack. *Lancet* 369:283–292

Justice AC, Covinsky KE, Berlin JA (1999). Assessing the generalizability of prognostic information. *Annals of Internal Medicine* 130:515–524

Kernan WN, Feinstein AR, Brass LM (1991). A methodological appraisal of research on prognosis after transient ischemic attacks. *Stroke* 22:1108–1116

Kim LG, Johnson TL, Marson AG for the MRC MESS Study Group (2006). Prediction of risk of seizure recurrence after a single seizure and early epilepsy: Further results from the MESS trial. *Lancet Neurology* 5:317–322

Laupacis A, Boysen G, Connolly S *et al.* (1994). Risk factors for stroke and efficacy of antithrombotic therapy in atrial fibrillation. Analysis of pooled data from five randomised controlled trials. *Archives of Internal Medicine* 154:1449–1457

Laupacis A, Sekar N, Stiell IG (1997). Clinical prediction rules. A review and suggested modifications of methodological standards. *Journal of the American Medical Association* 277:488–494

Lewis S (2007). Regression analysis. *Practical Neurology* 7:259–264

Li W, Boissel JP, Girard P *et al.* (1998). Identification and prediction of responders to a therapy: A model and its preliminary application to actual data. *Journal of Epidemiology and Biostatistics* 3:189–197

Lip GY, Nieuwlaat R, Pisters R *et al.* (2010). Refining clinical risk stratification for predicting stroke and thromboembolism in atrial fibrillation using a novel risk factor-based approach: The euro heart survey on atrial fibrillation. *Chest* **137**:263–272

Mackillop WJ, Quirt CF (1997). Measuring the accuracy of prognostic judgments in oncology. *Journal of Clinical Epidemiology* **50**:21–29

Mallett S, Royston P, Dutton S *et al.* (2010). Reporting methods in studies developing prognostic models in cancer: A review. *BMC Medicine* **8**:20

Medical Research Council Working Party (1985). MRC trial of treatment of mild hypertension: Principal results. *British Medical Journal* **291**:97–104

Morrow J, Russell A, Guthrie E *et al.* (2006). Malformation risks of antiepileptic drugs in pregnancy: A prospective study from the UK Epilepsy and Pregnancy Register. *Journal of Neurology, Neurosurgery Psychiatry* **77**:193–198

Pagliaro L, D'Amico G, Soronson TIA *et al.* (1992). Prevention of bleeding in cirrhosis. *Annals of Internal Medicine* **117**:59–70

Reilly BM, Evans AT (2006). Translating clinical research into clinical practice: Impact of using prediction rules to make decisions. *Annals of Internal Medicine* **144**:201–209

Rothwell PM (2003). Incidence, risk factors and prognosis of stroke and TIA: The need for high-quality, large-scale epidemiological studies and meta-analyses. *Cerebrovascular Diseases* **16** (Suppl 3):2–10

Rothwell PM, Mehta Z, Howard SC *et al.* (2005). From subgroups to individuals: General principles and the example of carotid endartectomy. *Lancet* **365**:256–265

Royston P, Sauerbrei W (2004). A new measure of prognostic separation in survival data. *Statistics in Medicine* **23**:723–748

Royston P, Altman DG, Sauerbrei W (2006). Dichotomizing continuous predictors in multiple regression: A bad idea. *Statistics in Medicine* **25**:127–141

Sackett DL, Whelan G (1980). Cancer risk in ulcerative colitis: Scientific requirements for the study of prognosis. *Gastroenterology* **78**:1632–1635

Sanmuganathan PS, Ghahramani P, Jackson PR *et al.* (2001). Aspirin for primary prevention of coronary heart disease: Safety and absolute benefit related to coronary risk derived from meta-analysis of randomised trials. *Heart* **85**:265–271

Schafer JL, Graham JW (2002). Missing data: Our view of the state of the art. *Psychological Methods* **7**:147–177

Schmoor C, Sauerbrei W, Schumacher M (2000). Sample size considerations for the evaluation of prognostic factors in survival analysis. *Statistics in Medicine* **19**:441–452

Schumacher M, Hollander N, Sauerbrei W (1997). Resampling and cross-validation techniques: a tool to reduce bias caused by model building? *Statistics in Medicine* **16**:2813–2827

Stevens DL, Matthews WB (1973). Cryptogenic drop attacks: An affliction of women. *British Medical Journal* **1**:439–442

Stroke Prevention in Atrial Fibrillation Investigators (1995). Risk factors for thromboembolism during aspirin therapy in patients with atrial fibrillation: The Stroke Prevention in Atrial Fibrillation study. *Journal of Stroke and Cerebrovascular Diseases 1995*; **5**:147–157

Sun GW, Shook TL, Kay GL (1996). Inappropriate use of bivariable analysis to screen risk factors for use in multivariable analysis. *Journal of Clinical Epidemiology.* **49**:907–916

Vach W (1997). Some issues in estimating the effect of prognostic factors from incomplete covariate data. *Statistics in Medicine* **16**:57–72

van Houwelingen HC, Thorogood J (1995). Construction, validation and updating of a prognostic model for kidney graft survival. *Statistics in Medicine* **14**:1999–2008

van Koningsveld R, Steyerberg EW, Hughes RA *et al.* (2007). A clinical prognostic scoring system for Guillain–Barré syndrome. *Lancet Neurology* **6**:589–594

Verweij PJ, van Houwelingen HC (1993). Cross-validation in survival analysis. *Statistics in Medicine* **12**:2305–2314

Walgaard C, Lingsma HF, Ruts L *et al.* (2011). Early recognition of poor prognosis in Guillain-Barré syndrome. *Neurology* **76**:968–975

West of Scotland Coronary Prevention Group (1996). West of Scotland Coronary Prevention

Study: Identification of high-risk groups and comparison with other cardiovascular intervention trials. *Lancet* **348**:1339–1342

Wyatt JC, Altman DG (1995). Commentary. Prognostic models: Clinically useful or quickly forgotten? *British Medical Journal* **311**:1539–1541

Yusuf S, Zucker D, Peduzzi P *et al.* (1994). Effect of coronary artery bypass graft surgery on survival: Overview of 10-year results from randomised trials by the Coronary Artery Bypass Graft Surgery Trialists' Collaboration. *Lancet* **344**:563–570

Short-Term Prognosis after Transient Ischemic Attack and Minor Stroke

The risk of stroke immediately after TIA or minor stroke is considerable (Giles and Rothwell 2007; Wu *et al.* 2007). However, this poses a challenge to clinical services because although the majority of patients will, by definition, have suffered a transient event with no immediate major sequelae, an important minority are at risk of a major stroke in the short term. Prognostic tools have, therefore, been developed to identify patients at high (and low) risk in order to inform public education, aid effective triage to secondary care, and direct secondary preventive treatment.

Early Risk of Stroke after Transient Ischemic Attack or Minor Stroke

Patients with major stroke often report earlier short-lived neurological symptoms, and data from population-based studies and trials suggest that approximately 20% of patients with stroke have a preceding TIA (Rothwell and Warlow 2005). A similar proportion of major strokes are probably preceded by a minor stroke. However, the prospective estimation of risk after TIA or minor stroke is challenging, and in the past the risk has been considered to be low (approximately 1–2% at 1 week and 2–4% at 1 month) (Hankey *et al.* 1991; Gubitz *et al.* 1999; Gubitz and Sandercock 2000; Warlow *et al.* 2001). However, these risks are now considered underestimates because they were calculated from cohort studies and clinical trials in which patients were recruited some time after their initial event and patients who experienced subsequent stroke before recruitment were excluded (Rothwell 2003).

Accurate estimation of the early risk of stroke after TIA or minor stroke requires particular study methods. First, potential patients must be recruited as rapidly as possible after the event so that strokes following very early after TIA are included. Second, patients should be assessed initially by an expert stroke physician to ensure that the diagnosis is made reliably and mimics are excluded. Third, follow-up should be in person and outcome events should be independently adjudicated to ensure correct identification of subsequent strokes. Lastly, patients should ideally be recruited from a defined population as opposed to a particular clinical setting in order to reduce selection bias.

A number of more recent studies have met most or all of these criteria. The first was published in 2000 (Johnston *et al.* 2000). All patients presenting to emergency departments (ED) with a diagnosis of TIA within a health maintenance organization in California, USA, were studied over a year, starting in February 1997. Of 1,707 patients, almost all presenting within 24 hours of the event, 180 (10.5%) returned to the ED within 90 days of the index TIA with a stroke, half of which occurred in the first 2 days after the TIA. Also, within the first 90 days, 2.6% of patients were hospitalized for cardiovascular events, 2.6% of patients died, and

12.7% suffered recurrent TIAs. In this study, patients were included if they had a diagnosis of TIA made by an ED physician, but these estimates of risk did not change substantially when the charts were examined by a neurologist and patients in whom the diagnosis was in doubt were excluded from the analysis.

Comparable risks of stroke after TIA were measured in population-based studies in Oxfordshire, UK (Lovett *et al.* 2003; Coull *et al.* 2004). In a cohort of 249 consecutive patients with a TIA ascertained in the Oxford Vascular Study (OXVASC) over a 30-month period, stroke risks at 2 and 7 days were 6.8% (95% confidence interval [CI], 3.7–10.0) and 12.0% (95% CI, 8.0–16.1), respectively (Rothwell *et al.* 2007). Although this cohort was smaller than the Californian cohort, it had the advantages of being population based and, therefore, included patients who were treated as inpatients, treated as outpatients, and managed solely in primary care; diagnoses were made by an experienced stoke physician; and follow-up was face-to-face with independent adjudication of outcome events.

In a systematic review of eighteen independent cohorts composed of 10,126 patients with TIA, the pooled stroke risks were 3.1% (95% CI, 2.0–4.1) at 2 days and 5.2% (95% CI, 3.9–6.5) at 7 days, but there was considerable heterogeneity between studies ($p <$ 0.0001), with risks ranging from 0% to 12.8% at 7 days (Giles and Rothwell 2007). However, the risks observed in individual studies over different intervals of follow-up were highly consistent, and the heterogeneity between studies was almost fully explained by study method, setting, and treatment. The lowest stroke risks at 7 days were seen in studies in specialist stroke services offering emergency access and treatment (0.9%; 95% CI, 0.0–1.9 [four studies]) and highest risks in population-based without urgent treatment (11.0%; 95% CI, 8.6–13.5 [three studies]). Intermediate risks were measured by studies recruiting from single EDs (5.8%; 95% CI, 3.7–8.0 [three studies]) and low risks in studies recruiting from routine neurovascular clinics (3.3%; 95% CI, 1.6–5.0 [two studies]) (Fig. 15.1). Findings were similar for stroke risks at 2 days. These differences in measured risk reflect a combination of patient selection by different care settings, with higher-risk patients being managed in emergency care; exclusion of high-risk individuals when there is a delay to recruitment; and modification of risk in patients who are urgently and aggressively treated with secondary preventive medication (Table 15.1).

The risk of stroke following minor stroke has not been studied in such depth. However, in a provisional report from the first year of OXVASC, the risk of stroke among 87 patients with minor stroke (defined as a score of ≤ 3 on the National Institutes of Health Stroke Scale [NIHSS]) was 11.5% (95% CI, 4.8–11.2) at 7 days and 18.5% (95% CI, 10.3–26.7) at 90 days (Coull *et al.* 2004). Among patients with minor stroke who were referred to the dedicated neurovascular clinic in the EXPRESS study and did not need immediate admission to hospital, the rates of recurrent stroke at 90 days were 10.8% (17/158) in phase 1, without urgent intervention, and 4.0% (5/125) in phase 2, with urgent intervention (Rothwell *et al.* 2007) (Chapter 20).

Identification of High-Risk Patients: Simple Risk Scores

Patients with TIA and minor stroke are very heterogeneous in terms of symptoms, risk factors, underlying pathology, and early prognosis. Effective management requires the reliable identification of patients at high (and low) risk in order to inform public education,

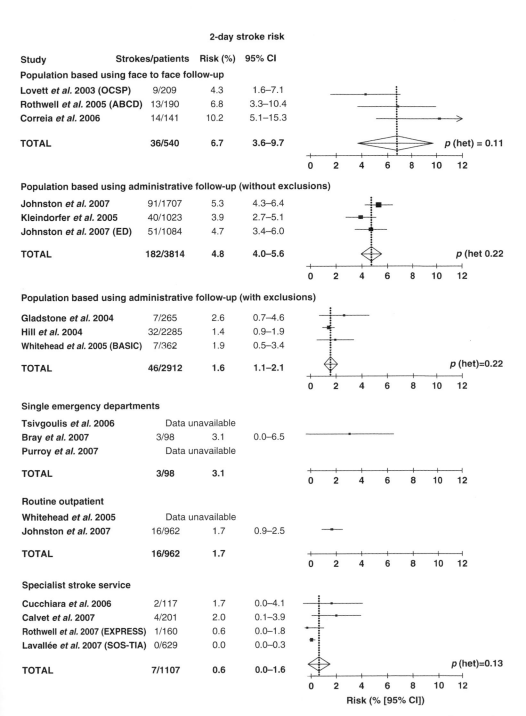

Fig. 15.1 Stroke risks at 2 and 7 days measured in a systematic review of independent cohorts, stratified according to study method and setting (Giles and Rothwell 2007). CI, confidence interval; p (het), p value for heterogeneity between studies; p (sig), p value for overall significance of the meta-analysis of comparisons between studies.

7-day stroke risk

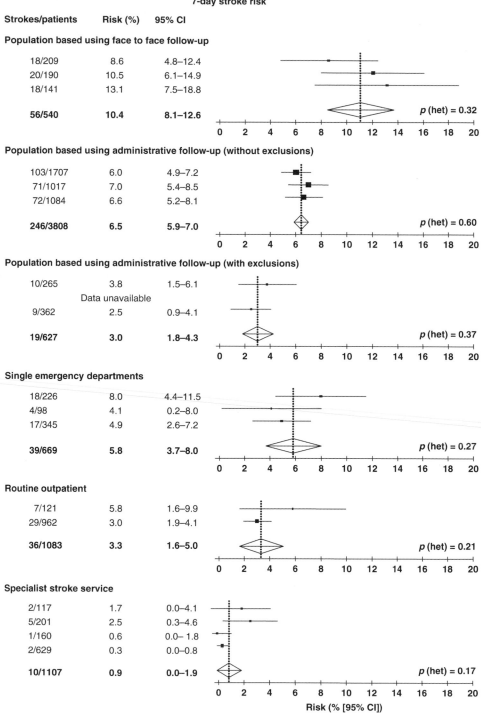

Strokes/patients	Risk (%)	95% CI
Population based using face to face follow-up		
18/209	8.6	4.8–12.4
20/190	10.5	6.1–14.9
18/141	13.1	7.5–18.8
56/540	**10.4**	**8.1–12.6**
p (het) = 0.32		
Population based using administrative follow-up (without exclusions)		
103/1707	6.0	4.9–7.2
71/1017	7.0	5.4–8.5
72/1084	6.6	5.2–8.1
246/3808	**6.5**	**5.9–7.0**
p (het) = 0.60		
Population based using administrative follow-up (with exclusions)		
10/265	3.8	1.5–6.1
	Data unavailable	
9/362	2.5	0.9–4.1
19/627	**3.0**	**1.8–4.3**
p (het) = 0.37		
Single emergency departments		
18/226	8.0	4.4–11.5
4/98	4.1	0.2–8.0
17/345	4.9	2.6–7.2
39/669	**5.8**	**3.7–8.0**
p (het) = 0.27		
Routine outpatient		
7/121	5.8	1.6–9.9
29/962	3.0	1.9–4.1
36/1083	**3.3**	**1.6–5.0**
p (het) = 0.21		
Specialist stroke service		
2/117	1.7	0.0–4.1
5/201	2.5	0.3–4.6
1/160	0.6	0.0–1.8
2/629	0.3	0.0–0.8
10/1107	**0.9**	**0.0–1.9**
p (het) = 0.17		

Risk (% [95% CI])

Fig. 15.1 (cont.)

Table 15.1 Advantages and disadvantages of different clinical settings in studies of early prognosis after transient ischemic attack or minor stroke

Setting	Advantages	Disadvantages
ED	Short delay between clinical event and presentation to medical attention	Selection bias: patients managed in alternative settings not studied
	Large cohorts in different departments can be identified and studied	Data collected retrospectively
	Computerized databases can be searched rapidly	Diagnosis and management by ED physician and may not be consistent/fully described
		Patients with a TIA and then a stroke before attending ED not included
		Non-standardized follow-up
Population-based	No selection bias	Costly and labor and time intensive
	Uniform diagnosis, management and follow-up	
	Sensitive follow-up to detect outcome events	
	Complete data available on patient cohort	
	Some data available on study population	
Outpatient clinic	Standardized diagnosis and management	Frequent delay between event and clinic attendance

Notes: ED, emergency department; TIA, transient ischemic attack.

aid effective triage to specialist services, and direct secondary preventive treatment. There is evidence that clinical features of a TIA provide substantial prognostic information, as do some other methods.

Five risk factors were found to be independently associated with high risk of recurrent stroke at 3 months in a large ED cohort of patients with TIA (Johnston *et al.* 2000). These included age over 60 years, symptom duration >10 minutes, motor weakness, speech impairment, and diabetes mellitus. Recurrent stroke risk at 3 months varied from 0% for those with none of these factors to 34% for those with all five factors. Isolated sensory or visual symptoms were associated with low risk.

These and other factors identified as being associated with early stroke risk (Gladstone *et al.* 2004; Hill *et al.* 2004) were used to derive the ABCD score, a predictive tool of stroke risk within 7 days after TIA (Rothwell *et al.* 2005). Briefly, all clinical features that had previously been found to be independently predictive of stroke after TIA were tested in a derivation cohort of 209 patients recruited from the Oxfordshire Community Stroke Project (OCSP, Lovett *et al.* 2003). Any variable that was a univariate predictor of the 7-day risk of stroke with a significance of $p \leq 0.1$

Table 15.2 The clinical features and scoring for the ABCD system of assessing risk of stroke in the 7 days after a transient ischemic attack

	Clinical feature	Category	Score
A	Age	≥ 60 years	1
		< 60 years	0
B	Blood pressure at assessment[a]	SBP ≥ 140 mmHg or DBP ≥ 90 mmHg	1
		Other	0
C	Clinical features	Unilateral weakness	2
		Speech disturbance (no weakness)	1
		Other	0
D	Duration	≥ 60 minutes	2
		10–59 minutes	1
		< 10 minutes	0
	Total(maximum)		6

Notes: SBP, systolic blood pressure; DBP, diastolic blood pressure.
[a] Measured at earliest assessment after the attack.
Source: From Rothwell et al. (2005).

assessed with the log rank test was incorporated into the score. The score was then validated in three further independent cohorts.

The score is based on four clinical features and is out of a total of 6 (Table 15.2). The score was found to be highly predictive with areas under the receiver operating characteristic (ROC) curves of 0.85 (95% CI, 0.78–0.91), 0.91 (95% CI, 0.86–0.95), and 0.80 (95% CI, 0.72–0.89) for each of the validation cohorts. In the OXVASC population-based validation cohort of all 377 referrals with suspected, possible, or definite TIA, there were 20 strokes at 7 days after the initial event: 19 (95%) of these occurred in the 101 patients (27%) with a risk score ≥ 5. The 7-day risks were 0.4% (95% CI, 0–1.1) in 274 patients (73%) with a score of < 5, 12.1% (95% CI, 4.2–20.0) in 66 patients (18%) with a score of 5, and 31.4% (95% CI, 16.0–46.8) in 35 patients (9%) with a score of 6.

The score was originally designed to facilitate triage between primary and secondary care and to inform public education of "high risk" scenarios in which medical attention should be sought urgently (Rothwell et al. 2005), although its use has been extended to treatment decisions (National Institute for Health and Clinical Excellence 2017).

The ABCD scoring system has since been refined in larger cohorts of patients with the subsequent addition of 1 point for diabetes to make the $ABCD^2$ score out of 7 (Rothwell et al. 2005; Johnston et al. 2007) (Table 15.3).

Both the ABCD and the $ABCD^2$ scores have been further validated in independent cohorts since publication in 2005 and 2007, respectively. In a systematic review, 20 cohorts were identified that reported the performance of one or both ABCD and $ABCD^2$ scores including 9808 subjects with 456 stroke at 7 days (Giles and Rothwell 2010). Pooled estimates of the areas under the ROC curves for the ABCD and $ABCD^2$ scores, respectively, were 0.72 (95% CI, 0.67–0.77) and 0.72 (95% CI, 0.63–0.80) for stroke risk at 7 days. Predictive power was independent of clinical setting (ED, specialist neurovascular units,

Table 15.3 The clinical features and scoring for the ABCD^2 system

	Clinical feature	Category	Score
A	Age	≥ 60 years	1
		< 60 years	0
B	Blood pressure at assessment^a	SBP ≥ 140 mmHg or DBP ≥ 90 mmHg	1
		Other	0
C	Clinical Features	Unilateral weakness	2
		Speech disturbance (no weakness)	1
		Other	0
D	Duration	≥ 60 minutes	2
		10–59 minutes	1
		< 10 minutes	0
D	Diabetes	Present	1
		Absent	0
	Total (maximum)		7

Notes: SBP, systolic blood pressure; DBP, diastolic blood pressure.
^{a} Measured at earliest assessment after the attack.
Sources: From Rothwell et al. (2005) and Johnston et al. (2007).

and population-based studies) but was greater in cohorts that included patients with both suspected and confirmed TIA than in cohorts of patients with confirmed TIA only. These findings imply that the scores work partly by providing diagnostic information, but this cannot fully explain their prognostic power.

In conclusion, the ABCD and ABCD^2 scores are reliable tools to predict the early risk of stroke after TIA. However, although they are sensitive and easily calculable using clinical information readily available at the time of assessment, they have a high false-positive rate and were deliberately designed to include only clinical data so that they could be used for initial triage. Further information may, therefore, be required to refine risk prediction.

Risk of Recurrence by Vascular Territory

The early risk of stroke after TIA also depends on the vascular territory of the event. Monocular events are associated with a low risk of subsequent cerebral stroke (Hankey et al. 1991; Benavente et al. 2001). Posterior circulation TIAs, which make up approximately 25% of all attacks, were thought for many years to be associated with a lower risk of stroke than carotid territory TIAs (Sivenius et al. 1991; Mohr et al. 1992; Caplan 1996). Correspondingly, they were often managed less aggressively.

However, a systematic review of 37 published cohort studies and five unpublished studies reporting the risk of stroke after a TIA or minor stroke by territory of presenting event found no major differences in prognosis between vertebrobasilar events and carotid events. In fact, studies that recruited during the acute phase after the presenting event found a higher risk of subsequent stroke in patients with vertebrobasilar events (odds ratio [OR], 1.47; 95% CI, 1.1–2.0; $p = 0.014$) (Flossman and Rothwell 2003; Gulli et al. 2013). Subsequent

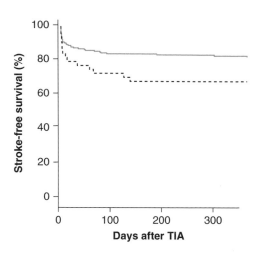

Fig. 15.2 Stroke-free survival curves for consecutive patients with transient ischemic attacks (TIAs) and anterior (—) versus posterior (–) circulation events in the Oxford Vascular Study (OXVASC) (log rank $p = 0.04$) (Flossman *et al.* 2006).

data from OXVASC suggest that TIAs attributable to the posterior circulation have higher rates of recurrent stroke than those attributable to the anterior circulation (Flossman *et al.* 2006). Among 256 consecutive patients with TIA, 44 (17.1%) with a posterior event and 212 (82.5%) with an anterior event, rates of stroke were 15.9% and 9.4%, respectively ($p = 0.22$), at 7 days and 31.8% and 17.0%, respectively ($p = 0.03$), at 1 year (Fig. 15.2). In a further series of patients with TIA and minor stroke in OXVASC, the rate of symptomatic large artery stenosis was higher among patients with posterior circulation events than among those with carotid territory events (Marquardt *et al.* 2009). More recent data from the St. George's Hospital study and OXVASC of 323 patients with a posterior circulation TIA/ischemic stroke revealed that the 90-day recurrent stroke risk was greater in patients with significant (> 50%) vertebrobasilar stenosis (24.6%) compared with those without (7.2%). The risk was greatest in patients with intracranial stenosis (33%) compared with those with extracranial stenosis (16%), while patients without significant stenosis had a 90-day recurrent stroke risk of 7% (Gulli *et al.* 2013). These findings have led to an increased interest in imaging the posterior circulation and in angioplasty or stenting any atherothrombotic stenosis detected in the vertebral or proximal basilar arteries (Markus *et al.* 2013) (see Chapter 26).

Risk by Underlying Pathology

Several population-based studies of stroke have shown that recurrent stroke risk is highest in those with large arterial territory stroke and lowest in those with lacunar stroke (Lovett *et al.* 2004a) (Fig. 15.3). Although large artery pathology accounted for only 14% of the initial strokes in a pooled analysis of data from four such studies, 37% of the recurrences at 7 days occurred in this group (Lovett *et al.* 2004a). Subtype differences in early recurrent risk are probably smaller in patients with TIA, where some patients with small vessel disease can have a very high risk of early stroke, for instance the "capsular warning syndrome" (Paul *et al.* 2012). Nevertheless, several other observations highlight the high early risk of stroke after large artery TIA, including the very high risk of stroke during delays to carotid endarterectomy in patients with recently symptomatic stenosis $\geq$ 50% of the carotid artery (Fairhead and Rothwell 2005; Rantner *et al.* 2005). Patients with cardioembolic TIA or stroke, predominantly

1-month risks

Subgroup	Events/ patients (%)	Events/ patients (%)	Odds ratio	95% CI
LAA vs. rest				
OXVASC	7/26 (26.9)	13/125 (10.4)	3.17	1.1–9.0
OCSP	5/78 (6.4)	15/499 (3.0)	2.21	0.8–6.3
Erlangen	2/71 (2.8)	9/460 (2.0)	1.45	0.3–6.9
Rochester	9/70 (12.9)	12/380 (3.2)	4.52	1.8–11.2
Subtotal	23/245 (9.4)	49/1464 (3.3)	2.91	1.7–4.9
				p (het) = 0.375
				p (sig) < 0.001
SMVD vs. rest				
OXVASC	2/33 (6.1)	18/118 (15.3)	0.36	0.1–1.6
OCSP	1/119 (0.8)	19/458 (4.1)	0.20	0.0–1.5
Erlangen	0/120 (0.1)	11/411 (2.7)	0.03	0.0–15.4
Rochester	1/72 (1.4)	20/378 (5.3)	0.25	0.0–1.9
Subtotal	4/344 (1.2)	68/1365 (5.0)	0.22	0.1–0.6
				p (het) = 0.964
				p (sig) = 0.003
CE vs. rest				
OXVASC	4/37 (10.8)	16/114 (14.0)	0.74	0.2–2.4
OCSP	3/127 (2.4)	17/450 (3.8)	0.62	0.2–2.1
Erlangen	5/143 (3.5)	6/388 (1.5)	2.31	0.7–7.7
Rochester	6/132 (4.5)	15/318 (4.7)	0.96	0.4–2.5
Subtotal	18/439 (4.1)	54/1270 (4.3)	0.97	0.6–1.7
				p (het) = 0.425
				p (sig) = 0.983
Undetermined vs. rest				
OXVASC	6/54 (11.1)	14/97 (14.4)	0.74	0.3–2.1
OCSP	11/220 (5.0)	9/357 (2.5)	2.04	0.8–5.0
Erlangen	4/188 (2.1)	7/343 (2.0)	1.04	0.3–3.6
Rochester	5/164 (3.0)	16/286 (5.6)	0.53	0.2–1.5
Subtotal	26/626 (4.2)	46/1083 (4.2)	0.98	0.6–1.6
				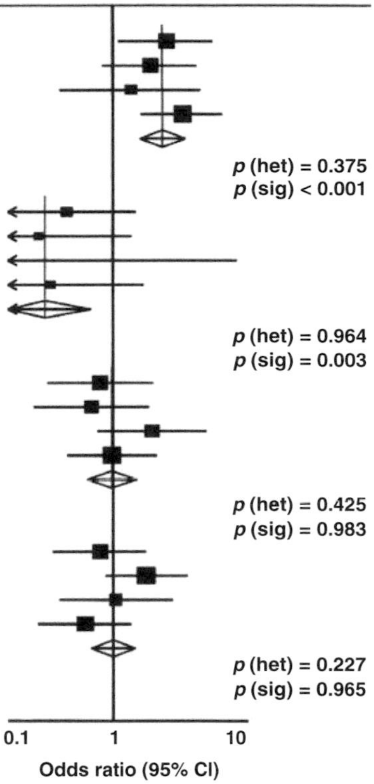 *p* (het) = 0.227
				p (sig) = 0.965

Odds ratio (95% CI) — 0.1 — 1 — 10

Fig. 15.3 Meta-analysis of population-based studies showing odds ratios for risk of recurrent stroke at 1 month according to pathological subtype (Lovett *et al.* 2004a). CI, confidence interval; *p* (het), *p* value for heterogeneity between studies; *p* (sig), *p* value overall significance of the meta-analysis of comparisons between studies; LAA, large vessel atherosclerotic stroke; SMVD, small vessel disease; CE, cardioembolic stroke. *Sources*: Flossman *et al.* (2006) (OXVASC); Lovett *et al.* (2003) (OCSP); Petty *et al.* (2000) (Rochester study); Kolominsky-Rabas *et al.* (2001) (Erlingen study).

consisting of patients with non-valvular atrial fibrillation, are at intermediate early risk of recurrence (Lovett *et al.* 2004b).

Imaging and Prognosis

Some early studies suggested that the presence of infarction on CT in patients with TIA or minor stroke predicts an increased risk of stroke recurrence (Evans *et al.* 1991; van Swieten *et al.* 1992; Dutch TIA Trial Study Group 1993), although others have failed to confirm this finding (Davalos *et al.* 1988; Dennis *et al.* 1990). Interpretation of these studies is difficult as scans were often performed some time after the clinical event and new and old infarction was not differentiated. A subsequent study of TIA patients who had CT scans performed within 48 hours of their clinical event showed that appearances consistent with recent infarction on CT predicted recurrent stroke (OR, 4.06; 95% CI, 1.16–14.14; $p = 0.028$) (Douglas *et al.* 2003), and it has been suggested that the presence of infarction detected by CT scanning after TIA may improve the prediction of early stroke (Sciolla and Melis 2008).

As reviewed in Chapter 10, diffusion-weighted MRI (DWI) is a particularly sensitive (although somewhat nonspecific) technique for identifying acute cerebral ischemia. It is, therefore, likely that the presence of abnormalities on DWI in a patient with TIA or minor stroke would suggest an active "vascular process" such as a source of emboli or large artery atheromatous disease and would, therefore, signify a high risk of further thromboembolism and so recurrent stroke (Tong and Caplan 2007). Focal motor weakness, speech disturbance, and symptoms lasting longer than 1 hour are all associated with DWI-detected lesions in patients with TIA (Redgrave *et al.* 2007a, b). Several studies have also demonstrated an association between abnormalities on DWI in the acute phase and the development of further abnormalities (Sylaja *et al.* 2007). However, although DWI technology has been available since the mid-1990s, the association between abnormalities on DWI in patients with TIA and minor stroke and those with recurrent stroke was not demonstrated until approximately 10 years later. This is partly because of the small size of studies in relation to the patient numbers required to demonstrate such an association, as illustrated by the main studies described in the following section.

In one cohort of 83 consecutive patients with a TIA attending an ED who were scanned with DWI, abnormalities were identified in 27. The combination of DWI abnormalities and symptoms lasting more than an hour was found to be predictive of a combined endpoint of stroke or other vascular event (Purroy *et al.* 2004). In another cohort of 120 patients with TIA or minor stroke, all of whom received DWI within 24 hours, the presence of abnormalities on DWI was associated with a higher risk of stroke at 90 days, as was vessel occlusion (Coutts *et al.* 2005). In a further cohort of 87 patients with TIA and 74 with ischemic stroke, the rate of recurrent stroke was highest in the group with TIA and infarction on DWI (Ay *et al.* 2005). Lastly, in a retrospective cohort study of 146 patients with TIA, 37 (25%) had abnormalities on DWI; the presence of these abnormalities was shown to be independently associated with a higher risk of in-hospital recurrent TIA or stroke (OR, 11.2; $p < 0.01$) (Prabhakaran *et al.* 2007).

Furthermore, the presence of solid microembolic signals in the middle cerebral artery detected by transcranial Doppler has been shown to be associated with a high risk of stroke following TIA or minor stroke in patients with recently symptomatic carotid stenosis, although this technique is not readily available in everyday clinical practice. In one study of 73 patients with minor stroke or TIA in whom transcranial Doppler imaging of the symptomatic cerebral artery was performed within 7 days, the presence of microembolic signals was a predictor of the early recurrence of ischemia after adjustment for the presence of carotid stenosis, antiplatelet therapy during follow-up, and other confounding variables (relative risk, 8.7; 95% CI, 2.0–38.2; $p = 0.0015$) (Valton *et al.* 1998). In another study of 111 subjects with both symptomatic and asymptomatic carotid stenosis > 60%, the presence of microembolic signals was predictive of TIA and stroke risk during follow-up (Molloy and Markus 1999). The role of perfusion imaging in short-term risk prediction after TIA and minor stroke is nevertheless uncertain (Latchaw *et al.* 2003).

In view of the high risk of early stroke after TIA in patients with a recent earlier TIA (e.g., in capsular warning syndrome) and in TIA patients with acute DWI hyperintensity or significant carotid stenosis, the $ABCD^3$ and $ABCD^3$-I scores were proposed (Table 15.4) (Merwick *et al.* 2010). Similar to the $ABCD^2$ score, the $ABCD^3$ score is also purely based on clinical information but allocates an extra 2 points to the $ABCD^2$

Table 15.4 The clinical features and scoring for the ABCD^3 and ABCD^3-I system

	Clinical feature	Category	ABCD^3 Score	ABCD^3-I Score
A	Age	≥ 60 years	1	1
		< 60 years	0	0
B	Blood pressure at assessment^a	SBP ≥ 140 mmHg or DBP ≥ 90 mmHg	1	1
		Other	0	0
C	Clinical Features	Unilateral weakness	2	2
		Speech disturbance (no weakness)	1	1
		Other	0	0
D	Duration	≥ 60 minutes	2	2
		10–59 minutes	1	1
		< 10 minutes	0	0
D	Diabetes	Present	1	1
		Absent	0	0
D	Dual TIA (TIA prompting medical attention plus at least one other TIA in the preceding 7 days)	Present	2	2
		Absent	0	0
I	Imaging (Ipsilateral ≥50% stenosis of internal carotid artery)	Present	NA	2
		Absent	NA	0
I	Imaging (acute DWI hyperintensity)	Present	NA	2
		Absent	NA	0
	Total (maximum)		9	13

Notes: SBP, systolic blood pressure; DBP, diastolic blood pressure; DWI, diffusion weighted imaging.
^{a} Measured at earliest assessment after the attack.
Source: Merwick *et al.* (2010).

score in TIA patients who had at least an additional TIA in the preceding 7 days (total score of 9). The ABCD^3-I score, however, further incorporates results from initial investigations and allocates another 2 points to TIA patients who have an underlying ipsilateral ≥ 50% stenosis of the internal carotid artery on vascular imaging and 2 more to those who also have an acute DWI hyperintense lesion on MRI (total score of 13). These two scores were derived from 3,886 patients with TIA, pooled from various centers, while these scores were validated initially in a combined cohort consisting of 1,232 TIA patients from OXVASC and Dublin. Both the ABCD^3 and ABCD^3-I scores significantly predicted early risk of recurrent stroke at 7, 28, and 90 days in the derivation and validation cohorts (Merwick *et al.* 2010). However, only the ABCD^3-I score resulted in a net reclassification improvement of 90-day stroke risk prediction compared with the ABCD^2 in both the derivation and validation cohorts, while the ABCD^3 score did not result in a net reclassification improvement in the validation cohort. Since the introduction of these two scores, the ABCD^3-I has been further validated in other cohorts (Song *et al.* 2013; Kelly *et al.* 2016) and was recently shown in 2,176 patients from 16 cohort studies to reliably identify patients at highest risk of an early stroke after TIA with improved risk prediction compared with the ABCD^2 (c-statistic 0.84 versus 0.64, $p < 0.001$) and also ABCD^2-I scores (c-statistic 0.84 vs. 0.74, $p < 0.001$) (Kelly *et al.* 2016). These results therefore provide further evidence of the importance of urgent assessment, vascular imaging, and MRI (where available) in patients presenting with a TIA.

References

Ay H, Koroshetz WJ, Benner T *et al.* (2005). Transient ischemic attack with infarction: A unique syndrome? *Annals of Neurology* 57:679–686

Benavente O, Eliasziw M, Streifler JY *et al.* (2001). For the NASCET Collaborators: Prognosis after transient monocular blindness associated with carotid artery stenosis. *New England Journal of Medicine* 345:1084–1090

Bray JE, Coughlan K, Bladin C (2007). Can the ABCD score be dichotomised to identify high-risk patients with transient ischaemic attack in the emergency department?, *Emergency Medicine Journal* 24:92–95

Calvet D, Lamy C, Touzé E *et al.* (2007). Management and outcome of patients with transient ischemic attack admitted to a stroke unit, *Cerebrovascular Diseases* 24:80–85

Caplan LR (1996). *Posterior Circulation Disease: Clinical Findings, Diagnosis and Management*, pp. 20–21. Boston, MA: Blackwell Science.

Correia M, Silva MR, Magalhaes R, Guimaraes L, Silva MC (2006). Transient ischemic attacks in rural and urban northern Portugal: Incidence and short-term prognosis. *Stroke* 37:50–55

Coull AJ, Lovett JK, Rothwell PM for the Oxford Vascular Study (2004). Population based study of early risk of stroke after transient ischaemic attack or minor stroke: Implications for public education and organisation of services. *British Medical Journal* 328:326

Coutts SB, Simon JE, Eliasziw M *et al.* (2005). Triaging transient ischemic attack and minor stroke patients using acute magnetic resonance imaging. *Annals of Neurology* 57:848–854

Cucchiara BL, Messe SR, Taylor RA *et al.* (2006). Is the ABCD score useful for risk stratification of patients with acute transient ischemic attack? *Stroke* 37:1710–1714

Davalos A, Matias-Guiu J, Torrent O *et al.* (1988). Computed tomography in reversible ischaemic attacks: Clinical and prognostic correlations in a prospective study. *Journal of Neurology* 235:155–158

Dennis M, Bamford J, Sandercock P *et al.* (1990). Computed tomography in patients with transient ischaemic attacks: When is a transient ischaemic attack not a transient ischaemic attack but a stroke? *Journal of Neurology* 237:257–261

Douglas CD, Johnston CM, Elkins J *et al.* (2003). Head computed tomography findings predict short-term stroke risk after transient ischemic attack. *Stroke* 34:2894–2899

Dutch TIA Trial Study Group (1993). Predictors of major vascular events in patients with a transient ischemic attack or nondisabling stroke: The Dutch TIA Trial Study Group. *Stroke* 24:527–531

Evans GW, Howard G, Murros KE *et al.* (1991). Cerebral infarction verified by cranial computed tomography and prognosis for survival following transient ischemic attack. *Stroke* 22:431–436

Fairhead JF, Rothwell PM (2005). The need for urgency in identification and treatment of symptomatic carotid stenosis is already established. *Cerebrovascular Diseases* 19:355–358

Flossman E, Rothwell PM (2003). Prognosis of vertebrobasilar transient ischaemic attack and minor ischaemic stroke. *Brain* **126**:1940–1954

Flossman E, Touze E, Giles MF *et al.* (2006). The early risk of stroke after vertebrobasilar TIA is higher than after carotid TIA. *Cerebrovascular Diseases* **21**(Suppl 4):6

Giles MF, Rothwell PM (2007). Risk of stroke early after transient ischaemic attack: A systematic review and meta-analysis. *Lancet Neurology* **6**:1063–1072

Giles MF, Rothwell PM (2008). Systematic review and pooled analysis of published and unpublished validations of the ABCD and ABCD^2 transient ischemic attack risk scores. *Stroke* **41**:667–673

Gladstone DJ, Kapral MK, Fang J Laupacis A, Tu JV (2004). Management and outcomes of transient ischaemic attacks in Ontario. *Canadian Medical Association Journal CMAJ* 1707:1099–1104

Gubitz G, Sandercock P (2000). Prevention of ischaemic stroke. *British Medical Journal* **321**:1455–1459

Gubitz G, Phillips S, Dwyer V (1999). What is the cost of admitting patients with transient ischaemic attacks to hospital? *Cerebrovascular Diseases* **9**:210–214

Gulli G, Marquardt L, Rothwell PM *et al.* (2013). Stroke risk after posterior circulation stroke/ transient ischemic attack and its relationship to site of vertebrobasilar stenosis: Pooled data analysis from prospective studies. *Stroke* **44**:598–604

Hankey GJ, Slattery JM, Warlow CP (1991). The prognosis of hospital-referred transient ischaemic attacks. *Journal of Neurology, Neurosurgery Psychiatry* **54**:793–802

Hill MD, Yiannakoulias N, Jeerakathil T *et al.* (2004). The high risk of stroke immediately after transient ischemic attack. A population-based study. *Neurology* **62**:2015–2020

Johnston SC, Gress DR, Browner WS *et al.* (2000). Short-term prognosis after emergency department diagnosis of TIA. *Journal of the American Medical Association* **284**:2901–2906

Johnston SC, Rothwell PM, Nguyen-Huynh MN *et al.* (2007). Validation and refinement of scores to predict very early stroke risk after transient ischaemic attack. *Lancet* **369**:283–292

Kelly PJ, Albers GW, Chatzikonstantinou A *et al.* (2016). Validation and comparison of imaging-based scores for prediction of early stroke risk after transient ischemic attack: A pooled analysis of individual-patient data from cohort studies. *Lancet Neurology* **15**:1238–1247

Kleindorfer D, Panagos P, Pancioli A *et al.* (2005). Incidence and short-term prognosis of transient ischemic attack in a population-based study, *Stroke* **36**:720–723

Kolominsky-Rabas PL, Weber M, Gefeller O, Neundoerfer B, Heuschmann PU (2001). Epidemiology of ischemic stroke subtypes according to TOAST criteria: Incidence, recurrence, and long-term survival in ischemic stroke subtypes: A population-based study. *Stroke* **32**:2735–2740

Latchaw RE, Yonas H, Hunter GJ *et al.* (2003). Guidelines and recommendations for perfusion imaging in cerebral ischemia: A scientific statement for healthcare professionals by the Writing Group on Perfusion Imaging, from the Council on Cardiovascular Radiology of the American Heart Association. *Stroke* **34**:1084–1104

Lavallée PC, Mesegaur E, Abboud F *et al.* (2007). A transient ischaemic attack clinic with round-the-clock access (SOS-TIA): Feasibility and effects. *Lancet Neurology* **6**:953–960

Lovett JK, Dennis MS, Sandercock PA *et al.* (2003). Very early risk of stroke after a first transient ischemic attack. *Stroke* **34**: e138–e140

Lovett JK, Coull AJ, Rothwell PM (2004a). Early risk of recurrence by subtype of ischemic stroke in population-based incidence studies. *Neurology* **62**:569–573

Lovett JK, Gallagher PJ, Hands LJ *et al.* (2004b). Histological correlates of carotid plaque surface morphology on lumen contrast imaging. *Circulation* **110**:2190–2197

Markus, HS, van der Worp HB, Rothwell PM (2013). Posterior circulation ischemic stroke and transient ischemic attack: Diagnosis, investigation, and secondary prevention. *Lancet Neurology* **12**:989–998

Marquardt L, Kuker W, Chandratheva A *et al.* (2009). Incidence and prognosis of ≥50% symptomatic vertebral or basilar artery stenosis: Prospective population-based study. *Brain* **132**:982–988

Merwick A, Albers GW, Amarenco P *et al.* (2010). Addition of brain and carotid imaging to the ABCD^2 score to identify patients at early risk of stroke after transient ischemic attack: A multicenter observational study. *Lancet Neurology* **9**:1060–1069

Mohr JP, Gautier JC, Pessin MS (1992). Internal carotid artery disease. In *Stroke*, Barnett HJM Mohr JP Stein BM Yatsu FM (eds.), p. 311. New York, NY: Churchill Livingstone

Molloy J, Markus HS (1999). Asymptomatic embolization predicts stroke and TIA risk in patients with carotid artery stenosis. *Stroke* **30**:1440–1443

National Institute for Health and Clinical Excellence (2017). *Stroke and Transient Ischemic Attack in Over 16s: Diagnosis and Initial Management.* London: NICE

Paul NL, Simoni M, Chandratheva A *et al.* (2012). Population-based study of capsular warning syndrome and prognosis after early recurrent TIA. *Neurology* **79**:1356–1362

Petty GW, Brown R-DJ, Whisnant JP *et al.* (2000). Ischemic stroke subtypes: A population-based study of functional outcome, survival, and recurrence. *Stroke* **31**:1062–1068

Prabhakaran S, Chong JY, Sacco RL (2007). Impact of abnormal diffusion-weighted imaging results on short-term outcome following transient ischemic attack. *Archives of Neurology* **64**:1105–1109

Purroy F, Montaner J, Rovira A *et al.* (2004). Higher risk of further vascular events among transient ischaemic attack patients with diffusion-weighted imaging acute lesions. *Stroke* **35**:2313–2319

Purroy F, Molina CA, Montaner J, Alvarez-Sabin J (2007). Absence of usefulness of ABCD score in the early risk of stroke of transient ischemic attack patients. *Stroke* **38**:855–856

Rantner B, Pavelka M, Posch L (2005). Carotid endarterectomy after ischemic stroke: Is there a justification for delayed surgery? *European Journal of Vascular Endovascular Surgery* **30**:36–40

Redgrave JN, Schulz UG, Briley D *et al.* (2007a). Presence of acute ischemic lesions on diffusion-weighted imaging is associated with clinical predictors of early risk of stroke after transient ischemic attack. *Cerebrovascular Diseases* **24**:86–90

Redgrave JN, Coutts SB, Schulz UG *et al.* (2007b). Systemic review of associations between the presence of acute ischemic lesions on diffusion-weighted imaging and clinical predictors of early stroke risk after transient ischemic attack. *Stroke* **38**:1482–1488

Rothwell PM (2003). Incidence, risk factors and prognosis of stroke and transient ischaemic attack: The need for high-quality large-scale epidemiological studies. *Cerebrovascular Diseases* **16**(Suppl 3):2–10

Rothwell PM, Warlow CP (2005). Timing of TIAs preceding stroke: Time window for prevention is very short. *Neurology* **64**:817–820

Rothwell PM, Giles MF, Flossmann E *et al.* (2005). A simple score (ABCD) to identify individuals at high early risk of stroke after transient ischaemic attack. *Lancet* **366**:29–36

Rothwell PM, Giles MF, Chandratheva A on behalf of the Early use of Existing Preventive Strategies for Stroke (EXPRESS) Study (2007). Major reduction in risk of early recurrent stroke by urgent treatment of TIA and minor stroke: EXPRESS Study. *Lancet* **370**:1432–1442

Sciolla R, Melis F for the SINPAC Group (2008). Rapid identification of high-risk transient ischemic attacks: Prospective validation of the ABCD score. *Stroke* **39**:297–302

Sivenius J, Riekkinen PJ, Smets P *et al.* (1991). The European Stroke Prevention Study (ESPS): Results by arterial distribution. *Annals of Neurology* **29**:596–600

Song B, Fang H, Zhao L *et al.* (2013). Validation of the ABCD^3-I score to predict stroke risk after transient ischemic attack. *Stroke* **44**:1244–1248

Sylaja PN, Coutts SB, Subramaniam S for the VISION Study Group (2007). Acute ischemic lesions of varying ages predict risk of ischemic events in stroke/TIA patients. *Neurology* **68**:415–419

Tong DC, Caplan LR (2007). Determining future stroke risk using MRI: New data, new questions. *Neurology* **68**:398–399

Tsivgoulis G, Spengos K, Manta P *et al.* (2006). Validation of the ABCD score in identifying individuals at high early risk of stroke after a transient ischemic attack: A hospital-based case series study. *Stroke* **37**:2892–2897

Valton L, Larrue V, le Traon AP (1998). Microembolic signals and risk of early recurrence in patients with stroke or transient ischemic attack. *Stroke* **29**:2125–2128

van Swieten JC, Kappelle LJ, Algra A *et al.* (1992). Hypodensity of cerebral white matter in patients with transient ischaemic attack or minor stroke: Influence on the rate of

subsequent stroke: Dutch TIA Study Group. *Annals of Neurology* **32**:177–183

Warlow CP, Dennis MS, van Gijn J *et al.* (2001). Preventing recurrent stroke and other serious vascular events. In *Stroke: A Practical Guide to Management*, pp. 653–722. Oxford: Blackwell

Whitehead MA, McManus J, McAlpine C, Langhorne P (2005). Early recurrence of cerebrovascular events after transient ischaemic attack. *Stroke* **36**:1

Wu CM, McLaughlin K, Lorenzetti DL *et al.* (2007). Early risk of stroke after transient ischemic attack: A systematic review and meta-analysis. *Archives of Internal Medicine* **167**:2417–2422

Chapter 16

Short-Term Prognosis after Major Stroke

The short-term prognosis after major stroke depends on stroke subtype (Table 16.1), the occurrence of stroke-associated complications, stroke extension, or recurrence. While stroke subtype is fixed, optimal acute stroke treatment can affect stroke morbidity and mortality through minimizing the likelihood of neurological deterioration and the occurrence of complications such as pulmonary embolus and pneumonia (Chapter 20) as well as through the administration of specific therapies (Chapter 21).

Mortality

The prognosis of hospitalized patients tends to be worse than that of patients in the population at large because those with mild strokes are more likely to be cared for as

Table 16.1 Outcomes at 30 days, 6 months, and 1 year by ischemic stroke subtype

	Outcome (No. [%])				
	LACI	TACI	PACI	POCI	All
30 Days					
Dead	3 (2)	36 (39)	8 (4)	9 (7)	56 (10)
Dep	49 (36)	52 (56)	73 (39)	40 (31)	214 (39)
Indep	85 (62)	4 (4)	104 (56)	80 (62)	273 (50)
6 Months					
Dead	10 (7)	52 (56)	19 (10)	18 (14)	99 (18)
Dep	36 (26)	36 (39)	64 (34)	23 (18)	159 (29)
Indep	91 (66)	4 (4)	102 (55)	88 (68)	285 (52)
1 Year					
Dead	15 (11)	55 (60)	30 (16)	24 (19)	124 (23)
Dep	39 (28)	33 (36)	52 (29)	26 (19)	150 (28)
Indep	83 (60)	4 (4)	103 (55)	79 (62)	269 (49)

Notes: LACI, lacunar infarct; TACI, total anterior circulation infarct; PACI, partial anterior circulation infarct; POCI, posterior circulation infarct; Dep, functionally dependent (Rankin 3–5); Indep, functionally independent (Rankin 0–2).
Source: From Bamford et al. (1991).

outpatients. In the community, about 20% of all patients with first-ever stroke are dead within a month. Deaths in the first few days are almost all caused by the brain lesion itself. Deaths after the first week are more likely to be indirect consequences of the brain lesion, such as bronchopneumonia, pulmonary embolism, coincidental cardiac disease, or recurrence.

The prognosis is much better for ischemic stroke overall than for intracranial hemorrhage, with approximately 10% and 50% dying, respectively (Bamford *et al.* 1990; Lovelock *et al.* 2007). Early characteristics predicting death in patients with primary intracerebral hemorrhage are:

- level of consciousness assessed by the Glasgow Coma Scale.
- age.
- volume of hematoma.
- intraventricular extension of hemorrhage.

So far predictive models are not sufficiently accurate to inform treatment decisions in routine clinical practice. The various subtypes of ischemic stroke have very different outcomes: patients with total anterior circulation infarction (TACI) have just as poor an outcome as those with primary intracerebral hemorrhage (Table 16.1). The best single predictor of early death is impaired consciousness, but many other predictors of survival have been identified (Table 16.2). Many of these variables are interrelated, but prognostic models based on independent variables do not provide much more information than an experienced clinician's estimate (Counsell and Dennis 2001; Counsell *et al.* 2002).

Table 16.2 Factors predictive of early death after major stroke

	Factors
Demographic factors	Increasing age Male sex
Previous medical/social history	Myocardial infarction Cardiac failure TIA or stroke Diabetes Atrial fibrillation Pre-stroke handicap
Clinical features at presentation	Reduced level of consciousness Fever High or low blood pressure Severe motor deficit
Investigation results	High plasma glucose High white blood cell count Visible infarction on brain imaging Large stroke lesion on brain imaging (hematoma or infarction) Intraventricular blood

Table 16.3 Neurological causes of deterioration after stroke

	Ischemic stroke	Primary intracerebral hemorrhage
Hemorrhagic transformation	+	−
Cerebral edema	+	(+)
Brain shift (mass effect)	+	+
"Vasospasm"	−	−
Thrombus propagation	+	−
Recurrent embolism	+	−
Hemorrhage growth/recurrence	−	+
Hydrocephalus	(+)	+
Epileptic seizures	+	+

Although stroke onset is usually abrupt, the neurological deficit often worsens over the following minutes, hours, and sometimes days. Deterioration may be caused by neurological factors (Table 16.3) or systemic factors (Table 16.4) (Karepov *et al.* 2006), but progressive non-stroke pathologies should also be reconsidered.

Disability and Dependency

Nearly all patients who do not die as a result of their stroke recover to some extent. The mechanisms of recovery are discussed further in Chapter 23. Table 16.1 shows the numbers of patients with ischemic stroke who are functionally dependent at 30 days, 6 months, and 1 year by subtype of ischemic stroke. The prognosis is poorest for those with TACI, with high rates of dependency, and best for those with a posterior circulation infarct. Patients with a lacunar infarct have lower rates of dependency than those with TACI, but within this group there is wide variation in outcome, with some patients remaining severely disabled. Rates of dependency are high overall for hemorrhagic stroke, but some of these patients do well. At present, it is difficult to predict outcome in an individual patient, and models using clinical criteria appear as good (or bad) as any other methods including brain imaging (Chapter 23).

Early Deterioration after Ischemic Stroke: Neurological Factors

Very early worsening after stroke is more likely to be caused by neurological factors than systemic ones. The mechanism of worsening may not be clear in an individual patient and is likely to be the result of complex interactions between hemodynamic and other physiological factors. High or low blood pressure, diabetes, coronary heart disease, early CT signs of infarction, and middle cerebral artery occlusion have all been associated with increased risk of early deterioration after stroke.

Table 16.4 Systemic causes of neurological deterioration after stroke

Factor	Sequelae
Hypoxia	Pneumonia Pulmonary embolism Cardiac failure Chronic respiratory disease
Hypotension	Pulmonary embolism Cardiac failure Cardiac arrhythmia Pneumonia Dehydration Septicemia Hypotensive drugs/vasodilators Bleeding peptic ulcer
Infection and fever	Pneumonia Urinary tract infection Septicemia
Others	Water and electrolyte imbalance Hypo/hyperglycemia Depression Sedative/hypnotic drugs Anticonvulsant drugs

Hemorrhage into Cerebral Infarcts or Hemorrhagic Transformation

At autopsy, spontaneous petechial hemorrhages are very common in infarcts. During life they are seen on brain CT in about 15% of patients in the absence of thrombolytic therapy (Fig. 16.1). However, incidence rates must be considered in the context of the timing and mode of imaging, the definition of clinically significant hemorrhagic transformation, and the fact that there is interobserver variability in identifying hemorrhage (Khatri *et al.* 2007). Hemorrhagic transformation is said to be more common in cardioembolic infarcts, particularly when associated with infective endocarditis (Alexandrov *et al.* 1997), perhaps because the infarcts are often large and patients are frequently receiving anticoagulation therapy (Chapter 6). Hemorrhagic transformation is not often symptomatic unless there is confluent hematoma (Larrue *et al.* 1997; Berger *et al.* 2001).

Hemorrhagic transformation is of particular interest in acute stroke therapy since thrombolysis is associated with increased risk (Whiteley *et al.* 2016). Other factors associated with an increased risk of hemorrhagic transformation include old age; uncontrolled blood pressure; fever; hyperglycemia; severe or large territorial strokes; low serum cholesterol concentration (especially low density lipoprotein cholesterol); use of aspirin or anticoagulants at presentation; presence of edema, mass effect, or severe leucoaraiosis on neuroimaging; intra-arterial use of thrombolytic treatment (especially in those with a high number of microcatheter injections, high dose of heparin used, and post-procedure evidence of contrast extravasation on CT); and late (> 6 hours) spontaneous recanalization after thrombolytic treatment (Álvarez-Sabín *et al.* 2013).

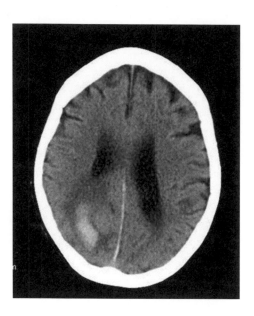

Fig. 16.1 A CT brain scan of a patient with stroke taken on day 3 after onset, illustrating the difficulty of distinguishing between primary intracerebral hemorrhage and hemorrhagic transformation of an infarct.

Abnormal permeability of the blood–brain barrier and microvascular damage leading to loss of vessel wall integrity are thought to be the cause of hemorrhage into an infarct. The mechanisms for this include plasmin-generated laminin degradation, activation of proteolytic enzymes (e.g., matrix metalloproteinase), and transmigration of leukocytes through the vessel wall (Álvarez-Sabín *et al.* 2013). It has been suggested that use of tissue plasminogen activator may increase the risk of hemorrhagic transformation not just by reperfusion but also through a direct effect on the molecular processes, such as promoting metalloproteinase release and neutrophil degranulation, leading to vessel damage (Cuadrado *et al.* 2008).

Peri-Infarct Edema

Peri-infarct edema reduces local cerebral blood flow and causes brain shift and herniation, the last being the most common "neurological" cause of death. This complication is a common explanation for worsening over the first few days and can often be detected by CT scan. Intravenous mannitol may reduce the deficit for a while but is unlikely to have a major impact on outcome. Early surgical decompression with decompressive hemicraniectomy for malignant middle cerebral artery territory infarction significantly reduces 12-month severe disability and mortality but is associated with a nonsignificantly higher major disability among survivors compared with conservative treatment (Frank *et al.* 2014; Yang *et al.* 2015) (Chapter 21).

Propagating Thrombosis

Propagating thrombosis proximal or distal to a thrombotic, embolic, or any other type of occlusion or within collateral vessels is often assumed to explain neurological deterioration if other causes have been excluded. However, direct evidence is almost impossible to obtain, except perhaps with transcranial Doppler ultrasound.

Recurrent Embolization

In theory, recurrent embolization may cause deterioration. However, the distinction between propagating thrombosis and embolization is very difficult. There is only anecdotal evidence that full anticoagulation with intravenous heparin slows progression and improves outcome if no other cause of deterioration is evident (Slivka *et al.* 1989).

Epileptic Seizures

Partial or generalized epileptic seizures occur for the first time in about 2% of those with acute strokes at around the time of onset, rising to approximately 10% at 5 years, more with large cortical infarcts or intracranial hemorrhage (Chapter 9) (Pitkänen *et al.* 2016). Seizures are more common with large strokes, especially if hemorrhagic, and with cortical as opposed to lacunar strokes. Cerebrovascular disease is the most common cause of epilepsy in the elderly, and late-onset epilepsy is a predictor of subsequent stroke (Cleary *et al.* 2004; Pitkänen *et al.* 2016). Seizures may cause neurological deterioration or be mistaken for recurrent stroke. Intractable recurrent seizures are distinctly unusual.

Early Deterioration after Ischemic Stroke: Systemic Factors

Systemic factors commonly causing deterioration after stroke are shown in Table 16.4 (Chapter 20). Systemic illness usually becomes important from 2 days or so after stroke onset. A history and careful general examination should reveal features such as confusion, shortness of breath, cough, hypoxia, or leg swelling. Simple investigations including full blood count, inflammatory markers, renal function, blood cultures, urine examination, and chest X-ray will usually be required to confirm a coexistent medical disorder. Close monitoring of patients with stroke, ideally on a stroke unit, should aim to enable rapid diagnosis of coexistent medical conditions so that treatment can be instituted (Chapter 20) and deterioration prevented.

It is important to note that systemic illness will make a given neurological syndrome worse: a patient with a lacunar infarction may become drowsy and confused such that the clinical features are more consistent with a TACI. This may result in a falsely pessimistic prognosis being given to the patient and family.

References

Alexandrov AV, Black SE, Ehrlich LE *et al.* (1997). Predictors of hemorrhagic transformation occurring spontaneously and on anticoagulants in patients with acute ischemic stroke. *Stroke* 28:1198–1202

Álvarez-Sabín J, Maisterra O, Santamarina E *et al.* (2013). Factors influencing hemorrhagic transformation in ischemic stroke. *Lancet Neurology* 12:689–705

Bamford J, Sandercock PAG, Dennis M *et al.* (1990). A prospective study of acute cerebrovascular disease in the community: The Oxfordshire Community Stroke Project 1981–86. 2. Incidence, case fatality rates and overall outcome at one year of cerebral infarction, primary intracerebral and subarachnoid haemorrhage. *Journal of Neurology, Neurosurgery and Psychiatry* 53:16–22

Bamford J, Sandercock P, Dennis M *et al.* (1991). Classification and natural history of clinically identifiable subtypes of cerebral infarction. *Lancet* 337:1521–1526.

Berger C, Fiorelli M, Steiner T *et al.* (2001). Hemorrhagic transformation of ischemic brain tissue: Asymptomatic or symptomatic? *Stroke* 32:1330–1335

Cleary P, Shorvon S, Tallis R (2004). Late-onset seizures as a predictor of subsequent stroke. *Lancet* 363:1184–1186

Counsell, Dennis M (2001). Systematic review of prognostic models in patients with acute stroke. *Cerebrovascular Diseases* **12**:159–170

Counsell C, Dennis M, McDowall M *et al.* (2002). Predicting outcome after acute and subacute stroke: Development and validation of new prognostic models. *Stroke* **33**:1041–1047

Cuadrado E, Ortega L, Hernández-Guillamon M *et al.* (2008). Tissue plasminogen activator (t-PA) promotes neutrophil degranulation and MMP-9 release. *Journal of Leukocyte Biology* **84**:207–214

Frank JI, Schumm LP, Wroblewski K *et al.* (2014). Hemicraniectomy and durotomy upon deterioration from infarction-related swelling trial: Randomized pilot clinical trial. *Stroke* **45**:781–787

Karepov VG, Gur AY, Bova I *et al.* (2006). Stroke-in-evolution: Infarct-inherent mechanisms versus systemic causes. *Cerebrovascular Diseases* **21**:42–46

Khatri P, Wechsler LR, Broderick JP (2007). Intracranial hemorrhage associated with revascularization therapies. *Stroke* **38**:431–440

Larrue V, von Kummer R, del Zoppo G *et al.* (1997). Haemorrhagic transformation in acute ischemic stroke. Potential contributing factors in the European Cooperative Acute Stroke Study. *Stroke* **28**:957–960

Lovelock CE, Molyneux AJ, Rothwell PM *et al.* (2007). Change in incidence and aetiology of intracerebral haemorrhage in Oxfordshire, UK, between 1981 and 2006: A population-based study. *Lancet Neurology* **6**:487–493

Pitkänen A, Roivainen R and Lukasiuk K (2016). Development of epilepsy after ischemic stroke. *Lancet Neurology* **15**:185–197

Slivka A, Levy D, Lapinski RH (1989). Risk associated with heparin withdrawal in ischaemic cerebrovascular disease. *Journal of Neurology, Neurosurgery and Psychiatry* **52**:1332–1336

Whiteley WN, Emberson J, Lees KR *et al.* (2016). Risk of intracerebral hemorrhage with alteplase after acute ischemic stroke: A secondary analysis of an individual patient data meta-analysis. *Lancet Neurology* **15**:925–933

Yang MH, Lin HY, Fu J et al. (2015). Decompressive hemicraniectomy in patients with malignant middle cerebral artery infarct: A systematic review and meta-analysis. *Surgeon* **13**:230–230

Long-Term Prognosis after Transient Ischemic Attack and Stroke

In the same way that data on the short-term risk of stroke following TIA are essential for informing the early management of patients, data on the medium-term (1 to 5 years) and long-term (5 years and beyond) prognosis are required to counsel patients and direct secondary prevention.

Medium- and Long-Term Stroke Risks after a Transient Ischemic Attack

Many studies have addressed the question of medium-term prognosis after TIA, but because the condition is heterogeneous and patients have been recruited in a number of different clinical settings, the findings have been difficult to interpret. For example, in 1991, a paper critically reviewed all studies after 1950 of the prognosis after TIA that included more than 50 patients and were published in English (Kernan *et al.* 1991). Eligible studies were tested against six key quality methodological principles:

- specified diagnostic criteria and procedures.
- "inception cohort" by inclusion of all patients at a specified time after the event (ideally as soon as possible after TIA).
- appropriate endpoints.
- adequate description of endpoint surveillance.
- adequate reporting and analysis of censored patients.
- multivariate analysis of predictive variables.

A total of 60 eligible papers were identified: 22 were observational studies of patients receiving specific treatment; 32 were observational studies, not based on specific treatments; six were randomized controlled trials. No studies adhered to all six methodological principles. When the principles were "relaxed" to include only an inception cohort with adequate reporting and analysis of censored patients and appropriate endpoints, only two reports met these criteria, both from the Oxfordshire Community Stroke Project (OCSP: 184 patients, follow-up over 3.7 years) (Dennis *et al.* 1989, 1990).

Since the publication of this review, two further high-quality, prospective, population-based studies of the medium-term prognosis of TIA have been published, one from Söderhamn, Sweden (97 patients, follow-up over 3 years) (Terent 1990), and the other from Perugia, Italy (94 patients, follow-up over 9 years) (Ricci *et al.* 1998). The mean age of patients in all three cohorts was 69 years.

In the Söderhamn cohort, the risk of stroke was approximately 5% per year, and the overall mortality was 24.7% over a mean of 3 years (Terent 1990). No data were reported on cardiovascular morbidity or mortality. In the Perugia cohort, the annual risk of stroke after

TIA was 2.4% (95% confidence interval [CI] 0.7–4.7) (Ricci *et al.* 1998). The actuarial risk of death was 28.6% (95% CI, 19.2–37.8) at 5 years and 49.5% (95% CI, 38.9–60.0) at 10 years, with roughly equal numbers of cerebrovascular, cardiovascular, and non-vascular deaths. In OCSP, the annual stroke risk was 4.4% (95% CI, 5.0–7.3) although this was "front-loaded" – being highest in the first year after initial TIA (Dennis *et al.* 1990). The risk of death at 5 years was 31.3% (95% CI, 23.3–39.3), and the annual risk of death was 6.3% (95% CI, 4.7–7.9). Again, there were roughly equal numbers of cerebrovascular, cardiovascular, and non-vascular deaths. The risk of either fatal or nonfatal myocardial infarction was 12.1% (95% CI, 5.8–18.4) at 5 years, and the approximate annual risk was 2.4%.

There are similarly few high-quality prospective hospital-based cohort studies of the medium-term prognosis of TIA (Hankey 2003). Of the four main studies that recruited patients with TIA from hospital as opposed to population-based recruitment, the mean age tended to be younger owing to referral bias, with elderly patients being less likely to be referred to secondary care services (Heyman *et al.* 1984; Hankey *et al.* 1991; Carolei *et al.* 1992; Howard *et al.* 1994). However, in these studies, the annual rate of stroke was 2.2–5.0% over 4–5 years, which is similar to the risk of myocardial infarction (1.1–4.6%) over the same period. Of note in these studies is the high early risk of stroke measured when patients are recruited very early after the event, which falls after a year or so, in contrast to a steady background risk of acute coronary disease (Hankey *et al.* 1991). It has been argued that the early risk of stroke reflects an active, unstable plaque, which heals with time, while the risk of coronary disease reflects the underlying "atherosclerotic burden" (Hankey 2003).

These studies indicate that the risk of stroke and other vascular events is appreciable in the medium term, but a question that has recently been addressed is the vascular risk in the longer term and whether there is a need for ongoing aggressive secondary prevention. Only two studies provide reliable data on prognosis up to 15 years after a TIA.

The first study examined the long-term vascular risk starting some time after the initial TIA (Clark *et al.* 2003). The study was composed of 290 patients with TIA, diagnosed by a neurologist, who had participated either in OCSP (Dennis *et al.* 1990) or a contemporaneous hospital-referred cohort study (Hankey *et al.* 1991). Patients were followed over a 10-year period starting in 1988, a median time of 3.8 years (interquartile range, 2.2–5.8) after their most recent TIA. Mean age at baseline was 69 years. At the end of the 10-year follow-up, the risk of stroke was 18.8% (95% CI, 13.6–23.7); the risk of myocardial infarction or death from coronary heart disease was 27.8% (95% CI, 21.8–33.3), and risk of death from any cause was 50.7% (95% CI not given) (Fig. 17.1). The risk of any first stroke, myocardial infarction, or vascular death was 42.8% (95% CI, 36.4–48.5). Compared with the rates in the general population standardized for age and sex, only the rate of fatal coronary events was significantly higher than expected (standardized mortality ratio 1.47; 95% CI, 1.10–1.93; $p = 0.009$). The risk of major vascular events was found to be constant throughout the follow-up.

The Life Long After Cerebral Ischemia (LILAC) study reported near complete follow-up on 2,473 participants from the Dutch TIA Trial (van Wijk *et al.* 2005). Mean age was 65 years, and 759 had a TIA while the remainder suffered a minor stroke (defined as a score on the modified Rankin scale ≤ 3) at enrollment. The trial recruited patients between 1986 and 1989, all of whom were assessed by a neurologist and randomized to two different dosages of aspirin. After a mean follow-up of 10.1 years, 1,489 (60%) had died and 1,336 (54%) had suffered at least one vascular event. At 10 years, the cumulative risk of recurrent stroke was 18.4% (95% CI, 16.7–20.1), of first major vascular event was 44.1% (95% CI,

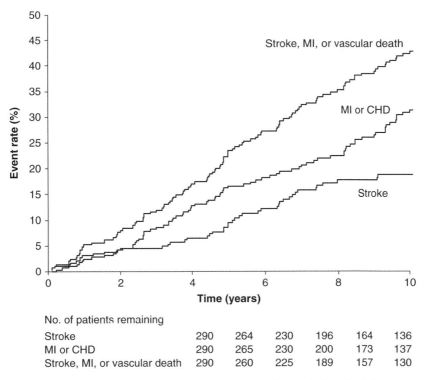

Fig. 17.1 Kaplan–Meier event rates for any stroke; any myocardial infarction (MI) or death from coronary heart disease (CHD); and any stroke, MI, or vascular death in a cohort of 290 patients with transient ischemic attack (Clark *et al.* 2003).

42.0–46.1), and of death was 46.6% (95% CI, 44.2–51.3). The corresponding figures for those presenting with TIA at inception (as opposed to minor stroke) were 35.8% (95% CI, 32.3–39.3) for first vascular event and 34.1% (95% CI, 30.7–37.4) for death. The 10-year risk of stroke for patients with TIA was not reported. Importantly, because of the inclusion criteria of the original trial, only 22% of patients were randomized within a week of the initial vascular event (median time to randomization was 18 days), so much of the very high acute risk described above was missed from these estimates.

These studies both reveal a high vascular risk compared with the "normal population", with this risk continuing up to 10 or 15 years and probably beyond following TIA. They, therefore, support the ongoing use of secondary preventive medication.

Medium- and Long-Term Stroke Risks after Stroke

The risks of stroke, other acute vascular events, and death after stroke have been studied in six population-based cohorts over a follow-up period of 5 or more years (Scmidt *et al.* 1988; Burn *et al.* 1994; Hankey *et al.* 2000; Petty *et al.* 2000; Brønnum-Hansen *et al.* 2001; Hartmann *et al.* 2001). Two of these studies included ischemic stroke only (Petty *et al.* 2000; Hartmann *et al.* 2001), and the remaining four included both ischemic and hemorrhagic stroke. One study included incident and recurrent events (Brønnum-Hansen *et al.* 2001), and the remaining five included incident stroke only. The risks of death at 5 years varied between 41% and 72%, while the proportion of deaths caused by acute coronary disease and stroke (either inception event or recurrent stroke) were similar. As in the TIA outcome studies, the risk of stroke tended to be highest early after the event and then fell, whereas the risk of coronary events was constant over the follow-up period (Hankey 2003).

Risks of Myocardial Infarction and Vascular Death after Transient Ischemic Attack and Stroke

In a systematic review and meta-analysis of studies of the risk of myocardial infarction and vascular death after TIA and ischemic stroke (Touzé et al. 2005), cohort studies including more than 100 patients with TIA or ischemic stroke and reporting risks of myocardial infarction or non-stroke vascular death over at least 1 year of follow-up published between 1980 and 2005 were identified. The analysis included 39 studies reporting outcomes in 65,996 patients. The ranges of annual risks reported in individual studies were 0.4–3.8% for non-stroke vascular death, 0.5–4.7% for total myocardial infarction, 0.4–3.2% for nonfatal myocardial infarction, and 0.2–3.7% for fatal myocardial infarction. The annual risks obtained through meta-regression were 2.1% (95% CI, 1.9–2.4) for non-stroke vascular death (29 studies), 2.2% (95% CI, 1.7–2.7) for total myocardial infarction (22 studies), 0.9% (95% CI, 0.7–1.2) for nonfatal myocardial infarction (16 studies), and 1.1% (95% CI, 0.8–1.5) for fatal myocardial infarction (19 studies) (Touzé et al. 2005) (Fig. 17.2).

The risk of non-stroke vascular death was lower in studies that enrolled patients after 1990 than in those that enrolled patients before 1990. However, there was no significant heterogeneity in the risk of nonfatal, fatal, and total myocardial infarction or non-stroke vascular death according to the other baseline study characteristics, including population-based studies versus randomized controlled trials and mean age of the cohort under 65 years versus more than 65 years. Perhaps surprisingly, the risks of myocardial infarction and non-stroke vascular death were similar in studies of patients with TIA or stroke caused specifically by atherosclerosis as in other studies. However, although several observations would support an association between stroke related to atherosclerosis and coronary artery disease, particularly the positive correlation between carotid, vertebral, and coronary vascular disease (Mathur et al. 1963; Solberg et al. 1968) and the correlation between asymptomatic carotid disease and coronary artery disease (Joakimsen et al. 2000), individual patient data were lacking to study this association in full.

Risk Prediction in the Medium and Long Term

Several published models have addressed risk prediction in the medium and long term following TIA, but many have methodological flaws (Hankey and Warlow 1994). Three models that have been proposed for use in the targeting of longer-term secondary prevention for patients after initial TIA are reviewed in this section (Table 17.1).

The first was derived from a cohort of 451 patients consecutively admitted to a hospital in North Carolina, USA, between 1977 and 1983 and predicts survival at 1 and 5 years (Howard et al. 1987). Using regression modeling to identify independent risk factors, age over 60 years, carotid territory TIA, cigarette smoking, previous contralateral stroke, ischemic heart disease, and diabetes mellitus were found to predict an increased risk of death. On internal validation, patients under 60 years of age with none of the listed risk

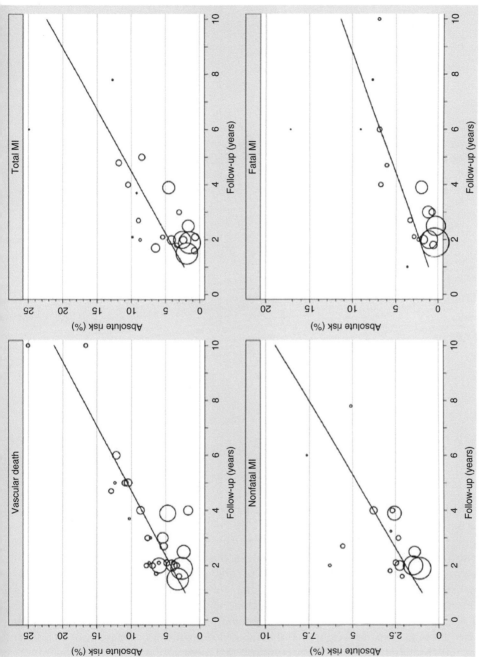

Fig. 17.2 Absolute risk of nonfatal myocardial infarction (MI), fatal MI, all MI, and any vascular death plotted against mean follow-up with fitted regression lines obtained through weighted meta-regressions from a systematic review of 39 studies reporting relevant risks in patients with transient ischemic attack and ischemic stroke. Each circle represents a study, and its size is inversely proportional to the within-trial variance (Touzé *et al.* 2005).

Table 17.1 Comparison of variables used in different prognostic models for medium- to long-term outcome after transient ischemic attack and stroke in the Hankey, Kernan (SPI-II), and Howard models

Risk factor	Model (outcome of interest)		
	Hankey (stroke)	Kernan (stroke or death)	Howard (death)
Demographic			
Increasing age	+	+	+
Previous medical history			
Cerebrovascular disease	+ (multiple TIAs)	+ (stroke)	+ (stroke)
Ischemic heart disease	–	+	+
Congestive cardiac failure	–	+	–
Left ventricular failure	+	–	–
Peripheral vascular disease	+	–	–
Diabetes	–	+	+
Hypertension	–	+	–
Smoking	–	–	+
Event			
Territory	TIA of brain (versus eye)	–	Anterior versus posterior
		–	

Note: TIA, transient ischemic attack.
Sources: From Hankey et al. (1992), Kernan et al. (2000), and Howard et al. (1987).

factors had a 5-year survival of over 95%, while patients over 60 years of age with all of these risk factors had a 5-year survival of less than 25%.

Hankey and colleagues (1992) studied 469 patients referred to a hospital in Oxfordshire, UK, with TIA between 1976 and 1986 and used regression modeling to identify independent risk factors for stroke, coronary events, and the combination of stroke, myocardial infarction, or vascular death at 1 and 5 years. Risk factors for stroke were an increasing number of TIAs in the 3 months before presentation, increasing age, peripheral vascular disease, left ventricular hypertrophy, and TIAs of the brain (compared with the eye). The contribution of each of these factors was weighted and combined in mathematical equations to predict relative and absolute risks for each endpoint at 1 and 5 years.

The Stroke Prognosis Instrument II (SPI-II) is a simple score for predicting risk of stroke or death within 2 years after TIA or non-disabling stroke (Kernan et al. 2000). It was derived in 525 patients participating in the Women's Estrogen for Stroke Trial (WEST) and validated in three other cohorts. Multivariate analysis was used to identify independent risk factors for stroke and death, and these were then combined into a risk score: congestive heart failure (3 points), diabetes (3 points), prior stroke (3 points), age > 70 years (2 points), stroke for the index event (as opposed to TIA) (2 points), hypertension (1 point), and coronary artery disease (1 point). Risk groups I, II, and III contained patients with 0–3, 4–7, and 8–15 points, respectively. On testing in pooled data from the validation cohorts, rates of stroke or death at 2 years were 10%, 19%, and 31%, respectively, for each of the different risk groups. In receiver operator characteristic analysis, the area under the curve was 0.63 (95% CI, 0.62–0.65).

From these studies, it appears that the medium- and long-term prognosis after TIA is more dependent on underlying vascular risk factors than characteristics of the event itself, in contrast to the prognosis in the short term. This observation is supported by independent predictors of vascular risk and modeling as reported in the LILAC study, in which models of increasing complexity were devised to predict longer-term risk (van Wijk *et al.* 2005) (Table 17.2). It is noteworthy that the predictive power of each model, as measured by the area and the curve for the receiver operator characteristic, is only minimally improved compared with model 1 (based on established demographics and vascular risk factors) first by the inclusion of clinical characteristics in model 2 and second by the inclusion of CT and electrocardiology findings in model 3.

Table 17.2 Independent predictors of long-term vascular event risk in 2,362 individuals with transient ischemic attack[a] or minor stroke

Risk factor	Hazard ratio (95% CI)		
	Model 1	Model 2	Model 3
Demographic characteristics			
Male	1·42 (1·26–1·60)	1·40 (1·25–1·58)	1·38 (1·22–1·56)
Age[b]	1·06 (1·05–1·06)	1·06 (1·05–1·06)	1·05 (1·05–1·06)
History			
Myocardial infarction	1·13 (1·05–1·22)	1·14 (1·06–1·23)	1·11 (1·02–1·21)
Intermittent claudication	1·68 (1·34–2·10)	1·73 (1·38–2·16)	1·77 (1·42–2·19)
Diabetes	2·19 (1·84–2·61)	2·11 (1·77–2·51)	2·05 (1·72–2·44)
Hypertension	1·12 (1·05–1·20)	1·11 (1·04–1·19)	1·09 (1·02–1·17)
Peripheral vascular surgery	1·39 (0·96–2·01)	1·39 (0·96–2·02)	–
Event characteristics			
Minor stroke versus TIA	–	1·22 (1·07–1·40)	1·14 (0·99–1·30)
Vertigo	–	0·75 (0·62–0·90)	0·77 (0·64–0·93)
Amaurosis fugax	–	0·71 (0·49–1·02)	–
Dysarthria	–	1·10 (0·97–1·25)	1·13 (1·00–1·28)
CT brain scan			
White matter lesions	–	–	1·42 (1·22–1·66)
Any infarct	–	–	1·28 (1·14–1·44)

Table 17.2 (cont.)

Risk factor	Hazard ratio (95% CI)		
	Model 1	Model 2	Model 3
12-lead ECG			
Q wave on ECG	–	–	1·38 (1·20–1·60)
Negative T wave	–	–	1·19 (1·00–1·42)
ST depression	–	–	1·15 (0·96–1·39)
AUC-ROC	0·70 (0·68–0·72)	0·70 (0·68–0·72)	0·72 (0·70–0·74)

Notes: CI, confidence interval; TIA, transient ischemic attack; CT, computed tomography; ECG, electrocardiography; AUC-ROC, area under the curve of the received operator characteristic.
[a] Model 1 includes baseline risk factor and demographic data; model 2 incorporates event characteristics; and model 3 adds investigation results. Note that the simplest model has very similar discriminatory power, as measured by the AUC-ROC, as the more complex models.
[b] Age was entered as a continuous variable; the increase in hazard is for every incremental year.
Source: From van Wijk et al. (2005).

Although intracerebral hemorrhage is rare, it is a potentially devastating condition. Patients with TIA are unlikely to be at much higher short-term risk of intracranial hemorrhage than age- and sex-matched controls, unlike patients with ischemic stroke, in whom hemorrhagic transformation of an ischemic lesion is more likely. Analysis of data from 12,648 individuals with TIA or minor stroke from the Cerebrovascular Cohort Studies Collaboration showed that the incidence of intracranial hemorrhage was 1% over a 5-year follow-up after the event (Ariesen et al. 2006). Independent risk factors for intracranial hemorrhage were age (> 60 years; hazard ratio [HR], 2.07), blood glucose level (> 7 mmol/L; HR, 1.33), systolic blood pressure (> 140 mmHg; HR, 2.17), and use of antihypertensive drugs (HR, 1.53). In addition, the Stroke Prevention in Reversible Ischemia Trial (SPIRIT) identified the presence of leukoaraiosis as a risk factor for intracranial hemorrhage in patients receiving anticoagulation (Stroke Prevention in Reversible Ischemia Trial [SPIRIT] Study Group 1997).

Risk Prediction in Specific Circumstances

Risk prediction in specific conditions following stroke or TIA using modeling is helpful in targeting secondary preventive treatments that might themselves be associated with benefit and harm. Models can provide data on the risk for a specific patient, which can then more reliably inform the risk–benefit ratio for that individual and guide decision making about treatment. Risk models have been developed in symptomatic carotid disease (Chapter 27) and atrial fibrillation (Chapters 14 and 24), and these will be discussed later.

Symptomatic Carotid Stenosis

The risk models described previously were derived and validated in populations with a low prevalence of symptomatic carotid disease and, therefore, did not include the degree of carotid stenosis. Given the importance of carotid stenosis in determining the risk of stroke in patients with recently symptomatic carotid disease, models are required for use in this specific clinical situation. This is particularly important because the treatment for carotid stenosis, carotid endarterectomy, itself has important risks associated with it. Risk models have, therefore, been derived to predict the risks associated with medical and surgical treatment in patients with carotid stenosis in order to inform decision making surrounding treatment options.

Risk prediction in carotid stenosis is more fully discussed in Chapter 27.

Atrial Fibrillation

Atrial fibrillation is a well-recognized risk factor for TIA and stroke, and many studies have identified independent prognostic factors for stroke in all patients with non-rheumatic atrial fibrillation (NRAF), irrespective of previous cerebrovascular disease (Stroke Prevention in Atrial Fibrillation Investigators 1992a, b; Atrial Fibrillation Investigators 1994). The CHADS2 and CHA_2DS_2-VASc score has been derived and validated to predict the risk of stroke for patients with atrial fibrillation and includes previous cerebrovascular disease as one of the independent risk factors (Gage et al. 2001; Lip et al. 2010a; Friberg et al. 2012) (Chapters 2, 14, and 24).

However, there is only one report specifically on which patients with a previous TIA or stroke and NRAF are at high (and low) risk, based on 375 patients with NRAF and TIA or non-disabling stroke treated in the placebo arm of the European Atrial Fibrillation Trial (van Latum et al. 1995). Independent risk factors for vascular death, stroke, and other major vascular events included increasing age, previous thromboembolism, ischemic heart disease, enlarged cardiothoracic ratio on chest radiograph, systolic blood pressure > 160 mmHg at study entry, NRAF for more than 1 year, and presence of an ischemic lesion on CT scan. There are no corresponding studies of predictors of risk in patients with previous TIA or stroke and NRAF who are treated with anticoagulation. However, as mentioned earlier, the SPIRIT trial identified the presence of leukoaraiosis as a risk factor for intracranial hemorrhage in patients receiving anticoagulation (Stroke Prevention in Reversible Ischemia Trial [SPIRIT] Study Group 1997), while a recent systematic review of anticoagulation-related bleeding complications in patients with atrial fibrillation irrespective of previous cerebrovascular disease identified advanced age, uncontrolled hypertension, history of ischemic heart disease, cerebrovascular disease, anemia or bleeding, and the concomitant use of antiplatelet agents as independently predictive (Hughes and Lip 2007). History of stroke is therefore also incorporated into the HAS-BLED score (Chapter 24 Box 24.3), which aims to stratify the risk of bleeding in patients with atrial fibrillation in whom use of vitamin K oral anticoagulants is considered (Lip et al. 2010b; Pisters et al. 2010).

References

Ariesen MJ, Algra A, Warlow CP et al. (2006). Predictors of risk of intracerebral haemorrhage in patients with a history of TIA or minor ischaemic stroke. *Journal of Neurology, Neurosurgery and Psychiatry* 77:92–94

Atrial Fibrillation Investigators (1994). Risk factors for stroke and efficacy of anti-thrombotic therapy in atrial fibrillation: analysis of pooled data from five randomized controlled trials.

Archives of International Medicine 154:1449–1457

Brønnum-Hansen H, Davidsen M, Thorvaldsen P et al. (2001). Long-term survival and causes of death after stroke. *Stroke* 32:2131–2136

Burn J, Dennis M, Bamford J et al. (1994). Long-term risk of recurrent stroke after a first-ever stroke. The Oxfordshire Community Stroke Project. *Stroke* 25:333–337

Carolei A, Candelise L, Fiorelli M et al. (1992). Long-term prognosis of transient ischemic attacks and reversible ischemic neurologic deficits: A hospital-based study. *Cerebrovascular Diseases* 2:266–272

Clark TG, Murphy MFG, Rothwell PM (2003). Long term risks of stroke, myocardial infarction, and vascular death in "low risk" patients with a non-recent transient ischaemic attack. *Journal of Neurology, Neurosurgery and Psychiatry* 74:577–580

Dennis MS, Bamford JM, Sandercock PAG et al. (1989). Incidence of transient ischemic attacks in Oxfordshire, England. *Stroke* 20:333–339

Dennis MS, Bamford J, Sandercock P et al. (1990). Prognosis of transient ischemic attacks in the Oxfordshire Community Stroke Project. *Stroke* 21:848–853

Friberg L, Rosenqvist M, Lip GY (2012). Evaluation of risk stratification schemes for ischemic stroke and bleeding in 182678 patients with atrial fibrillation: the Swedish Atrial Fibrillation cohort study. *European Heart Journal* 33:1500–1510

Gage BF, Waterman AD, Shannon W et al. (2001). Validation of clinical classification schemes for predicting stroke: results from the National Registry of Atrial Fibrillation. *Journal of the American Medical Association* 285:2864–2870

Hankey GJ (2003). Long term outcome after ischaemic stroke/transient ischaemic attack. *Cerebrovascular Diseases* 16(Suppl 1):14–19

Hankey GJ, Warlow CP (1994). *Major Problems in Neurology, Vol. 27: Transient Ischaemic Attacks of the Brain and Eye.* London: Saunders

Hankey GJ, Slattery JM, Warlow CP (1991). The prognosis of hospital-referred transient ischaemic attacks. *Journal of Neurology, Neurosurgery and Psychiatry* 54:793–802

Hankey GJ, Slattery JM, Warlow CP (1992). Transient ischaemic attacks: which patients are at high (and low) risk of serious vascular events? *Journal of Neurology, Neurosurgery and Psychiatry* 55:640–652

Hankey GJ, Jamrozik K, Broadhurst RJ et al. (2000). Five-year survival after first-ever stroke and related prognostic factors in the Perth Community Stroke Study. *Stroke* 31:2080–2086

Hartmann A, Rundek T, Mast H et al. (2001). Mortality and causes of death after first ischemic stroke. *Neurology* 57:2000–2005

Heyman A, Wilkinson WE, Hurwitz BJ et al. (1984). Risk of ischemic heart disease in patients with TIA. *Neurology* 34:626–630

Howard G, Toole JF, Frye-Pierson J et al. (1987). Factors influencing the survival of 451 transient ischemic attack patients. *Stroke* 18:552–557

Howard G, Evans GW, Rouse JR III et al. (1994). A prospective re-evaluation of transient ischemic attacks as a risk factor for death and fatal or nonfatal cardiovascular events. *Stroke* 25:342–345

Hughes M, Lip GY (2007). Guideline Development Group for the NICE national clinical guideline for management of atrial fibrillation in primary and secondary care. Risk factors for anticoagulation-related bleeding complications in patients with atrial fibrillation: A systematic review. *Quarterly Journal of Medicine* 100:599–607

Joakimsen O, Bonaa KH, Mathiesen EB et al. (2000). Prediction of mortality by ultrasound screening of a general population for carotid stenosis: The Tromso Study. *Stroke* 31:1871–1876

Kernan WN, Feinstein AR, Brass LM (1991). A methodological appraisal of research on prognosis after transient ischemic attacks. *Stroke* 22:1108–1116

Kernan WN, Viscoli CM, Brass LM et al. (2000). The Stroke Prognosis Instrument II (SPI II): A clinical prediction instrument for patients with transient ischaemia and non-disabling ischaemic stroke. *Stroke* 31:456–462

Lip GY, Nieuwlaat R, Pisters R et al. (2010a). Refining clinical risk stratification for predicting stroke and thromboembolism in atrial fibrillation using a novel risk factor-based approach: The Euro Heart Survey on Atrial Fibrillation. *Chest* 137:263–272

Lip GY, Frison L, Halperin JL et al. (2010b). Comparative validation of a novel risk score for predicting bleeding risk in anticoagulated patients with atrial fibrillation: The HAS-BLED (Hypertension, Abnormal Renal/Liver

Function, Stroke, Bleeding History or Predisposition, Labile INR, Elderly, Drug/Alcohol Concomitantly) score. *Journal of American College of Cardiology* **57**:173–180

Mathur KS, Kashyap SK, Kumar V (1963). Correlation of the extent and severity of atherosclerosis in the coronary and cerebral arteries. *Circulation* **27**:929–934

Petty GW, Brown RD Jr., Whisnant JP *et al.* (2000). Ischemic stroke subtypes. A population-based study of functional outcome, survival and recurrence. *Stroke* **31**:1062–1068

Pisters R, Lane DA, Nieuwlaat R *et al.* (2010). A novel user-friendly score (HAS-BLED) to assess 1-year risk of major bleeding in patients with atrial fibrillation: The Euro Heart Survey. *Chest* **138**:1093–1100

Ricci S, Cantisani AT, Righetti E *et al.* (1998). Long term follow up of TIAs: The SEPIVAC Study. *Neuroepidemiology* **17**:54

Scmidt EV, Smirnov VE, Ryabova VS (1988). Results of the seven-year prospective study of stroke patients. *Stroke* **19**:942–949

Solberg LA, McGarry PA, Moossy J *et al.* (1968). Severity of atherosclerosis in cerebral arteries, coronary arteries, and aortas. *Annals of the New York Academy of Sciences* **149**:956–973

Stroke Prevention in Atrial Fibrillation Investigators (1992a). Predictors of thromboembolism in atrial fibrillation, I:

Clinical features of patients at risk. *Annals of Internal Medicine* **116**:1–5

Stroke Prevention in Atrial Fibrillation Investigators (1992b). Predictors of thromboembolism in atrial fibrillation, II: Echocardiographic features of patients at risk. *Annals of Internal Medicine* **116**:6–12

Stroke Prevention in Reversible Ischemia Trial (SPIRIT) Study Group (1997). A randomized trial of anticoagulants versus aspirin after cerebral ischemia of presumed arterial origin. *Annals of Neurology* **42**:857–865

Terent A (1990). Survival after stroke and transient ischemic attacks during the 1970s and 1980s. *Stroke* **21**:848–853

Touzé E, Varenne O, Chatellier G *et al.* (2005). Risk of myocardial infarction and vascular death after transient ischemic attack and ischemic stroke: a systematic review and meta-analysis. *Stroke* **36**:2748–2755

van Latum JC, Koudstaal P, Venables GS *et al.* (1995). Predictors of major vascular events in patients with a transient ischemic attack or minor ischemic stroke and with non-rheumatic atrial fibrillation. *Stroke* **26**:801–806

van Wijk I, Kappelle LJ, van Gijn J *et al.* (2005) For the LILAC study group. Long-term survival and vascular event risk after transient ischaemic attack or minor stroke: a cohort study. *Lancet* **365**:2098–2104

Chapter 18

Methods of Assessing Treatments

It is clearly important that treatments used in neurological disease are properly assessed before being introduced into routine clinical practice. There are many examples throughout medicine of interventions that were considered beneficial on the basis of theory or uncontrolled observational studies but were subsequently shown to be harmful in randomized controlled trials (Table 18.1).

The justification for randomized trials is not that no worthwhile observations can be made without them but that important biases can occur in non-randomized comparisons that are particularly problematic if the benefits of treatment are, in reality, small or absent. For example, a non-randomized comparison of the effect of aspirin dosage on the operative risk of carotid endarterectomy (Table 18.2) reported a clinically and statistically significant lower operative risk in patients on high-dose aspirin (1,300 mg) than taking low-dose aspirin (325 mg or less) (Barnett *et al.* 1998); however, a subsequent randomized trial (Taylor *et al.* 1999), performed to confirm this observation, showed that high-dose aspirin was, in fact, harmful (Table 18.1). It is likely that the non-randomized comparison had been biased by unmeasured differences between the patients in the low-dose and high-dose aspirin groups.

Randomized trials and systematic reviews of trials, therefore, provide the most reliable data on the effects of treatment. That is not to say, however, that non-randomized studies

Table 18.1 Examples of interventions that were thought initially to be beneficial (or harmful) a view changed by randomized controlled trials

	Examples
Considered beneficial, shown to be harmful	High-dose oxygen therapy in neonates Antiarrhythmic drugs after myocardial infarction Fluoride treatment for osteoporosis Bed rest in twin pregnancy Hormone replacement therapy in vascular prevention Extracranial to intracranial arterial bypass surgery in stroke prevention High-dose aspirin for carotid endarterectomy
Considered harmful, shown to be beneficial	Beta-blockers in heart failure Digoxin after myocardial infarction

Source: From Rothwell (2005a).

Table 18.2 The relationship between aspirin dose and the risk of stroke and death within 30 days of carotid endarterectomy in a non-randomized comparison within the North American Symptomatic Carotid Endarterectomy Trial (Barnett *et al.* 1998) and in a subsequent randomized controlled trial (Taylor *et al.* 1999)

	Operative risk of stroke and death with aspirin dosage (%)		Relative risk	*P*-value
	< 650 mg	> 650 mg		
Non-randomized study	7.1	3.9	1.8	< 0.001
Randomized trial	3.7	8.2	0.45	0.002

cannot sometimes provide reliable evidence on the benefits of intervention. Few people would doubt the validity of the observational data on the benefits of antibiotic treatment in bacterial meningitis or the benefits of treatment with levodopa in Parkinson's disease. Similarly, clinical guidelines have been revised worldwide on the basis of the non-randomized evidence of the substantial reduction in the risk of early recurrent stroke (see Fig. 19.2) as a result of the urgent initiation of standard secondary prevention (Rothwell *et al.* 2007).

However, such large treatment effects are rare. Most treatments used in medicine have smaller effects that require assessment in randomized controlled trials if they are to be reliably quantified. Specifically, randomization has two main advantages over a non-randomized comparison. First, it ensures that clinicians do not know which treatment the patient will receive and cannot select certain types of patient for one particular treatment. Second, it tends to result in an equal balance of baseline risk across the treatment groups.

Assessment of the Internal Validity of a Randomized Controlled Trial

Randomized controlled trials have the potential to produce reliable estimates of the effects of treatments, but they will not inevitably do so. There are many potential sources of bias that must be addressed in the design and performance of a trial in order to ensure that results are reliable. The extent to which bias has been avoided is usually termed *internal validity*, the assessment of which is detailed in the following section. The extent to which the results of a trial can be generalized to other settings, usually meaning routine clinical practice, is termed *external validity* and is considered later in this chapter.

How Was Randomization Performed?

It is important that the method of randomization is actually *random*. Treatment allocation according to day of the week, date of birth, or date of admission or by alternate cases is not random. The investigator will often know what treatment the patient will get if they enter the trial, and so these methods are open to bias. Randomization must be based on tables of random numbers or computer-generated random allocation. It is also important that randomization is secure. Central telephone randomization is preferable to other methods, such as sealed envelopes containing the treatment allocation.

Table 18.3 Effect of sample size on the reliability of the result of a trial of a hypothetical treatment that is expected to reduce the risk of a poor outcome by 20%: From 10% to 8%

Total patients	P^a	Trial power (%)	Comments on trial size
200	0.99	1	Completely hopeless
400	0.98	2	Still hopeless
800	0.96	4	Completely inadequate
1,600	0.90	10	Still inadequate
3,200	0.75	25	Not really adequate
6,400	0.43	57	Barely adequate
12,800	0.09	91	Probably adequate
20,000	0.01	99	Definitely adequate

^{a} Probability of failing to achieve $p < 0.01$ significance if true relative risk reduction is 20%.

Were the Treatment Groups Balanced?

Randomization will not inevitably result in an adequate balance of clinical characteristics and prognostic factors between the treatment groups in a trial, particularly if the sample size is relatively small. Details of the important clinical characteristics of the patients should, therefore, be reported by treatment group. If a prognostic variable is particularly important, a relatively minor (and not necessarily statistically significant) imbalance between the treatment groups may have a major effect on the trial result.

Was the Trial Sufficiently Powered?

Sample sizes for randomized controlled trials in neurology may need to be large, either because treatment effects are relatively small or because the progression of disease is slow. Table 18.3 shows the effect of sample size on the reliability of the result of a trial of a hypothetical neurological treatment that is assumed to reduce the risk of a poor outcome by 20%, from 10% to 8%. The risk of getting the wrong result when a trial has an inadequate sample size is illustrated in Fig. 18.1. In this trial, there was considerable variability in the apparent effect of treatment until several hundred patients had been randomized. If the trial had been small, misleading trends in treatment effect could easily have been reported.

Was the Trial Stopped Early?

A trial may need to be stopped early if a treatment has serious adverse effects or if there is clear benefit. However, as is seen in Fig. 18.1, the chance fluctuations during the early stages of a trial can easily reach statistical significance at the $p = 0.05$ level. If the stopping rule is based on a p value of 0.05, it is quite possible that the trial will be stopped early and the wrong conclusions drawn. Stopping rules should be based on significance levels of $p < 0.01$ or ideally $p < 0.001$, and the evolving results should be assessed on only a limited number of prespecified occasions.

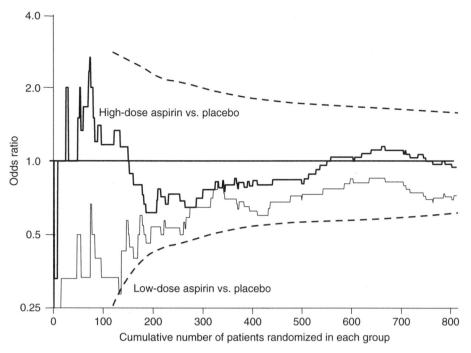

Fig. 18.1 The evolution of the estimates of treatment effect in the UKTIA-Aspirin Trial (Farrell *et al.* 1991) of high-dose aspirin versus low-dose aspirin versus placebo in patients with transient ischemic attack or minor stroke. The treatment effect (odds ratio) calculated at each point was based on the outcomes at final follow-up for patients randomized to that point (PM Rothwell, unpublished data). The dashed lines represent the level at which the apparent treatment effect approached statistical significance at the *p* = 0.05 level.

Was Outcome Assessment Blind to Treatment Allocation?

There are two main reasons for blinding the trial clinicians: first, so that the use of non-trial treatments and interventions is not influenced by a knowledge of whether the patients received the trial treatment; second, so that clinicians are not biased in their assessment of clinical outcomes. The potential for bias depends on the subjectivity of the trial outcome. Biased assessment of neurological impairment and disability was clearly demonstrated in a multiple sclerosis trial in which blind and non-blind outcome assessment produced very different results (Noseworthy *et al.* 1994). Trials with blind assessment should also report whether blinding was effective. It is, of course, sometimes impossible to blind clinical assessment, but non-blind trials should report data on non-trial treatments given to patients during follow-up to ensure that these were not biased.

Were Serious Complications of Treatment Included in the Main Outcome?

Some treatments have serious complications that should be included in the primary outcome rather than relegated to a table of "side effects," for example life-threatening gastrointestinal bleeding in trials of antiplatelet agents and anticoagulants.

Was the Main Analysis an Intention-to-Treat Analysis?

The primary analysis in any randomized trial should be an intention-to-treat analysis: that is, patients remain in the treatment group to which they were originally randomized irrespective of the treatment they eventually received. The alternative, an efficacy analysis (an analysis that is confined to patients who complied with the randomized treatment), is prone to bias. This was illustrated by the Coronary Drug Project (Coronary Drug Project Research Group 1980), a randomized trial comparing several different lipid-lowering regimens with placebo following myocardial infarction. By intention-to-treat analysis, the 5-year mortality in the clofibrate group was 20.0% versus 20.9% in the placebo group. However, when patients who complied with treatment in the clofibrate group were compared with non-compliers, the results seemed to suggest that there was a treatment effect: 5-year mortality was 15.0% in the compliers versus 24.6% in the non-compliers. Perhaps clofibrate was beneficial. However, the same analysis in patients in the placebo group showed the same trend: 15.1% mortality in compliers versus 28.2% mortality in non-compliers. The apparent effect of clofibrate in the treatment group was simply a bias generated by the fact that patients who do not comply with treatment tend to have a worse prognosis.

Were Any Patients Excluded from the Main Analysis?

It is not uncommon in reports of trials to find that a certain number of the patients who were randomized initially were excluded from the final analysis. Common reasons for exclusion are that following randomization it was found that a number of patients did not actually fit the eligibility criteria (so called *protocol violators*) or that some patients never received the randomized treatment because they developed a clear indication for a specific treatment or because they withdrew from the trial for other reasons. However, the interpretation of what is a protocol violation can be rather subjective, and since the decision will often be made toward the end of the trial and may not be blind to outcome, it is open to abuse. For example, 71 of 1,629 patients randomized in a trial of an antiplatelet agent following myocardial infarction were excluded from the final analysis, apparently because they did not meet the eligibility criteria (Anturane Reinfarction Trial Research Group 1980). It subsequently transpired that there was a large excess of deaths in the exclusions from the treatment group compared with the placebo group (Temple and Pledger 1980). Exclusion of these patients led to a bias that had contributed to the statistically significant apparent benefit in the treatment group. A second trial failed to confirm any benefit.

How Many Patients Were Lost to Follow-Up?

Another important potential cause of bias in the analysis of trial results is loss of patients to follow-up. Just as patients who comply with treatment are different from patients who do not, patients who are lost to follow-up are usually different from those who remain in the trial. For example, it may not be possible to contact patients because they are either incapacitated in some way or even dead. It is, therefore, very difficult to interpret the results of a trial with significant loss to follow-up.

Assessment of the External Validity of a Randomized Controlled Trial

Randomized controlled trials must be internally valid (i.e., design and conduct must eliminate the possibility of bias), but to be clinically useful, the result must also be relevant to a definable group of patients in a particular clinical setting (i.e., they must be externally valid). Lack of external validity is the most frequent criticism by clinicians of trials, systematic reviews, and guidelines and is one explanation for the widespread underuse in routine practice of many treatments that have been shown to be beneficial in trials and are recommended in guidelines (Rothwell 2005a). Yet medical journals, funding agencies, ethics committees, the pharmaceutical industry, and governmental regulators give external validity a low priority. Admittedly, whereas the determinants of internal validity are intuitive and can generally be worked out from first principles, understanding of the determinants of the external validity requires clinical rather than statistical expertise and often depends on a detailed understanding of the particular clinical condition under study and its management in routine clinical practice. However, reliable judgments about the external validity of randomized trials are essential if treatments are to be used correctly in as many patients as possible in routine clinical practice.

Whether the results of a trial can be applied in routine clinical practice depends to some extent on the type of trial. Generally speaking, explanatory (phase II) trials measure the *effectiveness* of treatment, whereas pragmatic (phase III) trials measure the *usefulness* of treatment. A treatment may be *effective*, but it may not be *useful* because it is too poorly tolerated, too expensive, or too complex to administer. Explanatory trials are often small, include a tightly defined group of patients, and frequently have nonclinical (surrogate) measures of outcome. Pragmatic trials seek to measure the usefulness of treatments in situations that, as far as possible, mimic normal clinical practice. However, it would be wrong to assume that a pragmatic trial will always have greater external validity than an explanatory trial. For example, although broad eligibility criteria, limited collection of baseline data, and inclusion of centers with a range of expertise and differing patient populations have many advantages, they can also make it very difficult to generalize the effect of treatment to a particular clinical setting. Moreover, no randomized trial or systematic review will ever be relevant to all patients and all settings. However, trials should be designed and reported in a way that allows clinicians to judge to whom the results can reasonably be applied. Table 18.4 lists some of the important potential determinants of external validity, each of which is reviewed briefly in the following section.

What Was the Setting of the Trial?

A detailed understanding of the setting in which a trial is performed, including any peculiarities of the healthcare system in particular countries, can be essential in judging external validity. The potential impact of differences between healthcare systems is illustrated by the analysis of the results of the European Carotid Surgery Trial, a randomized trial of endarterectomy versus medical treatment alone for recently symptomatic carotid stenosis (Rothwell 2005b). National differences in the speed with which patients were investigated, with a median delay from last symptoms to randomization of greater than 2 months in the UK (slow centers) compared with 3 weeks in Belgium and Holland (fast centers), resulted in very different treatment effects in these different healthcare systems – owing to the shortness of the time window for effective prevention of stroke (Fig. 18.2).

Table 18.4 Some of the factors that can affect external validity of randomized controlled trials and should be addressed in reports of the results and be considered by clinicians

	Factors
Setting of the trial	Healthcare system Country Recruitment from primary, secondary or tertiary care Selection of participating centers Selection of participating clinicians
Selection of patients	Methods of pre-randomization diagnosis and investigation Eligibility criteria Exclusion criteria Placebo run-in period Treatment run-in period "Enrichment" strategies Ratio of randomized patients to eligible non-randomized patients in participating centers Proportion of patients who declined randomization
Characteristics of randomized patients	Baseline clinical characteristics Racial group Uniformity of underlying pathology Stage in the natural history of their disease Severity of disease Comorbidity Absolute risks of a poor outcome in the control group
Differences between the trial protocol and routine practice	Trial intervention Timing of treatment Appropriateness/relevance of control intervention Adequacy of non-trial treatment: both intended and actual Prohibition of certain non-trial treatments Therapeutic or diagnostic advances since trial was performed
Outcome measures and follow-up	Clinical relevance of surrogate outcomes Clinical relevance, validity and reproducibility of complex scales Effect of intervention on most relevant components of composite outcomes Who measured outcome Use of patient-centered outcomes Frequency of follow-up Adequacy of the length of follow-up
Adverse effects of treatment	Completeness of reporting of relevant adverse effects Rates of discontinuation of treatment Selection of trial centers and/or clinicians on the basis of skill or experience Exclusion of patients at risk of complications Exclusion of patients who experienced adverse effects during a run-in period Intensity of trial safety procedures

Source: From Rothwell (2005a).

Moderate stenosis

Ipsilateral ischemic stroke or operative stroke/death

	Surgical	Medical	ARR (%)	95% CI
Fast centers	17/174	21/127	8.3	−0.1 to 16.7
Slow centers	29/206	11/139	−5.6	−12.6 to 1.4
TOTAL	46/380	32/266	0.9	−4.5 to 6.4

Any stroke or operative death

	Surgical	Medical	ARR (%)	95% CI
Fast centers	21/174	28/127	11.8	2.4 to 21.2
Slow centers	38/206	25/139	0.3	−8.6 to 9.3
TOTAL	59/380	53/266	5.7	−0.8 to 12.2

Severe stenosis

	Surgical	Medical	ARR (%)	95% CI
Fast centers	8/162	25/106	19.9	10.7 to 29.1
Slow centers	25/173	25/113	7.6	−2.0 to 17.1
TOTAL	33/335	50/219	13.5	6.9 to 20.2

	Surgical	Medical	ARR (%)	95% CI
Fast centers	11/162	31/106	23.6	13.7 to 33.5
Slow centers	35/173	30/113	6.2	−4.3 to 16.6
TOTAL	46/335	61/219	14.7	7.4 to 21.9

Absolute risk reduction (% [95% CI])

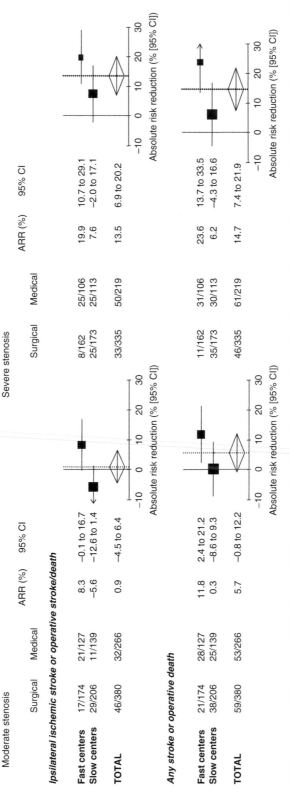

Fig. 18.2 The absolute risk reduction (ARR) at 5 years of ipsilateral ischemic stroke (top) and any stroke or death (bottom) with surgery in European Carotid Surgery Trial centers in which the median delay from last symptomatic event to randomization was ≤ 50 days (fast centers) compared with centers with a longer delay (slow centers) (Rothwell 2005a). Data are shown separately for patients with moderate (50–69%) and severe (70–99%) carotid stenosis. CI, confidence interval.

Similar differences in performance between healthcare systems will exist for other conditions, and there is, of course, the broader issue of how trials done in the developed world apply in the developing world. Moreover, other differences between countries in the methods of diagnosis and management of disease, which can be substantial, or important racial differences in pathology and natural history of disease also affect the external validity of trials. A good example is the heterogeneity of results of trials of bacille Calmette-Guérin (BCG) vaccine in prevention of tuberculosis, with a progressive loss of efficacy ($p < 0.0001$) with decreasing latitude (Fine 1995).

How Were Participating Centers Selected?

How centers and clinicians were selected to participate in trials is seldom reported, but it can also have important implications for external validity. For example, the Asymptomatic Carotid Atherosclerosis Study (ACAS) trial of endarterectomy for asymptomatic carotid stenosis only accepted surgeons with an excellent safety record, rejecting 40% of applicants initially and subsequently barring from further participation those who had adverse operative outcomes in the trial. The benefit from surgery in the trial was a result in major part of the consequently low operative risk (Asymptomatic Carotid Atherosclerosis Study Group 1995). A meta-analysis of 46 surgical case series that published operative risks during the 5 years after the trial found operative mortality to be eight times higher and the risk of stroke and death to be about three times higher than in ACAS (Rothwell 2005a). Trials should not include centers that do not have the competence to treat patients safely, but selection should not be so exclusive that the results cannot be generalized to routine clinical practice.

How Were Patients Selected and Excluded?

Concern is often expressed about highly selective trial eligibility criteria, but there are often several earlier stages of selection that are rarely recorded or reported but can be more problematic. For example, consider a trial of a new blood pressure–lowering drug, which like most such trials is performed in a hospital clinic. Fewer than 10% of patients with hypertension are managed in hospital clinics, and this group will differ from those managed in primary care. Moreover, only one of the ten physicians who see hypertensive patients in this particular hospital is taking part in the trial, and this physician mainly sees young patients with resistant hypertension. In this way, even before any consideration of eligibility or exclusion criteria, potential recruits are already very unrepresentative of patients in the local community. It is essential, therefore, that, where possible, trials record and report the pathways to recruitment.

Patients are then further selected according to trial eligibility criteria. Some trials exclude women and many exclude the elderly and/or patients with common comorbidities. One review of 214 drug trials in acute myocardial infarction found that more than 60% excluded patients older than 75 (Gurwitz et al. 1992), despite the fact that more than 50% of myocardial infarctions occur in this older age group. A review of 41 US National Institutes of Health randomized trials found an average exclusion rate of 73% (Charlson and Horwitz 1984), but rates can be much higher. One study of an acute stroke treatment trial found that of the small proportion of patients admitted to hospital sufficiently quickly to be suitable for treatment, 96% were ineligible based on the various other exclusion criteria (Jorgensen et al. 1999). One center in another acute stroke trial had to screen 192 patients over 2 years to find one eligible patient (LaRue et al. 1988). Yet highly selective recruitment is not inevitable.

The Gruppo Italiano per lo Studio della Streptochinasi nell'Infarto Miocardico GISSI-1 trial of thrombolysis for acute myocardial infarction, for example, recruited 90% of patients admitted within 12 hours of the event with a definite diagnosis and no contraindications (Gruppo Italiano per lo Studio della Streptochinasi nell'Infarto Miocardico [GISSI] 1986).

Strict eligibility criteria can limit the external validity of trials, but physicians should at least be able to select similar patients for treatment in routine practice. Unfortunately, however, reporting of trial eligibility criteria is frequently inadequate. A review of trials leading to clinical alerts by the US National Institutes of Health revealed that, of an average of 31 eligibility criteria, only 63% were published in the main trial report and only 19% in the clinical alert (Shapiro *et al.* 2000). Inadequate reporting is also a major problem in secondary publications, such as systematic reviews and clinical guidelines, where the need for a succinct message does not usually allow detailed consideration of the eligibility and exclusion criteria or other determinants of external validity.

Was There a Run-In Period?

Pre-randomization run-in periods are also often used to select or exclude patients. In a placebo run-in, all eligible patients receive placebo, and those who are poorly compliant are excluded. There can be good reasons for doing this, but high rates of exclusion will reduce external validity. Active treatment run-in periods in which patients who have adverse events or show signs that treatment may be ineffective are excluded are more likely to undermine external validity. For example, two trials of carvedilol, a vasodilatory beta-blocker, in chronic heart failure excluded 6% and 9% of eligible patients in treatment run-in periods, mainly because of worsening heart failure and other adverse events, some of which were fatal (Rothwell 2005a). In both trials, the complication rates in the subsequent randomized phase were much lower than in the run-in phase.

Trials also sometimes actively recruit patients who are likely to respond well to treatment (often termed "enrichment"). For example, some trials of antipsychotic drugs have selectively recruited patients who had a good response to antipsychotic drugs previously (Rothwell 2005a). Other trials have excluded non-responders in a run-in phase. One trial of a cholinesterase inhibitor, tacrine, in Alzheimer's disease recruited 632 patients to a 6-week "enrichment" phase in which they were randomized to different doses of tacrine or placebo (Davis *et al.* 1992). After a washout-period, only the 215 (34%) patients who had a measured improvement on tacrine in the "enrichment" phase were randomized to tacrine (at their best dose) versus placebo in the main phase of the trial. External validity is clearly undermined here.

What Were the Characteristics of the Randomized Patients?

Even in large pragmatic trials with very few exclusion criteria, recruitment of less than 10% of potentially eligible patients in participating centers is common. Those patients who are recruited generally differ from those who are eligible but not recruited in terms of age, sex, race, severity of disease, educational status, social class, and place of residence (Rothwell 2005a). The outcome in patients included in trials is also usually better than those not in trials, often markedly so, not because of better treatment but because of a better baseline prognosis. Trial reports usually include the baseline clinical characteristics of randomized patients, and so it is argued that clinicians can assess external validity by comparison with their own patient(s). However, recorded baseline clinical characteristics often say very little

Table 18.5 The baseline clinical characteristics and hemorrhage outcomes of patients randomized to anticoagulation with warfarin in the European Atrial Fibrillation Trial (EAFT) and the Stroke Prevention in Reversible Ischemia Trial (SPIRIT)

	SPIRIT ($n = 651$)	EAFT ($n = 225$)
Baseline clinical characteristics (%)		
Male sex	66	55
Age > 65 years	47	81
Hypertension	39	48
Angina	9	11
Myocardial infarction	9	7
Diabetes	11	12
Leukoaraiosis on CT brain scan	7	14
Outcomes during trial		
Mean INR during trial (SD)	3.3 (1.1)	2.9 (0.7)
Patient-years of follow-up	735	507
Intracranial hemorrhage (no.)	27	0^a
Extracranial hemorrhage (no.)	26	13
Adjusted hazard ratio (95% CI) for SPIRIT versus EAFT		
Intracranial hemorrhage	19.0 (2.4–250)	$p < 0.0001$
Extracranial hemorrhage	1.9 (0.8–4.7)	$p = 0.15$

Notes: INR, international normalized ratio; SD, standard deviation; CI, confidence interval.
^{a} There were no proven intracranial hemorrhages, but no CT scan was performed in two strokes. For the purpose of calculation of the adjusted hazard ratio for hemorrhage, these two strokes were categorized as having been caused by intracranial hemorrhage.
Source: From Gorter (1999).

about the real makeup of the trial population and can be misleading. For example, Table 18.5 shows the baseline clinical characteristics of the patients randomized to warfarin in two trials of secondary prevention of stroke. In one trial, patients were in atrial fibrillation, and in the other, they were in sinus rhythm, but the characteristics of the two cohorts were otherwise fairly similar. However, the risk of intracranial hemorrhage on warfarin was nineteen times higher ($p < 0.0001$) in the Stroke Prevention in Reversible Ischemia Trial than in the European Atrial Fibrillation Trial even after adjustment for differences in baseline clinical characteristics and the intensity of anticoagulation therapy (Gorter 1999). In judging external validity, an understanding of how patients were referred, investigated, and diagnosed (i.e. their pathway to recruitment) as well as how they were subsequently selected and excluded is often very much more informative than a list of baseline characteristics.

Was the Intervention, Control Treatment, and Pretrial or Non-Trial Management Appropriate?

External validity can also be affected if trials have protocols that differ from usual clinical practice. For example, prior to randomization in the trials of endarterectomy for symptomatic carotid stenosis, patients had to be diagnosed by a neurologist and to

Table 18.6 Examples where trials based on surrogate outcomes proved to be misleading predictors of the effect of treatment on clinical outcomes in subsequent pragmatic clinical trials

Treatment	Condition	Surrogate outcome	Clinical outcome
Fluoride	Osteoporosis	Increase in bone density	Major increase in fractures
Antiarrhythmic drugs	Post-MI	Reduction in ECG abnormalities	Increased mortality
Beta-interferon	Multiple sclerosis	70% reduction in new lesions brain MRI	No convincing effect on disability
Milrinone and epoprostanol	Heart failure	Improved exercise tolerance	Increased mortality
Ibopamine	Heart failure	Improved ejection fraction and heart rate variability	Increased mortality

Notes: MI, myocardial infarction; ECG, electrocardiography.
Source: From Rothwell (2005a).

have conventional arterial angiography, neither of which is routine in many centers. The trial intervention itself may also differ from that used in current practice, such as in the formulation and bioavailability of a drug or the type of anesthetic used for an operation. The same can be true of the treatment in the control group in a trial, which may use a particularly low dose of the comparator drug or fall short of best current practice in some other way. External validity can also be undermined by too stringent limitations on the use of non-trial treatments. Any prohibition of non-trial treatments should be reported in the main trial publications along with details of relevant non-trial treatments that were used. The timing of many interventions is also critical and should be reported when relevant.

Were the Outcome Measures Appropriate?

The external validity of a trial also depends on whether the outcomes were clinically relevant. Many trials use "surrogate" outcomes, usually biological or imaging markers that are thought to be indirect measures of the effect of treatment on clinical outcomes. Surrogate outcomes (e.g., infarct size on CT brain scan in an acute stroke trial or MRI activity in multiple sclerosis) can be useful in explanatory trials because they may be more sensitive to the effects of the treatment than clinical outcomes, and they are readily assessed blind to treatment allocation. However, they do not measure clinical effectiveness and may sometimes be highly misleading. There are many examples of treatments that had a major beneficial effect on a surrogate outcome, which had been shown to be correlated with a relevant clinical outcome in observational studies, but where the treatments proved ineffective or harmful in subsequent large trials that used these same clinical outcomes (Table 18.6). For example, a trial of three different antiarrhythmic drugs versus placebo after acute myocardial infarction assessed the frequency of ventricular extrasystoles on 24-hour ambulatory electrocardiographic monitoring (Cardiac Arrhythmia Suppression Trial [CAST] Investigators 1989). All three drugs produced a substantial reduction in the frequency of extrasystoles, but the trial was subsequently stopped because of a major excess of deaths in the treatment group (33 versus 9 in the control group; $p = 0.0003$). Similarly, reduced bone density, which is known to be a useful marker for risk of fractures, was used as a surrogate outcome in a trial of sodium fluoride in women with osteoporosis (Riggs *et al.* 1990). Sodium fluoride produced a highly statistically significant, and apparently clinically important, increase in bone density. However, further follow-up revealed a 30% increase in vertebral fractures and a threefold increase in non-vertebral fractures in the sodium fluoride group.

Complex scales, often made up of arbitrary combinations of symptoms and clinical signs, are also problematic. A review of 196 trials in rheumatoid arthritis identified more than 70 different outcome scales (Gøtzsche 1989). A review of 2,000 trials in schizophrenia identified 640 outcome scales, many of which were devised for the particular trial and had no supporting data on validity or reliability. These unvalidated scales were more likely to show statistically significant treatment effects than established scales (Marshall *et al.* 2000). Moreover, the clinical meaning of apparent treatment effects (e.g., a 2.7-point mean reduction in a 100-point outcome scale made up of various symptoms and signs) is usually impossible to discern. Simple clinical outcomes usually have most external validity, but even then only if they reflect the priorities of patients. For example, patients with epilepsy are much more interested in the proportion of individuals rendered free of seizures in trials of anticonvulsants than they are in changes in mean seizure frequency. Who actually measured the outcome can also be important. For example, the recorded operative risk of stroke in carotid endarterectomy is highly dependent on whether patients were assessed by a surgeon or a neurologist (Rothwell and Warlow 1995).

Many trials combine events in their primary outcome measure. This can produce a useful measure of the overall effect of treatment on all the relevant outcomes, and it usually affords greater statistical power, but the outcome that is most important to a particular patient may be affected differently by treatment than the combined outcome. Composite outcomes also sometimes combine events of very different severity, and treatment effects can be driven by the least important outcome, which is often the most frequent. Equally problematic is the composite of definite clinical events and episodes of hospitalization. The fact that a patient is in a trial will probably affect the likelihood of hospitalization, and it will certainly vary between different healthcare systems.

Was the Follow-Up Sufficient?

Another major problem for the external validity of trials is an inadequate duration of treatment and/or follow-up. For example, although patients with refractory epilepsy or migraine require treatment for many years, most trials of new drugs look at the effect of treatment for only a few weeks. Whether initial response is a good predictor of long-term benefit is unknown. This problem has been identified in trials in schizophrenia, with fewer than 50% of trials having greater than 6 weeks of follow-up and only 20% following patients for longer than 6 months (Thornley and Adams 1998). The contrast between beneficial effects of treatments in short-term trials and the less-encouraging experience of long-term treatment in clinical practice has also been highlighted by clinicians treating patients with rheumatoid arthritis (Pincus 1998).

How Were Adverse Effects of Treatment Assessed and Reported?

Reporting of adverse effects of treatment in trials and systematic reviews is often poor. In a review of 192 pharmaceutical trials, less than a third had adequate reporting of adverse clinical events or laboratory toxicology (Ioannidis and Contopoulos-Ioannidis 1998). Treatment discontinuation rates provide some guide to tolerability, but pharmaceutical trials often use eligibility criteria and run-in periods to exclude patients who might be prone to adverse effects.

Clinicians are usually most concerned about external validity of trials of potentially dangerous treatments. Complications of medical interventions are a leading cause of death in developed countries. Risks can be overestimated in trials, particularly during the introduction of new treatments when trials are often carried out with patients with very severe disease, but stringent selection of patients, confinement to specialist centers, and intensive safety monitoring usually lead to lower risks than in routine clinical practice. Trials of warfarin in non-rheumatic atrial fibrillation are a good example. Prior to 2007, all trials reporting benefit with warfarin had complication rates that were much lower than in routine practice, and consequent doubts about external validity were partly to blame for major underprescribing of warfarin, particularly in the elderly.

Applying the Results of Randomized Trials to Treatment Decisions for Individual Patients

Many treatments, such as blood pressure lowering in uncontrolled hypertension, are indicated in the vast majority of patients. However, a targeted approach is useful for treatments with modest benefits (e.g., lipid lowering in primary prevention of vascular disease), for costly treatments with moderate overall benefits (e.g., beta-interferon in multiple sclerosis), if the availability of treatment is limited (e.g., organ transplantation), in developing countries with very limited healthcare budgets, and, most importantly, for treatments that although of overall benefit in large trials are associated with a significant risk of harm. The crux of the problem faced by clinicians in these situations is how to use data from large randomized trials and systematic reviews, which provide the most reliable estimates of the overall average effects of treatment, to determine the likely effect of treatment in an individual.

When considering the likely effect of a treatment in an individual patient, it is important to consider the overall result of a trial or systematic review as an absolute risk reduction with treatment or the number needed to treat to prevent a poor outcome. An absolute risk reduction tells us what chance an individual has of benefiting from treatment; for example, an absolute risk reduction of 25% indicates that there is a 1:4 chance of benefit (four people need to be treated to ensure a good outcome in one). In contrast, a particular relative risk reduction gives absolutely no information about the likelihood of individual benefit. For example, the relative reductions in the risk of stroke were virtually identical in the Swedish Trial in Old Patients with hypertension (STOP-hypertension) (relative risk, 0.53; 95% confidence interval [CI], 0.33–0.86) (Dahlof *et al.* 1991) and the Medical Research

Council Trial (relative risk, 0.55; 95% CI, 0.25–0.60) (Medical Research Council Working Party 1985) of blood pressure lowering in primary prevention, but there was a twelvefold difference in absolute risk reduction. All other things being equal, 830 of the young hypertensives in the Medical Research Council trial would have to be treated for 1 year to prevent one stroke compared with 69 of the elderly hypertensives in the STOP-hypertension trial.

Trials should report subgroup analyses if there are potentially large differences between groups in the risk of a poor outcome with or without treatment; if there is potential heterogeneity of treatment effect in relation to pathophysiology; if there are practical questions about when to treat (e.g., stage of disease, timing of treatment); or if there are doubts about benefit in specific groups, such as the elderly, which are likely to lead to undertreatment (Rothwell 2005b). Analyses must be predefined, carefully justified, and limited to a few clinically important questions, and post hoc observations should be treated with skepticism irrespective of their statistical significance. Concerns about heterogeneity of treatment effects will often be unfounded, but if they are not addressed, they will restrict the use of treatment in routine practice. If important subgroup effects are anticipated, trials should either be powered to detect them reliably or pooled analyses of multiple trials should be undertaken.

Univariate subgroup analysis is of relatively limited value, even when done reliably, in situations where there are multiple determinants of the individual response to treatment. In this situation, targeting treatment using risk models can be useful, particularly in conditions or for interventions where benefit is likely to be very dependent on the absolute risk of a poor outcome with or without treatment. Stratification of trial results with independently derived and validated prognostic models can allow clinicians to systematically take into account the characteristics of an individual patient and their interactions, to consider the risks and benefits of interventions separately if required, and to provide patients with personalized estimates of their likelihood of benefit from treatment (Rothwell 2005b).

References

Anturane Reinfarction Trial Research Group (1980). Sulfinpyrazone in the prevention of sudden death after myocardial infarction. *New England Journal of Medicine* **302**:250–256

Asymptomatic Carotid Atherosclerosis Study Group (1995). Carotid endarterectomy for patients with asymptomatic internal carotid artery stenosis. *Journal of the American Medical Association* **273**:1421–1428

Barnett HJ, Taylor DW, Eliasziw M et al. (1998). The final results of the NASCET trial. *New England Journal of Medicine* **339**:1415–1425

Cardiac Arrhythmia Suppression Trial (CAST) Investigators (1989). Preliminary report: Effect of encainide and flecainide on mortality in a randomised trial of arrhythmia suppression after myocardial infarction. *New England Journal of Medicine* **321**:406–412

Charlson ME, Horwitz RI (1984). Applying results of randomised trials to clinical practice: Impact of losses before randomisation. *British Medical Journal* **289**:1281–1284

Coronary Drug Project Research Group (1980). Influence of adherence to treatment and response to cholesterol on mortality in the Coronary Drug Project. *New England Journal of Medicine* **303**:1038–1041

Dahlof B, Lindholm LH, Hansson L et al. (1991). Morbidity and mortality in the Swedish trial in old patients with hypertension (STOP-hypertension). *Lancet* **338**:1281–1285

Davis KL, Thal LJ, Gamzu ER *et al.* (1992). A double-blind, placebo-controlled multicenter study of tacrine for Alzheimer's disease. *New England Journal of Medicine* **321**:406–412

Farrell B, Godwin J, Richards S *et al.* (1991). The United Kingdom transient ischaemic attack (UK-TIA) aspirin trial: Final results. *Journal of Neurology, Neurosurgery and Psychiatry* **54**:1044–1054

Fine PEM (1995). Variation in protection by BCG: implications of and for heterologous immunity. *Lancet* **346**:1339–1345

Gorter JW for the Stroke Prevention in Reversible Ischaemia Trial (SPIRIT) and European Atrial Fibrillation Trial (EAFT) Groups (1999). Major bleeding during anticoagulation after cerebral ischaemia: Patterns and risk factors. *Neurology* **53**:1319–1327

Gøtzsche PC (1989). Methodology and overt and hidden bias in reports of 196 double-blind trials of nonsteroidal antiinflammatory drugs in rheumatoid arthritis. *Control in Clinical Trials* **10**:31–56

Gruppo Italiano per lo Studio della Streptochinasi nell'Infarto Miocardico (GISSI) (1986). Effectiveness of intravenous thrombolytic treatment in acute myocardial infarction. *Lancet* **i**:397–402

Gurwitz JH, Col NF, Avorn J (1992). The exclusion of elderly and women from clinical trials in acute myocardial infarction. *Journal of the American Medical Association* **268**:1417–1422

Ioannidis JP, Contopoulos-Ioannidis DG (1998). Reporting of safety data from randomised trials. *Lancet* **352**:1752–1753

Jorgensen HS, Nakayama H, Kammersgaard LP *et al.* (1999). Predicted impact of intravenous thrombolysis on prognosis of general population of stroke patients: Simulation model. *British Medical Journal* **319**:288–289

LaRue LJ, Alter M, Traven ND *et al.* (1988). Acute stroke therapy trials: Problems in patient accrual. *Stroke* **19**:950–954

Marshall M, Lockwood A, Bradley C *et al.* (2000). Unpublished rating scales: A major source of bias in randomised controlled trials of treatments for schizophrenia? *British Journal of Psychiatry* **176**:249–252

Medical Research Council Working Party (1985). MRC trial of treatment of mild hypertension: Principal results. *British Medical Journal* **291**:97–104

Noseworthy JH, Ebers GC, Vandervoort MK *et al.* (1994). The impact of blinding on the results of a randomized, placebo-controlled multiple sclerosis clinical trial. *Neurology* **44**:16–20

Pincus T (1998). Rheumatoid arthritis: Disappointing long-term outcomes despite successful short-term clinical trials. *Journal of Clinical Epidemiology* **41**:1037–1041

Riggs BL, Hodgson SF, O'Fallon WM *et al.* (1990). Effect of fluoride treatment on fracture rate in postmenopausal women with osteoporosis. *New England Journal of Medicine* **322**:802–809

Rothwell PM (2005a). External validity of randomised controlled trials: To whom do the results of this trial apply? *Lancet* **365**:82–93

Rothwell PM (2005b). Subgroup analysis in randomised controlled trials: Importance, indications and interpretation. *Lancet* **365**:176–186

Rothwell PM, Warlow CP (1995). Is self-audit reliable? *Lancet* **346**:1623

Rothwell PM, Giles MF, Chandratheva A *et al.* (2007). Major reduction in risk of early recurrent stroke by urgent treatment of TIA and minor stroke: EXPRESS Study. *Lancet* **370**:1432–1442

Shapiro SH, Weijer C, Freedman B (2000). Reporting the study populations of clinical trials. *Clear transmission or static on the line? Journal of Clinical Epidemiology* **53**:973–979

Taylor DW, Barnett HJM, Haynes RB *et al.* (1999). Low dose and high dose acetylsalicylic acid for patients undergoing carotid endarterectomy: A randomised controlled trial. *Lancet* **353**:2179–2184

Temple R, Pledger GW (1980). The FDA's critique of the Anturane Reinfarction Trial. *New England Journal of Medicine* **303**:1488–1492

Thornley B, Adams CE (1998). Content and quality of 2000 controlled trials in schizophrenia over 50 years. *British Medical Journal* **317**:1181–1184

Chapter 19

Acute Treatment of Transient Ischemic Attack and Minor Stroke

Although the acute treatment of TIA and minor and major stroke have many common elements, there are important differences. In the acute treatment of TIA and minor stroke, the aim is the secondary prevention of a disabling stroke, which might follow in the immediate hours and days after the initial event, as opposed to reversal of any neurological deficit caused by the stroke itself. Reduction of delays by improved public education and triage to secondary care and coordinated patient management in specialist units are vital aspects of treatment in TIA and minor and major stroke. However, there is a greater focus on urgent, effective secondary prevention for TIA and minor stroke.

Another important difference is the extent of the evidence base for treatments in major stroke compared with TIA and minor stroke. The concepts of stroke units and administration of thrombolysis have been researched, developed, and implemented since the 1980s for patients with major stroke. Yet, although the concept of TIA arose in the 1950s and treatments such as carotid endarterectomy, anticoagulation, antiplatelet therapy, and other risk factor management were subsequently proven effective, it was not until 2007 that the first reports were published on the feasibility and effectiveness of urgent assessment and treatment of TIA in specialist units (Lavallée *et al.* 2007; Rothwell *et al.* 2007).

This chapter will summarize the aspects of acute treatment that are specific to TIA and minor stroke.

Recognition of Symptoms and Delays to Management

The urgent management of patients with minor stroke or TIA depends upon the correct recognition of symptoms and appropriate action by patients and their swift triage to specialist care where investigation and treatment are rapidly initiated.

Public Awareness and Behavior

In contrast to major stroke, where extensive studies have examined knowledge among the general public (Pancioli *et al.* 1998; Reeves *et al.* 2002; Parahoo *et al.* 2003; Carroll *et al.* 2004) and individuals' immediate behavior (Salisbury *et al.* 1998; Smith *et al.* 1998; Evenson *et al.* 2001; Lacy *et al.* 2001; Harraf *et al.* 2002, Lecouturier *et al.* 2010), equivalent studies in minor stroke and TIA are lacking.

One study of knowledge among the general public indicated that 2.3% of a randomly selected sample of people in the USA have been told by a physician that they had a TIA, based on self-report in a telephone survey (Johnston *et al.* 2003). However, an additional 3.2% of respondents recalled symptoms consistent with TIA but had not sought medical attention at all and consequently had not been diagnosed by a doctor. Of those with "diagnosed" TIA, only 64% had seen a doctor within 24 hours of the event. Only 8.2% correctly related the definition of TIA, and 8.6% were able to identify a typical symptom.

In a study of 422 residents of Bern, Switzerland, who were interviewed in person about their knowledge of stroke and TIA, only 8.3% recognized TIA as symptoms of stroke resolving within 24 hours, and only 2.8% identified TIA as a disease requiring immediate medical help (Nedeltchev *et al.* 2007). One possible explanation for this paucity of knowledge may be the lack of public education programs targeting TIA. Most public-awareness messages regarding stroke warning signs do not emphasize that the occurrence of symptoms, whether transient or permanent, demands prompt medical attention and a call to emergency medical services.

However, more relevant to delays to treatment is actual behavior in the event of a TIA or minor stroke itself as opposed to knowledge among the general public. Data from Oxfordshire, UK, suggest that behavior is variable and significant delays are common (Giles *et al.* 2006; Chandratheva *et al.* 2010a). Consecutive patients with TIA or minor stroke participating in the Oxford Vascular Study (OXVASC) or attending dedicated hospital clinics were interviewed. Of 1,000 patients, 442 (44%) sought medical attention within 3 hours of the event and 700 (70%) did so on the same day (Chandratheva *et al.* 2010a). The majority (77%) of patients first sought medical attention through their primary care physician, and only 175 (18%) patients immediately attended the emergency department (ED). In patients with TIA, incorrect recognition of symptoms, absence of motor or speech symptoms, shorter duration of symptoms, lower $ABCD^2$ score, no prior history of stroke or atrial fibrillation, and presentation of TIA on weekends were associated with significantly longer delays in seeking medical attention (Chandratheva *et al.* 2010a). Age, sex, social class, and educational levels were all unrelated to correct recognition of symptoms or delay in seeking medical attention (Chandratheva *et al.* 2010a). These findings were supported from observations in a clinical trial of patients with asymptomatic carotid stenosis, in which only a third of those who had a TIA during follow-up reported it to medical attention within 3 days despite being regularly reminded to do so (Castaldo *et al.* 1997). These data suggest that frequent public education is required not only on the nature of a TIA but also on what to do in the event of one.

Recognition Tools

Several tools have been devised to aid the correct recognition of stroke and TIA symptoms (Table 19.1). In the pre-hospital setting, FAST (Face, Arm, Speech Test; Nor *et al.* 2004), LAPPS (Los Angeles Pre-hospital Stroke Scale; Kidwell *et al.* 2000) and CPSS (Cincinnati Pre-hospital Stroke Scale; Kothari *et al.* 1999) have been designed for use by emergency medical services to ensure rapid transport of appropriate patients to specialist care. In the ED setting, the Recognition of Stroke in the Emergency Department (ROSIER) score has been designed to aid emergency physicians in diagnosis and, therefore, referral of stroke patients (Nor *et al.* 2005) (Table 19.2). These tools are based mainly on features that discriminate both positively and negatively between stroke and stroke mimics and contain symptoms and signs.

The primary aim of these tools has been to increase the numbers of stroke patients presenting to hospital within 3 hours and, therefore, increase eligibility for thrombolysis. However, with increasing emphasis on rapid management for minor stroke and TIA, their use in informing public education and correct diagnosis of minor TIA and stroke is likely to

Table 19.1 Elements of early detection systems for transient ischemic attack and stroke

LAPSS	CPCC	FAST
Age > 45 years	Facial droop	Facial weakness
No previous seizure history	Arm drift	Arm and leg weakness
Onset within 24 hours	Slurred speech	Speech problems
Patient ambulant previously		
Blood glucose		
Asymmetry of:		
smile/grimace		
grip strength		
arm strength		

Notes: LAPSS, Los Angeles Pre-hospital Stroke Scale; CPCC, Cincinnati Pre-hospital Stroke Scale; FAST, Face, Arm, Speech Test.
Sources: From Kothari *et al.* (1999), Kidwell *et al.* (2000), and Nor *et al.* (2004).

Table 19.2 The Recognition of Stroke in the Emergency Department (ROSIER) score[a]

Feature	Score for answer	
	Yes	No
If blood glucose (BM) is < 3.5 mmol/L, treat urgently and then re-assess		
Has there been loss of consciousness or syncope?	−1	0
Has there been seizure activity?	−1	0
Is there a new acute onset (or awakening from sleep)?		
Asymmetrical facial weakness	+1	0
Asymmetrical arm weakness	+1	0
Asymmetrical leg weakness	+1	0
Speech disturbance	+1	0
Visual field defect	+1	0
Total (−2 to +5)		

[a] On validation in 343 patients with suspected stroke, the optimum cutoff point for stroke diagnosis was determined to be a total score of +1 or above. Using this cut point, the corresponding sensitivity and specificity were 92% (95% confidence interval [CI], 89–95) and 86% (95% CI, 82–90), respectively (Nor *et al.* 2005).

become more widespread. Indeed, data from OXVASC have shown that public education via the UK FAST TV campaign in 2009 was highly successful (Wolters *et al.* 2015). Stroke patients were more likely to present directly to emergency services and arrive at a hospital within 3 hours (median time to hospital arrival reduced from 185 to 119 minutes) during the 4-year period after the campaign (Wolters *et al.* 2015). Moreover, medical attention was sought by a bystander in 90% of these cases, illustrating the importance and success of mass-media public education (Wolters *et al.* 2015). Other risk stratification strategies such as the ABCD^2 score are also widely implemented to predict the early risk of stroke (especially severe events) following TIA, and one of their main uses has been in triage between primary and secondary care (Rothwell *et al.* 2005; Chandratheva *et al.* 2010b; National Institute for Health and Clinical Excellence 2017) (see Chapter 15).

Urgency and Clinical Setting for Treatment of Transient Ischemic Attack and Minor Stroke

A number of treatments have been shown to prevent stroke in the short and long term after a TIA or minor ischemic stroke (Chapter 24), including antiplatelet agents such as aspirin, clopidogrel, ticagrelor, and the combination of low-dose aspirin and extended-release dipyridamole or low-dose aspirin and clopidogrel (CAPRIE Steering Committee 1996; Diener *et al.* 1996; Antithrombotic Trialists Collaboration 2002; Halkes *et al.* 2006; Wong *et al.* 2013; Johnston *et al.* 2016; Rothwell *et al.* 2016); blood pressure–lowering drugs (Liu *et al.* 2009); statins (Amarenco *et al.* 2006); anticoagulation for atrial fibrillation (Hart *et al.* 2007; Ruff *et al.* 2014); and endarterectomy for symptomatic carotid stenosis ≥ 50% (Rothwell *et al.* 2003, 2004a). If the effects of these treatments are independent, combined use of all of these interventions in appropriate patients would be predicted to reduce the risk of recurrent stroke by 80–90% (Hackam and Spence 2007). However, although trials of treatment in acute stroke and acute coronary syndromes suggest that the relative benefits of several of these interventions are even greater in the acute phase, until recently there have been few reliable data on the benefits of acute treatment after TIA and minor stroke (Rothwell *et al.* 2007, 2016).

Guidelines suggest that assessment and investigation should be completed within 1 week of a TIA or minor stroke (Johnston *et al.* 2006; Kernan *et al.* 2014; National Institute for Health and Clinical Excellence 2017). However, perhaps unsurprisingly given the historical lack of evidence, there is considerable international variation in how patients with suspected TIA or minor stroke are managed in the acute phase. Some healthcare systems provide immediate emergency inpatient care, and others provide nonemergency outpatient clinic assessment.

Ranta and Barber (2016) reviewed seven different TIA service models from five countries (Lavallée *et al.* 2007; Rothwell *et al.* 2007; Wasserman *et al.* 2010; Olivot *et al.* 2011; Sanders *et al.* 2012; Ranta *et al.* 2015). In the traditional model, all patients with suspected TIA are admitted to a short-stay emergency department, medical assessment unit, or inpatient stroke unit with input from a stroke specialist. While this model has the advantage of being able to closely monitor all individuals in the early high risk period and hence maximize the chances of timely provision of intravenous thrombolytic therapy or endovascular therapy, this model will likely lead to admission of many non-vascular or low-risk patients. As these low-risk individuals would need to compete with other high-risk patients for investigations and inpatient assessments, hospital resources are not effectively utilized (Ranta and Barber 2016). Admitting all suspected TIA patients is therefore not cost-effective (Joshi *et al.* 2011).

Other TIA service models differ in their case identification (emergency department versus primary care versus 24-hour telephone hotline) and evaluation settings (emergency

Table 19.3 Summary of the study design for the Early Use of Existing Preventive Strategies for Stroke (EXPRESS) study

	Phase 1	Phase 2
Period	0–30 months	30–60 months
Appointment system	Daily appointment clinic	Emergency access clinic
Treatment initiation	Advice faxed to GP	Started immediately in clinic
Treatment protocol	Similar throughout	
Patient assessment	Similar throughout	
Follow-up	Similar throughout	
Outcome adjudication	Outcomes independently audited, blind to study period	

Note: GP, general practitioner.

department versus primary care practice versus specialist TIA outpatient clinic), triage and risk stratification algorithms, and personnel involved (stroke specialist, stroke team, and/or nurse specialist) (Burke and McDermott 2016; Ranta and Barber 2016). Implementation of these models has led to a significant 60–90% reduction in 90-day stroke risk, which is likely to be due to the timeliness of evaluation of patients (Ranta and Barber 2016). Although it remains unclear which model is superior or more cost-effective, the optimal model(s) to adopt would depend on the local needs and availability of resources. In the following section, we discuss two such TIA service models (Lavallée et al. 2007; Rothwell et al. 2007).

The Early Use of Existing Preventive Strategies for Stroke Study

The Early Use of Existing Preventive Strategies for Stroke (EXPRESS) study aimed to determine the effect of more rapid treatment after TIA and minor stroke in patients who were treated in a specialist neurovascular clinic (Rothwell et al. 2007) within OXVASC. In a prospective, population-based, sequential comparison study, the effect on the process of care and outcome of either urgent access and immediate treatment in a dedicated neuro-vascular clinic or an appointment-based access and routine treatment initiated in primary care was compared for all patients with TIA or minor stroke who did not need hospital admission. The primary outcome was the risk of stroke during the 90 days after first seeking medical attention.

The study was split into two 30-month phases lasting from April 2002 to September 2004 and from October 2004 to March 2007 (Table 19.3). Throughout the two phases, all patients in the study were ascertained and followed up in the same way, whether they were managed in the study's dedicated neurovascular clinic, admitted to the hospital, or managed at home by their general practitioner (primary care physician). During the first phase, the study clinic offered appointment-based access to patients and treatment recommendations were communicated by fax or telephone to the general practitioner, who would then initiate the prescription. In the second phase, patients were sent to the clinic urgently without the need for an appointment and treatment was started immediately in the clinic. The study clinic operated on weekdays but not on weekends. Importantly, throughout the study period, the

Table 19.4 Delay to seeking medical attention and subsequent delay in being seen in the clinic for all patients who were referred to the study clinic in the EXPRESS study[a]

Delay	Phase 1 (n = 310)	Phase 2 (n = 281)	p-value
First call for medical attention[b]			
≤ 12 hours	128 (41.3%)	105 (37.5%)	0.35
≤ 24 hours	184 (59.4%)	160 (57.1%)	0.62
First call for attention to assessment in study clinic[c]			
≤ 6 hours	5 (1.7%)	80 (29.0%)	< 0.0001
≤ 24 hours	70 (23.4%)	163 (59.1%)	< 0.0001

[a] See Table 19.3 for study details.
[b] Data unavailable for one patient in phase 2.
[c] Data unavailable for one patient in phase 1 and two patients in phase 2 and not applicable in a further 10 patients in phase 1 and three patients in phase 2 who were referred to the EXPRESS clinic but had a stroke and were admitted to hospital prior to the clinic assessment.
Source: From Rothwell *et al.* (2007).

treatment regimen used and methods of assessment, imaging, and follow-up did not change. If a recurrent vascular event was suspected at a follow-up visit, the patient was reassessed and investigated by a study physician, but all potential outcome events were independently adjudicated, blinded to study period (Table 19.3).

Of the 1,278 patients in the OXVASC population who presented with TIA or stroke throughout the study period, 607, predominantly with major stroke, were referred or presented directly to the hospital; 620 were referred for outpatient assessment with TIA or minor stroke; and 51 were not referred to secondary care. Of all outpatient referrals, 591 out of 620 (95%) were to the dedicated EXPRESS study neurovascular clinic. There were 634 events during phase 1 and 644 during phase 2.

Baseline characteristics and delays in seeking initial medical attention were similar in the two periods. However, median delay to assessment in the study clinic fell from 3 days (range, 2–5) in phase 1 to < 1 (range, 0–3) in phase 2 (p < 0.001) (Table 19.4), and the median delay to first prescription of treatment fell from 20 days (range, 8–53) to 1 day (range, 0–3) (p < 0.001). Fig. 19.1 shows the cumulative proportions of patients referred to the EXPRESS clinic in phases 1 and 2 and their resulting medication. The 90-day risk of recurrent stroke in all patients referred to the study clinic was 10.3% (32/310) in phase 1 versus 2.1% (6/281) in phase 2 (hazard ratio, 0.20; 95% confidence interval [CI], 0.08–0.48; p < 0.001) (Fig. 19.2). There was no significant change in risk in patients treated elsewhere. The 90-day risk of recurrent stroke after all TIA or stroke presentations in the whole population fell from 9.9% (63/635) in phase 1 to 4.4% (28/644) in phase 2 (p = 0.0002), while that for patients with TIA alone fell from 12.4% (29/233) in phase 1 to 4.4% (11/252) in phase 2 (p = 0.0015). This reduction in risk was independent of age and sex, and early treatment did not increase the risk of intracerebral hemorrhage or other bleeding.

Because the EXPRESS study was nested within OXVASC (Rothwell *et al.* 2004b), identical methods of case ascertainment, assessment, and follow-up for the entire study population during both phases ensured that there were no temporal changes in referral patterns, patient characteristics, or other potential sources of bias. The findings, therefore,

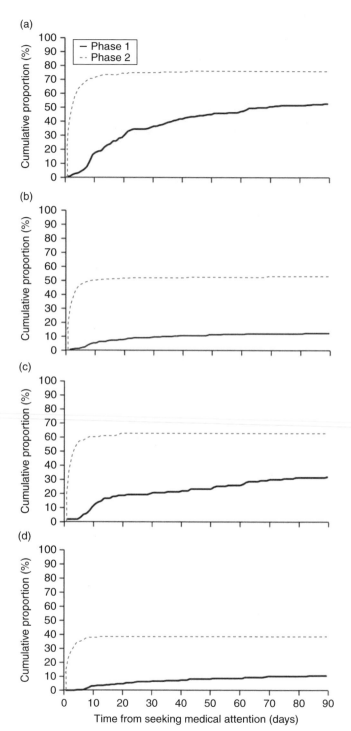

Fig. 19.1 Cumulative proportions of patients referred to the Early Use of Existing Preventive Strategies for Stroke (EXPRESS) study clinic in phases 1 (—) and 2 (–) prescribed new medication. (a) Any statin drug (in patients not already on a statin); (b) clopidogrel (usually in addition to aspirin); (c) initiation of a first blood pressure–lowering drug (in patients not already on such medication); (d) initiation of two blood pressure-lowering drugs (in patients previously on no or only one drug) (Rothwell *et al.* 2007).

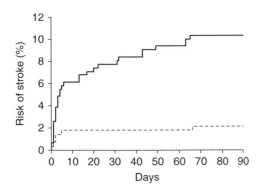

Fig. 19.2 The 90-day risk of recurrent stroke after first seeking medical attention in all patients with transient ischemic attack or stroke referred to the study clinic in the non-randomized Early Use of Existing Preventive Strategies for Stroke (EXPRESS) study (Rothwell *et al.* 2007). The continuous line represents phase 1 of the study (standard treatment), and the dotted line represents phase 2 (urgent treatment).

strongly suggested that the considerable impact on outcome was a consequence of more rapid assessment and treatment.

The SOS-TIA Study

The good prognosis associated with urgent and intensive treatment observed in the EXPRESS study was also highlighted by the results of the SOS-TIA study (Lavallée *et al.* 2007). In 2003, a dedicated emergency TIA clinic was set up in the Neurology Department of the Neurology and Stroke Center of Bichat Hospital in an administrative region of Paris. All 15,000 general practitioners, cardiologists, neurologists, and ophthalmologists in the region were sent information about the service, which offered emergency assessment of all patients with suspected TIA via a toll-free referral telephone number. The SOS-TIA service was available and accessible 24 hours a day, 7 days a week. It aimed to offer an evaluation by a vascular neurologist within 4 hours of referral: if a TIA was confirmed, further standardized investigations were performed including MRI, carotid Doppler, and transcranial Doppler ultrasound. Medical treatment was initiated immediately. Patients were discharged home unless they fulfilled predefined criteria for admission to the hospital's stroke unit (Table 19.5).

The study recorded the medical history, medications, symptom details, examination findings, final diagnosis, treatment plans, and 1-year outcomes (assessed by phone calls) of all referrals. In the first report of all 629 consecutive patients with definite TIA seen from January 2003 to December 2005, there were 3 strokes within 7 days and 12 strokes within 3 months of follow-up, giving risks of 0.3% and 1.9%, respectively. The expected risk of stroke at 3 months as calculated by the $ABCD^2$ score (Johnston *et al.* 2007) was 6%. Although there was no formal comparison arm of the study, the considerable reduction in observed rates of stroke compared with those expected by the $ABCD^2$ score was reasonably attributed to urgent access to and treatment in a dedicated specialist neurovascular unit. However, it should be noted that this study assessed stroke risk only among patients referred to the clinic and not all those within the population.

Specific Treatments in Transient Ischemic Attack and Minor Stroke

One potential criticism of the EXPRESS (Rothwell *et al.* 2007) and SOS-TIA (Lavallée *et al.* 2007) studies is that a "black box" intervention approach was used. All patients received a standardized treatment regimen of antiplatelet agents, antihypertensives, and statins plus,

Table 19.5 Criteria for admission to the stroke unit after assessment in the SOS-TIA clinic

	Criteria
Related to TIA cause (highly suspected or identified)	High-grade stenosis of intra- or extracranial brain arteries
	Intracranial hemodynamic compromise with low flow in the middle cerebral artery
	Suspected cardiac source at high risk of recurrent embolism: prosthetic mechanical heart valve, endocarditis, aortic dissection, acute coronary syndrome, overt congestive heart failure
Related to the TIA presentation	Crescendo TIA
Cardiac monitoring over 24 hours warranted	High level of suspicion for paroxysmal atrial fibrillation

Note: TIA, transient ischemic attack.

in selected cases, anticoagulation and carotid endarterectomy, which was administered rapidly in the context of an urgent-access dedicated neurovascular service. The relative benefit or even harm attributable to any particular part of the interventional package could not be determined. However, recent meta-analysis of 12 aspirin trials ($n = 15778$) showed that aspirin is the key intervention in reducing the risk of early recurrent stroke (Rothwell *et al.* 2016). In patients presenting with TIA or minor stroke, aspirin reduced the 6-week risk of recurrent ischemic stroke by 62% and the risk of disabling or fatal ischemic stroke by 81% (Rothwell *et al.* 2016).

Trials studying the efficacy of antiplatelet agents other than aspirin in patients with acute TIA or minor ischemic stroke are limited (see Chapter 24). Clopidogrel, for example, was studied in the Clopidogrel versus Aspirin in Patients at Risk of Ischemic Events (CAPRIE) trial among patients with occlusive vascular disease not limited to acute TIA or minor ischemic stroke (CAPRIE Steering Committee 1996), while cilostazol was investigated in patients who had an ischemic stroke within the past 6 months (Huang *et al.* 2008; Shinohara *et al.* 2010) (see Chapter 24). Ticagrelor is a newer-generation antiplatelet agent that reversibly binds and inhibits the P2Y12 receptor on platelets. However, in contrast to other thienopyridines that also block the P2Y12 receptor, such as clopidogrel, ticagrelor is orally active and does not require metabolic activation. Compared with clopidogrel, ticagrelor has also been shown to have a faster onset of action and more potent inhibition of platelet aggregation and hence is a promising new antiplatelet agent in patients with ischemic stroke (Husted *et al.* 2006; Storey *et al.* 2007). Recently, the Acute Stroke or Transient Ischemic Attack Treated with Aspirin or Ticagrelor and Patient Outcomes (SOCRATES) trial compared ticagrelor with aspirin in 13,199 patients with acute (onset within 24 hours) non-cardioembolic high-risk TIA or minor ischemic stroke (Johnston *et al.* 2016). Although the primary endpoint of stroke, myocardial infarction or death within 90 days, did not differ between ticagrelor (6.7%) and aspirin (7.5%) (hazard ratio 0.89; 95% CI, 0.78–1.01; $p = 0.07$), the secondary endpoint of recurrent ischemic stroke at 90 days was marginally significant in favor of ticagrelor use (5.8% versus 6.7%; hazard ratio 0.87, 95% CI, 0.76–1.00; p = 0.046). Furthermore, in a prespecified subgroup analysis of 3,081 patients with a potentially symptomatic ipsilateral atherosclerotic stenosis, a treatment-by-atherosclerotic stenosis interaction was noted (p = 0.017) (Amarenco et al. 2017). Fewer patients in the ticagrelor group with ipsilateral stenosis developed a stroke, myocardial infarction, or death within 90 days (6.7%), compared with 9.6% of patients in the aspirin group (hazard ratio 0.68, 95% CI 0.53–0.88; p = 0.003). In contrast, no significant differences in rate of stroke, myocardial infarction, or death at 90 days were noted in the 10,118 patients with no ipsilateral stenosis (p = 0.72). There were also no significant differences in risk of bleeding in patients treated with ticagrelor or aspirin (Johnston et al. 2016; Amarenco et al. 2017). Nevertheless, whether efficacy of ticagrelor is superior to combination antiplatelets (discussed later) in patients with high-risk TIA or ischemic stroke has yet to be studied.

Combination Antiplatelet Treatment

The FASTER randomized controlled pilot trial studied the benefit of clopidogrel versus placebo and simvastatin versus placebo initiated within 24 hours of symptom onset in patients with TIA or minor stroke, all of whom were treated with aspirin (Kennedy et al. 2007). The primary outcome was any stroke (ischemic and hemorrhagic) within 90 days. Minor stroke was defined as a score ≤ 3 on the National Institutes of Health Stroke Scale (NIHSS) at the time of randomization, and TIA was defined in the usual way. In addition, patients were excluded if they did not have weakness or speech disturbance or if symptom duration was less than 5 minutes.

The trial was stopped early owing to a failure to recruit patients, probably because of the increased use of statins during the study period. A total of 392 patients were included (mean age 68.1 years; 185 [47.1%] female) of whom 100 received clopidogrel and simvastatin, 98 received clopidogrel and placebo, 99 received simvastatin and placebo, and 95 received placebo only. In the patients taking clopidogrel, 14 (7.1%) had a stroke within 90 days, compared with 21 (10.8%) of those on placebo (risk ratio, 0.7 [95% CI, 0.3–1.2]; absolute risk reduction, −3.8% [95% CI, −9.4 to 1.9]; p = 0.19). Two patients on clopidogrel had intracranial hemorrhage compared with none on placebo (absolute risk increase, 1.0% [95% CI, −0.4 to 2.4]; p = 0.5). In the group taking simvastatin, 21 (10.6%) patients had a stroke within 90 days, compared with 14 (7.3%) patients taking placebo (risk ratio, 1.3 [95% CI, 0.7–2.4]; absolute risk increase, 3.3% [95% CI, −2.3 to 8.9]; p = 0.25), and there was no difference between groups for the simvastatin safety outcomes.

The study concluded that the combination of aspirin and clopidogrel started within 24 hours of symptom onset may be superior to aspirin alone in reducing the risk of stroke at 90 days after TIA or minor stroke, although at the expense of a higher rate of hemorrhage. These results were subsequently confirmed in the Clopidogrel in High-Risk Patients with Acute Non-disabling Cerebrovascular Events (CHANCE) trial (Wang et al. 2013), which demonstrated that use of clopidogrel (300 mg loading dose followed by 75 mg daily) and aspirin 75 mg daily within 24 hours of symptom onset for 21 days followed by clopidogrel 75 mg only was superior to aspirin 75 mg alone in reducing the 90-day risk of recurrent stroke (8.2% versus 11.7%) among patients with high-risk TIA or minor ischemic stroke (Wang et al. 2013). There were no differences in the risk of intracerebral hemorrhage in the two treatment arms (both 0.3%) (Wang et al. 2013). The Platelet-Oriented Inhibition in New TIA and minor ischemic stroke (POINT) trial is currently under way and similarly studies the benefits of dual antiplatelet therapy in prevention of early recurrent stroke in patients with minor ischemic stroke or TIA but aims to initiate antiplatelet treatment within 12 hours of symptom onset (Johnston *et al.* 2013). Duration of dual antiplatelet treatment is also longer (90 days) compared with the CHANCE trial (Johnston *et al.* 2013). The potential benefit of 30 days of triple antiplatelet agents (aspirin, clopidogrel plus dipyridamole) versus standard care (clopidogrel alone or combined aspirin and dipyridamole) in patients with high-risk TIA or ischemic stroke was also tested recently in the Triple Antiplatelets for Reducing Dependency in Ischemic Stroke trial (TARDIS) (Bath *et al.* 2017). Patients receiving triple antiplatelet therapy were not at reduced risk of recurrent TIA or ischemic stroke at 90 days (6% versus 7%) but were at significantly increased risk of more frequent and more severe bleeding (Bath *et al.* 2017).

References

Amarenco P, Bogousslavsky J, Callahan A III for the Stroke Prevention by Aggressive Reduction in Cholesterol Levels (SPARCL) Investigators (2006). High-dose atorvastatin after stroke or transient ischemic attack. *New England Journal of Medicine* 355:549–559

Amarenco P, Albers GW, Denison H *et al.* (2017). Efficacy and safety of ticagrelor versus aspirin in acute stroke or transient ischemic attack of atherosclerotic origin: A subgroup analysis of SOCRATES, a randomized, double-blind, controlled trial. *Lancet Neurology* 16:301–310

Antithrombotic Trialists Collaboration (2002). Collaborative meta-analysis of randomised trials of antiplatelet therapy for prevention of death, myocardial infarction, and stroke in high risk patients. *British Medical Journal* 324:71–86

Bath PM, Robson K, Woodhouse LJ *et al.* (2015). Statistical analysis plan for the 'Triple Antiplatelets for Reducing Dependency after Ischemic Stroke' (TARDIS) trial. *International Journal of Stroke* 10:449–451

Bath PM, Woodhouse LJ, Appleton JP *et al.* (2017). Antiplatelet therapy with aspirin, clopidogrel, and dipyridamole versus clopidogrel alone or aspirin and dipyridamole in patients with acute cerebral ischemic (TARDIS): A randomized, open-label, phase 3 superiority trial. *Lancet*. doi:10.1016/S0140-6736(17)32849-0 [Epub ahead of print]

Burke JF, McDermott M (2016). Pursuing "model care" of transient ischemic attacks. *Neurology* 86:888–889

CAPRIE Steering Committee (1996). A randomised, blinded, trial of clopidogrel versus aspirin in patients at risk of ischaemic events (CAPRIE). *Lancet* 348:1329–1339

Carroll C, Hobart J, Fox C *et al.* (2004). Stroke in Devon: Knowledge was good, but action was poor. *Journal of Neurology, Neurosurgery and Psychiatry* 75:567–571

Castaldo JE, Nelson JJ, Reed JF III *et al.* (1997). The delay in reporting symptoms of carotid artery stenosis in an at-risk population. The Asymptomatic Carotid Atherosclerosis Study experience: A statement of concern regarding watchful waiting. *Archives of Neurology* 54:1267–1271

Chandratheva A, Lasserson DS, Geraghty OC *et al.* (2010a). Population-based study of behavior immediately after transient ischemic attack and minor stroke in 1000 consecutive patients: Lessons for public education. *Stroke* 41:1108–1114

Chandratheva A, Geraghty OC, Luengo-Fernandez R *et al.* (2010b). ABCD² score predicts severity rather than risk of early recurrent events after transient ischemic attack. *Stroke* 41:851–856

Diener HC, Cunha L, Forbes C *et al.* (1996). European secondary prevention study 2: Dipyridamole and acetylsalicylic acid in the secondary prevention of stroke. *Journal of Neurology Science* 143:1–13

Evenson KR, Rosamond WD, Morris DL (2001). Prehospital and in-hospital delays in acute stroke care. *Neuroepidemiology* 20:65–76

Giles MF, Flossman E, Rothwell PM (2006). Patient behaviour immediately after transient ischemic attack according to clinical characteristics, perception of the event, and predicted risk of stroke. *Stroke* 37:1254–1260

Hackam DG, Spence JD (2007). Combining multiple approaches for the secondary prevention of vascular events after stroke: A quantitative modeling study. *Stroke* 38:1881–1885

Halkes PH, van Gijn J for the ESPRIT Study Group (2006). Aspirin plus dipyridamole versus aspirin alone after cerebral ischaemia of arterial origin (ESPRIT): Randomised controlled trial. *Lancet* 367:1665–1673

Harraf F, Sharma AK, Brown MM *et al.* (2002). A multicentre observational study of presentation and early assessment of acute stroke. *British Medical Journal* 325:17–22

Hart RG, Pearce LA, Aguilar MI (2007). Meta-analysis: Antithrombotic therapy to prevent stroke in patients who have nonvalvular atrial fibrillation. *Annals of Internal Medicine* 146:857–867

Huang Y, Cheng Y, Wu J *et al.* (2008). Cilostazol as an alternative to aspirin after ischemic stroke: A randomized, double-blind, pilot study. *Lancet Neurology* 7:494–499

Husted S, Emanuelsson H, Heptinstall S *et al.* (2006). Pharmacodynamics, pharmacokinetics, and safety of the oral reversible P2Y12 antagonist AZD6140 with aspirin in patients with atherosclerosis: A double-blind comparison to clopidogrel with aspirin. *European Heart Journal* 27:1038–1047

Johnston SC, Fayad PB, Gorelick PB *et al.* (2003). Prevalence and knowledge of transient ischemic attack among US adults. *Neurology* 60:1429–1434

Johnston SC, Nguyen-Huynh MN, Schwarz ME *et al.* (2006). National Stroke Association guidelines for the management of transient ischemic attacks. *Annals of Neurology* 60:301–313

Johnston SC, Rothwell PM, Nguyen-Huynh MN *et al.* (2007). Validation and refinement of scores to predict very early stroke risk after transient ischaemic attack. *Lancet* 369:283–292

Johnston SC, Easton JD, Farrant M *et al.* (2013). Platelet-oriented inhibition in new TIA and minor ischemic stroke (POINT) trial: Rationale

and design. *International Journal of Stroke* 8:479–483

Johnston SC, Amarenco P, Albers GW *et al.* (2016). Ticagrelor versus aspirin in acute stroke or transient ischemic attack. *New England Journal of Medicine* 375:35–43

Joshi JK, Ouyang B, Prabhakaran S (2011). Should TIA patients be hospitalized or referred to a same-day clinic?: A decision analysis. *Neurology* 77:2082–2088

Kennedy J, Hill MD, Ryckborst KJ *et al.* (2007). Fast Assessment of Stroke and Transient Ischaemic Attack to Prevent Early Recurrence (FASTER): A randomised controlled pilot trial. *Lancet Neurology* 6:961–969

Kernan WN, Ovbiagele B, Black HR *et al.* (2014). Guidelines for the prevention of stroke in patients with stroke and transient ischemic attack: A guideline for healthcare professionals from the American Heart Association/American Stroke Association. *Stroke* 45:2160–2236

Kidwell CS, Starkman S, Eckstein M *et al.* (2000). Identifying stroke in the field. Prospective validation of the Los Angeles prehospital stroke screen (LAPSS). *Stroke* 31:71–76

Kothari RU, Pancioli A, Liu T *et al.* (1999). Cincinnati Prehospital Stroke Scale: Reproducibility and validity. *Annals of Emergency Medicine* 33:373–378

Lacy CR, Suh DC, Bueno M *et al.* (2001). Delay in presentation and evaluation for acute stroke: Stroke Time Registry for Outcomes Knowledge and Epidemiology (STROKE). *Stroke* 32:63–69

Lavallée PC, Meseguer E, Abboud H *et al.* (2007). A transient ischaemic attack clinic with round-the-clock access (SOS-TIA): Feasibility and effects. *Lancet Neurology* 6:953–960

Lecouturier J, Murtagh MJ, Thomson RG *et al.* (2010). Response to symptoms of stroke in the UK: A systematic review. *BMC Health Services Research* 10:157

Liu L, Wang Z, Gong L *et al.* (2009). Blood pressure reduction for the secondary prevention of stroke: A Chinese trial and a systematic review of the literature. *Hypertension Research* 32:1032–1040

National Institute for Health and Clinical Excellence (2017). *Stroke and Transient Ischemic*

Attack in Over 16s: Diagnosis and Initial Management. London: NICE

Nedeltchev K, Fischer U, Arnold M *et al.* (2007). Low awareness of transient ischemic attacks and risk factors of stroke in a Swiss urban community. *Journal of Neurology* **254**:179–184

Nor A, Mc Allister C, Louw S *et al.* (2004). Agreement between ambulance paramedicand physician-recorded neurological signs using the Face Arm Speech Test (FAST) in acute stroke patients. *Stroke* **35**:1355–1359

Nor AM, Davis J, Sen B *et al.* (2005). The Recognition of Stroke in the Emergency Room (ROSIER) scale: Development and validation of a stroke recognition instrument. *Lancet Neurology* **4**:727–734

Olivot JM, Wolford C, Castle J *et al.* (2011). Two aces: Transient ischemic attack work-up as outpatient assessment of clinical evaluation and safety. *Stroke* **42**:1839–1843

Pancioli A, Broderick J, Kothari R *et al.* (1998). Public perception of stroke warning signs and knowledge of potential risk factors. *Journal of the American Medical Association* **279**:1288–1292

Parahoo K, Thompson K, Cooper M *et al.* (2003). Stroke: Awareness of the signs, symptoms and risk factors – a population-based survey. *Cerebrovascular Diseases* **16**:134–140

Ranta A, Dovey S, Weatherall M *et al.* (2015). Cluster randomized controlled trial of TIA electronic decision support in primary care. *Neurology* **84**:1545–1551

Ranta A, Barber PA (2016). Transient ischemic attack service provision: A review of available service models. *Neurology* **86**:947–953

Reeves MJ, Hogan JG, Rafferty AP (2002). Knowledge of stroke risk factors and warning signs among Michigan adults. *Neurology* **59**:1547–1552

Rothwell PM, Gutnikov SA, Eliasziw M for the Carotid Endarterectomy Trialists' Collaboration (2003). Pooled analysis of individual patient data from randomised controlled trials of endarterectomy for symptomatic carotid stenosis. *Lancet* **361**:107–116

Rothwell PM, Eliasziw M, Gutnikov SA for the Carotid Endarterectomy Trialists Collaboration (2004a). Effect of endarterectomy for symptomatic carotid stenosis in relation to clinical subgroups and to the timing of surgery. *Lancet* **363**:915–924

Rothwell PM, Coull A, Giles MF for the Oxford Vascular Study (2004b). Change in stroke incidence, mortality, case-fatality, severity, and risk factors in Oxfordshire, UK from 1981 to 2004 (Oxford Vascular Study). *Lancet* **363**:1925–1933

Rothwell PM, Giles MF, Flossman E *et al.* (2005). A simple score (ABCD) to identify individuals at high early risk of stroke after transient ischaemic attack. *Lancet* **366**:29–36

Rothwell PM, Giles MF, Chandratheva A *et al.* (2007). Effect of urgent treatment of transient ischaemic attack and minor stroke on early recurrent stroke (EXPRESS study): A prospective population-based sequential comparison. *Lancet* **370**:1432–1442

Rothwell PM, Algra A, Chen Z *et al.* (2016). Effects of aspirin on risk and severity of early recurrent stroke after transient ischemic attack and ischemic stroke: Time-course analysis of randomized trials. *Lancet* **388**:365–375

Ruff CT, Giugliano RP, Braunwald E *et al.* (2014). Comparison of the efficacy and safety of new oral anticoagulants with warfarin in patients with atrial fibrillation: A meta-analysis of randomized trials. *Lancet* **383**:955–962

Salisbury HR, Banks BJ, Footitt DR *et al.* (1998). Delay in presentation of patients with acute stroke to hospital in Oxford. *Quarterly Journal of Medicine* **97**:635–640

Sanders LM, Srikanth VK, Jolley DJ *et al.* (2012). Monash transient ischemic attack triaging treatment: Safety of a transient ischemic attack mechanism-based outpatient model of care. *Stroke* **43**:2936–2941

Shinohara Y, Katayama Y, Uchiyama S *et al.* (2010). Cilostazol for prevention of secondary stroke (CSPS 2): An aspirin-controlled, double-blind, randomized non-inferiority trial. *Lancet Neurology* **9**:959–968

Smith MA, Doliszny KM, Shahar E *et al.* (1998). Delayed hospital arrival for acute stroke: The Minnesota Stroke Survey. *Annals of International Medicine* **129**:190–196

Storey RF, Husted S, Harrington RA *et al.* (2007). Inhibition of platelet aggregation by

AZD6140, a reversible oral P2Y12 receptor antagonist, compared with clopidogrel in patient with acute coronary syndromes. *Journal of American College of Cardiology* **50**:1852–1856

Wang Y Wang Y, Zhao X *et al.* (2013). Clopidogrel with aspirin in acute minor stroke or transient ischemic attack. *New England Journal of Medicine* 369:11–19

Wasserman J, Perry J, Dowlatshahi D *et al.* (2010). Stratified, urgent care for transient ischemic attack results in low stroke rates. *Stroke* **41**:2601–2605

Wolters FJ, Paul NL, Li L *et al.* (2015). Sustained impact of UK FAST-test public education on response to stroke: A population-based time-series study. *International Journal of Stroke* **10**:1108–1114

Wong KS, Wang Y, Leng X *et al.* (2013). Early dual versus mono antiplatelet therapy for acute non-cardioembolic ischemic stroke or transient ischemic attack: An updated systematic review and meta-analysis. *Circulation* **128**:1656–1666

Chapter 20
Acute Treatment of Major Stroke: General Principles

The general treatments described in this chapter are applicable to all patients with acute major stroke regardless of etiology. Specific treatment for ischemic and hemorrhagic stroke is discussed in Chapters 21 and 22, respectively. Therapy for acute stroke can be divided into:

- treatment of the acute event in which the aim is to minimize mortality, impairment, and disability and reduce the complications of stroke.
- prevention of recurrent stroke.

For patients who have suffered a major disabling stroke, emphasis is placed, at least initially, on the former, whereas in patients with TIA or minor stroke, the emphasis is on the latter.

Non-Neurological Complications and Their Management

Non-neurological complications after acute stroke are more frequent with increasing age, pre-stroke disability, stroke severity, and poor general nursing and other care (Box 20.1).

BOX 20.1 General Medical Complications of Acute Stroke

Pneumonia

Venous thromboembolism

Urinary incontinence and infection

Pressure sores

Cardiac arrhythmias, failure, myocardial infarction

Fluid imbalance, hyponatremia

"Mechanical" problems

- spasticity
- contractures
- malalignment/subluxation/frozen shoulder
- falls and fractures
- osteoporosis
- ankle swelling
- peripheral nerve pressure palsies

Depression

Fatigue

Gastric ulceration and hemorrhage

Pain

Table 20.1 Routine monitoring in acute stroke

	Monitor
Vital signs	Respiratory rate and rhythm, blood gases Heart rate and rhythm (often with electrocardiographic monitor) Blood pressure (normal arm) Temperature (normal axilla)
Neurological	Conscious level (Glasgow Coma Scale) Pupils Limb weakness Epileptic seizures
General	Fluid balance Electrolytes and urea Blood glucose Hematocrit

To some extent, the site of the lesion may also be relevant; for instance, obstructive and central sleep apnea might occur more often in brainstem stroke (Davenport *et al.* 1996a; van der Worp and Kappelle 1998). Early detection and prevention of complications depend on clinical monitoring (Table 20.1).

Pneumonia

Pneumonia is a frequent complication after stroke and is the most common cause of fever during the first 2 days of an acute stroke (Kumar *et al.* 2010). It is also associated with a threefold increased risk of death compared with patients without pneumonia (Katzan *et al.* 2003). Post-stroke pneumonia is most commonly due to aspiration of bacteria that are seeded in the gingival crevices or have colonized the pharynx (Kumar *et al.* 2010). Risk factors for post-stroke pneumonia include: age > 65 years, more severe stroke, brainstem stroke, multi-territory stroke, dysphagia, speech or cognitive impairment, weakness of expiratory or facial muscles, impaired cough reflex, reduced level of consciousness, and mechanical ventilation (Kobayashi *et al.* 1994; Hilker *et al.* 2003; Martino *et al.* 2005; Sellars *et al.* 2007). The risk can be reduced by maintaining good dental hygiene and oral care, positioning patients who are unable to handle their own secretions in a semi-upright position with frequent oral suctioning, and use of oral antiseptics in ventilated patients (Yoneyama *et al.* 1999; Chan *et al.* 2007). Routine use of antibiotics was not shown to be effective in prevention of post-stroke pneumonia or improve functional outcome (Kalra *et al.* 2015; Westendorp *et al.* 2015).

Venous Thromboembolism

In the absence of thromboprophylaxis, approximately 50% of hemiparetic patients in hospital develop a deep vein thrombosis (DVT) in their paralyzed leg. However, a recent study conducted in a specialized stroke unit showed that only 2.5% of patients would develop a clinically apparent DVT during the first 3 months of stroke

(Indredavik *et al.* 2008). Nevertheless, a swollen and painful leg compromises rehabilitation, and a resultant pulmonary embolism (~1.2% of stroke patients) causes hypoxia and pneumonia, affects neurological recovery, and may cause death (Indredavik *et al.* 2008; Kumar *et al.* 2010). Risk factors for DVT include old age, severe stroke, and dehydration (Kumar *et al.* 2010). Subcutaneous heparin and aspirin are effective in reducing the risk of DVT (Andre *et al.* 2007; Sandercock *et al.* 2014). However, the benefit of prophylactic heparin in preventing symptomatic pulmonary embolism is outweighed by its risk of symptomatic intracerebral hemorrhage, and so it is not recommended for routine use (Geeganage *et al.* 2013; Hankey 2017). Aspirin should be given after ischemic stroke since this reduces the risk of recurrent stroke as well as venous thromboembolism (Sandercock *et al.* 2014; Rothwell *et al.* 2016). Graduated compression stockings do not reduce risk of DVT, pulmonary embolism, or mortality but are associated with a fourfold increased risk of skin ulcers and necrosis and a small increased risk in lower-limb ischemia (CLOTS Trials Collaboration 2009). Recently, it has been shown that in immobile patients, intermittent pneumatic compression with thigh-length sleeves worn on both legs for 30 days reduces proximal and symptomatic DVT and improves 6-month survival but does not improve functional outcome (CLOTS Trials Collaboration 2014).

Urinary Incontinence and Urinary Tract Infections

Urinary incontinence affects 40–60% of acute stroke patients and can be permanent in up to 15% (Barrett 2001). Older patients and those with diabetes, hypertension, prior disability, and more severe strokes are at increased risk (Nakayama *et al.* 1997; Brittain *et al.* 1998). Urinary incontinence is often due to damage to the corticospinal pathways resulting in detrusor hyper-reflexia (Gelber *et al.* 1993). Patients may also have overflow incontinence as a result of a hyporeflexic bladder secondary to neuropathy or medication use (e.g., anticholinergics) (Gelber *et al.* 1993). Urinary incontinence often affects the morale and self-esteem of patients, imposes a substantial burden on their caregivers, results in delays in hospital discharge, and can lead to institutionalized care (Patel *et al.* 2001). Although current trials are insufficient to guide continence care of adults after stroke due to a high degree of heterogeneity, systematic assessment and management of urinary symptoms with specialized professional input appear to be beneficial (Thomas *et al.* 2008). Catheterization is often required to maintain skin care, at least initially. Urinary infection is common owing to immobility and the use of urinary catheters (Kumar *et al.* 2010).

Pressure Sores

Patients with stroke, especially those who are bedridden, are susceptible to developing pressure sores, most often occurring at the sacrum, buttocks, and heels. Incontinence, malnourishment, and immobility increase the risk of skin breaks. Pressure sores may become infected and may take months to heal, thus delaying rehabilitation. They can be avoided by early mobilization, frequent turning of immobile patients, special attention to pressure areas, and use of padded heel boots and air mattresses (National Institute for Health and Care Excellence 2014).

Cardiac Complications

Patients with acute stroke are susceptible to a number of cardiac complications (Kumar *et al.* 2010). Indeed, stroke and ischemic heart disease share common risk factors, and cardiac diseases such as atrial fibrillation, valvular heart disease, and congestive heart failure increase the risk of stroke. Autonomic dysfunction is common after stroke and can also result in arrhythmias, myocardial injury with elevated serum troponin levels, acute coronary syndrome, stress cardiomyopathy (Takotsubo syndrome), and sudden death (Kumar *et al.* 2010; Sörös and Hachinski 2012).

Electrocardiographic ST depression, T wave flattening and inversion, U waves, and a prolonged Q–T interval are common after acute ischemic, and particularly after acute hemorrhagic stroke. They are often transient and seldom cause clinical problems. Some abnormalities may have preceded the stroke (Oppenheimer *et al.* 1990). However, recent data showed that a prolonged Q-T interval in patients with ischemic stroke is independently associated with an increased risk of cardiac death (Prosser *et al.* 2007).

The annual risks of non-stroke vascular death or an acute coronary syndrome in stroke patients are ~2% (Touzé *et al.* 2005). However, the early risks of non-stroke vascular death may be up to ~4%, likely due to the more immediate physiological consequences of stroke on the cardiovascular system (Prosser *et al.* 2007). The insula, in particular, is a crucial center for control of autonomic function, and strokes involving the right insula may result in parasympathetic overactivity, bradyarrhythmias, and asystole. On the other hand, strokes affecting the left insula may result in sympathetic overactivity, tachyarrhythmias, and ventricular fibrillation (Sörös and Hachinski 2012).

Fluid Imbalance

Patients unable to take sufficient fluids orally require fluid by nasogastric tube or intravenous hydration. Hyponatremia, probably reflecting salt wasting and the stress response, is particularly common after subarachnoid hemorrhage and, in general, should be treated by plasma volume expansion and not fluid restriction. Urinary tract infection and dehydration may cause renal failure.

Mechanical Problems

Spasticity, muscle contractures, painful shoulder and other joints of a paralyzed limb, malalignment or subluxation of the shoulder, falls, and fractures can all potentially be avoided by good nursing and physiotherapy. Osteoporosis in a paralyzed limb presumably increases the risk of fractures but may be unavoidable (Sato *et al.* 1998). As most fractures are the result of a fall, all stroke patients should receive a fall assessment. Those at high risk of falls include patients with cognitive or motor impairments, difficulties in balance, inattention, seizures, and white matter disease on brain imaging (Kumar *et al.* 2010). Use of hip protectors as shock absorbers in the nursing care or residential care setting reduces the risk of hip fractures in the elderly but does not reduce the risk of falls (Santesso *et al.* 2014). They are, however, not well accepted in general by users, and overall compliance is poor (Santesso *et al.* 2014).

Gastrointestinal Bleeding

Gastrointestinal bleeding occurs in approximately 1.5% of patients with ischemic stroke during the inpatient period (O'Donnell *et al.* 2008), but the incidence appears to be higher in patients of Asian ethnicity (Hsu *et al.* 2009). Predictors of gastrointestinal bleeding in stroke patients include more severe strokes, history of peptic ulcer disease, concomitant malignancy, renal failure, sepsis, and liver function derangement (Davenport *et al.* 1996b; O'Donnell *et al.* 2008; Hsu *et al.* 2009). Individuals receiving enteral nutrition via a nasogastric tube are also at higher risk compared with those feeding via a percutaneous endoscopic gastrostomy tube (Dennis *et al.* 2005). Patients with gastrointestinal hemorrhage are more likely to develop recurrent stroke, acute coronary syndrome, venous thromboembolism, and death, possibly due to hemodynamic instability or cessation of antithrombotic treatment (O'Donnell *et al.* 2008). Use of prophylactic antacids, H2-receptor antagonists, and proton-pump inhibitors is effective in reducing the risks of gastrointestinal bleeding and should be considered in patients at high risk of gastrointestinal bleeding (Cook *et al.* 1996).

Depression

A systematic review of observational studies of post-stroke depression produced an estimated overall prevalence of 33% among all stroke survivors (Hackett *et al.* 2005). Women, younger patients, and those with greater disability and cognitive impairment are at increased risk (Carota *et al.* 2005; Hackett and Andersen 2005). It has been postulated that left-sided brain lesions are more likely to cause depression, but this remains unproven (Bhogal *et al.* 2004). Depression may impede rehabilitation and contribute to disability and handicap but usually improves with time. Selective serotonin reuptake inhibitors appear to improve dependence, neurological impairment, anxiety, and depression after stroke (Mead *et al.* 2012). Psychotherapy may also prevent depression and improve mood (Hackett *et al.* 2008).

Pain

Up to a third of patients may experience moderate to severe pain in the first few months after stroke and are transient in most cases (Jönsson *et al.* 2006). Post-stroke pain mainly affects the limbs (particularly shoulders) and also the head. Central post-stroke pain syndrome, or "thalamic" pain, is a burning, severe, and paroxysmal pain exacerbated by touch and other stimuli. Such post-stroke pain is rare and usually occurs weeks or months after stroke (Nasreddine and Saver 1997; Frese *et al.* 2006). There are usually some sensory signs in the affected areas. The lesion is usually located in the contralateral thalamus but may lie elsewhere in the central sensory pathways. Treatments that have been shown to be effective include amitriptyline, lamotrigine, gabapentin, and pregabalin (Leijon and Boivie 1989; Vestergaard *et al.* 2001; Kim *et al.* 2011; Hesami *et al.* 2015).

Generic Treatment for Acute Stroke

Many of the interventions described in this chapter aim to prevent physiological changes such as hypotension, hyperglycemia, and pyrexia. These might result in secondary ischemic injury through exacerbating the flow/metabolism mismatch in the penumbral and oligemic areas surrounding the infarcted core, resulting in extension of infarction into these areas.

> **BOX 20.2** Core Features of Stroke Units Included by Stroke Unit Trialists' Collaboration
>
> Multidisciplinary team members (medical, nursing, and therapy staff – usually including physical therapy, occupational therapy, speech therapy, social work) that have a special interest in stroke or rehabilitation
>
> Coordinated multidisciplinary rehabilitation
>
> Coordinated multidisciplinary team care incorporating meetings at least once per week
>
> Routine involvement of caregivers in the rehabilitation process
>
> Regular programs of education and training
>
> *Source:* Stroke Unit Trialists' Collaboration (2013).

Stroke Units

The concept of a stroke unit as being a geographically defined service offering either acute or subacute (or both) care and rehabilitation delivered by a dedicated team is quite clear, although the exact definition of a stroke unit is less so. There is evidence that admission to an acute stroke unit providing certain core features (Box 20.2) reduces morbidity, mortality, and dependency (Stroke Unit Trialists' Collaboration 2013). The benefits are most apparent in units that are based in a discrete ward setting and are present regardless of age, sex and stroke severity (Stroke Unit Trialists' Collaboration 2013). Processes associated with reduced mortality include review by a stroke consultant within 24 hours of admission, formal swallowing assessment, adequate fluids and nutrition within 72 hours of admission, and antiplatelet therapy within 72 hours in patients with acute ischemic stroke (Bray *et al.* 2013). Stroke unit care also reduces length of stay and is cost-effective in comparison with care on general wards with or without mobile specialist team input and domiciliary care (Patel *et al.* 2004; Moodie *et al.* 2006). The beneficial effects of stroke unit care are also maintained long term (Fuentes *et al.* 2006).

Despite the evidence for the effectiveness of stroke units, many patients in the UK are not admitted to such a unit owing to lack of capacity, although the situation is improving (Intercollegiate Working Party on Stroke 2010).

Blood Pressure

The optimal management of blood pressure in acute stroke is uncertain. Ischemic and infarcted brain cannot autoregulate, and so relatively modest increases in cerebral perfusion pressure can cause hyperemia, which may subsequently lead to cerebral edema and hemorrhagic infarction, whereas a fall in cerebral perfusion pressure may exacerbate cerebral ischemia. Blood pressure is often elevated on admission but tends to fall spontaneously during the first few days (Bath and Bath 1997).

Lowering blood pressure in the first few days after ischemic or hemorrhagic stroke is not associated with improved functional outcome, and there is no urgency to resume pre-stroke antihypertensive medications until patients are medically and neurologically stable or unless there are concomitant comorbidities requiring anti-hypertensive use (Bath and Krishnan 2014; Bath *et al.* 2015).

Further details on blood pressure management in major acute ischemic and hemorrhagic stroke as well as for secondary prevention can be found in Chapters 21, 22, and 24

Hypoxia

Twenty to 60% of acute stroke patients develop some degree of oxygen desaturation during the acute phase of stroke (Sulter *et al.* 2000; Rowat et al. 2006). This can be due to a number of reasons including stroke-related impaired central regulation of respiration and complications such as pneumonia and pulmonary embolism (Kumar *et al.* 2010). Such a drop in oxygen saturation could worsen brain injury by further compromising delivery of oxygen to penumbral brain tissue and is associated with an increased risk of death (Rowat *et al.* 2006). Airway support and ventilator assistance are recommended for patients with acute stroke who have decreased consciousness or who have bulbar dysfunction that would compromise the airway (Jauch *et al.* 2013). Supplemental oxygen should be provided to maintain oxygen saturation > 94% if needed (Jauch *et al.* 2013). Routine supplemental oxygen has not been shown to improve clinical outcome, but further clinical trials are currently under way (Roffe *et al.* 2014).

Hyperglycemia

Hyperglycemia after acute stroke is common and is associated with an increased risk of death. However, recent meta-analysis has failed to show that administration of insulin with the objective of maintaining serum glucose within a specific range has any benefit in terms of improving functional outcome or reducing death (Bellolio *et al.* 2014). Many of the previous trials, however, were underpowered, and further large trials are currently under way (Bruno *et al.* 2014).

Fever

Fever may occur after stroke for a number of reasons (Box 20.3) and appears to be more common in patients with intracerebral hemorrhage or more severe stroke (Kumar *et al.* 2010). Animal studies and observational data in humans suggest that pyrexia can exacerbate neuronal injury by increasing metabolic demands on injured brain tissues, increases infarct size, and is associated with poor outcome (Reith *et al.* 1996). However, induced hypothermia is associated with hemorrhagic transformation of cerebral infarcts, venous thrombosis, cardiac arrhythmias, and infection, and has not been shown to reduce risk of dependency and death due to stroke (den Hertog *et al.* 2009a). Infection should be treated promptly. Current guidelines recommend antipyretic medications be administered to lower temperature in hyperthermic patients with stroke (Jauch *et al.* 2013), but findings from the Paracetamol (Acetaminophen) in Stroke (PAIS) trial do not support their routine use in all patients with acute stroke (den Hertog *et al.* 2009b). Nevertheless, post-hoc analysis

---

BOX 20.3 Causes of Fever after Stroke

Infection:
- urinary tract
- respiratory
- pressure sores
- septicemia
- intravenous access site

Deep vein thrombosis and pulmonary embolism

Infective endocarditis

Drug reaction

showed that paracetamol may have a beneficial effect on functional outcome in patients with a body temperature of 36.5°C or higher (den Hertog *et al.* 2009b), and PAIS 2 is currently under way to confirm this finding (de Ridder *et al.* 2015).

Dehydration

Dehydration should be corrected with intravenous fluid replacement and enteral feeding be instituted in those with significantly impaired swallowing function.

Impaired Swallowing

Dysphagia with risk of aspiration and pneumonia is present in 37–78% of patients with stroke and is particularly common in drowsy patients with severe hemispheric strokes and those with brainstem strokes (Martino *et al.* 2005). It almost always gets better in days or weeks (Hamdy *et al.* 1997). Assessment of swallowing before the patient begins eating, drinking, or receiving oral medications is recommended (Jauch *et al.* 2013) and is tested by asking the patient to sip some water and observing for any tendency to choke in the next minute or so and for added sensitivity using simple quantification (Mari *et al.* 1997; Hinds and Wiles 1998). However, further investigations, such as videofluoroscopic swallowing studies (VFSS) and fiberoptic endoscopic evaluation of swallowing (FEES), often performed by speech therapists, may be required for more accurate examination of swallowing function.

Nutrition

Feeding in the first few days may not be important, but later the patient should be kept well nourished since poor nutrition may be associated with worse outcome. Those who could not take solid food and liquids orally should receive a nasogastric tube or nasoduodenal or percutaneous endoscopic gastrostomy tube feeding to maintain hydration and nutrition while undergoing efforts to restore swallowing (Jauch *et al.* 2013).

Early Mobilization

Mobilization may reduce complications, including pneumonia, deep vein thrombosis, pulmonary embolism, and pressure ulcers. However, very early (within 24 hours of stroke onset), high-intensity, and frequent mobilization is associated with a less favorable outcome compared with patients receiving usual care, and hence, mobilization of patients in the first 24 hours of stroke onset should be cautious and restricted to only a few times a day, each less than 10 minutes (Bernhardt *et al.* 2015) (Ch. 23).

References

Andre C, de Freitas GR, Fukujima MM (2007). Prevention of deep venous thrombosis and pulmonary embolism following stroke: A systematic review of published articles. *European Journal of Neurology* 14:21–32

Barrett JA (2001). Bladder and bowel problems after a stroke. *Reviews in Clinical Gerontology* 12:253–267

Bath FJ, Bath PMW (1997). What is the correct management of blood pressure in acute stroke? The Blood Pressure in Acute Stroke Collaboration. *Cerebrovascular Diseases* 7:205–213

Bath PM, Krishnan K (2014). Interventions for deliberately altering blood pressure in acute stroke. *Cochrane Database of Systematic Reviews* 10:CD000039

Bath PM, Woodhouse L, Scutt P *et al.* (2015). Efficacy of nitric oxide, with or without continuing antihypertensive treatment, for management of high blood pressure in acute stroke (ENOS): A partial-factorial randomized controlled trial. *Lancet* **385**:617–628

Bellolio MF, Gilmore RM, Ganti L (2014). Insulin for glycemic control in acute ischemic stroke. *Cochrane Database of Systematic Reviews* 1:CD005346

Bernhardt J, Langhorne P, Lindley RI *et al.* (2015). Efficacy and safety of very early mobilization within 24 h of stroke onset (AVERT): A randomized controlled trial. *Lancet* **386**:46–55

Bhogal SK, Teasell R, Foley N *et al.* (2004). Lesion location and poststroke depression: Systematic review of the methodological limitations in the literature. *Stroke* **35**:794–802

Bray BD, Ayis S, Campbell J *et al.* (2013). Associations between the organization of stroke services, process of care, and mortality in England: Prospective cohort study. *British Medical Journal* **346**:f2827

Bruno A, Durkalski VL, Hall CE *et al.* (2014). The Stroke Hyperglycemia Insulin Network Effort (SHINE) trial protocol: A randomized, blinded, efficacy trial of standard vs. intensive hyperglycemia management in acute stroke. *International Journal of Stroke* **9**:246–251

Carota A, Berney A, Aybek S *et al.* (2005) A prospective study of predictors of poststroke depression. *Neurology* **64**:428–433

Chan EY, Ruest A, Meade MO *et al.* (2007) Oral decontamination for prevention of pneumonia in mechanically ventilated adults: Systematic review and meta-analysis. *British Medical Journal* **334**:889–893

CLOTS Trials Collaboration (2009). Effectiveness of thigh-length graduated compression stockings to reduce the risk of deep vein thrombosis after stroke (CLOTS trial 1): A multicenter, randomized controlled trial. *Lancet* **373**:1958–1965

CLOTS Trials Collaboration (2014). Effect of intermittent pneumatic compression on disability, living circumstances, quality of life, and hospital costs after stroke: Secondary analyses from CLOTS 3, a randomized trial. *Lancet Neurology* **13**:1186–1192

Cook DJ, Reeve BK, Guyatt GH *et al.* (1996). Stress ulcer prophylaxis in critically ill patients. Resolving discordant meta-analyses. *JAMA* **275**:308–314

Davenport RJ, Dennis MS, Wellwood I *et al.* (1996a). Complications after acute stroke. *Stroke* **27**:415–420

Davenport RJ, Dennis MS, Warlow CP (1996b). Gastrointestinal hemorrhage after acute stroke. *Stroke* **27**:421–424

de Ridder IR, de Jong FJ, den Hertog HM *et al.* (2015). Paracetamol (Acetaminophen) in stroke 2 (PAIS 2): Protocol for a randomized, placebo-controlled, double-blind clinical trial to assess the effect of high-dose paracetamol on functional outcome in patients with acute stroke and a body temperature of 36.5°C or above. *International Journal of Stroke* **10**:457–462

den Hertog HM, van der Worp HB, Tseng MC *et al.* (2009a). Cooling therapy for acute stroke. *Cochrane Database of Systematic Reviews* **1**: CD001247

den Hertog HM, van der Worp HB, van Gemert HM *et al.* (2009b). The Paracetamol (Acetaminophen) In Stroke (PAIS) trial: A multicenter, randomized, placebo-controlled, phase III trial. *Lancet Neurology* **8**:434: 440

Dennis MS, Lewis SC, Warlow C *et al.* (2005). Effect of timing and method of enteral tube feeding for dysphagic stroke patients (FOOD): A multicentre randomised controlled trial. *Lancet* **365**:764–772

Frese A, Husstedt IW, Ringelstein EB *et al.* (2006). Pharmacologic treatment of central post-stroke pain. *Clinical Journal of Pain* **22**:252–260

Fuentes B, Diez-Tejedor E, Ortega-Casarrubios MA *et al.* (2006). Consistency of the benefits of stroke units over years of operation: An 8-year effectiveness analysis. *Cerebrovascular Diseases* **21**:173–179

Geeganage CM, Sprigg N, Bath MW *et al.* (2013). Balance of symptomatic pulmonary embolism and symptomatic intracerebral hemorrhage with low-dose anticoagulation in recent ischemic stroke: A systematic review and meta-analysis of randomized controlled trials. *Journal of Stroke and Cerebrovascular Diseases* **22**:1018–1027

Gelber DA, Good DC, Laven LJ *et al.* (1993). Causes of urinary incontinence after acute hemispheric stroke. *Stroke* **24**:378–382

Hackett ML, Anderson CS (2005). Predictors of depression after stroke: A systematic review of observational studies. *Stroke* **36**:2296–2301

Hackett ML, Yapa C, Parag V et al. (2005). Frequency of depression after stroke: A systematic review of observational studies. *Stroke* **36**:1330–1340

Hackett ML, Anderson CS, House A et al. (2008). Interventions for treating depression after stroke. *Cochrane Database of Systematic Reviews* **8**:CD003437

Hamdy S, Aziz Q, Rothwell JC et al. (1997). Explaining oropharyngeal dysphagia after unilateral hemispheric stroke. *Lancet* **350**:686–692

Hankey GJ (2017). Stroke. *Lancet* **389**:641–654

Hesami O, Gharagozli K, Beladimoghadam N et al. (2015). The efficacy of gabapentin in patients with central post-stroke pain. *Iranian Journal of Pharmaceutical Research* **14**:95–101

Hilker R, Poetter C, Findeisen N et al. (2003). Nosocomial pneumonia after acute stroke: Implications for neurological intensive care medicine. *Stroke* **34**:975–981

Hinds NP, Wiles CM (1998). Assessment of swallowing and referral to speech and language therapists in acute stroke. *Quarterly Journal of Medicine* **91**:829–835

Hsu HL, Lin YH, Huang YC et al. (2009). Gastrointestinal hemorrhage after acute ischemic stroke and its risk factors in Asians. *European Neurology* **62**:212–218

Indredavik B, Rohweder G, Naalsund E et al. (2008). Medical complications in a comprehensive stroke unit and an early supported discharge service. *Stroke* **39**:414–420

Intercollegiate Working Party on Stroke (2010). *National Sentinel Audit*. London: Royal College of Physicians.

Kalra L, Irshad S, Hodsoll J et al. (2015). Prophylactic antibiotics after acute stroke for reducing pneumonia in patients with dysphagia (STROKE-INF): A prospective, cluster-randomised, open-label, masked endpoint, controlled clinical trial. *Lancet* **386**:1835–1844

Katzan IL, Cebul RD, Husak SH et al. (2003). The effect of pneumonia on mortality among patients hospitalized for acute stroke. *Neurology* **60**:620–625

Kim JS, Bashford G, Murphy TK et al. (2011). Safety and efficacy of pregabalin in patients with central post-stroke pain. *Pain* **152**:1018–1023

Kobayashi H, Hoshino M, Okayama K et al. (1994). Swallowing and cough reflexes after onset of stroke. *Chest* **105**:1623

Kumar S, Selim MH and Caplan LR (2010). Medical complications after stroke. *Lancet Neurology* **9**:105–108

Jauch EC, Saver JL, Adams HP Jr. et al. (2013). Guidelines for the early management of patients with acute ischemic stroke: A guideline for healthcare professionals from the American Heart Association/American Stroke Association. *Stroke* **44**:870–947

Jönsson AC, Lindgren I, Hallström B et al. (2006). Prevalence and intensity of pain after stroke: A population based study focusing on patients' perspectives. *Journal of Neurology, Neurosurgery and Psychiatry* **77**:590–595

Leijon G, Boivie J (1989). Central poststroke pain – a controlled trial of amitriptyline and carbamazepine. *Pain* **36**:27–36

Mari F, Matei M, Ceravolo MG et al. (1997). Predictive value of clinical indices in detecting aspiration in patients with neurological disorders. *Journal of Neurology, Neurosurgery and Psychiatry* **63**:456–460

Martino R, Foley N, Bhogal S et al. (2005). Dysphagia after stroke: Incidence, diagnosis, and pulmonary complications. *Stroke* **36**:2756–2763

Mead GE, Hsieh CF, Lee R et al. (2012). Selective serotonin reuptake inhibitors (SSRIs) for stroke recovery. *Cochrane Database of Systematic Reviews* **11**:CD009286

Moodie M, Cadilhac D, Pearce D et al. (2006). SCOPES Study Group. Economic evaluation of Australian stroke services: A prospective multicenter study comparing dedicated stroke units with other care modalities. *Stroke* **37**:2790–2795

Nakayama H, Jorgensen HS, Pedersen PM et al. (1997). Prevalence and risk factors of incontinence after stroke. *Stroke* **28**:58–62

Nasreddine ZS, Saver JL (1997). Pain after thalamic stroke: Right diencephalic predominance and clinical features in 180 patients. *Neurology* **48**:1196–1199

National Institute for Health and Care Excellence (2014). Pressure ulcers: Pressure and management. Clinical guideline [CG179]

O'Donnell MJ, Kapral MK, Fang J et al. (2008). Gastrointestinal bleeding after acute ischemic stroke. *Neurology* **71**:650–655

Oppenheimer SM, Cechetto DF, Hachinski VC (1990). Cerebrogenic cardiac arrhythmias. Cerebral electrocardiographic influences and their role in sudden death. *Archives of Neurology* **47**:513–519

Patel M, Coshall C, Rudd AG et al. (2001). Natural history and effects on 2-year outcomes of urinary incontinence after stroke. *Stroke* **32**:122–127

Patel A, Knapp M, Evans A et al. (2004). Training care givers of stroke patients: Economic evaluation. *British Medical Journal* **328**:1102

Prosser J, MacGregor L, Lees KR et al. (2007). Predictors of early cardiac morbidity and mortality after ischemic stroke. *Stroke* **38**:2295–2302

Reith J, Jorgensen HS, Pedersen PM et al. (1996). Body temperature in acute stroke: Relation to stroke severity, infarct size, mortality and outcome. *Lancet* **347**:422–425

Roffe C, Nevatte T, Crome P et al. (2014). The Stroke Oxygen Study (SO$_2$S) – a multi-center study to assess whether routine oxygen treatment in the first 72 hours after a stroke improves long-term outcome: Study protocol for a randomized controlled trial. *Trials* **15**:99

Rothwell PM, Algra A, Chen Z et al. (2016). Effects of aspirin on risk and severity of early recurrent stroke after transient ischaemic attack and ischaemic stroke: Time-course analysis of randomized trials. *Lancet* **388**:365–375

Rowat AM, Dennis MS, Wardlaw JM (2006). Hypoxemia in acute stroke is frequent and worsens outcome. *Cerebrovascular Diseases* **21**:166–172

Sandercock PA, Counsell C, Tseng MC et al. (2014). Oral antiplatelet therapy for acute ischaemic stroke. *Cochrane Database of Systematic Reviews* 3:CD000029

Santesso N, Carrasco-Labra A, Brignardello-Petersen R (2014). Hip protectors for preventing hip fractures in older people. *Cochrane Database of Systematic Reviews* 3:CD001255

Sato Y, Kuno H, Kaji M et al. (1998). Increased bone resorption during the first year after stroke. *Stroke* **29**:1373–1377

Sellars C, Bowie L, Bagg J et al. (2007). Risk factors for chest infection in acute stroke: A prospective cohort study. *Stroke* **38**:2284–2291

Sörös P, Hachinski V (2012). Cardiovascular and neurological causes of sudden death after ischaemic stroke. *Lancet Neurology* **11**:179–188

Stroke Unit Trialists' Collaboration (2013). Organised inpatient (stroke unit) care for stroke. *Cochrane Database of Systematic Reviews* **9**: CD000197

Sulter G, Elting JW, Stewart R et al. (2000). Continuous pulse oximetry in acute hemiparetic stroke. *Journal of the Neurological Sciences* **179**:65–69

Thomas LH, Cross S, Barrett J, et al. (2008). Treatment of urinary incontinence after stroke in adults. *Cochrane Database of Systematic Reviews* 1:CD004462

Touzé E, Varenne O, Chatellier G et al. (2005). Risk of myocardial infarction and vascular death after transient ischemic attack and ischemic stroke: A systematic review and meta-analysis. *Stroke* **36**:2748–2755

van der Worp HB, Kappelle LJ (1998). Complications of acute ischemic stroke. *Cerebrovascular Diseases* **8**:124–132

Vestergaard K, Andersen G, Gottrup H et al. (2001). Lamotrigine for central poststroke pain: A randomized controlled trial. *Neurology* **56**:184–190

Westendorp WF, Vermeij JD, Zock E, et al. (2015). The Preventive Antibiotics in Stroke Study (PASS): A pragmatic randomized open-label masked endpoint clinical trial. *Lancet* **385**:1519–1526

Yoneyama T, Yoshida M, Matsui T et al. (1999). Oral care and pneumonia. Oral Care Working Group. *Lancet* **354**:515

Specific Treatments for Major Acute Ischemic Stroke

Many of the trials of therapy in acute stroke did not distinguish between stroke subtypes other than by division into hemorrhagic and ischemic stroke. Therefore, there is little evidence for different effectiveness for most acute ischemic stroke treatments according to stroke subtype and location. However, stroke subtype determines patient selection for specific secondary preventive strategies. Therefore, better characterization of stroke will aid overall patient management (Chapter 6).

In patients with an anterior circulation ischemic stroke due to occlusion of a large artery, it has been estimated that with every minute that treatment is withheld, approximately 1.9 million neurons, 14 billion synapses, and 12 km of myelinated fibers are destroyed (Saver 2006). Therapies to reduce brain damage in ischemic stroke may therefore act by:

- recanalizing the occluded artery to restore blood flow and perfusion to salvageable tissue, thus reducing infarction within the penumbra: intravenous thrombolysis and endovascular therapy.
- prevention of thrombus extension: using antiplatelet and anticoagulant drugs.
- limiting the extent of brain ischemia: using neuroprotective agents.

Intravenous Thrombolysis

Thrombolysis aims to reduce the volume of infarcted brain by recanalizing the occluded vessel and restoring blood flow. Restoration of blood flow may not necessarily always be beneficial. First, studies in animals suggest that reperfusion of acutely ischemic brain may actually be harmful, through the release of free radicals and toxic products into the circulation. Second, thrombolysis will probably not be of benefit if infarction is completed or if the ischemic penumbra is small. Finally, thrombolysis may cause hemorrhagic transformation of the infarct or extracranial bleeding.

The first studies of intravenous thrombolysis in stroke were performed during 1950–1980 (Sussman and Fitch 1958; Meyer *et al.* 1963; Fletcher *et al.* 1976). Thrombolytic agents used at the time included fibrinolysin, plasmin, streptokinase, and urokinase. Many of these studies were, however, performed prior to the advent of computed tomography, and hence patients with hemorrhagic stroke were also treated. Most studies were also of small sample size, patients were often treated late into their course of cerebral ischemia, and few studies adhered to a rigorous randomized trial design. After the development of computed tomography scanners in the early 1980s, although studies showed improved outcomes for first-generation thrombolytics such as streptokinase and urokinase, the bleeding risks of these non-fibrin specific agents was unacceptably high with 21% of patients who received streptokinase subsequently developing a symptomatic intracerebral hemorrhage in the Multicenter Acute Stroke Trial – Europe (MAST-E) (MASTE-E Study Group 1996).

Also in the early 1980s, a second-generation thrombolytic – alteplase (a recombinant tissue plasminogen activator [rt-PA]) – was developed and, unlike its predecessors, was widely tested in preclinical studies to determine its efficacy and safety (Zivin *et al.* 1985; Lyden *et al.* 1990). Alteplase has a much higher fibrin specificity and is hence much more effective than first-generation thrombolytic agents (Collen 1987). Also, structurally, rt-PA is identical to human tissue-type plasminogen activator. Anaphylactic-type reactions that were previously seen with streptokinase are therefore extremely rare.

In the late 1980s, phase 1 dose-escalation studies using intravenous rt-PA at dosages ranging from 0.35 to 1.08 mg/kg were carried out in ischemic stroke patients < 90 and within 91–180 minutes of symptom onset (Brott *et al.* 1992; Haley *et al.* 1992). In these studies, only 1 out of 62 individuals (1.61%) who received rt-PA at a dose of ≤ 0.85 mg/kg developed an intracerebral hemorrhage, in contrast to 4 out of 32 individuals (12.5%) who were given a dose ≥ 0.95 mg/kg (Brott *et al.* 1992; Haley *et al.* 1992). These phase 1 studies led to the first positive randomized trial (National Institute of Neurological Disorders and Stroke [NINDS] rt-PA Stroke Study Group 1995) that demonstrated the efficacy of rt-PA in acute ischemic stroke. In the NINDS trial, ischemic stroke patients treated with rt-PA within 3 hours of symptom onset were approximately 30% more likely to have minimal or no disability at 3 months compared with those who received placebo (NINDS rt-PA Stroke Study Group 1995). However, 6.4% of patients treated with rt-PA developed an intracerebral hemorrhage compared with 0.6% in the placebo group (NINDS rt-PA Stroke Study Group 1995). These results were shortly followed by the US Food and Drug Administration (FDA) approving rt-PA as a treatment for acute ischemic stroke within 3 hours of symptom onset in 1996. A number of trials including Alteplase Thrombolysis for Acute Non-interventional Therapy in Ischemic Stroke (ATLANTIS); Echoplanar Imaging Thrombolysis Evaluation Trial (EPITHET); European Cooperative Acute Stroke Studies (ECASS) 1, 2, and 3; and IST-3 (International Stroke Trial) followed but showed mixed results (Hacke *et al.* 1995, 1998; Clark *et al.* 1999; Davis *et al.* 2008). However, these trials were heterogeneous with regard to the time window for which thrombolysis could be provided.

Meta-analysis of nine randomized clinical trials (*n* = 6756) from the Stroke Thrombolysis Trialists' Collaboration of rt-PA versus placebo (or untreated control) subsequently showed that the proportionate benefits of rt-PA was larger with earlier treatment (Emberson *et al.* 2014) (Fig. 21.1). When rt-PA was administered within 3 hours of symptom onset, 32.9% of patients did not have significant disability (mRS 0 or 1) compared with 23.1% of patients treated with placebo (or untreated controls). However, when patients were treated between 3 and 4.5 hours of symptom onset, 35.3% of individuals given rt-PA did not have significant disability compared with 30.1% of patients treated with placebo (Emberson *et al.* 2014). In other words, for every 100 patients with ischemic stroke treated with rt-PA within 3 hours of symptom onset, an additional 10 patients would make a full recovery; and if treated between 3 and 4.5 hours, an additional 5 would make a full recovery (Emberson *et al.* 2014). In patients treated after 4.5 hours of symptom onset, however, no differences in proportion of individuals with good outcome (32.6% versus 30.6%) were noted (Emberson *et al.* 2014). rt-PA was noted to be of no benefit if administered after 6.3 hours of symptom onset (Fig. 21.1). The beneficial effect of rt-PA was also similar for

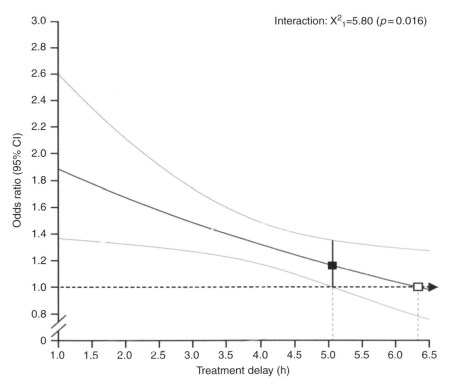

Fig. 21.1 Odds ratios of a favorable outcome at 3 months follow-up in patients treated with intravenous alteplase compared with controls by time from stroke onset to treatment, showing a decrease in benefit from treatment with time based on a pooled analysis of 6,756 patients from nine randomized controlled trials (Emberson *et al.* 2014). [Reprinted with permission from Elsevier (*Lancet*, 2014, volume 384, page 1931)]

patients greater or less than 80 years of age and regardless of stroke severity (Emberson *et al.* 2014) (Fig. 21.2).

Data from the Stroke Thrombolysis Trialists' Collaboration also showed that rt-PA was associated with a significant 6.8% risk of type 2 parenchymal hemorrhage (defined as a hematoma exceeding 30% of the infarct volume with a space-occupying effect seen on brain imaging, whether within or remote from the infarct), compared with 1.3% of patients receiving placebo or untreated control (Whiteley *et al.* 2016). Approximately 55% of intracerebral hemorrhages due to rt-PA resulted in a clinically significant (4 points or more) reduction in National Institutes of Health Stroke Scale (NIHSS) or led to death within 36 hours of treatment (Whiteley et al. 2016). Forty percent of rt-PA related type 2 parenchymal hemorrhages were fatal (Whiteley *et al.* 2016). The proportionate increase in intracerebral hemorrhage was similar regardless of treatment delay, patient age, or baseline stroke severity, although the absolute excess risk of intracerebral hemorrhage was greater with increasing stroke severity (Whiteley *et al.* 2016).

The third International Stroke Trial (IST-3) (*n* = 3035) is the largest trial to date that studied the benefits of rt-PA plus standard care versus standard care alone in patients older than 18 years of age within 6 hours of ischemic stroke (IST-3 Collaborative Group 2012). Importantly, 1,617 (53%) of study participants were > 80 years of age, whereas only 112

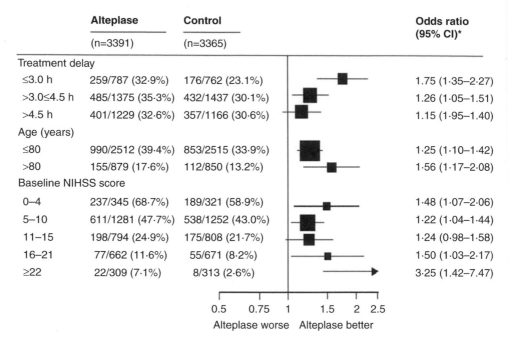

	Alteplase	Control		Odds ratio (95% CI)*
	(n=3391)	(n=3365)		
Treatment delay				
≤3.0 h	259/787 (32·9%)	176/762 (23.1%)		1.75 (1·35–2·27)
>3.0≤4.5 h	485/1375 (35·3%)	432/1437 (30·1%)		1.26 (1·05–1·51)
>4.5 h	401/1229 (32·6%)	357/1166 (30·6%)		1.15 (1·95–1.40)
Age (years)				
≤80	990/2512 (39·4%)	853/2515 (33·9%)		1·25 (1·10–1·42)
>80	155/879 (17·6%)	112/850 (13.2%)		1·56 (1·17–2·08)
Baseline NIHSS score				
0–4	237/345 (68·7%)	189/321 (58·9%)		1·48 (1·07–2·06)
5–10	611/1281 (47·7%)	538/1252 (43.0%)		1·22 (1·04–1·44)
11–15	198/794 (24·9%)	175/808 (21·7%)		1·24 (0·98–1·58)
16–21	77/662 (11·6%)	55/671 (8·2%)		1·50 (1·03–2·17)
≥22	22/309 (7·1%)	8/313 (2·6%)		3·25 (1.42–7.47)

0.5   0.75   1   1.5   2   2.5
Alteplase worse   Alteplase better

Fig. 21.2 Effect of intravenous alteplase on good stroke outcome (modified Rankin Scale 0–1), by treatment delay, age, and stroke severity. (Emberson *et al.* 2014). [Reprinted with permission from Elsevier (*Lancet*, 2014, volume 384, page 1931)]

patients within this age group were included in eight previous trials. Ninety-eight percent of patients received a CT scan prior to randomization. It was noted in IST-3 that in addition to rt-PA use, a higher NIHSS score, use of antiplatelets at the time of stroke, presence of a hyper-attenuated artery, and presence of old infarcts independently predicted risk of symptomatic intracerebral hemorrhage at 7 days after randomization (IST-3 Collaborative Group 2015). Increasing age, higher NIHSS score, large infarct, hyperattenuated artery, and presence of leukoaraiosis were also independently associated with a lower likelihood of being alive or independent at 6 months (IST-3 Collaborative Group 2015). Although none of the neuroimaging findings, alone or in combination, modified the effect of rt-PA on risk of symptomatic intracerebral hemorrhage or independence, the absolute increase in risk of symptomatic intracerebral hemorrhage after rt-PA with a combination of neuroimaging signs was highly significant. For example, patients with an old infarct and hyperattenuated artery on neuroimaging were at threefold increased odds of a symptomatic intracerebral hemorrhage compared with patients with neither signs present (absolute excess of events with rt-PA if both signs present: 13.8% versus 3.2% if both signs absent) (IST-3 Collaborative Group 2015). Meta-analysis of nine studies (*n* = 2479) that performed micro-bleed screening with MRI prior to rt-PA administration also showed that presence of microbleeds was associated with a 2.4-fold increased risk of symptomatic intracerebral hemorrhage compared with those with no microbleeds (Tsivgoulis *et al.* 2016). The risk increased steeply by burden of microbleeds such that in patients with > 10 microbleeds, the adjusted odds ratio of a symptomatic intracerebral hemorrhage was 18, compared to those with 0–10 microbleeds (Tsivgoulis *et al.* 2016).

In IST-3, 1,948 patients were followed up for 3 years, and among these, although patients treated with rt-PA had a significantly greater risk of death during the first 7 days (10% died in the rt-PA group versus 7% in the standard care alone group), patients in the rt-PA group were at significantly lower risk of death between 8 days and 3 years (41% versus 47%), suggesting that rt-PA also has long-term benefits in reduction of mortality (Berge *et al.* 2016).

In Japan, a lower dose of rt-PA at 0.6mg/kg is approved for patients with acute ischemic stroke. This was based on a prospective single-arm, open-label trial of 103 patients that showed equivalent clinical outcomes but a lower risk of symptomatic intracerebral hemorrhage (5.8%) compared with standard dose rt-PA (Yamaguchi *et al.* 2006). Other centers have tried replicating the results but have had inconsistent findings. Furthermore, in the United States, Asians treated with rt-PA were noted to have a higher risk of symptomatic intracerebral hemorrhage (Menon *et al.* 2012). It has therefore been postulated that low-dose rt-PA may be beneficial in reducing the risk of symptomatic intracerebral hemorrhage and may be useful, especially among Asians. Low-dose rt-PA would also cost less and may be an attractive safer option in some patient groups. These uncertainties led to the Enhanced Control of Hypertension and Thrombolysis Stroke Study (ENCHANTED) (Anderson *et al.* 2016). In this multicenter clinical trial, patients were randomized to receive low-dose (0.6 mg/kg) or standard-dose (0.9 mg/kg) rt-PA. Although patients receiving low-dose rt-PA had significantly fewer symptomatic intracerebral hemorrhages compared with standard-dose rt-PA, low-dose rt-PA did not result in an equivalent functional outcome improvement compared with standard-dose rt-PA at 90 days post-randomization (Anderson *et al.* 2016). These results remained similar after stratifying by age, sex, ethnicity, time from randomization, and baseline stroke severity (Anderson *et al.* 2016). Low-dose rt-PA therefore could not be recommended routinely at present. The second part of ENCHANTED, which aims to determine whether patients given rt-PA would benefit from an early intensive lowering of systolic blood pressure (130–140 mmHg) versus standard recommendations (systolic blood pressure < 180 mmHg), is due to be completed in 2018.

rt-PA, however, has a number of limitations besides its risk of intracerebral hemorrhage. These include a short half-life of 4–8 minutes, low recanalization rate (30–40% for proximal occlusions, < 5% for distal internal carotid artery occlusion), potential neurotoxicity, and a long list of absolute or relative contraindications (Table 21.1) (Bhatia *et al.* 2010; Jauch *et al.* 2013; Demaerschalk *et al.* 2016). Whether concomitant use of other treatment modalities such as hypothermia and transcranial Doppler ultrasound would increase the efficacy of rt-PA is currently being studied.

Tenecteplase, a fibrinolytic protein bioengineered from rt-PA, has a fifteen fold higher fibrin specificity, eighty fold reduced binding affinity to physiological plasminogen activator inhibitors, and sixfold longer half-life compared with rt-PA (i.e., single intravenous bolus administration possible compared with infusion for rt-PA) and therefore holds much promise as a future thrombolytic agent of choice in patients with acute ischemic stroke (Tanswell *et al.* 2002). In a phase 2b trial, tenecteplase was associated with significantly better reperfusion and clinical outcomes in ischemic stroke patients with intracranial large artery occlusion (Parsons *et al.* 2012). Further phase 3 clinical trials such as the Tenecteplase versus Alteplase for Stroke Thrombolysis Evaluation (TASTE) and Norwegian Tenecteplase Stroke Trial (NOR-TEST) are currently under way to confirm the efficacy of tenecteplase versus alteplase in ischemic stroke patients presenting within 4.5 hours of symptom onset.

Table 21.1 Absolute and relative contraindications to intravenous alteplase in acute ischemic stroke patients who present within 4.5 hours of symptom onset

Absolute contraindications
Significant head trauma or prior stroke in the previous 3 months
Symptoms suggest subarachnoid hemorrhage
Arterial puncture at a non-compressible site in previous 7 days
History of previous intracranial hemorrhage
Elevated blood pressure (systolic > 185 mmHg or diastolic > 110 mmHg)
Active internal bleeding
Acute bleeding diathesis, including but not limited to: <ul><li>Platelet count < 100 x 10^9/L.</li><li>Current use of warfarin with INR > 1.7 or PT > 15s.</li><li>Low molecular weight heparin use within the previous 24 hours.</li><li>Current use of direct thrombin inhibitors or direct factor Xa inhibitors with elevated sensitive laboratory tests (e.g., aPTT, INR, platelet count, ECT, TT, or appropriate factor Xa activity assays).</li></ul>
Blood glucose concentration <2.7mmol/L
Extensive regions of clear hypoattenuation on CT brain
N.B. There remains insufficient evidence to identify a threshold of hypoattenuation or extent that affects treatment response to rt-PA. Administrating rt-PA to patients whose CT brain exhibits extensive regions of clear hypoattenuation is nevertheless, not commended. Severe hypoattenuation represents irreversible injury and these patients will have a poor prognosis despite rt-PA.
Relative contraindications (treatment risks should be weighed against possible benefits)
Unruptured intracranial aneurysm
N.B. rt-PA is considered reasonable and probably recommended in patients with known small or moderate-sized (< 10 mm) unruptured and unsecured intracranial aneurysms. However, the usefulness and risks of rt-PA in patients with acute ischemic stroke who have a giant unruptured and unsecured intracranial aneurysm are not well established.
Intracranial vascular malformation
Intracranial neoplasms
N.B. rt-PA is probably recommended for patients with acute ischemic stroke who harbor an extra-axial intracranial neoplasm. However, in those with an intra-axial intracranial neoplasm, rt-PA is potentially harmful.
Minor, non-disabling stroke
Rapidly improving stroke symptoms (clearing spontaneously).
N.B. rt-PA should still be considered in patients with moderate-severe ischemic stroke who demonstrate early improvement but remain moderately impaired.
Pregnancy
Seizure at onset with postictal residual neurological impairments

Table 21.1 (cont.)

Relative contraindications (treatment risks should be weighed against possible benefits)
Major surgery or serious trauma within previous 14 days
Recent gastrointestinal or urinary tract hemorrhage (within 21 days)
Recent acute myocardial infarction (MI) (within 3 months).
N.B. rt-PA is considered reasonable if recent MI was a non-ST elevation MI or ST elevation MI involving the right or inferior myocardium. rt-PA may also be reasonable if the recent MI was a ST elevation MI involving the left anterior myocardium.

Notes: aPTT, activated partial thromboplastin time; INR, international normalized ratio; PT, prothrombin time; Ecarin clotting time; thrombin time; CT, computed tomography; NIHSS, National Institutes of Health Stroke Scale. *Source*: Adapted from the American Heart Association/American Stroke Association guidelines and scientific rationale for the inclusion and exclusion criteria for intravenous alteplase in acute ischemic stroke (Demaerschalk *et al.* 2016; Powers *et al.* 2018).

Desmoteplase, another fibrin-specific thrombolytic agent with longer half-life and less neurotoxicity than rt-PA, was noted to be efficacious and safe compared with placebo in two phase 2 trials – Desmoteplase in Acute Ischemic Stroke (DIAS) and Dose Escalation of Desmoteplase for Acute Ischemic Stroke (DEDAS) (Hacke *et al.* 2005; Furlan *et al.* 2006). However, desmoteplase did not improve functional outcome at 3 months in 2 phase 3 trials (DIAS 3 and 4) (Albers *et al.* 2015; von Kummer *et al.* 2016).

Other trials, such as Extending the Time for Thrombolysis in Emergency Neurological Deficits (EXTEND) and Efficacy and Safety of MRI-based Thrombolysis in Wake-up Stroke (WAKE-UP), are also ongoing to determine if patients presenting > 4.5 hours of symptom onset or with stroke of unknown time of onset (e.g., wake-up stroke) would also benefit from thrombolysis if noted to have a small ischemic core and substantial salvageable penumbra (e.g., by CT or MR perfusion) or a lesion that is DWI positive but normal on FLAIR imaging.

Finally, optimal management of acute ischemic stroke patients previously taking non-vitamin K antagonist oral anticoagulants (NOACs) such as direct thrombin inhibitors and factor Xa inhibitors remain uncertain. Current guidelines suggest that rt-PA is not recommended unless laboratory tests such as activated partial thromboplastin time (aPTT), international normalized ratio (INR), platelet count, Ecarin clotting time, thrombin time, or appropriate direct factor Xa activity assays are normal (Demaerschalk *et al.* 2016; Powers *et al.* 2018). However, traditional tests such as INR and aPTT are not reliable for measuring the anticoagulant effect of NOACs, and many of the more specialized hematological tests or specific tests to evaluate the plasma concentrations of NOACs either are not readily available or are still in development (Hankey *et al.* 2014). Alternatively, guidelines recommend that rt-PA may be administered if the patient did not receive a dose of NOAC for more than 48 hours (Demaerschalk *et al.* 2016; Powers *et al.* 2018), although experts consider rt-PA suitable unless they have missed their daily (or twice-daily) dose(s) of NOAC on the day of the stroke (Hankey *et al.* 2014), assuming renal function tests are normal. A specific reversal agent for dabigatran, idarucizumab (Pollack *et al.* 2015), is now available, and reversal agents for factor Xa inhibitors, such as andexanet alfa, are currently awaiting FDA approval (Connolly *et al.* 2016). However, experience of their use in patients on NOACs presenting with acute ischemic stroke remains very limited at present.

Endovascular Therapy

Intra-Arterial Thrombolysis

Intra-arterial thrombolysis has been proposed as a treatment for acute ischemic stroke since the 1980s and may potentially overcome many of the problems associated with patient selection for intravenous therapy:

- thrombolysis only after demonstration of vessel occlusion.
- higher rates of recanalization achieved.
- lower dosage of thrombolytic agent required, therefore lower risks of hemorrhage.
- therapeutic window for thrombolysis may be extended beyond 4.5 hours.

The first advantage is that it allows thrombolysis to be given only to those patients in whom vessel occlusion has been demonstrated. In 20% of patients presenting within 6 hours of stroke onset, no occlusion is identified. Second, recanalization rates appear to be higher for intra-arterial thrombolysis, approximately 70%, than for intravenous thrombolysis, approximately 34%, although there are no direct comparisons of the two techniques (Ma *et al.* 2015). Third, since intra-arterial thrombolysis involves the use of small amounts of thrombolytic agent applied directly to the site of occlusion, compared with the relatively high doses used systemically in intravenous thrombolysis, intra-arterial thrombolysis may offer the potential to treat patients at increased risk of hemorrhagic complications more safely.

In the late 1990s, two randomized controlled trials of intra-arterial thrombolysis were reported: the Prolyse in Acute Cerebral Thromboembolism trials PROACT I (del Zoppo *et al.* 1998) and PROACT II (Furlan *et al.* 1999). PROACT I remains the only placebo-controlled, double-blind, multicenter trial of intra-arterial thrombolysis with recombinant pro-urokinase in acute ischemic stroke. Recanalization rate was 58% in the active treatment group compared with 14% in the placebo group. Two doses of subsequent heparin were used, a high-dose 5000 U bolus followed by 100 U/hour, achieving a recanalization rate of 80% with a symptomatic intracranial hemorrhage rate of 27%. The equivalent rates in the low-dose heparin group were 47% and 6%, respectively. In PROACT II, 180 patients with a mean NIHSS of 17 were randomly assigned to receive either 9 mg of intra-arterial thrombolysis with recombinant pro-urokinase plus low-dose intravenous heparin or low-dose intravenous heparin alone. The median time from onset of symptoms to the initiation of intra-arterial thrombolysis was 5.3 hours. In the treated group, there was a 15% absolute benefit in the number of patients who achieved an mRS of ≤ 2 at 90 days ($p = 0.04$). On average, seven patients with middle cerebral artery occlusion would require intra-arterial thrombolysis for one to benefit. Symptomatic brain hemorrhage occurred in 10% of the thrombolysis group and 2% of the control group, but there was no excess mortality.

Mechanical Thrombectomy

The success of the PROACT trials led to the study of other endovascular techniques in the treatment of acute ischemic stroke. These included the Mechanical Embolus Removal in Cerebral Ischemia (MERCI) retriever, which was tested in the MERCI and multi-MERCI trials in 2005 and 2008 (Smith *et al.* 2005, 2008). These trials were prospective, single-arm, multicenter trials that aimed to test the safety and efficacy of the MERCI retriever to open occluded intracranial large vessels within 8 hours of symptom onset. Recanalization rates ranged from 48% in patients who received mechanical thrombectomy to 69.5% in patients who also received intra-arterial tissue plasminogen (Smith *et al.* 2005, 2008). In 2012, the FDA approved a number of second-generation mechanical thrombectomy devices, known as stent retrievers, which included Solitaire (Medtronic) and Trevo (Stryker Neurovascular), for treatment of acute ischemic stroke. These non-detachable devices enable the stent to be deployed within the clot, resulting in the thrombus to be embedded within the stent upon deployment. Retrieval of the stent would ideally lead to removal of thrombus and restoration of blood flow. Recanalization rates for stent retrievers ranged from 61% to 87.5% for Solitaire and was ~92% for Trevo (Pierot *et al.* 2015).

With these new mechanical thrombectomy devices, several trials such as the Interventional Management of Stroke (IMS) III, Synthesis Expansion: A Randomized Controlled Trial on IA Versus IV Thrombolysis in Acute Ischemic Stroke (SYNTHESIS) and Mechanical Retrieval and Recanalization of Stroke Clots using Embolectomy (MR RESCUE) were conducted that aimed to determine whether endovascular therapy was superior to intravenous thrombolysis in patients with acute ischemic stroke (Broderick *et al.* 2013; Ciccone *et al.* 2013; Kidwell *et al.* 2013). All three trials were negative, and no differences were noted with respect to clinical outcomes in patients who received endovascular treatment compared with those who received intravenous thrombolysis alone. However, these trials mainly utilized first-generation mechanical thrombectomy devices, and indeed, second-generation mechanical thrombectomy devices have been shown to be superior to the MERCI device in successfully recanalizing the occluded artery and are associated with better clinical outcomes (Nogueira *et al.* 2012; Saver *et al.* 2012). IMS III, SYNTHESIS, and MR RESCUE are further limited as these trials did not utilize imaging to confirm the presence of large artery occlusion nor did they exclude patients with a large infarct core and hence did not select the patient group in which mechanical thrombectomy is most likely to be beneficial.

In view of these limitations, further trials were initiated. The Multicenter Randomized Clinical Trial of Endovascular Treatment for Acute Ischemic Stroke in the Netherlands (MR CLEAN) randomized 500 patients with acute ischemic stroke with proximal middle cerebral (M1 or M2) or anterior cerebral (A1 or A2) artery occlusion identified on vascular imaging (CTA, MRA, or DSA) to endovascular treatment plus usual care ($n = 233$) or usual care alone ($n = 267$) (Berkhemer *et al.* 2015). Patients receiving endovascular treatment could be treated up to 6 hours from symptom onset. rt-PA was used in 89% of patients prior to randomization, and among patients randomized to the endovascular treatment arm, mechanical thrombectomy was performed in 195/233 (83.7%) patients, 190/195 (97.4%) of which were stent retrievers and other devices used in the remaining 5/195 (2.6%) of patients receiving mechanical thrombectomy. Concomitant intra-arterial thrombolytic agents were administered in 24/195 patients, 1/233 (0.4%) received intra-arterial thrombolysis alone, and no intervention was given in 37/233 (15.9%) of patients. A total of 32.6% of patients in the endovascular treatment arm were functionally independent (mRS 0–2) at 90 days compared with 19.1% of patients randomized to usual care alone (absolute difference 13.5%) (Berkhemer *et al.* 2015). There were, however, no differences in mortality or risk of symptomatic intracerebral hemorrhage between the two arms.

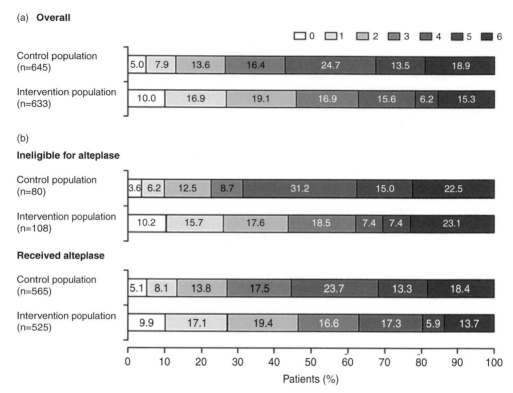

Fig. 21.3 Distribution of modified Rankin Scale scores at 90 days in the intervention and control groups in the overall trial populations (a) and for patients treated with or ineligible for intravenous alteplase (b). (Goyal *et al.* 2016). [Reprinted with permission from Elsevier (*Lancet*, 2016, volume 387, page 1726)]

The positive results of MR CLEAN led to an early interim analysis of several similar trials including the Endovascular Treatment for Small Core and Anterior Circulation Proximal Occlusion with Emphasis on Minimizing CT to Recanalization Times (ESCAPE), Randomized Trial of Revascularization with Solitaire FR Device versus Best Medical Therapy in the Treatment of Acute Stroke Due to Anterior Circulation Large Vessel Occlusion Presenting within Eight Hours of Symptom Onset (REVASCAT), Extending the Time for Thrombolysis in Emergency Neurological Deficits – Intra-Arterial (EXTEND-IA), and Solitaire with the Intention for Thrombectomy as Primary Endovascular Treatment (SWIFT PRIME) trials (Campbell *et al.* 2015; Goyal *et al.* 2015; Jovin *et al.* 2015; Saver *et al.* 2015a). All four trials were subsequently stopped due to positive results in favor of mechanical thrombectomy.

An individual patient data meta-analysis of these five trials (Highly Effective Reperfusion evaluated in Multiple Endovascular Stroke Trials [HERMES] collaboration) ($n = 1287$) subsequently confirmed that endovascular thrombectomy is of benefit to most patients with acute ischemic stroke caused by occlusion of the proximal anterior circulation (Goyal *et al.* 2016). Pooled data from HERMES showed that patients receiving mechanical thrombectomy were at significantly lower chance of disability at 90 days (adjusted OR 2.49, 95% CI 1.76–3.53, $p < 0.0001$) (Fig. 21.3) (Goyal *et al.* 2016). The number needed to treat for

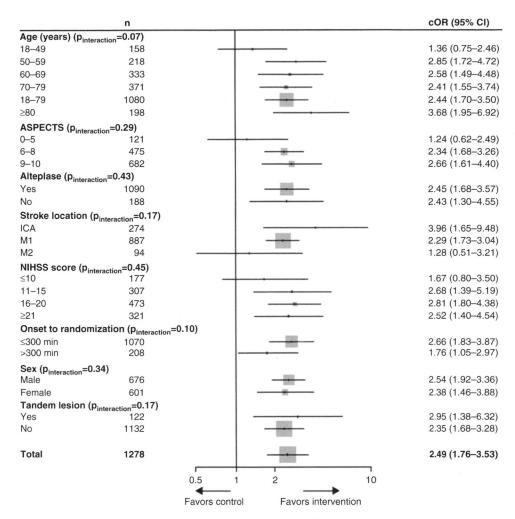

Fig. 21.4 Forrest plot showing adjusted treatment effect for modified Rankin Scale at 90 days in patients receiving mechanical thrombectomy versus intravenous alteplase only, stratified by age, sex, Alberta Stroke Program Early CT score (ASPECTS), concomitant intravenous alteplase use, stroke location, stroke severity, time from symptom onset to randomization, and presence of tandem lesion (Goyal *et al.* 2016). [Reprinted with permission from Elsevier (*Lancet*, 2016, volume 387, page 1728)]

one patient to have at least a 1-point reduction in disability on mRS was 2.6. A total of 26.9% of patients who received mechanical thrombectomy had an mRS of 0–1 at 90 days compared with 12.9% of patients who received usual care (risk difference 14%), and 46% of patients who received mechanical thrombectomy had an mRS of 0–2 at 90 days compared with 26.5% of patients who received usual care (risk difference 19.5%) (Goyal *et al.* 2016). No heterogeneity was present in subgroup analysis of mRS distribution shift at 90 days when patients were stratified by age, sex, NIHSS, site of intracranial occlusion, presence of tandem cervical carotid occlusion, Alberta Stroke Program Early CT score (ASPECTS), time from onset to randomization, and whether rt-PA was received (Goyal *et al.* 2016) (Fig. 21.4).

No differences in rate of symptomatic intracranial hemorrhage (4.4% versus 4.3%) were noted, nor were there any differences in mortality at 90 days (15.3% versus 18.9%) between patients who received endovascular therapy versus standard care (Goyal *et al.* 2016).

These five trials had a number of similarities, including the following: (1) majority of patients had a good premorbid functional status with mRS < 2; (2) majority of patients had a moderate-severe stroke severity with median NIHSS of 17; (3) only patients with anterior circulation ischemic strokes were recruited; (4) imaging evidence of large vessel occlusion was required (majority were internal carotid artery or M1 branch of middle cerebral artery); (5) in four of the trials, evidence of potentially salvageable brain tissue was required (by either perfusion imaging showing evidence of penumbra or exclusion of patients with ASPECTS < 6); (6) stent retrievers were used in the majority of patients; (7) most patients in the interventional arm also received intravenous rt-PA; and (8) time from stroke onset to endovascular treatment (groin puncture) was short, ranging from ~165 to 380 minutes. As a result of the significant positive results of these trials, the American Heart Association/ American Stroke Association revised its guidelines to include a number of Class I recommendations as listed out in Table 21.2 (Powers *et al.* 2018).

Table 21.2 Summary recommendations from the American Heart Association/American Stroke Association guidelines for the early management of patients with acute ischemic stroke

Class I	LOE
Patients eligible for intravenous rt-PA should receive intravenous rt-PA even if endovascular treatments are being considered.	A
In patients under consideration for mechanical thrombectomy, observation after intravenous rt-PA to assess for clinical response should not be performed	B-R
If endovascular therapy is contemplated, a noninvasive intracranial vascular study is strongly recommended during the initial imaging evaluation of the acute stroke patients but should not delay intravenous rt-PA if indicated. For patients who qualify for intravenous rt-PA, initiating intravenous rt-PA before noninvasive vascular imaging is recommended. Noninvasive intracranial vascular imaging should then be obtained as quickly as possible.	A
Patients should receive endovascular therapy with a stent retriever if they meet all the following criteria: • Pre-stroke modified Rankin Scale score < 2. • Causative occlusion of the internal carotid artery or proximal M1 branch of middle cerebral artery. • Age ≥ 18 years. • NIHSS score of ≥ 6. • ASPECTS ≥ 6. • Treatment can be initiated (groin puncture) within 6 hours of symptom onset.	A
Use of stent retrievers is indicated in preference to the MERCI device.	A
In selected patients with acute ischemic stroke within 6 to 24 hours of last known normal who have large vessel occlusion in the anterior circulation, obtaining CT	A

Table 21.2 (cont.)

Class I	LOE
perfusion, DW-MRI, or MR perfusion is recommended to aid patient selection for mechanical thrombectomy.	
In selected patients with acute ischemic stroke within 6 to 16 hours of last known normal who have large vessel occlusion in the anterior circulation and meet other DAWN or DEFUSE 3 eligibility criteria, mechanical thrombectomy is recommended	A
In selected patients with acute ischemic stroke within 6 to 24 hours of last known normal who have large vessel occlusion in the anterior circulation and meet other DAWN eligibility criteria, mechanical thrombectomy is reasonable	B-R
To maximize the probability of a good function outcome with endovascular therapy, reperfusion to TICI grade 2b/3 should be achieved as early as possible.	B-R
Regional stroke system of stroke care consisting of (1) healthcare facilitates that provide initial emergency care, including administration of rt-PA (e.g., primary stroke center) and (2) centers capable of performing endovascular stroke treatment with comprehensive periprocedural care (e.g., comprehensive stroke centers) should be developed.	A
Endovascular therapy requires the patients to be at an experienced stroke center with rapid access to cerebral angiography and qualified neurointerventionalists. Systems should be designed, executed, and monitored to emphasize expeditious assessment and treatment. Outcomes of all patients should be tracked. Facilities are encouraged to define criteria that can be used to credential individuals who can perform safe and timely intra-arterial revascularization procedures.	E

Notes: LOE, level of evidence; rt-PA, recombinant tissue plasminogen activator; NIHSS, National Institute of Health Stroke Scale; ASPECTS, Alberta Stroke Program Early CT score.
Source: Adapted from the 2018 American Heart Association/American Stroke Association Guidelines for the early management of patients with acute ischemic stroke (Powers *et al.* 2018).

Endovascular therapy (with stent retrievers and completed within 6 hours of stroke onset) without intravenous rt-PA is also considered reasonable in patients who have contraindications to intravenous rt-PA, e.g., severe head trauma, hemorrhagic coagulopathy, or receiving anticoagulant medications (Class IIa; Level of Evidence C) (Powers *et al.* 2015). However, there remain patient groups that have yet to be studied (or have not been extensively studied) by randomized controlled trials, including (1) patients < 18 years of age and (2) patients who have a causative occlusion of the M2 or M3 portion of the middle cerebral artery, anterior cerebral arteries, vertebral arteries, basilar artery, or posterior cerebral arteries and patients with premorbid mRS > 1, ASPECTS < 6, or NIHSS score < 6 and causative occlusion of the ICA or M1 branch of MCA. In these instances, the benefits of endovascular therapy have not been established or are uncertain, but treatment may be reasonable in carefully selected patients in whom treatment can be initiated (groin puncture) within 6 hours of symptom onset (Powers *et al.* 2015). Indeed, given the poor outcome of basilar artery occlusion, many clinicians believe mechanical thrombectomy is justified, even beyond 6 hours of symptom onset, particularly as there is some evidence that the brainstem and cerebellum are more resilient to ischemia; hence the window for revascularization therapy may extend for few more hours in patients with posterior circulation infarcts. This is mainly due to the rich collateral circulation (e.g., those from the anterior circulation via the posterior communicating arteries as well as other arteries from the posterior circulation) that may continue perfusing the brainstem and cerebellum despite a basilar artery occlusion. Nevertheless, clinical trials such as Acute Basilar Artery Occlusion: Endovascular Interventions versus Standard Medical Treatment (BEST) are currently under way to determine if endovascular treatment within 8 hours of acute basilar artery occlusions provides superior outcomes to standard medical therapy alone.

Recently, the DAWN (Diffusion weighted imaging or computerized tomography perfusion assessment with clinical mismatch in the triage of wake up and late presenting strokes undergoing neurointervention with Trevo) trial demonstrated that, in carefully selected acute ischemic stroke patients presenting between 6 and 24 hours from symptom onset, who had moderate-severe stroke due to intracranial internal carotid artery and/or M1 middle cerebral artery occlusion, affecting < 1/3 of the middle cerebral artery territory and with mismatch shown on MRI DWI or CT perfusion, mechanical thrombectomy significantly prevented disability compared with medical treatment alone (Nogueira *et al.* 2018). The DEFUSE 3 (Endovascular therapy following imaging evaluation for ischemic stroke) trial showed similar benefits of mechanical thrombectomy in acute stroke patients who had moderate-severe stroke due to internal carotid artery or M1 middle cerebral artery occlusion and with significant mismatch on CT or MR perfusion, who presented within 6 to 16 hours of symptom onset (Albers *et al.* 2018; Table 21.2).

Antiplatelet Therapy

Patients with acute stroke should be treated with aspirin as soon as practicable after brain imaging has excluded hemorrhage. In patients in whom intravenous thrombolysis or mechanical thrombectomy is considered, however, antiplatelets should be withheld until repeat neuroimaging the following day does not show any significant hemorrhagic transformation of infarct. One systematic review (Sandercock *et al.* 2003), including two very large randomized controlled trials (International Stroke Trial Collaborative Group 1997; Chinese Acute Stroke Trial [CAST] Collaborative Group 1997), has clearly established that starting aspirin therapy within the first 48 hours of acute ischemic stroke avoids death or disability at 6 months for approximately 10 patients per 1,000 patients treated. A further 10 patients per 1,000 treated will make a complete recovery. Both intracranial and extracranial hemorrhage are reported with aspirin therapy, but the rates are low and are offset by the benefit of extra lives saved.

More recently, an updated meta-analysis of 12 trials ($n = 15778$) of aspirin versus control in secondary prevention after TIA or ischemic stroke clearly demonstrated the benefits of aspirin use in preventing early risk of recurrent ischemic stroke (Rothwell *et al.* 2016). Compared with placebo, aspirin reduced the 6-week risk of recurrent ischemic stroke by about 60%. The benefit was greatest at 0–6 weeks, but further benefit accrued up to 12 weeks follow-up (Rothwell *et al.* 2016). Aspirin also reduced the severity of recurrent ischemic stroke during the 6 weeks after randomization by reducing the risk of disabling or fatal (modified Rankin Score [mRS] >2) ischemic stroke by ~70% and the risk of very severe (mRS 4–6) ischemic stroke by ~75% (Rothwell *et al.* 2016). Furthermore, aspirin also reduced the 6-week risk of acute myocardial infarction by about 80% (Rothwell *et al.* 2016).

In patients who are ineligible for thrombolysis or mechanical thrombectomy, there is no clear consensus about whether aspirin should be given prior to brain imaging. This applies to situations where access to imaging is delayed or where drugs could be administered by ambulance staff. Analysis of outcome in the subgroup of patients who were randomized and who received treatment prior to brain imaging, some of whom subsequently turned out to have primary intracerebral hemorrhage, did not show any obvious difference in risk and benefit from those in the rest of the trial (International Stroke Trial Collaborative Group 1997).

There is no clear evidence that any particular dose of aspirin is more effective than others. However, the symptoms of aspirin toxicity, such as dyspepsia and constipation, are dose related, so the smallest effective dose should be used. A starting dosage of 150–300 mg per day is advised for the acute phase of ischemic stroke followed by long-term treatment with 75–150 mg per day. Patients intolerant of aspirin should be treated with clopidogrel if available or if not with dipyridamole. These newer agents cost significantly more than aspirin. The use of combination antiplatelet therapy is discussed further in Chapter 24.

Anticoagulation

Immediate therapy with systemic anticoagulants including unfractionated heparin, low-molecular-weight heparin, heparinoids, or specific thrombin inhibitors in patients with acute ischemic stroke is not associated with net short- or long-term benefit (International Stroke Trial Collaborative Group 1997; Berge 2007; Wong et al. 2007). These agents reduce the risk of deep venous thrombosis and pulmonary embolus, but they are associated with a significant risk of intracranial hemorrhage, which is dose dependent. Patients in atrial fibrillation after presumed ischemic stroke or TIA benefit from anticoagulation in the long term to prevent further stroke. However, the best time to start therapy after an ischemic stroke is unclear as the risk of hemorrhagic transformation is difficult to predict (International Stroke Trial Collaborative Group 1997; O'Donnell et al. 2006). The use of anticoagulants for the secondary prevention of stroke is discussed further in Chapter 24.

Surgical Decompression for Malignant Middle Cerebral Artery Infarction

Malignant middle cerebral artery territory infarction is defined as a large middle cerebral artery infarct with marked edema and swelling, leading to raised intracranial pressure and a high risk of coning (Fig. 21.5; see also Figs. 5.1 and 11.2). Malignant middle cerebral artery infarction has a mortality rate of approximately 80% with medical treatment. Meta-analysis of randomized controlled trials showed that decompressive surgery (hemi-craniectomy and duroplasty) in patients with severe middle cerebral artery territory infarction within 96 hours of stroke onset is associated with an 81% reduction in risk of death at 12 months compared with best medical treatment (30% versus 71%, OR 0.19, 95% CI 0.12–0.30, $p < 0.0001$), the effect of which was significant in both patients less than or greater than 60 years of age (Yang et al. 2015). However, among stroke survivors, there were no significant differences in proportion of patients who had major disability (mRS 4–5) in those who received decompressive surgery versus best medical care (62% versus 55%, OR 1.71, 95% CI 0.78–3.74, $p = 0.18$), the effect of which was again similar regardless of age (Yang et al. 2015).

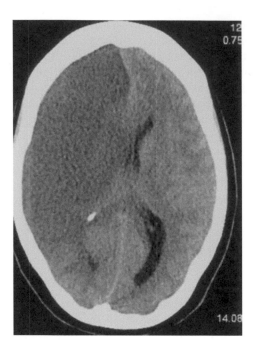

Fig. 21.5 A CT brain scan showing the development of malignant middle cerebral artery infarction in a young woman who subsequently underwent hemicraniectomy.

Neuroprotective Interventions

Neuroprotection is an attractive concept that is theoretically complementary to reperfusion strategies such as intravenous thrombolysis and endovascular therapy discussed earlier. Potential neuroprotective agents include metalloprotease inhibitors, anti-inflammatory drugs, antioxidants, and agents that reduce excitotoxicity. These compounds may act by interrupting toxic cellular, biochemical, and metabolic processes that mediate ischemic injury during stroke, therefore potentially limiting the infarct core but also salvaging the penumbra and extending the time that reperfusion strategies can be provided. Several neuroprotective agents have shown promising results in animal studies, but this has not, in general, translated into benefit in trials in humans (Sutherland *et al.* 2012). The many possible reasons for the discrepancy in results between animals and humans include length of time to treatment, the heterogeneity of stroke in humans (e.g., variations in age, underlying comorbidities, stroke etiology, and duration of vessel occlusion) compared with animal stroke models, and the small numbers and bias in animal studies (Sutherland *et al.* 2012). The current consensus is that neuroprotective agents require more rigorous testing in appropriate clinically relevant animal models before testing in humans with appropriate time windows and outcome measures (Sutherland *et al.* 2012). Moreover, variation in the outcome measurements used in acute stroke trials makes comparison between studies difficult, and reanalysis of data using different methods may yield different results.

Furthermore, many of the previous neuroprotection clinical trials have been criticized due to significant delays in administering the neuroprotective drug studied. While these agents are often injected within the first 2 hours of middle cerebral artery occlusion in animal models, these are often administered many hours after stroke onset in clinical trials (up to 72 hours in some studies), by which stage the cerebral infarct has already been well established with little or no penumbra that could be salvageable. Recently, the Field Administration of Stroke Therapy-Magnesium (FAST-MAG) trial tested whether magnesium sulfate, which has vasodilatory and direct neuroprotective and glioprotective effects (Muir 2001), improved functional outcome when administered by paramedics to acute ischemic stroke patients within 2 hours of symptom onset (Saver *et al.* 2015b). The trial recruited 1,700 patients (857 in the magnesium group and 843 in the placebo group), and while the trial did succeed by delivering the study agent to patients with a suspected stroke faster than any previous clinical trial (median time interval between patient last known to be symptom-free and start of study drug being 45 minutes), there was no significant shift in the distribution of 90-day disability outcomes on mRS between patients in the magnesium group and those receiving placebo ($p = 0.28$) (Saver *et al.* 2015b). Potential reasons for the neutral results of this trial included a potential delay in drug administration and peak drug concentration in the cerebrospinal fluid and, secondly, that neuroprotective agents that act on multiple biological pathways of ischemic injury may be more effective than agents that act on a single pathway alone (Saver *et al.* 2015b).

Hypothermia causes a variety of responses in ischemic brain that might confer neuroprotection, including significant alterations in metabolism, glutamate release and reuptake, inflammation, and free radical generation (Krieger and Yenari 2004). This, together with the observation that children and adults have survived prolonged immersion in cold water without neurological sequelae, has led to the proposal that induced hypothermia may improve stroke outcome. Hypothermia may also lengthen the time window for thrombolysis. In animal models, hypothermia improves outcome in temporary cerebral vessel occlusion, but effects after permanent occlusion are less consistent. In humans, two randomized trials have shown that mild hypothermia improves mortality and neurological outcome in patients who suffer cardiac arrest (Bernard *et al.* 2002; Hypothermia After Cardiac Arrest Study Group 2002). Pilot studies of hypothermia for stroke have been published, but there are no large randomized trials, and there is no consensus regarding timing, depth, and method of induction of hypothermia: surface or endovascular (Hemmen and Lyden 2007). Anesthetized patients have tolerated hypothermia for as long as 72 hours, but few awake patients have been treated, partly because awake patients do not tolerate deep hypothermia. Complications such as hypotension, cardiac arrhythmias, electrolyte disturbances, and infections are also common.

Systems of Care and Incorporating Telemedicine and Mobile Stroke Units

As discussed previously, mechanical thrombectomy is now an established treatment for selected patients with acute stroke due to large artery occlusion (Goyal *et al.* 2016). However, as mechanical thrombectomy can only be performed by highly specialized vascular neuro-interventionalists and good clinical outcome is dependent on case volume (Gupta *et al.* 2013), mechanical thrombectomy is only available in larger tertiary medical centers at present. Worldwide, many regional acute ischemic stroke care services have been restructured in the recent years such that only a limited number of tertiary centers have been designated as centers where mechanical thrombectomy can be provided. However, in many of these centers, mechanical thrombectomy is only available during limited times of the day.

It may take a few years for more neuro-interventionalists to be trained before mechanical thrombectomy can be made widely available.

The majority of other primary stroke care centers are now able to provide intravenous rt-PA as usual but not mechanical thrombectomy. Paramedics encountering patients with an acute ischemic stroke would therefore need to decide whether the patient should be transported to a primary stroke care center for consideration of rt-PA or whether the patient has exceeded (or is soon to exceed) the time window for rt-PA but may be a potential candidate for mechanical thrombectomy and transfer the patient directly to a center that could provide such a service. Nowadays, telemedicine is available in some countries, and this has allowed stroke neurologists working in distant primary stroke or tertiary stroke centers to assess patients (e.g., by performing an NIHSS) on the ambulance and to instruct paramedics as to which stroke center the patient should be transferred to. Mobile stroke units, which are ambulances equipped with portable CT imaging as well as paramedics, nurses, and/or clinicians specializing in stroke, have also been introduced in certain countries. These mobile stroke units have the advantage of being able to rapidly scan any patient with suspected acute stroke and also to provide intravenous rt-PA on the ambulance if needed.

References

Albers GW, von Kummer R, Truelsen T et al. (2015) Safety and efficacy of desmoteplase given 3–9 h after ischemic stroke in patients with occlusion or high-grade stenosis in major cerebral arteries (DIAS-3): A double-blind, randomized, placebo-controlled phase 3 trial. *Lancet Neurology* 14:575–584

Albers GW, Marks MP, Kemp S et al. (2018). Thrombectomy for stroke at 6 to 16 hours with selection by perfusion imaging. *New England Journal of Medicine* 378:708–718

Anderson CS, Robinson T, Lindley RI et al. (2016). Low-dose versus standard-dose intravenous alteplase in acute ischemic stroke. *New England Journal of Medicine* 374:2313–2323

Berge E (2007). Heparin for acute ischemic stroke: A never-ending story? *Lancet Neurology* 6:381–382

Berge E, Cohen G, Roaldsen MB et al. (2016). Effects of alteplase on survival after ischemic stroke (IST-3): 3 year follow-up of a randomized, controlled, open-label trial. *Lancet Neurology* 15:1028–1034

Berkhemer OA, Fransen PS, Beumer D et al. (2015). A randomized trial of intraarterial treatment for acute ischemic stroke. *New England Journal of Medicine* 372:11–20

Bernard SAGT, Buist MD, Jones BM et al. (2002). Treatment of comatose survivors of out-of-hospital cardiac arrest with induced hypothermia. *New England Journal of Medicine* 346:557–563

Bhatia R, Hill MD, Shobha N et al. (2010). Low rates of acute recanalization with intravenous recombinant tissue plasminogen activator in ischemic stroke: Real-world experience and a call for action. *Stroke* 41:2254–2258

Broderick JP, Palesch YY, Demchuck AM et al. (2013). Endovascular therapy after intravenous t-PA versus t-PA alone for stroke. *New England Journal of Medicine*. 368:893–903

Brott TG, Haley EC Jr., Levy DE et al. (1992). Urgent therapy for stroke. Part I. Pilot study of tissue plasminogen activator administered within 90 minutes. *Stroke* 23:632–640

Campbell BC, Mitchell MJ, Kleinig TJ et al. (2015). Endovascular therapy for ischemic stroke with perfusion-imaging selection. *New England Journal of Medicine* 372:1009–1018

Chinese Acute Stroke Trial (CAST) Collaborative Group (1997). CAST: Randomised placebo-controlled trial of early aspirin use in 20 000 patients with acute ischemic stroke. *Lancet* 349:1641–1649

Ciccone A, Valvassori L, Nichelatti M et al. (2013). Endovascular treatment for acute ischemic stroke. *New England Journal of Medicine* 368:904–913

Clark WM, Wissman S, Albers GW et al. (1999). Recombinant tissue-type plasminogen activator (Alteplase) for ischemic stroke 3 to 5 hours after symptom onset. The ATLANTIS Study: A randomized controlled trial. Alteplase Thrombolysis for acute Noninterventional Therapy in Ischemic Stroke. *JAMA* **282**:2019–2026

Collen D. (1987) Molecular mechanisms of fibrinolysis and their application to fibrin-specific thrombolytic therapy. *Journal of Cellular Biochemistry* **33**:77–86

Connolly SJ, Milling TJ Jr., Eikelboom JW *et al.* (2016). Andexanet alfa for acute major bleeding associated with factor Xa inhibitors. *New England Journal of Medicine* **375**:1131–1141

Davis SM, Donnan GA, Parsons MW *et al.* (2008) Effects of alteplase beyond 3h after stroke in the Echoplanar Imaging Thrombolytic Evaluation Trial (EPITHET): A placebo-controlled randomized trial. *Lancet Neurology* **7**:299–309

del Zoppo GJ, Higashida RT, Furlan AJ *et al.* (1998). PROACT: A phase II randomized trial of recombinant pro-urokinase by direct arterial delivery in acute middle cerebral artery stroke. PROACT Investigators Prolyse in Acute Cerebral Thromboembolism. *Stroke* **29**:4–11

Demaerschalk BM, Kleindorfer DO, Adeoye OM *et al.* (2016). Scientific rationale for the inclusion and exclusion criteria for intravenous alteplase in acute ischemic stroke: A statement for healthcare professionals from the American Heart Association/American Stroke Association. *Stroke* **47**:581–641

Emberson J, Lee KR, Lyden P *et al.* (2014). Effect of treatment delay, age, and stroke severity on the effects of intravenous thrombolysis with alteplase for acute ischemic stroke: A meta-analysis of individual patient data from randomized trials. *Lancet* **384**:1929–1935

Fletcher AP, Alkjaersig N, Lewis M *et al.* (1976). A pilot study of urokinase therapy in cerebral infarction. *Stroke* **7**:135–142

Furlan A, Higashida R, Wechsler L *et al.* (1999). Intra-arterial prourokinase for acute ischemic stroke. The PROACT II study: A randomized controlled trial. Prolyse in Acute Cerebral Thromboembolism. *Journal of the American Medical Association* **282**:2003–2011

Furlan AJ, Eyding D, Albers GW *et al.* (2006). Dose Escalation of Desmoteplase for Acute Ischemic Stroke (DEDAS): Evidence of safety and efficacy 3 to 9 hours after stroke onset. *Stroke* **37**:1227–1231

Goyal M, Demchuk AM, Menon BK *et al.* (2015). Randomized assessment of rapid endovascular treatment of ischemic stroke. *New England Journal of Medicine* **372**:1019–1030

Goyal M, Menon BK, van Zwam WH *et al.* (2016). Endovascular thrombectomy after large-vessel ischemic stroke: A meta-analysis of individual patient data from five randomized trials. *Lancet* **387**:1723–1731

Gupta R, Horev A, Nguyen T *et al.* (2013). Higher volume endovascular stroke centers have faster times to treatment, higher reperfusion rates and higher rates of good clinical outcomes. *Journal of NeuroInterventional Surgery* **5**:294–297

Hacke W, Kaste M, Fieschi C *et al.* (1995). Intravenous thrombolysis with recombinant tissue plasminogen activator for acute hemispheric stroke. The European Coorperative Acute Stroke Study (ECASS). *JAMA* **274**:1017–1025

Hacke W, Kaste M, Fieschi C *et al.* (1998). Randomised double-blind placebo-controlled trial of thrombolytic therapy with intravenous alteplase in acute ischemic stroke (ECASS II). Second European–Australasian Acute Stroke Study Investigators. *Lancet* **352**:1245–1251

Hacke W, Albers G, Al-Rawi Y *et al.* (2005). The Desmoteplase in Acute Ischemic Stroke Trial (DIAS): A phase II MRI-based 9-hour window acute stroke thrombolysis trial with intravenous desmoteplase. *Stroke* **36**:66–73

Haley EC Jr., Levy DE, Brott TG *et al.* (1992). Urgent therapy for stroke. Part II. Pilot study of tissue plasminogen activator administered 91–180 minutes from onset. *Stroke* **23**:641–645

Hankey GJ, Norrving B, Hacke W *et al.* (2014). Management of acute stroke in patients taking novel oral anticoagulants. *International Journal of Stroke* **9**:627–632

Hemmen TM, Lyden PD (2007). Induced hypothermia for acute stroke. *Stroke* **38**:794–799

Hypothermia After Cardiac Arrest Study Group (2002). Mild therapeutic hypothermia to improve the neurologic outcome after cardiac arrest. *New England Journal of Medicine* **346**:549–556

International Stroke Trial Collaborative Group (1997). The International Stroke Trial (IST): A randomised trial of aspirin subcutaneous heparin both or neither among 19435 patients with acute ischemic stroke. *Lancet* **349**:1569–1581

IST-3 Collaborative Group (2012). The benefits and harms of intravenous thrombolysis with recombinant tissue plasminogen activator within 6 h of acute ischemic stroke [the third International Stroke Trial (IST-3)]: A randomized controlled trial. *Lancet* **379**:2352–2363

IST-3 Collaborative Group (2015). Association between brain imaging signs, early and late outcomes, and response to intravenous alteplase after acute ischemic stroke in the third International Stroke Trial (IST-3): Secondary analysis of a randomized controlled trial. *Lancet Neurology* **14**:485–496

Jauch EC, Saver JL, Adams HP *et al.* (2013). Guidelines for the early management of patients with acute ischemic stroke: A guideline for healthcare professionals from the American Heart Association/American Stroke Association. *Stroke* **44**:870–947

Jovin TG, Chamorro A, Cobo E *et al.* (2015). Thrombectomy within 8 hours after symptom onset in ischemic stroke. *New England Journal of Medicine.* **372**:2296–2306

Kidwell CS, Jahan R, Gornbein J *et al.* (2013). A trial of imaging selection and endovascular treatment for ischemic stroke. *New England Journal of Medicine* **368**:914–923

Krieger DW, Yenari MA (2004). Therapeutic hypothermia for acute ischemic stroke: What do laboratory studies teach us? *Stroke* **35**:1482–1489

Lyden PD, Madden KP, Clark WM *et al.* (1990). Incidence of cerebral hemorrhage after treatment with tissue plasminogen activator or streptokinase following embolic stroke in rabbits. *Stroke* **21**:1589–1593

Ma QF, Chu CB, Song HQ (2015). Intravenous versus intra-arterial thrombolysis in ischemic stroke: A systematic review and meta-analysis. *PLoS One* **10**:e0116120

Menon BK, Saver JL, Prabhakaran S *et al.* (2012). Risk score for intracranial hemorrhage in patients with acute ischemic stroke treated with

intravenous tissue-type plasminogen activator. *Stroke* **43**:2293–2299

Meyer JS, Gilroy J, Barnhart MI *et al.* (1963). Therapeutic thrombolysis in cerebral thromboembolism. Double-blind evaluation of intravenous plasmin therapy in carotid and middle cerebral arterial occlusion. *Neurology* **13**:927–937

Muir KW (2001). Magnesium for neuroprotection in ischemic stroke: Rationale for use and evidence of effectiveness. *CNS Drugs* **15**:921–930

Multicenter Acute Stroke Trial – Europe Study Group (1996). Thrombolytic therapy with streptokinase in acute ischemic stroke. *New England Journal of Medicine* **335**:145–150

National Institute of Neurological Disorders and Stroke rt-PA Stroke Study Group (1995). Tissue plasminogen activator for acute ischemic stroke. *New England Journal of Medicine* **333**:1581–1588

Nogueira RG, Lutsep HL, Gupta R *et al.* (2012). Trevo versus Merci retrievers for thrombectomy revascularization of large vessel occlusion in acute ischemic stroke (TREVO 2): A randomized trial. *Lancet* **38**:1231–1240

Nogueira RG, Jadhav AP, Haussen DC *et al.* (2018). Thrombectomy 6 to 24 hours after stroke with a mismatch between deficit and infarct. *New England Journal of Medicine* **378**:11–21

O'Donnell MJ, Berge E, Sandset PM (2006). Are there patients with acute ischemic stroke and atrial fibrillation that benefit from low molecular weight heparin? *Stroke* **37**:452–455

Parsons M, Spratt N, Bivard A *et al.* (2012). A randomized trial of tenecteplase versus alteplase for acute ischemic stroke. *New England Journal of Medicine* **366**:1099–1107

Pierot L, Soize S, Benaissa A *et al.* (2015). Techniques for endovascular treatment of acute ischemic stroke: From intra-arterial fibrinolytics to stent-retrievers. *Stroke* **46**:909–914

Pollack CV Jr., Reilly PA, Eikelboom J *et al.* (2015). Idarucizumab for dabigatran reversal. *New England Journal of Medicine* **373**:511–520

Powers WJ, Derdeyn CP, Biller J et al. (2015). 2015 American Heart Association/American Stroke Association focused updated of the 2013 guidelines for the early management of patients with acute ischemic stroke regarding endovascular treatment: A guideline for healthcare professionals from the American Heart Association/American Stroke Association. *Stroke* **46**:3020–3035

Powers WJ, Rabinstein AA, Ackerson T *et al.* (2018). Guidelines for the early management of patients with acute ischemic stroke: A guideline for healthcare professionals from the American Heart Association/American Stroke Association. *Stroke* **49**:e46–e110

Rothwell PM, Algra A, Chen Z *et al.* (2016). Effects of aspirin on risk of severity of early recurrent stroke after transient ischemic attack and ischemic stroke: Time-course analysis of randomized trials. *Lancet* **388**:365–375

Sandercock P, Gubitz G, Foley P *et al.* (2003). Antiplatelet therapy for acute ischemic stroke. *Cochrane Database of Systematic Reviews* 2: CD000024

Saver JL (2006). Time is brain-quantified. *Stroke* **37**:263–266

Saver JL, Jahan R, Levy EI *et al.* (2012). Solitaire flow restoration device versus the Merci Retriever in patients with acute ischemic stroke (SWIFT): A randomized, parallel-group, non-inferiority trial. *Lancet* **380**:1241–1249

Saver JL, Goyal M, Bonafe A *et al.* (2015a). Stent-retriever thrombectomy after intravenous t-PA vs. t-PA alone in stroke. *New England Journal of Medicine* **372**:2285–2295

Saver JL, Starkman S, Eckstein M *et al.* (2015b). Prehospital use of magnesium sulfate as neuroprotection in acute stroke. *New England Journal of Medicine* **372**:528–536

Smith WS, Sung G, Starkman S *et al.* (2005). Safety and efficacy of mechanical embolectomy in acute ischemic: Results of the MERCI trial. *Stroke* **35**:1432–1438

Smith WS, Sung G, Saver J *et al.* (2008). Mechanical thrombectomy for acute ischemic stroke: Final results of the Multi MERCI trial. *Stroke* **39**:1205–1212

Sussman BJ, Fitch TS (1958). Thrombolysis with fibrinolysin in cerebral arterial occlusion. *JAMA* **167**:1705–1709

Sutherland BA, Minnerup J, Balami JS *et al.* (2012). Neuroprotection for ischemic stroke: Translation from the bench to the bedside. *International Journal of Stroke* **7**:407–418

Tanswell P, Modi N, Combs D *et al.* (2002). Pharmacokinetics and pharmacodynamics of tenecteplase in fibrinolytic therapy in acute myocardial infarction. *Clinical Pharmacokinetics* **41**:1229

Tsivgoulis G, Zand R, Katsanos AH *et al.* (2016). Risk of symptomatic intracerebral hemorrhage after intravenous thrombolysis in patients with acute ischemic stroke and high cerebral microbleed burden: A meta-analysis. *JAMA Neurology* **73**:675–683

von Kummer R, Mori E, Truelsen T *et al.* (2016). Desmoteplase 3 to 9 hours after major artery occlusion stroke: The DIAS-4 Trial (Efficacy and Safety Study of Desmoteplase to Treat Acute Ischemic Stroke). *Stroke* **47**:2880–2887

Whiteley WN, Emberson JE, Lees KR *et al.* (2016). Risk of intracerebral hemorrhage with alteplase after acute ischemic stroke: A secondary analysis of an individual patient data meta-analysis. *Lancet Neurology* **15**:925–933

Wong KS, Chen C, Ng PW *et al.* (2007). Low-molecular-weight heparin compared with aspirin for the treatment of acute ischemic stroke in Asian patients with large artery occlusive disease: A randomised study. *Lancet Neurology* **6**:407–413

Yamaguchi T, Mori E, Minematsu K *et al.* (2006). Alteplase at 0.6mg/kg for acute ischemic stroke within 3 hours of onset: Japan Alteplase Clinical Trial (J-ACT). *Stroke* **37**:1810–1815

Yang MH, Lin HY, Fu J *et al.* (2015). Decompressive hemicraniectomy in patients with malignant middle cerebral artery infarction: A systematic review and meta-analysis. *The Surgeon* **13**:230–240

Zivin JA, Fisher M, DeGirolami U *et al.* (1985). Tissue plasminogen activator reduces neurological damage after cerebral embolism. *Science* **230**:1289–1292

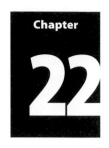

Specific Treatment of Acute Intracerebral Hemorrhage

Brain imaging using CT has a high sensitivity for intracerebral hemorrhage (ICH). The location, characteristics, and number of hemorrhages can aid in the diagnosis of the underlying cause and, thus, may influence subsequent patient management. For instance, the presence of multiple lobar hemorrhages may suggest cerebral amyloid angiopathy or an underlying metastatic tumor, whereas a basal ganglia hemorrhage in a hypertensive elderly person is unlikely to require further investigation. Repeat CT scanning is indicated if there is clinical deterioration, which may be caused by rebleeding or by hydrocephalus. If there are no changes, the search for systemic disorders should be intensified.

It is vital to instigate the correct management of patients with cerebellar hemorrhage as soon as possible owing to the high risk of hydrocephalus and brainstem compression.

Non-Surgical Treatments

Blood Pressure Management

Optimal blood pressure management in patients with ICH remains uncertain. Although aggressive lowering of systolic blood pressure, e.g., to < 140 mmHg compared with < 180 mmHg in the acute stage of ICH has been associated with a greater attenuation of hematoma growth (Tsivgoulis et al. 2014), intensive lowering of systolic blood pressure within 6 hours of ICH onset has not resulted in a lower risk of death or disability at 90 days in a meta-analysis of previous trials (Tsivgoulis et al. 2014) and also in the recent Antihypertensive Treatment of Acute Cerebral Hemorrhage II (ATACH-2) trial (Qureshi et al. 2016). On the other hand, however, aggressive lowering of blood pressure may lead to cerebral and renal hypoperfusion and was associated with more renal adverse events in the ATACH-2 trial (Qureshi et al. 2016) and possibly with cerebral ischemic injury detected on diffusion-weighted MRI in other studies (Menon et al. 2012). While current international stroke guidelines recommend that acute lowering of systolic blood pressure to 140 mmHg is safe (Hemphill et al. 2015), more studies that aim to differentiate individuals who are at high risk of hematoma expansion versus cerebral ischemic injury would be important in identifying individuals who would benefit most from aggressive blood pressure lowering in the acute stage of ICH.

Recombinant Factor VIIa

Recombinant factor VIIa is known to decrease the severity of hemorrhage in certain surgical settings. Since primary ICH has a tendency to enlarge over the first few hours, it has been proposed that agents promoting hemostasis may be beneficial in treating primary ICH.

However, although the use of recombinant factor VIIa has been shown to reduce hematoma growth in non-coagulopathic patients with ICH, it has not been shown to improve patient survival or functional outcome (Yuan *et al.* 2010). Furthermore, use of recombinant activated factor VIIa increases the incidence of arterial thromboembolic adverse events (Yuan *et al.* 2010). Recombinant activated factor VIIa is therefore not recommended in patients with primary ICH (Hemphill *et al.* 2015).

Cerebrospinal Fluid Drainage

Hydrocephalus is associated with a worse outcome in ICH. Insertion of a ventricular catheter can be life-saving in patients with cerebellar hemorrhage and hydrocephalus. In patients with supratentorial hemorrhage and hydrocephalus, however, the benefits of cerebrospinal fluid (CSF) diversion are less certain. In patients with intraventricular hemorrhage and acute obstructive hydrocephalus who subsequently receive an external ventricular drain, irrigation with alteplase is not associated with an improved functional outcome compared with irrigation with saline (Hanley *et al.* 2017).

Hyperventilation

Hyperventilation decreases intracranial pressure because hypocapnia, usually down to values of the order of 4 kPa, causes vasoconstriction. However, this will not necessarily be beneficial in patients with ICH since brain ischemia caused by compression is exchanged for ischemia caused by vasoconstriction (Stocchetti *et al.* 2005). In patients with head injury, the single randomized controlled trial of prolonged hyperventilation not only failed to show any benefit but also raised concerns about potential harm (Muizelaar *et al.* 1991; Schierhout and Roberts 2000). There are no controlled trials of hyperventilation in patients with intracerebral hematomas.

Osmotic Agents

Mannitol or hypertonic saline has been widely used in patients with primary ICH and a depressed level of consciousness to decrease intracranial pressure and alleviate the space-occupying effect of the hematoma in a deteriorating patient (Kamel *et al.* 2011). Although meta-analysis has shown that hypertonic saline is more effective than mannitol, current evidence is based on only a few trials of small sample size (Kamel *et al.* 2011), and large multicenter randomized trials are required before definitive recommendations could be made.

Surgical Treatment

Supratentorial Hemorrhage

There are five possible surgical procedures to treat intracerebral hematoma: simple aspiration, craniotomy with open surgery, decompressive craniectomy, endoscopic evacuation, and stereotactic aspiration. Craniotomy with open surgery remains the technique of choice at present.

In patients with large ICH and mass effect (Fig. 22.1), it might be thought that surgical removal would improve outcome. Craniotomy with open surgery was studied in the

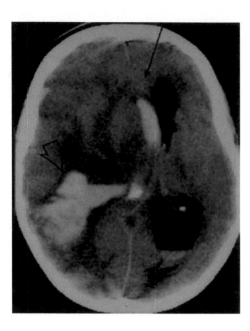

Fig. 22.1 A CT brain scan showing a primary ICH with rupture into the ventricular system (open arrow) and considerable mass effect (black arrow).

multicenter Surgical Trial in Intracerebral Hemorrhage (STICH; Mendelow *et al.* 2005). Nine preceding small randomized trials had produced conflicting results. The STICH trial randomized 1,033 patients, all with supratentorial hemorrhages, four times as many patients as in all previous trials taken together. Patients with a hematoma of at least 2 cm in diameter and a Glasgow Coma Score of ≥ 5 were randomized to initial conservative treatment versus early surgery if the admitting surgeon was uncertain of the benefit of surgery. Patients initially randomized to medical treatment could undergo surgery at a later time point if this was felt to be indicated. Surgical technique was left to the discretion of the surgeon.

The STICH trial reported no difference in outcome between those consigned to initial conservative or surgical management. In a prespecified subgroup analysis, patients with superficial hematomas within 1 cm of the cortical surface were more likely to have a favorable outcome than those with deep hematomas, and there was a nonsignificant relative benefit for surgery in this group. On the basis of these findings, STICH II (Mendelow *et al.* 2013) was conducted, specifically testing the hypothesis that early craniotomy within 48 hours of symptom onset improves clinical outcome in patients with superficial lobar ICH (10–100 cm^3 within 1 cm of the cortical surface and without intraventricular hemorrhage). There were nevertheless no differences in outcome in patients who were operated on compared with those who received conservative management. This result remained similar in an updated meta-analysis incorporating the two STICH trials (Mendelow *et al.* 2013). Nevertheless, in a non-prespecified analysis, the investigators of STICH II demonstrated that patients with a poor prognosis (GCS 9–12) did better with early surgery, while those with a good prognosis did not (Mendelow *et al.* 2013). Hence, although the benefit of early surgery in patients with supratentorial ICH remains unclear, current guidelines suggest that craniotomy in these instances may be considered in deteriorating patients (Hemphill *et al.* 2015).

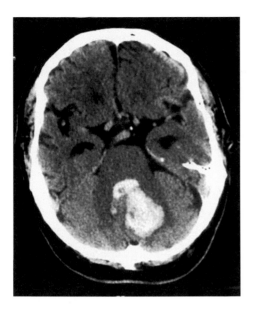

Fig. 22.2 A CT scan of a cerebellar hemorrhage.

Cerebellar Hemorrhage

Over the past few decades, surgical evacuation has been felt to be life-saving and relatively complication-free in patients with cerebellar hematomas who have clinical evidence of progressive brainstem compression (Fig. 22.2). Consequently, a randomized trial is unlikely to occur. Certain patients can be managed conservatively, but there is uncertainty about the selection criteria. Indications for evacuation of cerebellar hematoma include a depressed level of consciousness, signs of brainstem compression, hematoma size greater than 3 cm, hematoma volume greater than 7 cm^3, and obliteration of the fourth ventricle (Wijdicks *et al.* 2000; Cohen *et al.* 2002; Jensen and St. Louis 2005, Hankey 2017). Where all brainstem reflexes have been lost for more than a few hours, outcome is uniformly fatal. An external ventricular drain is usually inserted as well if there is associated hydrocephalus, but ventriculostomy alone in patients with cerebellar hemorrhage who have brainstem compression and/or hydrocephalus is not recommended (Hemphill *et al.* 2015).

Other Surgical Approaches

Decompressive craniectomy with or without hematoma evacuation might reduce mortality in patients with supratentorial ICH who are in coma, have large hematomas with significant midline shift, or have elevated intracranial pressure refractory to medical treatment (Takeuchi *et al.* 2013).

Aspiration not accompanied by any other intervention was attempted mainly in the 1950s but was subsequently abandoned because only small amounts of clot could be obtained and because the procedure could precipitate rebleeding. Since the 1990s, stereotactic aspiration of supratentorial hemorrhage without endoscopy, mostly combined with instillation of fibrinolytic agents, has been reported in several observational studies. Although a recent meta-analysis suggested superiority of these minimally invasive approaches over craniotomy, methodological flaws of this analysis have been raised (Zhou *et al.* 2012; Gregson *et al.* 2013). Since then, the Minimally Invasive Surgery Plus Recombinant Tissue-Type Plasminogen Activator for ICH Evacuation Trial II (MISTIE II) was conducted and demonstrated that minimally invasive surgery plus alteplase significantly reduces peri-hematomal edema with a trend of improved clinical outcomes and hence shows promise in treatment of deep hematomas (Mould *et al.* 2013). MISTIE III is currently under way, aiming to confirm these findings in a larger number of patients. In the meantime, the effectiveness of minimally invasive clot evacuation with stereotactic or endoscopic aspiration with or without thrombolytic usage remains uncertain (Hemphill *et al.* 2015).

Treatment of Specific Types of Intracerebral Hemorrhage

Pontine Hemorrhages

Pontine hemorrhages are fatal in around 50% of patients (Wijdicks and St. Louis 1997). Those caused by cavernomas or arteriovenous malformations have a better outcome (Rabinstein *et al.* 2004). The management of patients with "hypertensive" pontine hemorrhage is usually conservative, but some case reports have documented successful stereotactic aspiration. However, there is likely publication bias, and the natural history of the condition is difficult to predict since patients with small hemorrhages do well with conservative management.

Lobar Hemorrhage from Presumed Amyloid Angiopathy

In patients with lobar hemorrhage from amyloid angiopathy and with an impaired level of consciousness, the prognosis is poor after surgical intervention (McCarron *et al.* 1999). It remains unclear whether the outcome would have been better without surgery (Greene *et al.* 1990; Izumihara *et al.* 1999). Given these uncertainties and the danger that the operation provokes new hemorrhages from brittle vessels at distant sites (Brisman *et al.* 1996), conservative treatment seems the best option.

Cerebral Cavernous Malformations (Also Known as Cavernous Angiomas or Cavernomas)

There is little doubt that hemorrhages, which may be recurrent, from cerebral cavernous malformations (CCMs) are less destructive than brainstem hemorrhages from an arterial source (Rabinstein *et al.* 2004). However, although microsurgical resection or stereotactic "gamma knife" radiosurgery is regularly performed, these therapies have not been supported by randomized controlled trials. Furthermore, some CCMs may spontaneously regress (Yasui *et al.* 2005), and microsurgical resection may result in worse clinical outcome compared with conservative management alone (Moultrie *et al.* 2014). While stereotactic radiotherapy is likely to be associated with fewer adverse events compared with microsurgical resection, the long-term prognosis of patients receiving stereotactic radiotherapy also remains uncertain. Current guidelines are therefore unable to make specific recommendations regarding definitive management of CCMs (Samarasekera *et al.* 2012). Only recently has the clinical course of CCMs been fully understood (Horne *et al.* 2016). In an individual patient data meta-analysis of 1,620 patients, the 5-year estimated risk of ICH in patients who presented without ICH or focal neurological deficit was 3.8% for patients with non-brainstem CCMs and 8% for those with brainstem CCMs (Horne *et al.* 2016). In contrast, among patients who presented with ICH or focal neurological deficit, the 5-year risk of ICH was 18.4% for non-brainstem CCMs and 30.8% for brainstem CCMs (Horne *et al.* 2016). While microsurgical resection may therefore appear justified for symptomatic supratentorial CCMs (pooled post-operative adverse event risk ~7.7%) but probably not for symptomatic brainstem CCMs (pooled post-operative adverse event risk ~50.4%) or asymptomatic CCMs, further studies and randomized controlled trials which aim to determine the benefits and risks of conservative management versus microsurgical resection versus stereotactic radiosurgery in symptomatic and asymptomatic brainstem versus non-brainstem CCMs would be required before definitive recommendations could be made.

Dural Arteriovenous Fistulae

Arteriovenous fistulae in the dura are heterogeneous. They may or may not be secondary to occlusion of a major sinus. Abnormal venous drainage from meningeal arteries may be channeled into a dural sinus or into superficial veins of the surface of the brain, cerebellum, or brainstem. Accordingly, different methods are required to occlude the fistula. Surgical techniques include selective ligation of leptomeningeal draining veins, resection of fistulous sinus tracts, and a cranial base approach with extradural bone removal. Endovascular techniques may consist of an approach from the arterial or venous side, recanalization and stenting of a venous sinus, or venous embolization via a craniotomy (Tomak *et al.* 2003). Finally, stereotactic cobalt-generated radiation "gamma knife" therapy is also used for obliterating arteriovenous fistulae (O'Leary *et al.* 2002; Pan *et al.* 2002), sometimes in conjunction with an endovascular approach (Friedman *et al.* 2001).

Moyamoya Syndrome Associated Hemorrhage

Moyamoya syndrome (Chapter 6) causes gradual stenosis or occlusion of the terminal portions of the internal carotid arteries or middle cerebral arteries. This leads to formation of an abnormal collateral network of fragile vessels, which occasionally rupture. It has been proposed that constructing a bypass to relieve the pressure on the collaterals would be beneficial, for example between the superficial temporal artery and the middle cerebral artery (Kawaguchi *et al.* 2000), but whether this procedure prevents bleeding remains uncertain. In fact, an aneurysm may form and rupture at the site of the arterial bypass (Nishimoto *et al.* 2005).

Iatrogenic Intracerebral Hemorrhage

Anticoagulation

Vitamin K antagonists (warfarin) are associated with an increased rate of ICH (~0.2% per year) (Hart *et al.* 2007), while the risk of ICH in patients on non-vitamin K antagonist anticoagulants (NOACs) is about 50% lower (Verheugt and Granger 2015).

In patients with warfarin-related ICH, rapid correction of the international normalized ratio (INR) to < 1.3 and reduction of systolic blood pressure to < 160 mmHg within 4 hours are associated with reduced hematoma enlargement (Kuramatsu *et al.* 2015). Warfarin should be withheld and intravenous vitamin K (5–10 mg) given (Hemphill *et al.* 2015). However, administration of intravenous vitamin K alone is inadequate due to its slow onset of action (~2 hours after administration). Fresh frozen plasma (FFP) has traditionally been used to further lower the INR. However, FFP administration has many disadvantages including the need to thaw and cross-match, carries a potential risk of allergic and infectious transfusion reaction, often requires large volumes for full INR correction (and hence poses a risk of fluid overload), and has a slow onset of action. In contrast, prothrombin complex concentrate (PCC) does not require cross-matching, has been processed to inactivate infectious agents, could be administered quickly in small volumes (20–40 ml), and has been shown to rapidly normalize INR within minutes. PCC, however, may potentially increase the risk of thromboembolic events. Three-factor PCC contains factors II, IX, and X, while four-factor PCC also contains factor VII. Recently, the INCH trial compared the efficacy and safety of FFP versus four-factor PCC in patients with warfarin-associated ICH (Steiner *et al.* 2016). Results from this trial favored use of four-factor PCC over FFP and demonstrated a faster normalization of INR (67% versus 9% reached target INR < 1.3 within 3 hours of treatment) and lower risk of hematoma expansion (Steiner *et al.* 2016). As recombinant factor VIIa does not replace all clotting factors, it is not recommended for warfarin-associated ICH (Hemphill *et al.* 2015).

In patients with atrial fibrillation on warfarin who subsequently develop a lobar ICH, current guidelines do not recommend warfarin be resumed in view of the high risk of recurrent ICH (Hemphill *et al.* 2015). NOACs or left atrial appendage occlusion devices may have a role in these patients. Should anticoagulation be restarted, avoidance of oral anticoagulation for at least 4 weeks, in patients without mechanical heart valves, is recommended to decrease the risk of recurrent ICH (Hemphill *et al.* 2015). Anticoagulation might be reconsidered in those with deep ICH (Hemphill *et al.* 2015).

It remains uncertain when to reintroduce anticoagulants in patients with a strong indication for this treatment, such as those with artificial heart valves, since only anecdotal experience is available. In the Mayo Clinic series, only one ischemic stroke occurred in 52 patients with artificial heart valves in whom anticoagulants were discontinued for a median period of 10 days (Phan *et al.* 2000). In contrast, of seven similar patients from Heidelberg, three had large ischemic strokes within a comparable period after stopping anticoagulation (Bertram *et al.* 2000). Reintroduction of anticoagulation between one and two weeks after the hemorrhage is probably reasonable (Estol and Kase 2003) and is supported by evidence of low rates of rebleeding (Wijdicks *et al.* 1998; Leker and Abramsky 1998).

Patients on NOACs who develop ICH should similarly discontinue the NOAC immediately and receive PCC infusion (Heidbuchel *et al.* 2015). Activated charcoal could be provided in those with intake of NOAC within 2 hours (Hemphill *et al.* 2015). In patients previously on the direct thrombin inhibitor dabigatran, 5g of intravenous idarucizumab, a specific reversal agent of dabigatran that is able to completely reverse the anticoagulant effect of dabigatran within minutes (Pollack *et al.* 2015), should be given as soon as possible (Heidbuchel *et al.* 2015). Reversal agents for factor Xa inhibitors (e.g., rivaroxaban, apixaban, and edoxaban) such as andexanet alfa have similarly been shown to reduce factor Xa activity quickly and are currently awaiting FDA approval before their routine clinical use (Connolly *et al.* 2016). Antidotes for potential reversal of a range of anticoagulants (direct thrombin inhibitors, factor Xa inhibitors, and heparin), such as aripazine (also known as ciraparantag or PER977), are currently being developed and tested (Ansell *et al.* 2014, 2016).

Aspirin

Aspirin treatment is associated with a small risk of intracerebral hemorrhage (0.2 events per 1,000 patient-years) (Gorelick and Weisman 2005). Compared with individuals not on antiplatelets, antiplatelet use at the time of ICH is independently associated with increased mortality but not with poor functional outcome (Thompson *et al.* 2010). Although it was suggested in small case series that platelet transfusion within 12 hours of ICH symptom onset may possibly be associated with better functional outcome (Naidech *et al.* 2012), the recent PATCH (Platelet transfusion versus standard care after acute stroke due to spontaneous cerebral hemorrhage associated with antiplatelet therapy) trial have demonstrated the opposite (Baharoglu *et al.* 2016). Platelet transfusion in antiplatelet-associated ICH was associated with an increased risk of death or dependence at 3 months, most probably due to a pro-thrombotic state as a result of platelet transfusion (Baharoglu *et al.* 2016). While antiplatelets should be stopped during the acute phase of ICH, whether the benefits of restarting antiplatelets outweigh its risks of recurrent ICH remains uncertain. Recent observational studies have suggested that the increase in coronary and cerebral ischemic events secondary to stopping aspirin may outweigh the risks of recurrent ICH (Chong *et al.* 2012), although the underlying location and burden of cerebral microbleeds would also need to be considered. The REstart or STop Antithrombotics Randomized Trial (RESTART) is currently under way to address this question.

Thrombolytic Therapy

Thrombolytic therapy for myocardial infarction is rarely complicated by intracerebral hemorrhage, but the case fatality is high. The risk of symptomatic ICH in acute ischemic stroke patients receiving thrombolysis is approximately 6.4%. Treatment includes stopping the infusion of fibrinolytic drugs and other anti-thrombotic drugs, control of hypertension, and administration of FFP. Use of anti-fibrinolytic drugs is controversial. Surgical treatment is of unproven value and may be especially hazardous given that amyloid angiopathy may be a contributing factor.

References

Ansell JE, Bakhru SH, Laulicht BE *et al.* (2014). Use of PER977 to reverse the anticoagulant effect of edoxaban. *New England Journal of Medicine* **371**:2141–2142

Ansell JE, Laulicht BE, Bakhru SH *et al.* (2016). Ciraparantag safely and completely reverses the anticoagulant effects of low molecular weight heparin. *Thrombosis Research* **146**:113–118

Baharoglu MI, Cordonnier C, Salman RA *et al.* (2016). Platelet transfusion versus standard care after acute stroke due to spontaneous cerebral hemorrhage associated with antiplatelet therapy (PATCH): A randomized, open-label, phase 3 trial. *Lancet* **387**:2605–2613

Bertram M, Bonsanto M, Hacke W *et al.* (2000). Managing the therapeutic dilemma: patients with spontaneous intracerebral hemorrhage and urgent need for anticoagulation. *Journal of Neurology* **247**:209–214

Brisman MH, Bederson JB, Sen CN *et al.* (1996). Intracerebral hemorrhage occurring remote from the craniotomy site. *Neurosurgery* **39**:1114–1121

Chong BH, Chan KH, Pong V *et al.* (2012). Use of aspirin in Chinese after recovery from primary intracerebral hemorrhage. *Thrombosis and Hemostasis* **107**:241–247

Cohen ZR, Ram Z, Knoller N *et al.* (2002). Management and outcome of non-traumatic cerebellar haemorrhage. *Cerebrovascular Diseases* **14**:207–213

Connolly SJ, Milling TJ Jr., Eikelboom JW *et al.* (2016). Andexanet alfa for acute major bleeding associated with factor Xa inhibitors. *New England Journal of Medicine* 375:1131–1141

Estol CJ, Kase CS (2003). Need for continued use of anticoagulants after intracerebral hemorrhage. *Current Treatment Options in Cardiovascular Medicine* 5:201–209

Friedman JA, Pollock BE, Nichols DA et al. (2001). Results of combined stereotactic, radiosurgery and transarterial embolization for dural arteriovenous fistulas of the transverse and sigmoid sinuses. *Journal of Neurosurgery* 94:886–891

Gorelick PB and Weisman SM. (2005). Risk of hemorrhagic stroke with aspirin use: an update. *Stroke* 36:1801–1807

Greene GM, Godersky JC, Biller J et al. (1990). Surgical experience with cerebral amyloid angiopathy. *Stroke* 21:1545–1549

Gregson BA, Rowan EN and Mendelow AD (2013). Letter to the editor by Gregson et al. regarding article, "Minimally invasive surgery for spontaneous supratentorial intracerebral hemorrhage: A meta-analysis of randomized controlled trials." *Stroke* 44:e45

Hanley DF, Lane K, McBee N et al. (2017). Thrombolytic removal of intraventricular hemorrhage in treatment of severe stroke: Results of the randomized, multicenter, multiregion, placebo-controlled CLEAR III trial. *Lancet* 389:603–611

Hankey GJ (2017). Stroke. *Lancet* 389:641–654

Hart RG, Pearce LA and Aguilar MI. (2007) Adjusted-dose warfarin versus aspirin for preventing stroke in patients with atrial fibrillation. *Annals of Internal Medicine* 147:590–592

Heidbuchel H, Verhamme P, Alings M et al. (2015). Updated European Heart Rhythm Association Practical Guide on the use of non-vitamin K antagonist anticoagulants in patients with non-valvular atrial fibrillation. *Europace* 17:1467–1507

Hemphill JC III, Greenberg SM, Anderson CS et al. (2015). Guidelines for the management of spontaneous intracerebral hemorrhage: A guideline for healthcare professionals from the American Heart Association/American Stroke Association. *Stroke* 46:2032–2060

Horne MA, Flemming KD, Su I-C et al. (2016). Clinical course of untreated cerebral cavernous malformations: A meta-analysis of individual patient data. *Lancet Neurology* 15:166–173

Izumihara A, Ishihara T, Iwamoto N et al. (1999). Postoperative outcome of 37 patients with lobar intracerebral hemorrhage related to cerebral amyloid angiopathy. *Stroke* 30:29–33

Jensen MB, St. Louis EK (2005). Management of acute cerebellar stroke. *Archives of Neurology* 62:537–544

Kamel H, Navi BB, Nakagawa K et al. (2011) Hypertonic saline versus mannitol for the treatment of elevated intracranial pressure: A meta-analysis of randomized clinical trials. *Critical Care Medicine* 39:554–559

Kawaguchi S, Okuno S, Sakaki T (2000). Effect of direct arterial bypass on the prevention of future stroke in patients with the hemorrhagic variety of moyamoya disease. *Journal of Neurosurgery* 93:397–401

Kuramatsu JB, Gerner ST, Schellinger PD et al. (2015). Anticoagulant reversal, blood pressure levels, and anticoagulant resumption in patients with anticoagulation-related intracerebral hemorrhage. *JAMA* 313:824–836

Leker RR, Abramsky O (1998). Early anticoagulation in patients with prosthetic heart valves and intracerebral hematoma. *Neurology* 50:1489–1491

McCarron MO, Nicoll JA, Love S et al. (1999). Surgical intervention biopsy and APOE genotype in cerebral amyloid angiopathy-related haemorrhage. *British Journal of Neurosurgery* 13:462–467

Mendelow AD, Gregson BA, Fernandes HM et al. (2005). Early surgery versus initial conservative treatment in patients with spontaneous supratentorial intracerebral hematomas in the international Surgical Trial in Intracerebral Hemorrhage (STICH): A randomized trial. *Lancet* 365:387–397

Mendelow AD, Gregson BA, Rowan EN et al. (2013). Early surgery versus initial conservative treatment in patients with spontaneous supratentorial lobar intracerebral hematomas (STITCH II): A randomized trial. *Lancet* 382:397–408

Menon RS, Burgess RE, Wing JJ et al. (2012). Predictors of highly prevalent brain ischemia in intracerebral hemorrhage. *Annals of Neurology* **71**:199–205

Mould WA, Carhuapoma JR, Muschelli J et al. (2013). Minimally invasive surgery plus recombinant tissue-type plasminogen activator for intracerebral hemorrhage evacuation decreases perihematomal edema. *Stroke* **44**:627–634

Moultrie F, Horne MA, Josephson CB et al. (2014). Outcome after surgical or conservative management of cerebral cavernous malformations. *Neurology* **83**:582–589

Muizelaar JP, Marmarou A, Ward JD et al. (1991). Adverse effects of prolonged hyperventilation in patients with severe head injury: A randomized clinical trial. *Journal of Neurosurgery* **75**:731–739

Naidech AM, Liebling SM, Rosenberg NF et al. (2012). Early platelet transfusion improves platelet activity and may improve outcomes after intracerebral hemorrhage. *Neurocritical Care* **16**:82–87

Nishimoto T, Yuki K, Sasaki T et al. (2005). A ruptured middle cerebral artery aneurysm originating from the site of anastomosis 20 years after extracranial-intracranial bypass for moyamoya disease: Case report. *Surgical Neurology* **64**:261–265

O'Leary S, Hodgson TJ, Coley SC et al. (2002). Intracranial dural arteriovenous malformations: Results of stereotactic radiosurgery in 17 patients. *Clinical Oncology of the Royal College of Radiologists* **14**:97–102

Pan DH, Chung WY, Guo WY et al. (2002). Stereotactic radiosurgery for the treatment of dural arteriovenous fistulas involving the transverse-sigmoid sinus. *Journal of Neurosurgery* **96**:823–829

Phan TG, Koh M, Wijdicks EFM (2000). Safety of discontinuation of anticoagulation in patients with intracranial hemorrhage at high thromboembolic risk. *Archives of Neurology* **57**:1710–1713

Pollack CV Jr., Reilly PA, Eikelboom J et al. (2015). Idarucizumab for dabigatran reversal. *New England Journal of Medicine* **373**:511–520

Qureshi AI, Palesch YY, Barsan WG et al. (2016). Intensive blood-pressure lowering in patients with acute cerebral hemorrhage. *New England Journal of Medicine* **375**:1033–1043

Rabinstein AA, Tisch SH, McClelland RL et al. (2004). Cause is the main predictor of outcome in patients with pontine hemorrhage. *Cerebrovascular Diseases* **17**:66–71

Samarasekera N, Poorthuis M, Kontoh K et al. (2012). *Guidelines for the Management of Cerebral Cavernous Malformations in Adults.* London: Genetic Alliance UK and Cavernoma Alliance UK.

Schierhout G and Roberts I (2000). Hyperventilation therapy for acute traumatic brain injury. *Cochrane Database of Systematic Reviews* **2**:CD000566

Steiner T, Poli S, Griebe M et al. (2016). Fresh frozen plasma versus prothrombin complex concentrate in patients with intracerebral hemorrhage related to vitamin K antagonists (INCH): A randomized trial. *Lancet* **15**:566–573

Stocchetti N, Maas AI, Chieregato A et al. (2005). Hyperventilation in head injury: A review. *Chest* **127**:1812–1827

Takeuchi S, Wada K, Nagatani K et al. (2013). Decompressive hemicraniectomy for spontaneous intracerebral hemorrhage. *Neurosurgical Focus* **345**:E5

Thompson BB, Béjot Y, Caso V et al. (2010). Prior antiplatelet therapy and outcome following intracerebral hemorrhage: a systematic review. *Neurology* **75**:1333–1342

Tomak PR, Cloft HJ, Kaga A et al. (2003). Evolution of the management of tentorial dural arteriovenous malformations. *Neurosurgery* **52**:750–760

Tsivgoulis G, Katsanos AH, Butcher KS et al. (2014). Intensive blood pressure reduction in acute intracerebral hemorrhage: A meta-analysis. *Neurology* **83**:1523–1529

Verheugt FWA and Granger GB (2015). Oral anticoagulants for stroke prevention in atrial fibrillation: current status, special situations, and unmet needs. *Lancet* **386**:303–310

Wijdicks EF, St. Louis E (1997). Clinical profiles predictive of outcome in pontine hemorrhage. *Neurology* **49**:1342–1346

Wijdicks EFM, Schievink WI, Brown RD et al. (1998). The dilemma of discontinuation of anticoagulation therapy for patients with intracranial hemorrhage and mechanical heart valves. *Neurosurgery* **42**:769–773

Wijdicks EFM, Louis EKS, Atkinson JD et al. (2000). Clinician's biases toward surgery in cerebellar hematomas: An analysis of decision-making in 94 patients. *Cerebrovascular Diseases* **10**:93–96

Yasui T, Komiyama M, Iwai Y et al. (2005). A brainstem cavernoma demonstrating a dramatic spontaneous decrease in size during follow-up: case report and review of the literature. *Surgical Neurology* **63**:170–173

Yuan ZH, Jiang JK, Huang WD et al. (2010). A meta-analysis of the efficacy and safety of recombinant activated factor VII for patients with acute intracerebral hemorrhage without hemophilia. *Journal of Clinical Neuroscience* **17**:685–693

Zhou X, Chen J, Li Q et al. (2012). Minimally invasive surgery for spontaneous supratentorial intracerebral hemorrhage: a meta-analysis of randomized controlled trials. *Stroke* **43**:2923–2930

Chapter 23

Recovery and Rehabilitation after Stroke

Some degree of recovery occurs in the majority of patients after stroke, and complete recovery is possible, although the prognosis is difficult to predict in an individual patient. Rehabilitation to aid recovery and enable the patient to develop strategies for coping with disability forms the mainstay of treatment after the acute stroke period.

Recovery after Stroke

Approximately two-thirds of stroke survivors become independent at 1 year, with little difference between ischemic or hemorrhagic strokes. However, within the ischemic group, only about 5% of patients with infarction of the whole middle cerebral artery territory are alive and independent at a year post-stroke compared with 50% of those with more restricted infarcts (Table 16.1) (Bamford *et al.* 1990). Approximately 90% of stroke survivors return home, leaving only a small proportion in institutional care, but because stroke is so common, their absolute number is large (Legh-Smith *et al.* 1986; Chuang *et al.* 2005).

The mechanisms of recovery are incompletely understood. Acute resolution of edema and recanalization of occluded vessels leading to resolution of penumbral dysfunction may contribute. In the subacute phase, changes in neuronal networks and neuronal plasticity are important (Kreisel *et al.* 2007; Nudo 2007). The mechanisms share similarities with those involved in learning and memory. The rate of recovery of all impairments is maximal in the first few weeks, slows down after 2 or 3 months, and probably stops at about 6–12 months post-stroke (Pedersen *et al.* 1995; Kreisel *et al.* 2007). Other factors that may play a role in the plateau of recovery include limited or absence of therapy, often resulting in learned disuse and hindering further improvement; post-stroke depression; side effects of medications such as excessive benzodiazepine use; and other concomitant comorbidities. Bodily functions that have bihemispheric representation in the cortex such as swallowing, facial movement, and gait tend to demonstrate better and faster recovery than other deficits that are more lateralized in functional anatomy such as language, spatial attention, and dominant hand movement (Hamdy *et al.* 1998; Cramer and Crafton 2006). Later improvement in functional abilities, and particularly in social activities, probably has more to do with adaptation to disability and minimizing handicap rather than further recovery of physical impairments. Impaired quality of life is common even when patients appear to have little disability.

Prediction of functional outcome for individuals immediately after stroke onset is difficult, and clinical features predict outcome as well as or better than conventional neuroradiological findings (Hand *et al.* 2006). Studies have shown that motor recovery tends to start in the proximal upper and lower limb muscles and then progress distally.

The Early Prediction of Functional Outcome After Stroke (EPOS) study found that recovery of upper limb function could be predicted based on the presence or absence of voluntary extension of the fingers and abduction of the hemiplegic shoulder (Nijland *et al.* 2010). Those who had some regain in power in extending the fingers and abducting the hemiplegic shoulder on the second day after stroke had a 98% chance of regaining some dexterity of the upper limb at 6 months, defined as an action research arm test (ARAT) score $\geq$ 10 (Lyle 1981; van der Lee *et al.* 2001; Yozbatiran *et al.* 2008; Nijland et al. 2010). Sixty percent of patients who had some recovery in voluntarily extending the fingers reached the maximum ARAT score at 6 months. However, the probability of regaining dexterity of the upper limb at 6 months in patients who could not voluntarily extend the fingers nor abduct the hemiplegic shoulder on day 2 reduced to 25% and further reduced to 14% if patients continued to have absence of these movements by day 9 post-stroke (Nijland *et al.* 2010).

In addition to upper limb paresis, a systematic review of prognostic studies also identified age and stroke severity as predictors of functional outcome, but sex and vascular risk factors were not (Veerbeek *et al.* 2011). However, due to insufficient methodological quality of most prognostic studies, the predictive value of many clinical determinants for outcome of activities of daily living remains unclear (Veerbeek *et al.* 2011). Various prognostic scores using a combination of clinical factors have been developed (e.g., Bologna Outcome Algorithm for Stroke [BOAS] scale – age, stroke severity, need of urinary catheter, oxygen administration, upper limb paralysis upon discharge; Acute Stroke Registry and Analysis of Lausanne [ASTRAL] – age, stroke severity, stroke onset to admission time, range of visual fields, acute glucose, level of consciousness), and these have shown good prediction of dependency after ischemic stroke (Muscari *et al.* 2011; Ntaios *et al.* 2012).

About 2 weeks after stroke, good prognostic signs include young age, initially mild deficit, normal conscious level, good sitting balance, lack of cognitive impairment, lack of urinary continence, and rapid improvement. Independent living is often also contingent on a high level of social support.

Strategies for Rehabilitation

Stroke rehabilitation attempts to restore patients to their previous physical, mental, and social capability (Langton Hewer 1990; Brandstater 2005). Rehabilitation approaches include restoration of previous function, compensation by increasing function for a given impairment, environmental modification, prevention of complications such as recurrent stroke or shoulder pain, and maintenance or prevention of deterioration. Achieving optimal quality of life is the ultimate goal. Although there is good evidence that increased time undergoing therapy is beneficial (Langhorne *et al.* 1996; Kwakkel *et al.* 2004; Kwakkel 2006), in general, patients spend very little of their time awake receiving therapy, only around 5% in one study (Bernhardt *et al.* 2004). As little as 5 hours a week of extra therapy results in clinically important improvements in walking (Blennerhassett and Dite 2004). Rehabilitation should not necessarily be confined to patients in the hospital, and early discharge with multidisciplinary support achieves as good of or better outcome (Langhorne and Holmqvist 2007).

The optimum time to start rehabilitation after stroke is not known, but some early rehabilitation within the first week is probably beneficial due to the following reasons: (1) bed rest may negatively affect cardiorespiratory function and musculoskeletal and immune systems and hence might slow recovery (Allen *et al.* 1999); (2) immobility after stroke may lead to an increased risk of complications (Langhorne *et al.* 2000; Bernhardt *et al.* 2004); and (3) there might be a narrow window of opportunity early after stroke for brain plasticity and repair (Murphy and Corbett 2009; Krakauer *et al.* 2012).

Recently, a large randomized trial (AVERT, A Very Early Rehabilitation Trial) compared the effectiveness of frequent, higher-dose, and very early mobilization versus usual care after stroke (Lynch *et al.* 2014; AVERT Trial Collaborative Group 2015). In AVERT, 1,054 patients with ischemic or hemorrhagic stroke were randomized to receive frequent, high-dose, and very early mobilization within 24 hours of stroke, and 1,050 patients were randomized to receive usual care. In was noted that compared with usual care, a higher-dose, very early mobilization protocol was associated with a reduction in odds of a favorable outcome (modified Rankin Scale < 3) at 3 months (AVERT Trial Collaborative Group 2015). However, in a subsequent prespecified dose-response analysis of all patients irrespective of treatment arm, a poor outcome was mainly accounted by increasing the minutes of out-of-bed activity (Bernhardt *et al.* 2016). In contrast, shorter but more frequent mobilization early after stroke was associated with a favorable outcome, independent of age and stroke severity, such that a 13% improvement in the odds of a favorable outcome was noted with each additional session of out-of-bed activity per day (Bernhardt *et al.* 2016). Nevertheless, the optimal timing to start out-of-bed activity remains uncertain (Bernhardt *et al.* 2016), although animal studies suggest that activity within 24–48 hours of ischemic stroke onset might be helpful (Austin *et al.* 2014; Egan *et al.* 2014). Clinical trials in patients with intracerebral hemorrhage have also shown that early rehabilitation starting within 48 hours of stroke onset demonstrated benefit in 6-month survival and functional outcome (Liu *et al.* 2014). The optimal "dose" of rehabilitation is also uncertain, and like AVERT, the Very Early Constraint-Induced Movement during Stroke Rehabilitation (VECTORS) trial showed that in patients with stroke, high-intensity constraint-induced movement therapy had significantly less improvement at day 90 compared with patients who received a less intensive regimen (Dromerick *et al.* 2009). The reason why early intensive therapy appears to be detrimental is uncertain but may be because intensive therapy may worsen any underlying ischemic injury due to an increased demand for oxygenated blood.

There is insufficient data to determine which patient groups benefit most from rehabilitation. Although severely affected patients benefit from rehabilitation, and in fact receive the most inpatient and outpatient therapy, they have the worst functional outcomes (Alexander *et al.* 2001). Therefore, it is unclear at present how best to target the available rehabilitation resources most efficiently.

The evidence base to support particular rehabilitation strategies is limited owing to a lack of large randomized trials. Yet it is clear that multidisciplinary input facilitates recovery and reduces handicap (Bayley *et al.* 2007). Key components of inpatient rehabilitation have been identified (Stroke Unit Trialists' Collaboration 1997; Langhorne and Duncan 2001; Langhorne and Dennis 2004) as:

- coordinated, multidisciplinary care with regular team meetings.
- early institution of rehabilitation within 1 to 2 weeks.
- goal setting.
- early assessment of impairments and function.
- discharge planning with early assessment of discharge needs.
- staff with a specialist interest in stroke or rehabilitation.
- routine involvement of caregivers.

- close linking of nursing with other multidisciplinary care.
- regular programs of education and training for staff.
- information provided about stroke, stroke recovery, and available services.

A systematic review of randomized control trials of inpatient multidisciplinary stroke rehabilitation has shown the benefits of rehabilitation, beyond 7 days after stroke, as distinct from the acute medical management aspects of acute stroke care in the first week after stroke (Langhorne and Duncan 2001), with a reduction in death (odds ratio [OR] 0.66; 95% confidence interval [CI], 0.49–0.88) and death or dependency (OR, 0.65; 95% CI, 0.50–0.85). For every 20 patients with stroke treated in a post-acute (beyond 7 days) multidisciplinary rehabilitation unit, one additional person returns home independent in activities of daily living.

There is also evidence that outpatient (Outpatient Service Trialists 2003) and home-based (Early Supported Discharge Trialists 2005; Langhorne and Holmqvist 2007) rehabilitation are effective for patients who have returned to the community in preventing death, deterioration, and dependency and may allow earlier hospital discharge.

Assessment Tools Used in Rehabilitation

Assessment tools identify, measure, and record impairments, disabilities, handicaps, and quality of life. Assessment is the first step in rehabilitation, and measurement of outcome is crucial for clinical trials, audit, and comparison of different institutions. Patients' present levels of functioning must be compared with their premorbid levels, taking account of the numerous comorbidities often present in the elderly (Collen and Wade 1991).

For clinical trial and audit purposes in large samples, three simple questions group patients into those who are completely recovered, those who are still symptomatic but independent, and those who are dependent or dead (Dennis *et al.* 1997a, b). Various more detailed assessment instruments are available that are designed to test different domains (Lyden and Hantson 1998; Warlow *et al.* 1996):

- motricity index and trunk control test (Collin and Wade 1990).
- action research arm test (Lyle 1981).
- walking speed test (Wade *et al.* 1987; Collen *et al.* 1990).
- Rivermead mobility index (Collen *et al.* 1991).
- Frenchay Aphasia Screening Test for aphasia (Enderby *et al.* 1986).
- Star Cancellation Test for neglect (Jehkonen *et al.* 1998).
- Barthel Activities of Daily Living Index.
- modified Rankin Scale (Oxford Handicap Scale) – may be more useful than the Barthel Index (Table 23.1) (Bamford *et al.* 1989).
- Frenchay Activity Index for social functioning (Wade *et al.* 1985).

It is important to try to assess mood after stroke, even though this is often difficult since the risk is high and depression contributes to poor cognitive function and outcome. The Short Form-36 is the most widely used generic instrument for assessment of "quality of life", but the EuroQol is also used. Neither is reliable enough to monitor individuals over time, but they may be used to compare groups of patients (de Haan *et al.* 1993; Dorman *et al.* 1998).

Interventions

Stroke rehabilitation teams usually consist of physical therapists, occupational therapists, speech therapists, and social workers as well as nursing staff. The stroke rehabilitation team

Table 23.1 Modified Rankin scale

Grade	Symptoms
0	No symptoms
1	Minor symptoms that do not interfere with lifestyle
2	Minor handicap; symptoms that lead to some restriction in lifestyle but do not interfere with patients' ability to look after themselves
3	Moderate handicap; symptoms that significantly restrict lifestyle and prevent totally independent existence
4	Moderately severe handicap; symptoms that clearly prevent independent existence although not needing constant care and attention
5	Severe handicap; totally dependent, requiring constant attention day and night
6	Dead

provides a range of interventions and is also able to advise regarding return to work, driving, finance, benefits, and sexual activity. Information about local stroke clubs and other voluntary organizations should be given to patients and carergivers. The latter may also need care and support since they may experience high levels of burden (van Heugten *et al.* 2006).

Physical therapy improves functional recovery after stroke by strengthening patients' muscles used in movement (reaching and manipulation, sitting to standing, walking) and balance (sitting, standing, walking). Several approaches are often incorporated into the training program, consisting of a mixture of functional task training and active and passive musculoskeletal, cardiopulmonary, and neurophysiological interventions, although there is limited evidence to suggest that one modality is better than another (Pollock *et al.* 2014a). Cardiorespiratory training involving walking improves walking speed, endurance, and balance after stroke, but its effect on dependence and death are unclear (Saunders *et al.* 2013). In stroke patients who are able to walk, treadmill training, with or without body weight support, may improve walking speed and endurance (Mehrholz *et al.* 2014). Electromechanical-assisted gait training in combination with physical therapy may increase the chances of independent walking after stroke (Mehrholz *et al.* 2017). In particular, patients in the first three months after stroke and those who are not able to walk appear to benefit most. However, the duration and frequency of gait training that is most effective remains uncertain (Mehrholz *et al.* 2017). Physical therapists also assist with the use of foot-drop splints, canes, and wheelchairs, and they instruct carers in transferring, lifting, walking, and exercises. They are also able to advise on the care of the hemiplegic arm, particularly the shoulder. There is good evidence that functional electric stimulation reduces shoulder pain, prevents shoulder subluxation, maintains range of movement, and improves upper limb activity (Foley *et al.* 2006). Routine corticosteroid injection or ultrasound for shoulder pain has not been shown to be beneficial, and overhead arm pulleys and positional shoulder static stretches are harmful and should not be used (Gustafsson and McKenna 2006).

Occupational therapy prevents deterioration after stroke and facilitates patient independence by teaching stroke patients strategies to cope with activities of daily living such as eating, dressing, bathing, and cooking. However, the exact nature of the occupational therapy intervention to achieve maximum benefit remains to be defined (Legg *et al.* 2006). Evidence of moderate quality has shown that constraint-induced movement therapy, mental practice, mirror therapy, interventions for sensory impairment, virtual reality, and frequent repetitive task practice might improve upper limb function and that unilateral arm training may be more effective than bilateral arm training (Pollock *et al.* 2014b; Laver *et al.* 2015). However, the ideal dose and timing of training remain uncertain, and recent randomized controlled trials showed that a structured, intensive, high-dose, task-oriented motor training program of the upper limbs did not improve motor function of the upper limb compared with usual care (Winstein *et al.* 2016). Electromechanical and robotic-assisted arm and hand training after stroke might improve arm and hand function, muscle strength, and activities of daily living, but quality of evidence is limited at present (Mehrholz *et al.* 2015). Evidence on the effectiveness for transcranial direct current stimulation in improving activities of daily living after stroke is also of low-moderate quality, and it remains uncertain whether arm and leg function, muscle strength, and cognitive function might be improved with transcranial direct current stimulation (Elsner *et al.* 2016).

Speech therapy is effective for post-stroke aphasia and improves functional communication, reading, writing, and expressive language compared with no therapy (Brady *et al.* 2016). Therapy of higher intensity and higher dose lasting over a longer period is beneficial, even in patients with onset of stroke more than 6 months before (Brady *et al.* 2016; Breitenstein *et al.* 2017). However, transcranial direct current stimulation has not been shown to be effective in improving functional communication, language impairment and cognition in stroke patients with aphasia (Elsner *et al.* 2015). There is also insufficient evidence to support or refute possible benefits of speech therapy after stroke for speech apraxia (West *et al.* 2005), although patients and carers value such input and stroke-care guidelines recommend speech therapy. Speech therapists also have a role in the management of dysarthria and swallowing, although, again, there are currently no definitive, adequately powered trials of intervention for patients with dysarthria (Mitchell *et al.* 2017) (see Chapter 20 for management of impaired swallowing and nutrition).

Neglect is one of the most disabling impairments for patients after stroke. Although individual studies of cognitive rehabilitation interventions specifically for neglect have shown benefit, a systematic review and meta-analysis of 23 such studies demonstrated no overall effect of these interventions in reducing long-term disability (Bowen *et al.* 2013). Similarly, cognitive rehabilitation interventions have not been proven to be effective in reducing attentional impairments or executive dysfunction (Chung *et al.* 2013; Loetscher and Lincoln 2013).

Spasticity, if moderate to severe, may impede rehabilitation after stroke. In the chronic phase of stroke, spasticity has been shown to result in worse functional outcomes compared with patients without spasticity (Welmer *et al.* 2006; Lundström *et al.* 2008). Treatment of spasticity includes oral medications (e.g., baclofen), nerve blocks, and serial casting. However, these treatments are limited by their side effects. Intramuscular injection of botulinium toxin has an acceptable safety profile and is effective in reducing tone and pain due to spasticity (Gracies *et al.* 2015). However, whether botulinium toxin improves upper limb function and is cost-effective is uncertain. Intrathecal baclofen is also highly effective in reducing post-stroke spasticity at lower dosages compared with its oral form and is associated with fewer systemic side effects. It, too, has been shown to improve mobility, activities of daily living, and quality of life in stroke patients with spasticity (Dvorak *et al.* 2011). Finally, recent systematic reviews have demonstrated that neuromuscular electric stimulation is effective in reducing spasticity and increasing range of motion (Stein *et al.* 2015).

Other Interventions

Secondary consequences of neurological disability include painful shoulder, shoulder–hand syndrome, contractures, and falls. Physical therapists and other members of the multi-disciplinary team should have expertise in managing these problems. **Fatigue** after stroke is common. However, current trials on prevention and treatment of post-stroke fatigue have been small and heterogeneous (Wu *et al.* 2015). There is therefore, at present, insufficient evidence to support the use of any particular intervention to treat or prevent post-stroke fatigue (Wu *et al.* 2015). **Selective serotonin receptor inhibitors** appear to improve dependence, neurological impairment, anxiety, and depression after stroke (Mead *et al.* 2012) (see Chapter 20 for further discussion on post-stroke depression and pain). **Acupuncture** may have beneficial effects in improving dependency in patients with stroke without significant adverse events (Yang *et al.* 2016). However, current evidence is of low quality, and there is a lack of randomized trials of adequate quality and size. **Stem cell therapy** have the potential of stimulating endogenous repair processes such as angiogenesis and neurogenesis. The Pilot Investigation of Stem Cells in Stroke (PISCES) demonstrated that stereotactic intracerebral transplantation of human neural stem cells in 13 patients 6–60 months after ischemic stroke was safe and was associated with an improved neurological outcome (Kalladka *et al.* 2016). However, while the intravenous administration of bone marrow mononuclear stem cells in stroke patients has also been shown to be safe, no beneficial effect on stroke outcome was noted (Prasad *et al.* 2014).

Brain Imaging and Recovery after Stroke

The relationship between radiological findings and functional outcome has been examined in a number of studies using different imaging modalities and outcome measures. The importance of these studies from the point of view of acute stroke management is that they may allow identification of those patients who have the potential for good functional recovery. Rehabilitative and therapeutic strategies, such as neuroprotection agents, could then be targeted to those patients and rehabilitation strategies "personalized." The majority of studies have correlated lesion size in the acute or subacute period, using conventional CT or MRI, with outcome measured using a variety of scales of impairment or disability or combinations of these measures. Although a significant relationship between infarct size and outcome has been demonstrated in most studies, this is not invariably the case. The major reasons for a lack of correlation relate to lack of sensitivity in detection of infarcts but, more importantly, to the fact that these studies ignore the importance of lesion location in determining outcome from stroke.

Structural Imaging and Functional Outcome

In an analysis of more than 1,800 patients with ischemic stroke or intracerebral hemorrhage from the Virtual International Stroke Trials Archive (VISTA) Database, lesion volume assessed using CT at baseline was a predictor of functional outcome at 90 days (Vogt *et al.* 2012). Similarly, the Alberta Stroke Program Early CT Score (ASPECTS), a 10-point score that aims to estimate the infarct volume of ischemic strokes affecting the middle cerebral artery (MCA) territory, predicts functional outcome at 3 months and is now widely used before consideration of intravenous thrombolysis and/or endovascular therapy (Barber *et al.* 2000; Ryu *et al.* 2017). MRI techniques such as T_2 and diffusion weighted imaging (DWI) are more sensitive than CT at detecting infarction, especially small lesions and those affecting the posterior circulation, and studies have also shown that ischemic stroke patients with a larger infarct volume had better functional outcomes (Schiemanck *et al.* 2006). However, incorporating lesion volume, even with DWI, has not been shown to significantly predict functional outcome beyond clinical variables such as age and stroke severity (Hand *et al.* 2006; Johnston *et al.* 2007).

Nevertheless, significant methodological shortcomings from previous studies that have studied the relationship of lesion volume and functional outcome exist, as the majority have not studied the implications of lesion location and outcome. Involvement of the corticospinal tracts, for example, is an important factor limiting motor recovery (Lindenberg *et al.* 2010). In the Intensive Blood Pressure Reduction in Acute Cerebral Hemorrhage Trial (INTERACT2), lesions identified on CT affecting the posterior limb of the internal capsule, thalamus, and infratentorial regions were associated with the worst functional outcomes and quality of life measures at 90 days after stroke (Delcourt *et al.* 2017). Recently, researchers have used voxel-based lesion-symptom mapping on MRI to locate characteristic lesion patterns in areas of motor control and areas involved in lateralized brain functions that have been shown to influence functional outcome after a MCA territory infarct (Cheng *et al.* 2014). Similarly, voxel-based lesion-symptom mapping on MRI has been used to identify brain regions associated with aphasia, somatosensory deficits, and neglect after stroke (Phan *et al.* 2010; Meyer *et al.* 2016).

New MRI techniques such as tractography using diffusion tensor imaging (DTI) have also been developed recently. DTI aims to visualize white matter pathways not normally visible with CT or conventional MRI sequences. Damage to the corticospinal tract, for example, could be assessed using DTI during the acute stage of stroke and has been shown to be a more sensitive predictor of long-term motor impairment than infarct volume and stroke severity scores (Cho *et al.* 2007; Jang *et al.* 2010; Radlinska *et al.* 2010; Puig *et al.* 2011). DTI parameters of individual tracts or tracts in combination may also represent recovery potential in patients with stroke and hence may be used to developed personalized rehabilitation regimens in the future (Lindenberg *et al.* 2012).

Magnetic Resonance Spectroscopy and Functional Outcome

Cerebral damage following stroke has also been assessed by MR spectroscopy. This technique uses the same methods as MRI, but the signal obtained is converted into chemical as opposed to spatial information. Proton MR spectroscopy allows in vivo measurement of N-acetyl-containing compounds, creatine, choline, and lactate. The majority of the N-acetyl signal comes from N-acetyl aspartate (NAA), which is present in high concentrations in the brain. NAA is thought to play an osmoregulatory role in the central nervous system (Baslow 2003) and is of particular interest in studies of the brain since it is located almost exclusively in neurons in the adult. Decreases in the NAA resonance peak in vivo indicate neuronal or axonal injury or loss.

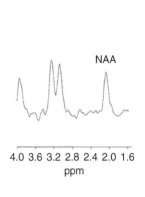
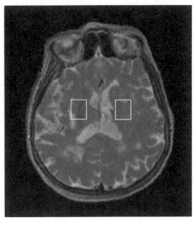
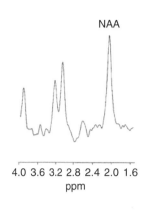

Fig. 23.1 Axial T_2-weighted image showing location of a spectroscopy voxel over the posterior limb of the internal capsule of each hemisphere together with the spectra obtained from the right and left internal capsules of a patient with subcortical stroke (Pendlebury *et al.* 1999). The *N*-acetyl aspartate (NAA) peak is reduced on the side of the affected right hemisphere consistent with damage to the descending motor pathways.

Early studies of MR spectroscopy in stroke showed increased lactate and decreased NAA within the stroke lesion (Berkelbach van der Sprenkel *et al.* 1988; Bruhn *et al.* 1989). Subsequently, it was shown that the magnitude of neuronal damage as measured by NAA loss from the infarcted region correlated with disability and impairment in stroke patients (Ford *et al.* 1992; Federico *et al.* 1998). It remains unclear whether NAA loss is a better prognostic indicator than other factors such as infarct volume as measured on imaging or indeed simple clinical tests. However, one study (Parsons *et al.* 2000) suggested that acute lactate/choline ratios correlate better with outcome than NAA/choline ratios or infarct volume. In all the studies described previously, metabolite changes were measured from the center of the infarcted region and, therefore, were not representative of the total infarct damage. Also the chosen outcome measures were not necessarily relevant to the area of brain under study. These points were addressed in a study in which NAA loss was measured in the descending motor pathways and correlated to a scale designed to measure motor impairment (Fig. 23.1) (Pendlebury *et al.* 1999). This study showed that NAA loss in the descending motor pathways was significantly associated with motor deficit and with the maximum proportion of the descending motor pathway cross-sectional area occupied by stroke, as described previously.

Recovery after Stroke and Functional Imaging

After a stroke, destroyed brain tissue usually cannot be replaced or regenerated. Recovery of neurological deficits can be achieved only either by reactivation of structurally intact but functionally disturbed neurons or by recruitment of unaffected pathways within the functional network. These compensatory mechanisms and changes in brain activation after stroke could be detected by measuring underlying alterations in blood flow or metabolism, such as via electrical or magnetic brain stimulation of pathways or imaging using positron emission tomography or functional MRI (fMRI).

Functional MRI relies on the fact that deoxyhemoglobin is paramagnetic whereas oxyhemoglobin is not. During neuronal activation, the neuronal oxygen demand and local cerebral blood flow rises, but to a level in excess of that required to supply the increased metabolic demand. Hence activation results in a reduced concentration of deoxyhemoglobin and thus an increased signal on MRI. Alterations in blood flow and metabolic demand of a functional network can be measured at rest (resting state fMRI), by correlating the location of activation to neurological deficit, or during activation tasks, where changes in activation patterns are compared with functional performance. Functional MRI therefore aims to identify brain territories or functional networks that are affected with altered patterns of blood flow and metabolism and hence provides a means to study the physiological correlates of neuroplasticity and recovery noninvasively.

However, fMRI studies are technically demanding to perform, and those that require patients to perform tasks during imaging require awake and cooperative subjects and assume that the normal relationship between metabolism and blood flow is maintained in normal aging and after a stroke. In fact, there are age-related decreases in cerebral blood flow and metabolic rate, and blood flow/metabolism coupling is impaired within ischemic tissue, although blood flow increases have been reported to occur in the remaining tissue in response to brain activation (Weiller *et al.* 1992). However, this does not necessarily indicate that the blood flow/metabolism coupling is normal in non-infarcted tissue. Certainly, there are widespread changes in the resting metabolic rate and perfusion of the brain after stroke, which persist into the chronic phase and may affect areas remote from the infarct.

Despite the limitations of fMRI outlined previously, fMRI studies have shown similar findings to those of positron emission tomography studies in recovery after stroke (Yozbatiran and Cramer 2006; Rijntjes 2006). Motor recovery, for example, depends on a number of mechanisms such as perilesional motor reorganization, recruitment of motor pathways in subcortical structures, recruitment of collateral pathways in the ipsilateral and contralateral hemisphere, and possibly development of new networks (Thirumala *et al.* 2002). Increased ipsilateral primary sensorimotor cortical activity with posterior displacement of the ipsilesional focus of activity, bilateral supplementary motor area activation, and premotor cortical activation have been shown to occur after stroke with use of the affected hand in comparison with use of the unaffected hand (Weiller *et al.* 1992; Cramer *et al.* 1997; Cao *et al.* 1998; Pineiro *et al.* 2001). Specifically, in patients with capsular or other subcortical stroke, good recovery is related to enhanced recruitment of the lateral premotor cortex of the lesional hemisphere and lateral premotor and, to a lesser extent, primary sensorimotor and parietal cortex of the contralateral hemisphere (Gerloff *et al.* 2006).

The mechanisms of motor recovery vary according to location of the lesion: cortical infarcts are associated with activation of the contralateral primary sensorimotor cortex, whereas subcortical infarcts appear to activate both primary sensorimotor cortices (Kwon *et al.* 2007). Several studies indicate that worse motor performance is related to a greater amount of contralesional activation (Calautti *et al.* 2007) and that patients who activate the ipsilesional primary motor cortex early had a better recovery of hand function (Loubinoux *et al.* 2007). Repetitive peripheral magnetic stimulation increases the activation of the ipsilesional parieto-premotor network and thereby might have a positive conditioning effect for treatment (Struppler *et al.* 2007). Inhibitory repetitive transcranial magnetic stimulation of the contralateral hemisphere may also aid recovery by reducing the transcallosal inhibition effects exerted by the contralateral hemisphere (Shimizu *et al.* 2002; Murase *et al.* 2004; Hsu *et al.* 2012).

In addition to changes in the activation pattern of the motor network, different activation patterns have been observed in the proprioceptive system, where the initially observed blood flow increases in sensory areas I and II of the noninfarcted hemisphere vanished during successful rehabilitation and the normal activation patterns were restored, indicating an interhemispheric shift of attention associated with recovery (Thiel *et al.* 2007).

Cortical functions such as post-stroke aphasia have too been heavily studied using fMRI. Changes in functional activities of the left fronto-temporal cortex have been correlated with language improvement in aphasic patients, and right inferior frontal gyrus activity is also frequently identified, although the underlying implications of this remains uncertain (Winhuisen *et al.* 2007; Crinion and Leff 2015). It also appears from functional imaging studies that non-language cognitive processes may also play a role in the recovery from aphasia (Crinion and Leff 2015). Nevertheless, many of the current functional imaging studies on post-stroke aphasia have not been well controlled, rendering it difficult to correlate changes on neuroimaging with various therapeutic interventions tested (Crinion and Leff 2015).

References

Alexander H, Bugge C, Hagen S (2001). What is the association between the different components of stroke rehabilitation and health outcomes? *Clinical Rehabilitation* 15:207–215

Allen C, Glasziou P, del Mar C (1999). Bed rest: A potentially harmful treatment needing more careful evaluation. *Lancet* 354:1229–1233

Austin MW, Ploughman M, Glynn L *et al.* (2014). Aerobic exercise effects on neuroprotection and brain repair following stroke: A systematic review and perspective. *Neuroscience Research* 87:8–15

AVERT Trial Collaboration Group (2015). Efficacy and safety of very early mobilization within 24 h of stroke onset (AVERT): A randomized controlled trial. *Lancet* 386:46–55

Bamford J, Sandercock PAG, Warlow CP *et al.* (1989). Interobserver agreement for the assessment of handicap in stroke patients. *Stroke* 20:828

Bamford J, Sandercock PAG, Dennis M *et al.* (1990). A prospective study of acute cerebrovascular disease in the community: The Oxfordshire Community Stroke Project 1981–86. 2. Incidence, case fatality rates and overall outcome at one year of cerebral infarction, primary intracerebral and subarachnoid haemorrhage. *Journal Neurology, Neurosurgery and Psychiatry* 53:16–22

Barber PA, Demchuk AM, Zhang J *et al.* (2000). Validity and reliability of a quantitative computed tomography score in predicting outcome of hyperacute stroke before thrombolytic therapy. ASPECTS Study Group. Alberta Stroke Program Early CT Score. *Lancet* 355:1670–1674

Baslow MH (2003). N-acetylaspartate in the vertebrate brain: Metabolism and function. *Neurochemical Research* 28:941–953

Bayley MT, Hurdowar A, Teasell R *et al.* (2007). Priorities for stroke rehabilitation and research: Results of a 2003 Canadian Stroke Network consensus conference. *Archives of Physical and Medical Rehabilitation* 88:526–528

Berkelbach van der Sprenkel JW, Luyten PR, van Rijen PC *et al.* (1988). Cerebral lactate detected by regional proton magnetic resonance spectroscopy in a patient with cerebral infarction. *Stroke* 19:1556–1560

Bernhardt J, Dewey H, Thrift A *et al.* (2004). Inactive and alone: Physical activity within the first 14 days of acute stroke unit care. *Stroke* 35:1005–1009

Bernhardt J, Churilov L, Ellery F *et al.* (2016). Prespecified dose-response analysis for A Very Early Rehabilitation Trial (AVERT). *Neurology* 86:1–8

Blennerhassett J, Dite W (2004). Additional task-related practice improves mobility and upper limb function early after stroke: A randomised controlled trial. *Australian Journal of Physiotherapy* 50:219–224

Bowen A, Hazelton C, Pollock A et al. (2013). Cognitive rehabilitation for spatial neglect following stroke. *Cochrane Database and Systematic Reviews* 7:CD00

Brady MC, Kelly H, Godwin J et al. (2016). Speech and language therapy for aphasia following stroke. *Cochrane Database of Systematic Reviews* 6:CD000425

Brandstater ME (2005). Stroke rehabilitation. In *Physical Medicine and Rehabilitation: Principles and Practice*, De Lisa JA, Gans BM, Walsh NE (eds.), pp. 1165–1169. Philadelphia, PA: Lippincott Williams & Wilkins

Breitenstein C, Grewe T, Flöel A et al. (2017). Intensive speech and language therapy in patients with chronic aphasia after stroke: A randomized, open-label, blinded-endpoint, controlled trial in a health-care setting. *Lancet* 389:1528–1538

Bruhn H, Frahm J, Gyngell ML et al. (1989). Cerebral metabolism in man after acute stroke: New observations using localized proton NMR spectroscopy. *Magnetic Resonance Medicine* 9:126–131

Calautti C, Naccarato M, Jones PS et al. (2007). The relationship between motor deficit and hemisphere activation balance after stroke: A 3T fMRI study. *Neuroimage* 34:322–331

Cao Y, D'Olhaberriague L, Vikingstad EM et al. (1998). Pilot study of functional MRI to assess cerebral activation of motor function after poststroke hemiparesis. *Stroke* 29:112–122

Cheng B, Forkert ND, Zavaglia M et al. (2014). Influence of stroke infarct location on functional outcome measured by the modified Rankin Scale. *Stroke* 45:1695–1702

Chuang KY, Wu SC, Yeh MC et al. (2005). Exploring the associations between longterm care and mortality rates among stroke patients. *Journal of Nursing Research* 13:66–74

Chung CS, Pollock A, Campbell T et al. (2013). Cognitive rehabilitation for executive dysfunction in adults with stroke or other adult non-progressive acquired brain damage. *Cochrane Database of Systematic Reviews* 4: CD008391

Cho SH, Kim DG, Kim DS et al. (2007). Motor outcome according to the integrity of the corticospinal tract determined by diffusion tensor tractography in the early stage of corona radiata infarct. *Neuroscience Letters* 426:123–127

Collen FM, Wade DT (1991). Residual mobility problems after stroke. *International Disability Studies* 13:12–15

Collen FM, Wade DT, Bradshaw CM (1990). Mobility after stroke: Reliability of measures of impairment and disability. *International Disability Studies* 12:6–9

Collen FM, Wade DT, Robb GF et al. (1991). The Rivermead Mobility Index: A further development of the Rivermead Motor Assessment. *International Disability Studies* 13:50–54

Collin C, Wade D (1990). Assessing motor impairment after stroke: A pilot reliability study. *Journal of Neurology, Neurosurgery and Psychiatry* 53:576–579

Cramer SC, Nelles G, Benson RR et al. (1997). A functional MRI study of subjects recovered from hemiparetic stroke. *Stroke* 28:2518–2527

Cramer SC, Crafton KR (2006). Somatotopy and movement representation sites following cortical stroke. *Experimental Brain Research* 168:25–32

Crinion JT, Leff AP (2015). Using functional imaging to understand therapeutic effects in poststroke aphasia. *Current Opinions in Neurology* 28:330–337

de Haan R, Aaronson N, Limburg M et al. (1993). Measuring quality of life in stroke. *Stroke* 24:320–327

Delcourt C, Sato S, Zhang S et al. (2017). Intracerebral hemorrhage location and outcome among INTERACT2 participants. *Neurology* 88:1408–1414

Dennis M, Wellwood I, Warlow C (1997a). Are simple questions a valid measure of outcome after stroke? *Cerebrovascular Diseases* 7:22–27

Dennis M, Wellwood I, O'Rourke S et al. (1997b). How reliable are simple questions in assessing outcome after stroke? *Cerebrovascular Diseases* 7:19–21

Dorman P, Slattery J, Farrell B et al. (1998). Qualitative comparison of the reliability of health status assessments with the EuroQol and SF-36 questionnaires after stroke. *Stroke* 29:63–68

Dromerick AW, Lang CE, Birkenmeier RL *et al.* (2009). Very Early Constraint-Induced Movement during Stroke Rehabilitation (VECTORS). *Neurology* **73**:195–201

Dvorak EM, Ketchum NC, McGuire JR (2011). The underutilization of intrathecal baclofen in poststroke spasticity. *Topics in Stroke Rehabilitation* **18**:195–202

Early Supported Discharge Trialists (2005). Services for reducing duration of hospital care for acute stroke patients. *Cochrane Database of Systematic Reviews* 1:CD000443

Egan K, Janssen H, Sena E *et al.* (2014). Exercise reduces infarct volume and facilitates neurobehavioral recovery: A systematic review and meta-analysis of exercise models in ischemic stroke. *Neurorehabilitation and Neural Repair* **28**:800–812

Elsner B, Kugler J, Pohl M *et al.* (2016). Transcranial direct current stimulation (tDCS) for improving activities of daily living, and physical and cognitive functioning, in people with stroke. *Cochrane Database of Systematic Reviews* 3:CD009645

Elsner B, Kugler J, Pohl M *et al.* (2015). Transcranial direct current stimulation (tDCS) for improving aphasia in patients with aphasia after stroke. *Cochrane Database of Systematic Reviews* 5:CD009760

Enderby PM, Wood VA, Wade DT *et al.* (1986). The Frenchay Aphasia Screening Test: A short simple test for aphasia appropriate for non-specialists. *International Rehabilitation Medicine* **8**:166–170

Federico F, Simone IL, Lucivero V *et al.* (1998). Prognostic value of proton magnetic resonance spectroscopy in ischemic stroke. *Archives of Neurology* **55**:489–494

Foley N, Bhogal S, Foley N (2006). Painful hemiplegic shoulder. In *Canadian Stroke Network Evidence-Based Reviews of Stroke Rehabilitation* http://ebrsrcom/index_ho mehtml (accessed 10 May 2007)

Ford CC, Griffey RH, Matwiyoff NA *et al.* (1992). Multivoxel 1H-MRS of stroke. *Neurology* **42**:1408–1412

Gerloff C, Bushara K, Sailer A *et al.* (2006). Multimodal imaging of brain reorganization in motor areas of the contralesional hemisphere of well recovered patients after capsular stroke. *Brain* **129**:791–808

Gracies JM, Brashear A, Jech R *et al.* (2015). Safety and efficacy of abobotulinumtoxinA for hemiparesis in adults with upper limb spasticity after stroke or traumatic brain injury: A double-blind randomized controlled trial. *Lancet Neurology* **14**:992–1001

Gustafsson L, McKenna K (2006). A programme of static positional stretches does not reduce hemiplegic shoulder pain or maintain shoulder range of motion: A randomized controlled trial. *Clinical Rehabilitation* **20**:277

Hamdy S, Aziz Q, Rothwell JC *et al.* (1998). Recovery of swallowing after dysphagic stroke relates to functional reorganization in the intact motor cortex. *Gastroenterology* **115**:1104–1112

Hand PJ, Kwan J, Lindley RI *et al.* (2006). Distinguishing between stroke and mimic at the bedside: The brain attack study. *Stroke* **37**:769–775

Hsu WY, Cheng CH, Liao KK *et al.* (2012). Effects of repetitive transcranial magnetic stimulation on motor functions in patients with stroke: A meta-analysis. *Stroke* **43**:1849–1857

Jang SH (2010) Prediction of motor outcome for hemiparetic stroke patients using diffusion tensor imaging: A review. *NeuroRehabilitation* **27**:367–372

Jehkonen M, Ahonen JP, Dastidar P *et al.* (1998). How to detect visual neglect in acute stroke. *Lancet* **351**:727–728

Johnston KC, Wagner DP, Wang XQ *et al.* (2007). Validation of an acute ischemic stroke model: Does diffusion-weighted imaging lesion volume offer a clinically significant improvement in prediction of outcome? *Stroke* **38**:1820–1825

Kalladka D, Sinden J, Pollock K *et al.* (2016). Human neural stem cells in patients with chronic ischemic stroke (PISCES): A phase 1, fist-in-man study. *Lancet* **388**:787–796

Krakauer JW, Carmichael ST, Corbett D *et al.* (2012). Getting neurorehabilitation right: What can be learned from animal models? *Neurorehabilitaiton and Neural Repair* **26**:923–931

Kreisel SH, Hennerici MG, Bazner H (2007). Pathophysiology of stroke rehabilitation:

The natural course of clinical recovery, use-dependent plasticity and rehabilitative outcome. *Cerebrovascular Diseases* 23:243–255

Kwakkel G (2006). Impact of intensity of practice after stroke: Issues for consideration. *Disability and Rehabilitation* 28:823–830

Kwakkel G, van Peppen R, Wagenaar RC *et al.* (2004). Effects of augmented exercise therapy time after stroke: A meta-analysis. *Stroke* 35:2529–2536

Kwon YH, Lee MY, Park JW *et al.* (2007). Differences of cortical activation pattern between cortical and corona radiata infarct. *Neuroscience Letters* 417:138–142

Langhorne P, Dennis MS (2004). Stroke units: The next 10 years. *Lancet* 363:834–835

Langhorne P, Duncan P (2001). Does the organization of postacute stroke care really matter? *Stroke* 32:268–274

Langhorne P, Holmqvist LW (2007). Early Supported Discharge Trialists. Early supported discharge after stroke. *Journal of Rehabilitation Medicine* 39:103–108

Langhorne P, Wagenaar R, Partridge C (1996). Physiotherapy after stroke: More is better? *Physiotherapy Research International* 1:75–88

Langhorne P, Stott D, Robertson L *et al.* (2000). Medical complications after stroke: A multicenter study. *Stroke* 31:1223–1229

Langton Hewer R (1990). Rehabilitation after stroke. *Quarterly Journal of Medicine* 76:659–674

Laver KE, George S, Thoomas S *et al.* (2015). Virtual reality for stroke rehabilitation. *Cochrane Database of Systematic Reviews* 10: CD008349

Legg LA, Drummond AE, Langhorne P (2006). Occupational therapy for patients with problems in activities of daily living after stroke. *Cochrane Database of Systematic Reviews* 4: CD0030585

Legh-Smith J, Wade DT, Langton-Hewer R (1986). Services for stroke patients one year after stroke. *Journal of Epidemiology Community Health* 40:161–165

Lindenberg R, Renga V, Zhu LL *et al.* (2010). Structural integrity of corticospinal motor fibers predicts motor impairment in chronic stroke. *Neurology* 74:280–287

Lindenberg R, Zhu LL, Rüber T *et al.* (2012). Predicting functional motor potential in chronic stroke patients using diffusion tensor imaging. *Human Brain Mapping* 33:1040–1051

Liu N, Cadilhac DA, Andrew NE *et al.* (2014). Randomized controlled trial of early rehabilitation after intracerebral hemorrhage: Difference in outcomes within 6 months of stroke. *Stroke* 45:3502–3507

Loetscher T, Lincoln NB (2013). Cognitive rehabilitation for attention deficits following stroke. *Cochrane Database of Systematic Reviews* 5:CD002842

Loubinoux I, Dechaumont-Palacin S, Castel-Lacanal E *et al.* (2007). Prognostic value of fMRI in recovery of hand function in subcortical stroke patients. *Cerebral Cortex* 17:2980–2987

Lyden PD, Hantson L (1998). Assessment scales for the evaluation of stroke patients. *Journal of Stroke and Cerebrovascular Diseases* 7:113–127

Lundström E, Terént A, Borg J (2008). Prevalence of disability spasticity 1 year after first-event stroke. *European Journal of Neurology* 15:533–539

Lyle RC (1981). A performance test for assessment of upper limb function in physical rehabilitation treatment and research. *International Journal of Rehabilitation Research* 4:483–492

Lynch E, Hillier S, Cadilhac D (2014). When should physical rehabilitation commence after stroke: A systematic review. *International Journal of Stroke* 9:468–478

Mead GE, Hsieh CF, Lee R *et al.* (2012). Selective serotonin reuptake inhibitors (SSRIs) for stroke recovery. *Cochrane Database of Systematic Reviews* 11:CD009286

Mehrholz J, Pohl M, Elsner B (2014). Treadmill training and body weight support for walking after stroke. *Cochrane Database of Systematic Reviews* 1:CD002840

Mehrholz J, Pohl M, Platz T *et al.* (2015). Electromechanical and robot-assisted arm training for improving activities of daily living, arm function, and arm muscle strength after stroke. *Cochrane Database of Systematic Reviews* 11:CD006876

Mehrholz J, Thomas S, Werner C *et al.* (2017). Electromechanical-assisted training for walking after stroke. *Cochrane Database of Systematic Reviews* 5:CD006185

Meyer S, Kessner SS, Cheng B *et al.* (2016). Voxel-based lesion-symptom mapping of stroke lesions underlying somatosensory deficits. *NeuroImage: Clinical* 10:257–266

Mitchell C, Bowen A, Tyson S *et al.* (2017). Interventions for dysarthria due to stroke and other adult-acquired, non-progressive brain injury. *Cochrane Database of Systematic Reviews* 1:CD002088

Murase N, Duque J, Mazzocchio R *et al.* (2004). Influence of interhemispheric interactions on motor function in chronic stroke. *Annals of Neurology* 55:400–409

Murphy TH, Corbett D (2009). Plasticity during stroke recovery: From synapse to behavior. *Nature Reviews Neuroscience* 10:861–872

Muscari A, Puddu GM, Santoro N *et al.* (2011). A simple scoring system for outcome prediction of ischemic stroke. *Acta Neurologica Scandinavica* 124:334–342

Nijland RH, van Wegen EE, Harmeling-van der Wel BC *et al.* (2010). Presence of finger extension and shoulder abduction within 72 hours after stroke predicts functional recovery: Early prediction of functional outcome after stroke: The EPOS cohort study. *Stroke* **41**:745–750

Ntaios G, Faouzi M, Ferrari J *et al.* (2012). An integer-based score to predict functional outcome in acute ischemic stroke: The ASTRAL score. *Neurology* 78:1916–1922

Nudo RJ (2007). Post infarct cortical plasticity and behavioural recovery. *Stroke* **38**:840–845

Outpatient Service Trialists (2003). Therapy-based rehabilitation services for stroke patients at home *Cochrane Database of Systematic Reviews* 1:CD002925

Parsons MW, Li T, Barber PA *et al.* (2000). Combined (1) H MR spectroscopy and diffusion-weighted MRI improves the prediction of stroke outcome. *Neurology* 55:498–505

Pedersen PM, Jorgensen HS, Nakayama H *et al.* (1995). Aphasia in acute stroke: Incidence determinants and recovery. *Annals of Neurology* 38:659–666

Pendlebury ST, Blamire AM, Lee MA *et al.* (1999). Axonal injury in the internal capsule correlates with motor impairment after stroke. *Stroke* **30**:956–962

Phan TG, Chen J, Donnan G *et al.* (2010). Development of a new tool to correlate stroke outcome with infarct topography: A proof-of-concept study. *Neuroimage* 49:127–133

Pineiro R, Pendlebury ST, Smith S *et al.* (2000). Relating MRI changes to motor deficit after ischemic stroke by segmentation of functional motor pathways. *Stroke* 31:672–679

Pineiro R, Pendlebury S, Johansen-Berg H *et al.* (2001). Functional MRI detects posterior shifts in primary sensorimotor cortex activation after stroke: Evidence of local adaptive reorganization? *Stroke* **32**:1134–1139

Pollock A, Baer G, Campbell P *et al.* (2014a). Physiotherapy rehabilitation approaches for the recovery of function and mobility following stroke. *Cochrane Database of Systematic Reviews* 4:CD001920

Pollock A, Farmer SE, Brady MC *et al.* (2014b). Interventions for improving upper limb function after stroke. *Cochrane Database of Systematic Reviews* 11:CD010820

Prasad K, Sharma A, Garg A *et al.* (2014). Intravenous autologous bone marrow mononuclear stem cell therapy for ischemic stroke: A multicentric, randomized trial. *Stroke* 45:3618–3624

Puig J, Pedraza S, Blasco G *et al.* (2011). Acute damage to the posterior limb of the internal capsule on diffusion tensor tractography as an early imaging predictor of motor outcome after stroke. *American Journal of Neuroradiology* 32:857–863

Radlinska B, Ghinani S, Leppert IR *et al.* (2010). Diffusion tensor imaging, permanent pyramidal tract damage, and outcome in subcortical stroke. *Neurology* 75:1048–1054

Rijntjes M (2006). Mechanisms of recovery in stroke patients with hemiparesis or aphasia: New insights, old questions and the meaning of therapies. *Current Opinions in Neurology* **19**:76–83

Ryu CW, Shin HS, Park S *et al.* (2017). Alberta Stroke Program Early CT Score in the prognostication after endovascular treatment for ischemic stroke: A meta-analysis. *Neurointervention* **12**:20–30

Saunders DH, Sanderson M, Brazzelli M *et al.* (2013). Physical fitness training for stroke patients. *Cochrane Database of Systematic Reviews* 10:CD003316

Schiemanck SK, Kwakkel G, Post MWM *et al.* (2006). Predictive value of ischemic lesion volume assessed with magnetic resonance imaging for neurological deficits and functional outcome poststroke: A critical review of the literature. *Neurorehabilitation and Neural Repair* **20**:492–502

Shimizu T, Hosaki A, Hino T et al. (2002). Motor cortical disinhibition in the unaffected hemisphere after unilateral cortical stroke. *Brain* **125**:1896–1907

Stein C, Fritsch CG, Robinson C *et al.* (2015). Effects of electrical stimulation in spastic muscles after stroke: Systematic review and meta-analysis of randomized controlled trial. *Stroke* **46**:2197–2205

Stroke Unit Trialists' Collaboration (1997). Collaborative systematic review of the randomised trials of organised inpatient (stroke unit) care after stroke. *British Medical Journal* **314**:1151–1159

Struppler A, Binkofski F, Angerer B *et al.* (2007). A fronto-parietal network is mediating improvement of motor function related to repetitive peripheral magnetic stimulation: A PET-H2O15 study. *Neuroimage* **36**(Suppl 2): T174–T186

Thiel A, Aleksic B, Klein J *et al.* (2007). Changes in proprioceptive systems activity during recovery from post-stroke hemiparesis. *Journal of Rehabilitation Medicine* **39**:520–525

Thirumala P, Hier DB, Patel P (2002). Motor recovery after stroke: Lessons from functional brain imaging. *Neurological Research* **24**:453–458

van der Lee JH, De Groot V, Beckerman H *et al.* (2001). The intra- and interrater reliability of the action research arm test: A practical test of upper extremity function in patients with stroke. *Archives of Physical Medicine and Rehabilitation* **82**:14–19

van Heugten C, Visser-Meily A, Post M *et al.* (2006). Care for carers of stroke patients: Evidence-based clinical practice guidelines. *Journal of Rehabilitation Medicine* **38**:153–158

Veerbeek JM, Kwakkel G, van Wegen EE *et al.* (2011). Early prediction of outcome of activities of daily living after stroke: A systematic review. *Stroke* **42**:1482–1488

Vogt G, Laage R, Shuaib A *et al.* (2012). Initial lesion volume is an independent predictor of clinical stroke outcome at day 90: An analysis of the Virtual International Stroke Trials Archive (VISTA) Database. *Stroke* **43**:1266–1272

Wade DT, Legh-Smith J, Langton Hewer R (1985). Social activities after stroke: Measurement and natural history using the Frenchay Activities Index. *International Rehabilitation Medicine* **7**:176–181

Wade DT, Wood VA, Heller A *et al.* (1987). Walking after stroke. Measurement and recovery over the first 3 months. *Scandinavian Journal of Rehabilitation Medicine* **19**:25–30

Warlow CP, Dennis MS, van Gijn J *et al.* (1996). What are this person's problems? A problem-based approach to the general management of stroke. In *Stroke: A Practical Guide to Management*, pp. 477–544. Oxford: Blackwell

Weiller C, Chollet F, Friston KJ *et al.* (1992). Functional reorganization of the brain in recovery from striatocapsular infarction in man. *Annals of Neurology* **31**:463–472

Welmer AK, von Arbin M, Widén Holmqvist L *et al.* (2006). Spasticity and its association with functioning and health-related quality of life 18 months after stroke. *Cerebrovascular Diseases* **21**:247–253

West C, Hesketh A, Vail A *et al.* (2005). Interventions for apraxia of speech following stroke. *Cochrane Database of Systematic Reviews* 4:CD004298

Winhuisen L, Thiel A, Schumacher B *et al.* (2007). The right inferior frontal gyrus and post stroke aphasia: A follow-up investigation. *Stroke* **38**:1286–1292

Winstein CJ, Wolf SL, Dromerick AW *et al.* (2016). The ICARE randomized clinical trial. *JAMA* **315**:571–581

Wu S, Kutlubaev MA, Chun HY *et al.* (2015). Interventions for post-stroke fatigue. *Cochrane Database of Systematic Reviews* 7:CD007030

Yang A, Wu HM, Tang JL *et al.* (2016). Acupuncture for stroke rehabilitation. *Cochrane Database of Systematic Reviews* 8: CD004131

Yozbatiran N, Cramer SC (2006). Imaging motor recovery after stroke. *Neuroradiology* 3:482–488

Yozbatiran N, Der-Yeghiaian L, Cramer SC (2008). A standardized approach to performing the action research arm test. *Neurorehabilitation and Neural Repair* 22:78–90

24

Medical Therapies

As shown in Chapters 15 and 19, the early risk after TIA and minor stroke is high, but rapid treatment of TIA and minor stroke can prevent up to 80% of recurrent strokes (Rothwell *et al.* 2007). There is considerable evidence relating to the effectiveness of various treatments to reduce the medium- and long-term risk of vascular events after TIA and stroke, which is detailed in this chapter.

Antiplatelet Therapy for Non-Cardioembolic TIA or Ischemic Stroke

Antiplatelet therapy reduces the risk of recurrent vascular events after TIA and ischemic stroke, although few trials have distinguished between different etiological subtypes (Table 24.1). Most trial data concern aspirin, but other antiplatelet agents such as clopidogrel (Sudlow *et al.* 2009), extended-release dipyridamole (Leonardi-Bee *et al.* 2005), cilostazol (Kamal *et al.* 2011), and ticagrelor (Johnston *et al.* 2016) have also been shown to be effective, although mechanisms of action may differ (Table 24.2).

Table 24.1 Major trials and meta-analyses contributing to the evidence base for medical treatment in secondary prevention after non-cardioembolic TIA and ischemic stroke

Drug	Trial	Treatment
Aspirin	CAST	Aspirin versus placebo within 48 hours of major ischemic stroke
	IST	Aspirin versus placebo (and subcutaneous heparin versus placebo) acutely after major ischemic stroke
	Anti-thrombotic Trialists' Collaboration	Meta-analysis of trials studying antiplatelet agents in patients at high risk of occlusive vascular disease
Dipyridamole	ESPS-2	Aspirin and modified-release dipyridamole versus placebo in a 2 × 2 factorial design started within 3 months of TIA or ischemic stroke
	ESPRIT	Aspirin versus aspirin plus dipyridamole started within 6 months of TIA or minor stroke
	PRoFESS	Aspirin plus modified-release dipyridamole versus clopidogrel started within 3 months of ischemic stroke

Table 24.1 (cont.)

Drug	Trial	Treatment
Clopidogrel	CAPRIE	Clopidogrel versus aspirin in patients with occlusive vascular disease
Cilostazol	CASISP	Cilostazol versus aspirin started within 6 months of ischemic stroke
	CSPS2	Cilostazol versus aspirin started within 6 months of ischemic stroke
Ticagrelor	SOCRATES	Ticagrelor versus aspirin within 24 hours of TIA or minor ischemic stroke
Aspirin and clopidogrel	MATCH	Aspirin plus clopidogrel versus clopidogrel within 3 months of ischemic stroke or TIA
	CHARISMA	Aspirin versus aspirin plus clopidogrel in patients with cardiovascular disease or multiple risk factors (including ischemic stroke)
	FASTER	Aspirin versus aspirin plus clopidogrel within 24 hours of TIA or minor ischemic stroke
	SPS3	Aspirin versus aspirin plus clopidogrel within 6 months of MRI-proven, clinically evident subcortical stroke
	CHANCE	Aspirin versus aspirin plus clopidogrel within 24 hours of TIA or minor ischemic stroke
	SAMMPRIS	Aspirin plus clopidogrel and aggressive risk factor modification versus percutaneous transluminal angioplasty and stenting within 30 days of TIA or ischemic stroke with 70–99% stenosis of a major intracranial artery
Warfarin	SPIRIT	Warfarin (target INR 3.0–4.5) versus aspirin in TIA or ischemic stroke
	WARSS	Warfarin (target INR 1.4–2.8) versus aspirin within 30 days of ischemic stroke
	WASID	Warfarin (target INR 2.0–3.0) versus aspirin within 90 days of TIA or ischemic stroke with intracranial stenosis 50–99%
	ESPRIT	Warfarin (target INR 2.0–3.0) versus aspirin within 6 months of TIA or minor ischemic stroke

Notes: CAPRIE, Clopidogrel versus Aspirin in Patients at Risk of Ischemic Events; CASISP, Cilostazol versus Aspirin for Secondary Ischemic Stroke Prevention; CAST, Chinese Acute Stroke Trial; CHANCE, Clopidogrel in High-Risk Patients with Acute Non-disabling Cerebrovascular Events; CHARISMA, Clopidogrel for High Risk Atherothrombotic Risk and Ischemic Stabilization, Management and Avoidance; CSPS2, Cilostazol for Prevention of Secondary Stroke; ESPRIT, European/Australasian Stroke Prevention in Reversible Ischemia Trial; ESPS, European Stroke Prevention Study; FASTER, Fast Assessment of Stroke and Transient Ischemic Attack to Prevent Early Recurrence; IST, International Stroke Trial; MATCH, Management of Atherothrombosis with Clopidogrel in High-risk patients; PRoFESS, The Prevention Regimen for Effectively Avoiding Second Strokes; SOCRATES, Acute Stroke or Transient Ischemic Attack Treated with or Ticagrelor and Patients Outcomes; SPIRIT, Stroke Prevention in Reversible Ischemia Trial; TIA, transient ischemic attack; WASID, Warfarin-Aspirin Symptomatic Intracranial Disease Trial; WARSS, Warfarin-Aspirin Recurrent Stroke Study; see text for other trials.

Table 24.2 Mechanisms of action of commonly used antiplatelet agents

Agent	Mechanism of action
Antiplatelet agents in general	Prevention of propagation of arterial thrombus Prevent platelet aggregation in the microcirculation Prevent re-embolization from embolic source Reduce the release of eicosanoids and other neurotoxic agents
Aspirin	Inhibition of cyclooxygenase-1, reducing the breakdown of arachidonic acid to thromboxane A_2 and platelet granule release
Dipyridamole and cilostazol	Inhibition of phosphodiesterase, causing elevation of intracellular platelet cyclic AMP and a consequent inhibition of platelet activation and granule release
Clopidogrel, other thienopyridines, and ticagrelor	Blockade of platelet membrane ADP receptors, inhibiting ADP-dependent platelet activation and granule release

In the acute stage of TIA or ischemic stroke, early use of aspirin reduces the 6-week risk of recurrent ischemic stroke by about 60% and the risk of disabling or fatal ischemic stroke by about 70% (Rothwell *et al.* 2016). Clopidogrel without aspirin has not been studied in acute TIA or ischemic stroke. However, in patients with a history of occlusive vascular disease, clopidogrel was not superior to aspirin in prevention of recurrent strokes but was associated with a small but significant reduction in risk of overall recurrent vascular events (CAPRIE trial; CAPRIE Steering Committee 1996). Ticagrelor is as safe as but not superior to aspirin in prevention of recurrent vascular events at 90 days in patients with acute TIA or ischemic stroke (SOCRATES trial; Johnston *et al.* 2016;). A short course of aspirin and clopidogrel is more effective than aspirin alone in reducing the early risk of recurrent stroke but is not associated with an increased risk of major bleeding (CHANCE trial; Wang *et al.* 2013; Wong *et al.* 2013).

For long-term prevention of recurrent ischemic stroke, the combination of aspirin and dipyridamole is more effective than aspirin alone (ESPS-2 and ESPRIT trials; Diener *et al.* 1996; Halkes *et al.* 2006) and as effective as clopidogrel monotherapy (PRoFESS trial; Sacco *et al.* 2008). Long-term use of aspirin and clopidogrel combined in stable patients, however, is associated with an increased risk of bleeding and is not recommended (CHARISMA and MATCH trials; Diener *et al.* 2004; Berger *et al.* 2010). Cilostazol was mainly studied in the Asian populations and has been shown to be as effective as aspirin in prevention of recurrent ischemic strokes and is associated with a lower risk of intra- and extracranial bleeds (CASISP and CSPS2 trials; Kamal *et al.* 2011).

Few trials of antiplatelet agents have distinguished between different vascular territories or mechanisms of stroke. The Secondary Prevention of Small Subcortical Strokes Trial (SPS3 investigators 2012) randomized patients with subcortical infarcts within 6 months to aspirin or aspirin and clopidogrel. There was no significant difference in recurrent stroke risk between the two groups (Benavente *et al.* 2012). However, patients with aspirin and clopidogrel were at higher risk of major hemorrhage and all-cause mortality (Benavente *et al.* 2012). In a subgroup analysis of the SOCRATES trial, it was noted that among patients with acute ischemic stroke or TIA with associated ipsilateral atherosclerotic stenosis, ticagrelor was superior to aspirin at preventing stroke, myocardial infarction, or death at 90 days (Amarenco *et al.* 2017).

The Canadian Cooperative Study Group (1978) showed that aspirin reduced recurrent episodes of cerebral ischemia and death in patients with vertebrobasilar events. The European Stroke Prevention Study (ESPS; Sivenius *et al.* 1991) of aspirin and immediate-release dipyridamole versus placebo appeared to show that patients with posterior circulation TIA benefited more than those with carotid disease, but the numbers of events were too small to be certain. Recently, the Antiplatelet treatment compared with anticoagulation treatment for cervical artery dissection (CADISS) trial showed that there was no difference in efficacy of antiplatelet and anticoagulant drugs in preventing stroke and death in patients with symptomatic carotid and vertebral artery dissection (CADISS Trial Investigators 2015).

Warfarin is not effective in secondary prevention of patients with non-cardioembolic TIA or ischemic stroke but is associated with a significantly greater risk of major bleeding, especially intracerebral hemorrhage (ESPRIT, SPIRIT, WASID, and WARSS trials; SPIRIT Study Group 1997; Mohr *et al.* 2001; Chimowitz *et al.* 2005; ESPRIT Study Group *et al.* 2007).

In patients with recent TIA or ischemic stroke due to severe (70–99%) intracranial atherosclerosis, aspirin and clopidogrel for 90 days, together with intensive risk factor management, significantly reduces the 30-day recurrent stroke risk compared with percutaneous transluminal angioplasty and stenting using a Wingspan stent system (5.8% versus 12.5%) (SAMMPRIS trial; Chimowitz *et al.* 2011). Compared with high-dose aspirin, warfarin is associated with a significantly greater risk of adverse events in patients with TIA or ischemic stroke due to intracranial atherosclerosis but does not reduce the risk of recurrent stroke (WASID trial; Chimowitz *et al.* 2005).

Anticoagulation for Cardioembolic TIA or Ischemic Stroke

Patients in atrial fibrillation who have a TIA or ischemic stroke should be given anticoagulation therapy if there are no contraindications (Kernan *et al.* 2014). In patients with atrial fibrillation, oral anticoagulation with vitamin K antagonists (e.g., warfarin) with an international normalized ratio (INR) maintained at 2–3 reduces the risk of ischemic stroke or systemic embolism by 64% and all-cause mortality by 26% compared with placebo (Hart *et al.* 2007). Although aspirin was once considered to be a potential alternative to warfarin, especially in the elderly for whom the bleeding risks was perceived to be high, pooled analyses have shown that aspirin, when compared with placebo, is associated with a non-significant 19% reduction in risk of stroke (Hart *et al.* 2007). These results were mainly driven by a single positive trial that is considered to have significant methodological flaws (Stroke Prevention in Atrial Fibrillation Investigators 1991; Freedman *et al.* 2015). Subsequent clinical trials have also shown that warfarin is as safe as aspirin in elderly patients with atrial fibrillation (Mant *et al.* 2007; Rash *et al.* 2007). Aspirin is therefore not recommended for stroke prevention in patients with atrial fibrillation (Kirchhof *et al.* 2016). Similarly, the combination of aspirin and clopidogrel remains inferior to warfarin in prevention of vascular events, with similar major bleeding rates as warfarin (ACTIVE Writing Group of the ACTIVE Investigators 2006).

Warfarin is, however, limited by its relatively narrow therapeutic window and variable dose-effect response, accounted for by differences in warfarin metabolism due to genetic variations and many food and drug interactions. Use of warfarin therefore requires close INR monitoring. Nevertheless, studies have shown that patients on long-term warfarin therapy spend less than two-thirds of the time within the therapeutic INR window of 2–3 (Verheugt and Granger 2015). Many patients are hence at risk of recurrent thrombo-embolic events or bleeding secondary to a sub- or supra-therapeutic INR. The risk of intracerebral hemorrhage with warfarin use is approximately 0.5% per year.

In view of the limitations of warfarin, several non-vitamin K antagonist oral antic-oagulants (NOACs; also known as direct oral anticoagulants, DOACs) have been developed over the past decade for atrial fibrillation patients without hemodynamically significant mitral stenosis or mechanical valves. These include direct thrombin inhibitors (dabigatran) (RE-LY trial; Connolly *et al.* 2009; Diener *et al.* 2010) and factor Xa inhibitors, including rivaroxaban (ROCKET-AF trial; Patel *et al.* 2011; Hankey *et al.* 2012), apixaban (AVEROES and ARISTOTLE trials; Connolly *et al.* 2011; Granger *et al.* 2011; Easton *et al.* 2012), and edoxaban (ENGAGE AF-TIMI 48; Giugliano *et al.* 2013; Rost *et al.* 2016) (Table 24.3). Compared with warfarin, the pharmacological effects of NOACs are much more predict-able, with a fast onset of action (2–3 hours to peak effect) and a short half-life of approxi-mately 12 hours (compared with a mean of ~40 hours for warfarin) (Verheugt *et al.* 2015).

Table 24.3 Major trials demonstrating the effectiveness of non-vitamin K antagonist oral anticoagulants in patients with atrial fibrillation

Drug	Trial	Treatment
Direct thrombin inhibitor (dabigatran)	RE-LY	Dabigatran 110 mg or 150 mg twice daily versus warfarin in patients with atrial fibrillation
	RE-ALIGN	Dabigatran versus warfarin in patients with mechanical heart valves (patients without atrial fibrillation also included)
Factor Xa inhibitors	ROCKET-AF	Rivaroxaban 20 mg or 15 mg daily versus warfarin in patients with atrial fibrillation
	AVERROES	Apixaban 5 mg or 2.5mg twice daily versus aspirin in patients with atrial fibrillation not suitable for warfarin
	ARISTOTLE	Apixaban 5 mg or 2.5mg twice daily versus warfarin in patients with atrial fibrillation
	ENGAGE AF-TIMI 48	Edoxaban 30 mg or 60 mg daily versus warfarin in patients with atrial fibrillation

Notes: ARISTOTLE, Apixaban for Reduction in Stroke and Other Thromboembolic Events in Atrial Fibrillation; AVERROES, Apixaban Versus Acetylsalicylic Acid to Prevent Stroke in Atrial Fibrillation Patients Who Have Failed or Are Unsuitable for Vitamin K Antagonist Treatment; ENGAGE AF-TIMI 48, Effective Anticoagulation with Factor Xa Next Generation in Atrial Fibrillation – Thrombolysis in Myocardial Infarction 48; RE-ALIGN, Randomized, Phase II Study to Evaluate the Safety and Pharmacokinetics of Oral Dabigatran Etexilate in Patients after Heart Valve Replacement; RE-LY, Randomized Evaluation of Long-Term Anticoagulation Therapy; ROCKET-AF, Rivaroxaban Once Daily Oral Direct Factor Xa Inhibition Compared with Vitamin K Antagonism for Prevention of Stroke and Embolism Trial in Atrial Fibrillation

Drug and food interactions with NOACs are much fewer compared with warfarin, and patients do not require routine INR monitoring (Verheugt *et al.* 2015).

Among TIA or ischemic stroke patients with atrial fibrillation, dabigatran, rivaroxaban, apixaban, and edoxaban are all non-inferior to warfarin in prevention of recurrent ischemic stroke (Diener *et al.* 2010; Easton *et al.* 2012; Hankey *et al.* 2012; Rost *et al.* 2016). They are, however, associated with a ~50% reduction in risk of intracerebral hemorrhage compared with warfarin (Ruff *et al.* 2014). High-dose dabigatran or edoxaban appears to be more effective than low-dose dabigatran or edoxaban in prevention of thrombo-embolic events but is associated with more major gastrointestinal bleeds (Connolly *et al.* 2009; Diener *et al.* 2010; Giugliano *et al.* 2013). NOACs have been shown to be equally effective as warfarin in patients with valvular heart disease (Siontis *et al.* 2017) and appear to be safe in patients with a remote bioprosthetic valve implantation (Carnicelli *et al.* 2017). NOACs are, however, not licensed in patients with hemodynamically significant mitral stenosis or mechanical heart valves as clinical trials either have not included this group of patients (ARISTOTLE, AVEROES, ENGAGE AF-TIMI 48, and ROCKET-AF trials; Connolly *et al.* 2011; Granger *et al.* 2011; Patel *et al.* 2011; Giugliano *et al.* 2013) or have not been able to show its efficacy or safety in this subgroup of patients (RE-ALIGN trial; Eikelboom *et al.* 2013). Clinical trials to determine the effectiveness of NOACs versus aspirin in patients with embolic stroke of undetermined source are currently under way.

Choice of warfarin or NOACs should be individualized and would depend on patients' renal function (currently dabigatran is licensed for patients with creatinine clearance $\geq$ 30 ml/min while rivaroxaban, apixaban, and edoxaban are licensed for patients with creatinine clearance $\geq$ 15 ml/min), potential for drug interactions, patient preference, and cost. Patients' potential to be within therapeutic range of INR 2–3 if started on warfarin should also be assessed. Risk scores such as the SAMe-TT_2R_2 (Apostolakis *et al.* 2013; Chan *et al.* 2016; Box 24.1) can serve this purpose. Individuals with a score > 2 are more likely to

---

BOX 24.1 SAMe-TT_2R_2 Score

Risk factor	Points
Sex (female)	1
Age < 60 years	1
Medical history (two of the following: hypertension, diabetes, history of acute coronary syndrome, congestive heart failure, peripheral vascular disease, stroke, pulmonary hepatic, or renal disease)	1
Treatment (interacting medications with warfarin)	1
Tobacco use within 2 years	2
Race (non-Caucasians)	2

Interpretation of score:

0–2: patient is likely to achieve a high time in therapeutic range and hence warfarin is likely to be beneficial

> 2: patient is less likely to achieve a high time in therapeutic range and an NOAC may be a better treatment option than warfarin

Source: From Apostolakis *et al.* (2013).

have a poor time in therapeutic range if started on warfarin, and hence NOACs could be considered in this subset of patients. In the past, a lack of an available antidote to rapidly reverse the action of NOACs in the event of a major bleeding episode was of concern. However, intravenous idarucizumab, a specific reversal agent that can completely reverse the anticoagulant effect of dabigatran within minutes, is now available (Pollack et al. 2015). Other reversal agents for factor Xa inhibitors, such as andexanet alfa, have similarly been shown to reduce factor Xa activity quickly and are currently awaiting FDA approval before their routine clinical use (Connolly et al. 2016) (see Chapter 22 for management of antic-oagulant-related intracerebral hemorrhage).

In patients in whom NOACs are to be considered, head-to-head comparisons of individual NOACs in patients with TIA or ischemic stroke are limited, but choice and dosing of NOACs would depend on patient's preference, age, renal function, risk of gastrointestinal bleeding, and route of administration (i.e., whether the patient requires tube-feeding) (Verheugt et al. 2015). Rivaroxaban and edoxaban are taken once a day, and dabigatran 150 mg has been associated with an excess risk of bleeding in patients age 80 and older. Apixaban is the only NOAC that has a lower gastrointestinal bleeding risk compared with warfarin. Only rivaroxaban and apixaban have been deemed suitable for use via feeding tubes. In a meta-analysis of real-world observational studies in patients with atrial fibrilla-tion, rivaroxaban and dabigatran appeared to be equally effective in prevention of ischemic stroke, thrombo-embolic events, and ICH, but rivaroxaban was associated with a higher risk of gastrointestinal bleeding compared with warfarin (Bai et al. 2017).

The optimal time to start warfarin after TIA or ischemic stroke remains uncertain. While it is normally considered safe to start warfarin upon diagnosis of TIA, in patients with ischemic stroke, a balance between the risk of early recurrent stroke (e.g., from CHA_2DS_2-VASc score, Box 24.2) and risk of hemorrhagic transformation from the infarcted brain (as determined from infarct size and stroke severity) would need to be made. It has been suggested that NOACs could be started 1 day after TIA, 3 days after a mild stroke (NIH Stroke Scale, NIHSS < 8), 6 days after a moderate stroke (NIHSS 8–16) if hemorrhagic transformation has been excluded by repeat neuroimaging, and 12 days after a severe (NIHSS > 16) stroke if hemorrhagic transformation has been excluded by repeat neuroima-ging (Heidbuchel et al. 2015).

Addition of antiplatelets to anticoagulation in TIA or ischemic stroke patients with atrial fibrillation and stable coronary artery disease does not reduce risk of recurrent coronary events or thromboembolism but is associated with an increased risk of bleeding (Lamberts et al. 2014) and is therefore not recommended (Kernan et al. 2014; Lip et al. 2014). However, in TIA or ischemic stroke patients with atrial fibrillation who also have concomitant acute coronary syndrome or require insertion of a stent, use and duration of additional single or dual antiplatelet therapy would depend on bleeding risk (e.g., as determined by the HAS-BLED score, Box 24.3), choice of drug-eluting stents versus bare metal stents, and future risk of coronary event (Kernan et al. 2014; Lip et al. 2014).

Blood Pressure Control

There is good evidence from randomized trials to show that blood pressure lowering is effective for secondary prevention of stroke. In a meta-analysis of 10 clinical trials involving patients with a history of TIA or stroke, sustained lowering of blood pressure by 5.1 mmHg systolic and 2.5 mmHg diastolic with anti-hypertensive medications reduced the risk of

BOX 24.2 CHA$_2$DS$_2$-VASc Score	
Risk factor	**Points**
Congestive heart failure (signs or symptoms of left or right heart failure or both, with investigations showing objective evidence of cardiac dysfunction)	1
Hypertension (systolic blood pressure >140 mmHg and/or diastolic blood pressure > 90 mmHg)	1
Age	
65–74 years	1
≥ 75 years	2
Diabetes mellitus (fasting blood glucose ≥ 7.0 mmol/L and/or treatment with oral hypoglycemic agent and/or insulin)	1
Stroke/TIA/thrombo-embolism	2
Vascular disease (prior angina, intermittent claudication, myocardial infarction, venous thrombosis, or previous intervention to coronary, peripheral, or aortic vascular beds)	1
Sex (female)	1

Points (maximum score of 9)	**Adjusted stroke rate (%/year)**
0	0%
1	1.3%
2	2.2%
3	3.2%
4	4.0%
5	6.7%
6	9.8%
7	9.6%
8	6.7%
9	15.2%

Source: From Lip *et al.* (2010a).

recurrent stroke by 22% (Liu *et al.* 2009). The optimal blood pressure target, however, remains uncertain. In the SPS3 trial, patients with lacunar infarct with a blood pressure of 120–128 mmHg systolic and 65–70 mmHg diastolic were at lowest risk of a recurrent stroke (Odden *et al.* 2016). In another meta-analysis of all large-scaled blood pressure lowering trials, every 10 mmHg reduction in systolic blood pressure in patients with known cardiovascular disease was associated with a 26% reduction in risk of stroke and 10% reduction in risk of death (Ettehad *et al.* 2016). Blood pressure lowering to < 130 mmHg systolic was associated with better outcomes compared with patients who had a systolic blood pressure

BOX 24.3 Hypertension, Abnormal Renal/Liver Function, Stroke, Bleeding History or Redisposition, Labile INR, Elderly, Drugs/Alcohol Concomitantly (HAS-BLED) Score

Risk factor	Point
Hypertension (uncontrolled, systolic blood pressure > 160 mmHg)	1
Renal disease (renal replacement therapy or creatinine > 200μmol/L)	1
Liver disease (cirrhosis or bilirubin 2x upper limit normal with AST/ALT/ALP >3x upper limit normal)	1
Stroke history	1
Prior major bleeding or predisposition to bleeding	1
Labile INR (unstable / high INR, time in therapeutic range < 60%)	1
Age >65	1
Drug usage predisposing to bleeding (e.g., antiplatelet agents or NSAIDs)	1
Alcohol (≥ 8 drinks per week)	1

Points (maximum score of 9)	Bleeds/100 patient years
0	1.13
1	1.12
2	1.88
3	3.74
4	8.70
5	12.50

Sources: From Lip *et al.* (2010b) and Pisters *et al.* (2010).

≥ 130 mmHg (Ettehad *et al.* 2016). However, many physicians may be cautious in lowering blood pressure to this target in patients with bilateral severe carotid stenosis or severe basilar or bilateral vertebral artery disease. Such patients may be at risk of border-zone infarction if their existing poor cerebral blood flow is further compromised by reduction in systemic blood pressure. Current guidelines make no recommendations in these patients (Kernan *et al.* 2014) but suggest that in TIA or ischemic stroke patients with intracranial atherosclerosis (50–99%), maintaining a systolic blood pressure target below 140 mmHg is recommended (Kernan *et al.* 2014).

The optimal drug regimen to achieve the target blood pressure control also remains uncertain due to limited direct comparisons between anti-hypertensive agents (Kernan *et al.* 2014). Current guidelines suggest that use of diuretics or the combination of diuretics and an angiotensin-converting enzyme inhibitor is useful (Kernan *et al.* 2014). These results are mainly driven by two large blood pressure–lowering trials (Post-stroke Antihypertensive

Treatment Study [PATS] and Perindopril PrOtection Against Recurrent Stroke Study [PROGRESS]; PROGRESS Collaborative Group 2001; Liu *et al.* 2009), which, together with other smaller trials, showed that TIA or stroke patients treated with indapamide with or without an angiotensin-converting enzyme inhibitor reduced the risk of recurrent stroke by 37% (Liu *et al.* 2009). In contrast, use of renin angiotensin system inhibitors alone was associated with a 7% reduction in risk of recurrent stroke (Liu *et al.* 2009).

Visit-to-visit systolic blood pressure variability is reduced in a dose-dependent fashion, most significantly with calcium channel blockers and to a lesser extent with non-loop diuretics, and hence calcium channel blockers are also likely to be effective in prevention of stroke (Webb *et al.* 2010; Webb and Rothwell 2011). However, although visit-to-visit blood pressure variability is a strong predictor of stroke, independent of mean systolic blood pressure (Rothwell *et al.* 2010), clinical trials that aim to determine the effect of reducing visit-to-visit blood pressure in patients with TIA or ischemic stroke are lacking.

Cholesterol

There is a positive association between cholesterol and risk of ischemic stroke, although the relationship is weaker compared with coronary heart disease due to the heterogeneous nature of ischemic stroke (Lewington *et al.* 2007). The Stroke Prevention by Aggressive Reduction in Cholesterol Levels (SPARCL) trial evaluated the benefits of statins (atorvastatin 80 mg daily versus placebo) in secondary prevention of patients with non-cardioembolic stroke and TIA within 6 months (Amarenco *et al.* 2006). Use of statins was associated with a 16% reduction in risk of recurrent stroke and 20% reduction in risk of major cardiovascular events (Amarenco *et al.* 2006). Benefit of statins in the SPARCL trial was greater in patients who had underlying large artery atherosclerosis or diabetes or were < 65 years of age (Sillesen *et al.* 2008). When results of the SPARCL trial were combined with other clinical trials of patients with cardiovascular diseases, lowering of LDL cholesterol concentration by about 1 mmol/L with statins was associated with a 12% lower risk of recurrent stroke (Amarenco and Labreuche 2009). Current guidelines therefore recommend use of statins with an intensive lipid-lowering effect (> 50% LDL reduction) in patients with TIA or ischemic stroke presumed to be of atherosclerotic origin (Kernan *et al.* 2014).

The optimal LDL target of patients with TIA or ischemic stroke on statins remains uncertain. Post-hoc analysis of the SPARCL trial showed that a reduction of LDL to ≤ 1.8 mmol/L was associated with a 28% relative risk reduction for recurrent stroke compared with patients with LDL > 2.6 mmol/L (Amarenco *et al.* 2007). The Treat Stroke to Target (TST) trial is currently under way to determine whether use of statins with or without ezetimibe in TIA or ischemic stroke patients to reach target LDL of 1.8 mmol/L or below is associated with a lower risk of recurrent vascular events compared with an LDL target of 2.6 mmol/L.

Use of other LDL-lowering medications such as fibrates and resins has not been shown to be effective in reducing the risk of stroke (Corvol *et al.* 2003). Indeed, statins have a number of pleotropic, cholesterol-independent properties such as anti-inflammatory and anti-thrombotic effects. Statins also reduce endothelial dysfunction and oxidative stress, which, taken together, would result in an improved stability of atherosclerotic plaques and, in some instances, may also lead to atherosclerotic plaque regression (Amarenco *et al.* 2004; Migrino *et al.* 2011).

However, in secondary prevention trials, use of statins was associated with a significantly increased risk of hemorrhagic stroke (Heart Protection Study and SPARCL; Collins *et al.* 2004; Amarenco *et al.* 2006), although this risk was not seen in primary prevention trials (Amarenco *et al.* 2009). Risk of intracerebral hemorrhage was independently associated with male sex, increased age, history of hemorrhagic stroke, and stage II hypertension but was not associated with degree of LDL reduction (Goldstein *et al.* 2008). Therefore, in patients with previous history of intracerebral hemorrhage, the potential hemorrhagic risks of statins should be balanced with their benefits in preventing an atherothrombotic event. Should statins be deemed beneficial in patients with a history of intracerebral hemorrhage, blood pressure should be controlled as much as possible.

In the recent few years, a new class of lipid-lowering agents that inhibit proprotein convertase subtilisin-kexin type 9 (PCSK9) have emerged (Giugliano and Sabatine 2015). Evolocumab, a PCSK9 inhibitor, was subsequently studied in the FOURIER trial, where 27,564 patients with atherosclerotic cardiovascular disease (19% with a history of nonhemorrhagic stroke) who were receiving statin therapy, but with LDL cholesterol levels of 1.8mmol/L or higher, were studied (Sabatine *et al.* 2017). Patients were randomized to receive subcutaneous evolocumab (140mg every 2 weeks or 420mg monthly) or placebo. After a median follow-up of 2.2 years, patients receiving evolocumab had an overall 59% reduction in LDL cholesterol levels. Risk of major adverse cardiovascular events was significantly lower in patients receiving evolocumab compared with placebo (9.8% versus 11.3%, hazard ratio 0.85, 95% confidence interval 0.79 to 0.92, $p<0.001$). Use of evolocumab was also associated with a significantly lower risk of ischemic stroke (1.2% versus 1.6%, hazard ratio 0.75, 95% confidence interval 0.62–0.92) (Sabatine *et al.* 2017). PCSK9 inhibitors may therefore be useful in further lowering of LDL cholesterol levels in ischemic stroke patients who are already on an optimal regimen of statin therapy but with suboptimal LDL cholesterol levels (Powers *et al.* 2018). However, based on the FOURIER trial, the number needed to treat to prevent 1 cardiovascular death, myocardial infarction, or stroke over a period of 2 years will be 74, with an estimated 2-year cost of US$2.1 million (Sabatine *et al.* 2017).

No trials on the benefits of triglyceride lowering in patients with stroke have been performed, although in the Veterans Affairs HDL Intervention Trial (VA-HIT), triglyceride reduction with gemfibrozil in patients with coronary artery disease led to a 33% reduction in risk of first stroke (Bloomfield *et al.* 2001). Plasma triglycerides reduced by 31% and HDL increased by 10% in the treatment arm, but there was no significant effect on LDL levels with use of gemfibrozil (Bloomfield *et al.* 2001).

Glucose Lowering

In patients with type 2 diabetes, intensive glucose lowering alone does not reduce the risk of non-fatal stroke compared with standard care (Seidu *et al.* 2016). In contrast, multi-factorial interventions incorporating additional blood pressure– and lipid-lowering strategies had much greater impact in reducing the risk of non-fatal stroke (Seidu *et al.* 2016). In patients with insulin resistance with TIA or ischemic stroke within 6 months, use of pioglitazone in the Insulin Resistance Intervention after Stroke (IRIS) trial was associated with a reduced risk of recurrent stroke or myocardial infarction, possibly related to pioglitazone's action in improving insulin sensitivity as well as reducing blood pressure, cholesterol, and inflammation (Kernan *et al.* 2016).

Secondary Prevention after Primary Intracerebral Hemorrhage

Much less is known about the long-term risk of recurrence after primary intracerebral hemorrhage than after ischemic stroke. In patients with primary intracerebral hemorrhage, approximately 25–50% of recurrent strokes are further hemorrhages, depending on the underlying disease process. The absolute risk also depends on the various underlying causes, such as arteriovenous malformation, cerebral amyloid angiopathy, poorly controlled hypertension, or coagulopathy. Although patients with primary intracerebral hemorrhage are at increased risk of ischemic stroke as well as further hemorrhage, most clinicians do not recommend antiplatelet therapy unless there is a particularly high risk of coronary or other ischemic vascular events. In contrast, most patients with primary intracerebral hemorrhage require blood pressure–lowering medication, with the possible exception of those elderly patients with hemorrhages secondary to amyloid angiography in whom blood pressure is sometimes already rather low.

References

ACTIVE Writing Group of the ACTIVE Investigators (2006). Clopidogrel plus aspirin versus oral anticoagulation for atrial fibrillation in the Atrial fibrillation Clopidogrel Trial with Irbesartan for prevention of Vascular Events (ACTIVE W): A randomized controlled trial. *Lancet* **367**:1903–1912

Amerenco P, Labreuche J, Lavallee P *et al.* (2004). Statins in stroke prevention and carotid atherosclerosis: Systematic review and up-to-date meta-analysis. *Stroke* **35**:2902–2909

Amarenco P, Bogousslavsky J, Callahan A III *et al.* (2006). High-dose atorvastatin after stroke or transient ischemic attack. *New England Journal of Medicine* **355**:549–559

Amarenco P, Goldstein LB, Szarek M *et al.* (2007). Effects of intense low-density lipoprotein cholesterol reduction in patients with stroke or transient ischemic attack: The Stroke Prevention by Aggressive Reduction in Cholesterol Levels (SPARCL) trial. *Stroke* **38**:3198–3204

Amarenco P, Labreuche J (2009). Lipid management in the prevention of stroke: Review and updated meta-analysis of statins for stroke prevention. *Lancet Neurology* **8**:453–463

Amarenco P, Albers GW, Denison H *et al.* (2017). Efficacy and safety of ticagrelor versus aspirin in acute stroke or transient ischemic attack of atherosclerotic origin: A subgroup analysis of SOCRATES, a randomised, double-blind, controlled trial. *Lancet Neurology* **16**:301–310

Antithrombotic Trialists' (ATT) Collaboration (2009). Aspirin in the primary and secondary prevention of vascular disease: Collaborative meta-analysis of individual participant data from randomized trials. *Lancet* **373**:1849–1860

Apostolakis S, Sullivan RM, Olshansky B *et al.* (2013). Factors affecting quality of anticoagulation control among patients with atrial fibrillation on warfarin: The SAMe-TT$_2$R$_2$ score. *Chest* **144**:1555–1563

Bai Y, Deng H, Shantsila A *et al.* (2017). Rivaroxaban versus dabigatran or warfarin in real-world studies of stroke prevention in atrial fibrillation: Systematic review and meta-analysis. *Stroke* (epub ahead of print)

Berger PB, Bhatt DL, Fuster V *et al.* (2010). Bleeding complications with dual antiplatelet therapy among patients with stable vascular disease or risk actors for vascular disease: Results from the Clopidogrel for High Atherothrombotic Risk and Ischemic Stabilization, Management and Avoidance (CHARISMA) trial. *Circulation* **121**:2575–2583

Bhatt DL, Flather MD, Hacke W *et al.* (2007). Patients with prior myocardial infarction, stroke, or symptomatic peripheral arterial disease in the CHARISMA trial. *Journal of the American College of Cardiologists* **49**:1982–1988

Bloomfield RH, Davenport J, Babikian V *et al.* (2001). Reduction in stroke with gemfibrozil in men with coronary heart disease and low HDL cholesterol: The Veterans Affairs HDL Intervention Trial (VA-HIT). *Circulation* **103**:2828–2833

CADISS Trial Investigators (2015). Antiplatelet treatment compared with anticoagulation treatment for cervical artery dissection

(CADISS): A randomised trial. *Lancet Neurology* **14**:361–367

Canadian Cooperative Study Group (1978). A randomized trial of aspirin and sulfinpyrazone in threatened stroke. *New England Journal of Medicine* **299**:53–59

CAPRIE Steering Committee (1996). A randomised blinded trial of clopidogrel versus aspirin in patients at risk of ischaemic events (CAPRIE). *Lancet* **348**:1329–1339

Carnicelli AP, Caterina RD, Halperin JL *et al.* (2017). Edoxaban for the prevention of thromboembolism in patients with atrial fibrillation and bioprosthetic valves. *Circulation* (epub ahead of print)

Chan PH, Chan EW, Li WH *et al.* (2016). Use of the SAMe-TT2R2 Score to predict good anticoagulation control with warfarin in Chinese patients with atrial fibrillation: relationship to ischemic stroke incidence. *PLoS One* **11**:e0150674

Chimowitz MI, Lynn MJ, Howlett-Smith H *et al.* (2005). Comparison of warfarin and aspirin for symptomatic intracranial arterial stenosis. *New England Journal of Medicine* **352**:1305–1316

Chimowitz MI, Lynn MJ, Derdeyn CP *et al.* (2011). Stenting versus aggressive medical therapy for intracranial artery stenosis. *New England Journal of Medicine* **365**:993–1003

Collins R, Armitage J, Parish S *et al.* (2004). Effects of cholesterol-lowering with simvastatin on stroke and other major vascular events in 20 536 people with cerebrovascular disease or other high-risk conditions. *Lancet* **363**:757–767

Connolly SJ, Ezekowitz MD, Yusuf S *et al.* (2009). Dabigatran versus warfarin in patients with atrial fibrillation. *New England Journal of Medicine* **361**:1139–1151

Connolly SJ, Eikelboom J, Joyner C *et al.* (2011). Apixaban in patients with atrial fibrillation. *New England Journal of Medicine* **364**:806–817

Connolly SJ, Milling TJ Jr, Eikelboom JW *et al.* (2016). Andexanet alfa for acute major bleeding associated with factor Xa inhibitors. *New England Journal of Medicine* **375**:1131–1141

Corvol JC, Bouzamondo A, Sirol M *et al.* (2003). Differential effects of lipid-lowering therapies on stroke prevention: A meta-analysis of randomized trials. *Archives of Internal Medicine* **163**:669–676

Diener HC, Cunha L, Forbes C *et al.* (1996). European Stroke Prevention Study. 2. Dipyridamole and acetylsalicylic acid in the secondary prevention of stroke. *Journal of the Neurological Sciences* **143**:1–13

Diener HC, Bogousslavsky J, Brass LM *et al.* (2004). Aspirin and clopidogrel compared with clopidogrel alone after recent ischaemic stroke or transient ischaemic attack in high-risk patients (MATCH): Randomised double-blind placebo-controlled trial. *Lancet* **364**:331–337

Diener HC, Connolly S, Ezekowitz MD *et al.* (2010). Dabigatran compared with warfarin in patients with atrial fibrillation and previous transient ishemic attack or stroke: A subgroup analysis of the RE-LY trial. *Lancet Neurology* **9**:1157–1163

Easton JD, Lopes RD, Bahit MC *et al.* (2012) Apixaban compared with warfarin in patients with atrial fibrillation and previous stroke or transient ischemic attack: A subgroup analysis of the ARISTOTLE trial. *Lancet Neurology* **11**:503–511

Eikelboom JW, Connolly SJ, Brueckmann M *et al.* (2013). Dabigatran versus warfarin in patients with mechanical heart valves. *New England Journal of Medicine* **369**:1206–1214

ESPRIT Study Group, Halkes PH, van Gijn J *et al.* (2007). Medium intensity oral anticoagulants versus aspirin after cerebral ischemic of arterial origin (ESPRIT): A randomized controlled trial. *Lancet Neurology* **6**:115–124

Ettehad D, Emdin CA, Kiran A *et al.* (2016). Blood pressure lowering for prevention of cardiovascular disease and death: A systematic review and meta-analysis. *Lancet* **387**:957–967

Freedman B, Gersh BJ, Lip GY (2015). Misperceptions of aspirin efficacy and safety may perpetuate anticoagulant underutilization in atrial fibrillation. *European Heart Journal* **36**:653–656

Giugliano RP, Ruff CT, Braunwald E *et al.* (2013). Edoxaban versus warfarin in patients with atrial fibrillation. *New England Journal of Medicine* **369**:2093–2104

Giugliano RP, Sabatine MS (2015). Are PCSK9 inhibitors the next breakthrough in the cardiovascular field? *Journal of the American College of Cardiology* 65:2638–2651

Goldstein LB, Amarenco P, Szarek S *et al.* (2008). Hemorrhagic stroke in Stroke Prevention by Aggressive Reduction in Cholesterol Levels study. *Neurology* 70:2364–2370

Granger GB, Alexander JH, McMurray JJ *et al.* (2011). Apixaban versus warfarin in patients with atrial fibrillation. *New England Journal of Medicine* 365:981–992

Halkes PH, van Gijn J for the ESPRIT Study Group (2006). Aspirin plus dipyridamole versus aspirin alone after cerebral ischaemia of arterial origin (ESPRIT): Randomised controlled trial. *Lancet* 367:1665–1673 [Erratum in *Lancet* (2007) 369:274]

Hankey GJ, Patel MR, Stevens SR *et al.* (2012). Rivaroxaban compared with warfarin in patients with atrial fibrillation and previous stroke or transient ischemic attack: A subgroup analysis of ROCKET AF. *Lancet Neurology* 11:315–322

Hart RG, Pearce LA, Aguilar MI (2007). Meta-analysis: Antithrombotic therapy to prevent stroke in patients who have nonvalvular atrial fibrillation. *Annals of Internal Medicine* 146:857–867

Heidbuchel H, Verhamme P, Alings M *et al.* (2015). Updated European Heart Rhythm Association Practical Guide on the use of non-vigtmain K antagnoist anticoagulants in patients with non-valvular atrial fibrillation. *Europace* 17:1467–1507

Kamal AK, Naqvi I, Husain MR *et al.* (2011). Cilostazol versus aspirin for secondary prevention of vascular events after stroke of arterial origin. *Cochrane Database of Systematic Reviews* 1:CD008076

Kernan WN, Ovbiagele B, Black HR *et al.* (2014). Guidelines for the prevention of stroke in patients with stroke and transient ischemic attack: A guideline for healthcare professionals from the American Heart Association/American Stroke Association. *Stroke* 45:2160–2236

Kernan WN, Viscoli CM, Furie KL *et al.* (2016). Pioglitazone after ischemic stroke or transient ischemic attack. *New England Journal of Medicine* 374:1321–1331

Kirchhof P, Benussi S, Kotecha D *et al.* (2016). 2016 ESC Guidelines for the management of atrial fibrillation developed in collaboration with EACTS. *European Heart Journal* 37:2893–2962

Johnston SC, Amarenco P, Albers GW *et al.* (2016). Ticagrelor versus aspirin in acute stroke or transient ischemic attack. *New England Journal of Medicine* 375:35–43

Lamberts M, Gislason GH, Lip GY *et al.* (2014). Antiplatelet therapy for stable coronary artery disease in atrial fibrillation patients taking an oral anticoagulant: A nationwide cohort study. *Circulation* 129:1577–1585

Leonardi-Bee J, Bath PM, Bousser MG *et al.* (2005) Dipyridamole for preventing recurrence ischemic stroke and other vascular events: A meta-analysis of individual patient data from randomized controlled trials. *Stroke* 36:162–168

Lewington S, Whitlock G, Clarke R *et al.* (2007). Blood cholesterol and vascular mortality by age, sex, and blood pressure: A meta-analysis of individual data from 61 prospective studies with 55,000 vascular deaths. *Lancet* 370:1829–1839

Lip GY, Nieuwlaat R, Pisters R *et al.* (2010a). Refining clinical risk stratification for predicting stroke and thromboembolism in atrial fibrillation using a novel risk factor-based approach: The Euro Heart Survey on Atrial Fibrillation. *Chest* 137:263–272

Lip GY, Frison L, Halperin JL *et al.* (2010b). Comparative validation of a novel risk score for predicting bleeding risk in anticoagulated patients with atrial fibrillation: The HAS-BLED (Hypertension, Abnormal Renal/Liver Function, Stroke, Bleeding History or Predisposition, Labile INR, Elderly, Drug/Alcohol Concomitantly) score. *Journal of American College of Cardiology* 57:173–180

Lip GY, Windecker S, Huber K *et al.* (2014). Management of antithrombotic therapy in atrial fibrillation patients presenting with acute coronary syndrome and/or undergoing percutaneous coronary or valve interventions: A joint consensus document of the European Society of Cardiology Working Group on Thrombosis, European Heart Rhythm Association (EHRA), European Association of Percutaneous Cardiovascular Interventions (EAPCI) and European Association of Acute Cardiac Care (ACCA) endorsed by the Heart Rhythm Society (HRS) and Asia-Pacific Heart

Rhythm Society (APHRS). *European Heart Journal* 35:3155–3179

Liu L, Wang Z, Gong L et al. (2009). Blood pressure reduction for the secondary prevention of stroke: A Chinese trial and a systematic review of the literature. *Hypertension Research* 32:1032–1040

Mant J, Hobbs FD, Fletcher K et al. (2007) Midland Research Practices Network (MidReC). Warfarin versus aspirin for stroke prevention in an elderly community population with atrial fibrillation (the Birmingham Atrial Fibrillation Treatment of the Aged Study, BAFTA): A randomised controlled trial. *Lancet* 370:493–503

Migrino RQ, Bowers M, Harmann L et al. (2011). Carotid plaque regression following 6-month statin therapy assessed by 3 T cardiovascular magnetic resonance: Comparison with ultrasound intima media thickness. *Journal of Cardiovascular Magnetic Resonance* 13:37

Mohr JP, Thompson JL, Lazar RM et al. (2001). A comparison of warfarin and aspirin for the prevention of recurrent ischemic stroke. *New England Journal of Medicine* 345:1444–1451

Odden MC, McClure LA, Sawaya BP et al. (2016). Achieved blood pressure and outcomes in the Secondary Prevention of Small Subcortical Strokes Trial. *Hypertension* 67:63–69

Patel MR, Mahaffey KW, Garg J et al. (2011). Rivaroxaban versus warfarin in nonvalvular atrial fibrillation. *New England Journal of Medicine* 365:883–891

Pisters R, Lane DA, Nieuwlaat R et al. (2010). A novel user-friendly score (HAS-BLED) to assess 1-year risk of major bleeding in patients with atrial fibrillation: The Euro Heart Survey. *Chest* 138:1093–1100

Pollack CV Jr., Reilly PA, Eikelboom J et al. (2015). Idarucizumab for dabigatran reversal. *New England Journal of Medicine* 373:511–520

Powers WJ, Rabinstein AA, Ackerson T et al. (2018). 2018 Guidelines for the early management of patients with acute ischemic stroke: A guideline for healthcare professionals from the American Heart Association/American Stroke Association. *Stroke* 49:e46–e110

PROGRESS Collaborative Group (2001). Randomised trial of a perindopril-based blood-pressure-lowering regimen among 6,105 individuals with previous stroke or transient ischaemic attacks. *Lancet* 358:1033–1041

Rash A, Downes T, Portner R et al. (2007). A randomised controlled trial of warfarin versus aspirin for stroke prevention in octogenarians with atrial fibrillation (WASPO). *Age Ageing* 36:151–156

Rost NS, Giugliano RP, Ruff CT et al. (2016). Outcomes with edoxaban versus warfarin in patients with previous cerebrovascular events: Findings from Effective Anticoagulation with Factor Xa Next Generation in Atrial Fibrillation-Thrombolysis in Myocardial Infarction. *Stroke* 47:2075–2082

Rothwell PM, Giles MF, Chandratheva A et al. (2007). Effect of urgent treatment of transient ischaemic attack and minor stroke on early recurrent stroke (EXPRESS study): A prospective population-based sequential comparison. *Lancet* 370:1432–1442

Rothwell PM, Howard SC, Dolan E et al. (2010). Prognostic significance of visit-to-visit variability, maximum systolic blood pressure, and episodic hypertension. *Lancet* 375:895–905

Rothwell PM, Algra A, Chen Z et al. (2016). Effects of aspirin on risk and severity of early recurrent stroke after transient ischemic attack and ischemic stroke: Time-course analysis of randomized trials. *Lancet* 388:365–375

Ruff CT, Giugliano RP, Braunwald E et al. (2014). Comparison of the efficacy and safety of new oral anticoagulants with warfarin in patients with atrial fibrillation: A meta-analysis of randomized trials. *Lancet* 383:955–962

Sabatine MS, Giugliano RP, Keech AC et al. (2017). Evolocumab and clinical outcomes in patients with cardiovascular disease. *New England Journal of Medicine* 376:1713–1722

Sacco RL, Diener HC, Yusuf S et al. (2008). Aspirin and extended-release dipyridamole versus clopidogrel for recurrent stroke. *New England Journal of Medicine* 359:1238–1251

Seidu S, Achana FA, Gray LJ et al. (2016). Effects of glucose-lowering and multifactorial interventions on cardiovascular and mortality outcomes: A meta-analysis of randomized control trials. *Diabetic Medicine* 33:280–289

Siontis KC, Yao X, Gersh BJ *et al.* (2017). Direct oral anticoagulants in patients with atrial fibrillation and valvular heart disease other than significant mitral stenosis and mechanical valves. *Circulation* **135**:714–716

Sillesen H, Amarenco P, Hennerici MG *et al.* (2008). Atorvastatin reduces the risk of cardiovascular events in patients with carotid atherosclerosis: A secondary analysis of the Stroke Prevention by Aggressive Reduction in Cholesterol Levels (SPARCL) Trial. *Stroke* **39**:3297–3302

Sivenius J, Riekkinen PJ, Smets P *et al.* (1991). The European Stroke Prevention Study (ESPS): Results by arterial distribution. *Annals of Neurology* **29**:596–600

SPS3 Investigators (2012). Effects of clopidogrel added to aspirin in patients with recent lacunar stroke. *New England Journal of Medicine* **367**:817–825

Stroke Prevention in Atrial Fibrillation Investigators (1991). Stroke prevention in atrial fibrillation study: Final results. *Circulation* **84**:527–539

Stroke Prevention in Reversible Ischemic Trial (SPIRIT) Study Group (1997). A randomized trial of anticoagulants versus aspirin after cerebral ischemic of presumed arterial origin. *Annals of Neurology* **42**:857–865

Sudlow CL, Mason G, Maurice JB *et al.* (2009). Thienopyridine derivatives versus aspirin for preventing stroke and other serious vascular events in high vascular risk patients. *Cochrane Database of Systematic Reviews* **4**: CD001246

Verheugt FW, Granger CB (2015). Oral anticoagulants for stroke prevention in atrial fibrillation: Current status, special situations, and unmet needs. *Lancet* **386**:303–310

Wang Y, Wang Y, Zhao X *et al.* (2013). Clopidogrel with aspirin in acute minor stroke or transient ischemic attack. *New England Journal of Medicine* **369**:11–19

Webb AJ, Fischer U, Mehta Z *et al.* (2010). Effects of antihypertensive-drug class on interindividual variation in blood pressure and risk of stroke: A systematic review and meta-analysis. *Lancet* **375**:906–915

Webb AJ, Rothwell PM (2011). Effect of dose and combination of antihypertensives on interindividual blood pressure variability: A systematic review. *Stroke* **42**:2850–2865

Wong KS, Wang Y, Leng X *et al.* (2013). Early dual versus mono antiplatelet therapy for acute non-cardioembolic ischemic stroke or transient ischemic attack: An updated systematic review and meta-analysis. *Circulation* **128**:1656–1666

Chapter 25

Carotid Endarterectomy

The surgical removal of atheromatous plaque from within the carotid artery is termed *carotid endarterectomy*. The operation was first performed in an attempt to improve the flow of blood to the brain, although no systematic attempt was made to assess the risks and benefits of the procedure. Subsequently, randomized trials were performed in patients with a history of recent symptomatic stroke, and also in those with asymptomatic disease, to determine whether the operation was beneficial and, if so, what the predictors of benefit would be. As a result of these trials, carotid endarterectomy has been proven to be an effective treatment for the secondary prevention of stroke in selected patients.

History

Knowledge of the relationship between atheromatous disease of the extracranial carotid and vertebral arteries and the occurrence of ischemic stroke goes back to the nineteenth century. In 1856, Virchow described carotid thrombosis in a patient with sudden-onset ipsilateral visual loss in whom the ophthalmic and retinal arteries were patent (Gurdjian 1979). In 1888, Penzoldt reported a patient who developed sudden permanent loss of vision in the right eye and later sustained a left hemiplegia (Penzoldt 1891). At autopsy, the patient was found to have thrombotic occlusion of the right distal common carotid artery and a large area of cerebral softening in the right cerebral hemisphere. In 1905, Chiari performed a number of pathological studies that led him to suggest that emboli could break away from ulcerated carotid plaques in the neck and cause cerebral infarction. This mechanism of stroke was reemphasized 50 years later by Miller Fisher (1951, 1954).

Several operations were developed in the 1950s and 1960s in which the aim of surgery was to restore the flow of blood to the brain in patients with stenosis or occlusion of the extracranial carotid or vertebral circulations (Thompson 1996). One of the main contributions leading up to this was the development of cerebral arteriography by Egas Moniz in 1927 and the subsequent demonstration of stenosis and occlusion of the carotid arteries in life (Moniz *et al.* 1937). The subsequent development of extracranial/intracranial bypass surgery and carotid endarterectomy are described in this chapter. Several other surgical techniques have been tried, although unlike endarterectomy and extracranial/intracranial bypass they have not been tested in randomized controlled trials. These include various bypass procedures for occlusion of the proximal neck and aortic arch vessels; vertebral artery endarterectomy, reconstruction, or bypass; and various arterial transpositions involving anastomosis of the subclavian and vertebral arteries into the common carotid artery. These procedures will not be discussed further here (see Chapter 26).

The first operations on the carotid artery were ligation procedures for trauma or hemorrhage. The first report was in Benjamin Bell's *Surgery* in 1793 (Wood 1857). However, most early ligations resulted in the death of the patient. The first successful ligation was performed by a British naval surgeon, David Fleming, in 1803 (Keevil 1949). This operation was performed for late carotid rupture following neck trauma in an attempted suicide. The first successful ligation for carotid aneurysm was performed 5 years later in London by Astley Cooper (Cooper 1836). By 1868, Pilz was able to collect 600 recorded cases of carotid ligation for cervical aneurysm or hemorrhage, with an overall mortality of 43% (Hamby 1952). In 1878, an American surgeon named John Wyeth reported a 41% mortality in a collected study of 898 common carotid ligations and contrasted this with a 4.5% mortality for ligation of the external carotid artery.

There were relatively few developments for the next 70 years. However, in 1946, a Portuguese surgeon, Cid Dos Santos, introduced thrombo-endarterectomy for restoration of flow in peripheral vessels (Dos Santos 1976). The first successful reconstruction of the carotid artery was performed by Carrea, Molins, and Murphy in Buenos Aires in 1951 (Carrea *et al.* 1955). However, this was not an endarterectomy. Rather, they performed an end-to-end anastomosis of the left external carotid artery and the distal internal carotid artery (ICA) in a 41-year-old man with a recently symptomatic severe carotid stenosis.

In 1954, Eastcott, Pickering, and Rob published a case report detailing a carotid resection performed in May 1954 on a 66-year-old woman with recurrent left carotid TIAs and a severe stenosis on angiography. The patient made an uneventful recovery and was relieved of her TIAs. In 1975, DeBakey reported that he had performed a carotid endarterectomy on a 53-year-old man in August 1953, but it was the report by Eastcott and colleagues (1954) that provided the impetus for the further development of carotid surgery. Over the next 5 years, there were numerous other reports of the operation being performed, and several technical improvements were suggested (Thompson 1996). Occlusion of the ICA generally came to be regarded as inoperable, and surgical attempts to correct carotid coils, kinks, and fibromuscular dysplasia were not generally supported.

By the early 1980s, there were more than 100,000 procedures per year in the USA alone (Pokras and Dyken 1988; Gillum 1995; Tu *et al.* 1998). However, other than innumerable surgical case series and two small inconclusive randomized trials (Fields *et al.* 1970; Shaw *et al.* 1984), there was no good evidence that the operation was of any value. This prompted several eminent clinicians in the early 1980s to question the widespread use of the operation (Barnett *et al.* 1984; Chambers and Norris 1984; Warlow 1984; Jonas 1987; Winslow *et al.* 1988), which led to a fall in the number of operations being performed and set the scene for a number of large randomized controlled trials. The first results in patients with symptomatic stenosis began to appear in the early 1990s (European Carotid Surgery Trialists' Collaborative Group 1991; Mayberg *et al.* 1991; North American Symptomatic Carotid Endarterectomy Trial Collaborators 1991). Surgery clearly did prevent stroke in patients with recently symptomatic severe ICA stenosis.

The Operation

The carotid bifurcation is exposed and mobilized and slings are placed around the internal, external, and common carotid arteries. After applying clamps to these arteries, away from any atheromatous plaque, the bifurcation is opened through a longitudinal incision, the entire stenotic lesion cored out, the distal intimal margin secured, the arteriotomy closed, and the clamps released to restore blood flow to the brain. Most patients should already be taking antiplatelet drugs before surgery, and these should be continued afterward because the patients are still at high risk of ischemic stroke in the territory of other arteries and of coronary events. In addition, most surgeons give patients heparin during the procedure itself. Controlling systemic blood pressure before, during, and after surgery is crucial to avoid hypotension, which will make any cerebral ischemia worse, and hypertension, which may cause cerebral edema or even intracerebral hemorrhage. Operative damage to the nerve to the carotid sinus, or changes in the carotid sinus itself, may make control of postoperative blood pressure more of a problem but in the long term has little if any effect (Eliasziw *et al.* 1998).

Eversion endarterectomy is a popular variation to conventional endarterectomy (Loftus and Quest 1987; Darling *et al.* 1996; Cao *et al.* 1998; Brothers 2005; Demirel *et al.* 2012). A systematic review of five randomized controlled trials (2,590 operations) compared eversion endarterectomy versus conventional endarterectomy performed with either primary closure or patch angioplasty (Cao *et al.* 2002). Overall, there was no significant difference in the rates of perioperative stroke, stroke or death, and local complication rates, but the absolute risks were rather low (risk of stroke or death was 1.7% with eversion and 2.6% with conventional endarterectomy).

Shunting

In theory, it should be possible to prevent low cerebral blood flow during carotid clamping, and possible ischemic stroke, by inserting a temporary intraluminal shunt (usually in the form of a silicon tube) from the common carotid artery to the ICA distal to the operation site. This serves as a temporary bypass that theoretically reduces the length of time the blood flow to the brain is interrupted during the operation. Some surgeons routinely shunt for this reason and to allow more time to teach trainees, but there are problems, including arterial wall damage leading to arterial dissection and transmission of emboli from thrombus in the common carotid artery as well as an increase in the duration of surgery and possibly in local operation site complications. A compromise is to use a shunt only in selected patients (e.g., identified by various cerebral monitoring techniques such as ultrasound) who are likely to develop or who actually are experiencing cerebral ischemia as a result of low flow. However, efforts to identify the patients who need shunts have been inconclusive (Ferguson 1986; Ojemann and Heros 1986; Naylor *et al.* 1992; Belardi *et al.* 2003), and there is considerable variation in routine practice (Bond *et al.* 2002a). Unfortunately, randomized trials of different shunting policies have been too small and too few to provide reliable answers (Bond *et al.* 2002b; Chongruksut *et al.* 2014). As a result, there is no standard policy for either operative monitoring or the use of shunts.

Restenosis and Patch Angioplasty

After carotid endarterectomy, the long-term risk of ischemic stroke ipsilateral to the operated artery is so low (Cunningham *et al.* 2002; Babu *et al.* 2013) that recurrent stenosis cannot be of any great clinical concern, in the sense of causing stroke. If stenosis does recur, then a second endarterectomy is more difficult and more risky (Bond *et al.* 2003a), and angioplasty or stenting may be preferable, although there is no randomized evidence for either procedure in symptomatic or asymptomatic restenosis (Yadav *et al.* 1996). In fact, the reported rate of restenosis varies enormously depending on whether the study was prospective or retrospective, the completeness and length of follow-up, the sensitivity and specificity of the imaging method used, and the definition of restenosis (Frericks *et al.* 1998). Certainly, recurrent atherothrombotic stenosis can occur, but usually not for some years, while early restenosis (within a year or so) is more likely to be caused by neointimal hyperplasia (Hunter *et al.* 1987). On balance, therefore, there is little point in repeated clinical or ultrasonographic follow-up to detect asymptomatic restenosis, but if a restenosis becomes symptomatic, then a repeat carotid endarterectomy or stenting is reasonable.

Many surgeons routinely use a patch of autologous vein or synthetic material to close the artery, enlarge the lumen, and so reduce the risk of restenosis and, more importantly, of stroke. A meta-analysis of randomized trials of primary closure, vein patch, or synthetic patch included data on 1,967 patients undergoing 2,157 operations in 10 trials (Rerkasem and Rothwell 2009). Carotid patch angioplasty was associated with an approximately 70% reduction in the operative risks of ipsilateral stroke during the perioperative period ($p = 0.001$) and long-term follow-up ($p = 0.001$). Patching was also associated with an 80% reduction in risk of perioperative arterial occlusion ($p < 0.0001$) and a 75% reduction in risk of restenosis during long-term follow-up ($p < 0.00001$). Although it was previously thought that patching may be associated with a higher risk of arterial hemorrhage and infection, especially with use of synthetic grafts, no significant difference in risks was identified between patching and primary closure in this meta-analysis. In fact, patching was associated with a 65% lower risk of re-operation within 30 days for complications such as occlusion, hemorrhage, or infection ($p = 0.01$).

Some surgeons who use carotid patching favor using a patch made from an autologous vein, while others prefer to use synthetic materials such as Dacron and PTFE. Recent meta-analysis of randomized trials of different types of patch included data on 2,083 operations (Rerkasem and Rothwell 2010). In studies that had more than 1-year follow-up, no differences were shown between patients receiving vein versus synthetic patch for the risk of stroke, death, or arterial restenosis. However, there were significantly fewer pseudoaneurysms associated with use of synthetic patches than vein (odds ratio [OR], 0.09; 95% confidence interval [CI], 0.02–0.49), although this was only based on 15 events in 776 patients and the clinical significance of this finding is uncertain. Compared with other synthetic patches such as PTFE, Dacron was associated with a higher risk of stroke or death ($p = 0.02$) and arterial restenosis ($p < 0.0001$). However, the number of outcomes was again small in this analysis.

General versus Regional Anesthesia

Surgery has traditionally been performed under general rather than regional anesthesia, but surgery under locoregional anesthesia has gained popularity in the recent years. With regional anesthesia, there is a much lower shunt rate because it is immediately obvious when a shunt is needed to restore blood flow distal to the carotid clamps; elaborate intraoperative monitoring is unnecessary. However, some patients will not tolerate the procedure, and a quick change to general anesthesia may be required. A detailed systematic review and meta-analysis of randomized studies has provided some useful information (Vaniyapong *et al.* 2013). Fourteen randomized trials involving 4,596 operations, including a European multicenter randomized trial (General Anesthetic versus Local Anesthetic for Carotid Surgery) (GALA Trial Collaborative Group 2008) that contributed 3,526 patients, were included. There were no statistically significant

BOX 25.1 Potential Complications of Carotid Endarterectomy

Death

Perioperative stroke caused by:

- temporary interruption of carotid blood flow during clamping.
- embolism from operative site.

Postoperative stroke caused by:

- embolism from residual atheromatous plaque.
- thrombus formation on the endarterectomized surface.
- thrombus formation on the suture lines.
- thrombus formation from an arterial dissection.

Cerebral hyperperfusion injury and cerebral hemorrhage

Cardiovascular complications (arrhythmia, myocardial infarction)

Respiratory complications (pulmonary embolism, pneumonia)

Cranial and peripheral nerve injuries

Bleeding or infection at wound site

Headache

Facial pain

differences in the risk of peri-operative stroke or death rate (3.6% versus 4.2%) nor the risk of operative complications between patients who received local versus general anesthesia. A nonsignificant trend toward lower operative mortality in the local anesthetic group (0.9% versus 1.5%) was observed. However, none of the trials nor the pooled analyses were adequately powered to reliably detect an effect on mortality. Choice of anesthetic technique should therefore be based on the surgeon's and anesthetist's assessment of patient suitability.

The Risks of Carotid Endarterectomy

Carotid endarterectomy is associated with a variety of potential complications (Naylor and Ruckley 1996; Bond *et al.* 2002c) (Box 25.1). The most important of these are stroke and death.

Death

Death within a few days of surgery occurs in approximately 1–2% of patients and is generally caused by stroke, myocardial infarction, or some other complication of the frequently associated coronary heart disease or, rarely, by pulmonary embolism (Rothwell *et al.* 1996a). Higher rates can be found in "administrative datasets," which may be a more realistic reflection of routine practice than large randomized trials, but any comparisons are confounded by variation in case mix, particularly the proportion of patients with asymptomatic stenosis, who have a lower case fatality (Rothwell *et al.* 1996b; Wennberg *et al.* 1998; Bond *et al.* 2003a, b).

Stroke

The main complication of surgery is perioperative stroke (Naylor and Ruckley 1996; Ferguson *et al.* 1999; Bond *et al.* 2002c) (see Chapter 27 for further discussion). The reported risk ranges from an implausibly low 1% or less to an unacceptably high 20% or more (Bond *et al.* 2004). This variation (Campbell 1993; Rothwell *et al.* 1996b) may be explained by differences in:

- the definition of stroke.
- whether all or only some strokes are included.
- the accuracy of stroke diagnosis.
- the completeness of the clinical details.
- whether the study was retrospective or prospective.
- whether the diagnosis of stroke was based on patient observation or just medical record review.
- variation in case mix and surgical and anesthetic skills.
- chance variation.
- publication bias.

No more than 20% of perioperative strokes are likely to be fatal, and so reports of less than four times as many non-fatal as fatal strokes suggest undercounting of mild strokes, a tendency that may well be a result of surgeons reporting their own results without the "help" of any neurologists (Rothwell and Warlow 1995). Despite the obvious implications for service planning, it has been all but impossible to sort out whether there really is a systematic difference in risk between surgeons. This is largely because of problems of adjusting for case mix as well as chance effects owing to the inevitably rather small numbers operated on by each surgeon (Rothwell *et al.* 1999). Indeed, in a large retrospective cohort study of 454,717 carotid endarterectomies performed during 2001–2008, surgeons who had a past-year case-volume of less than 10 were consistently associated with a higher 30-day mortality during the study period (Kumamaru *et al.* 2015).

There are several causes for perioperative stroke, but these are often difficult to identify when it occurs during general anesthesia or even afterward. It is difficult to be sure whether any stroke is caused by embolism or low flow (Steed *et al.* 1982; Krul *et al.* 1989; Riles *et al.* 1994; Spencer 1997). Clearly, temporary reduction in ICA blood flow during carotid clamping may cause ipsilateral ischemic stroke if the collateral supply is inadequate, particularly if there is already maximal cerebral vasodilatation (i.e., cerebrovascular reserve is exhausted). However, embolism from the operation site is probably the most common cause of stroke during surgery. Atherothrombotic debris may be released while the carotid bifurcation is being mobilized, as the carotid clamps are applied, when any shunt is inserted, and when the clamps are removed. Indeed, air bubbles or particulate emboli during surgery are very commonly detected by transcranial Doppler ultrasound, although most seem to be of little clinical consequence (Gaunt *et al.* 1993; Jansen *et al.* 1994a).

Postoperative ischemic stroke is usually caused by embolism from residual but disrupted atheromatous plaque, thrombus forming on the endarterectomized surface or on suture lines or more probably on a loose distal intimal flap where the lesion has been carelessly snapped off, thrombus complicating damaged arterial wall as a result of the clamps, and thrombus complicating arterial dissection starting at a loose intimal flap of the ICA or as a result of shunt damage to the arterial wall. A high rate of postoperative microembolic signals on transcranial Doppler monitoring may predict ischemic stroke (Levi *et al.* 1997).

Cerebral Hemorrhage and Hyperperfusion Syndrome

Intracranial hemorrhage accounts for approximately 5% of perioperative strokes (Bond *et al.* 2002c; Wilson and Ammar 2005). It can occur during surgery or up to about 1 week later, almost always ipsilateral to the operated artery. It may be a result of the increase in perfusion pressure and cerebral blood flow that occurs after removal of a severe ICA stenosis, particularly if cerebral autoregulation is defective as a consequence of a recent cerebral infarct (Ouriel *et al.* 1999). Antithrombotic drugs and uncontrolled hypertension may also play a part (Solomon *et al.* 1986; Hafner *et al.* 1987; Piepgras *et al.* 1988; Jansen *et al.* 1994b; Wilson and Ammar 2005).

Transient cerebral hyperperfusion, ipsilateral but sometimes bilateral, lasting some days is quite common after carotid endarterectomy (Adhiyaman and Alexander 2007), particularly if the lesion is severely stenosing and cerebrovascular reserve is already poor with impaired autoregulation. This may be the cause of the occasional case of ipsilateral transhemispheric cerebral edema, intracerebral hemorrhage, focal epileptic seizures, and headache, which can all occur a few days after surgery. Clearly, this syndrome is different from ischemic stroke caused by low flow or embolism, and it is distinguished by the slower onset as well as by brain and arterial imaging (Andrews *et al.* 1987; Schroeder *et al.* 1987; Naylor *et al.* 1993a; Chambers *et al.* 1994; Breen *et al.* 1996; van Mook *et al.* 2005; Adhiyaman and Alexander 2007). To complicate matters, a very similar clinical syndrome has been described as a result of cerebral vasoconstriction (Lopez-Valdes *et al.* 1997).

Cardiovascular and Respiratory Complications

Myocardial infarction during or in the early days after surgery occurs in 1–2% of patients (Bond *et al.* 2002c), more often if there is symptomatic coronary heart disease and particularly if myocardial infarction has occurred in the previous few months or if the patient has unstable angina. Perioperative myocardial infarction can be painless, so clues to the diagnosis are unexplained hypotension, tachycardia, and dysrhythmias. Congestive cardiac failure, angina, and cardiac dysrhythmias are also occasional concerns (Riles *et al.* 1979; North American Symptomatic Carotid Endarterectomy Trial Collaborators 1991; Urbinati *et al.* 1994; Paciaroni *et al.* 1999; Bond *et al.* 2002c). Postoperative hypertension and hypotension may be a problem, perhaps owing to operative interference with the carotid baroreceptors, but they are transient. Postoperative chest infection occurs in less than 1%.

Cranial and Peripheral Nerve Injuries

Nerve injuries result from traction, pressure, or transection and occur in up to 20% of patients, depending on how hard one looks. However, these injuries seldom have any long-term consequence (Cunningham *et al.* 2004). Damage to the recurrent and superior laryngeal branches of the vagus nerve, or more probably the vagus itself, causes change of voice quality, hoarseness, difficulty coughing, and sometimes dyspnea on exertion owing to vocal cord paralysis. If a simultaneous or staged bilateral carotid endarterectomy is done and causes bilateral vocal cord paralysis, then airway obstruction can occur. Hypoglossal nerve injury causes ipsilateral weakness of the tongue, which can lead to temporary or even permanent dysarthria, difficulty with mastication, or dysphagia. Again, bilateral damage causes much more serious speech and swallowing problems and sometimes even upper airway obstruction. Therefore, if a patient has symptoms referable to both severely stenosed carotid arteries requiring bilateral carotid endarterectomy, it is probably safer to do the operations a few weeks apart rather than under the same anesthetic, mostly because of the dangers of bilateral hypoglossal or vagal nerve damage.

Damage to the marginal mandibular branch of the facial nerve causes rather trivial weakness at the corner of the mouth. Spinal accessory nerve injury is rare and causes pain and stiffness in the shoulder and neck along with weakness of the sternomastoid and trapezius muscles. A high incision can cut the greater auricular nerve to cause numbness over the earlobe and angle of the jaw, which may persist and be irritating for the patient. Damage to the transverse cervical nerves is almost inevitable and causes numbness around the scar area, which is seldom a problem. Clearly, however, permanent disability from a nerve injury can be as bad as a mild stroke and needs to be taken into account when considering the risks and benefits of surgery (Gutrecht and Jones 1988; Maniglia and Han 1991; Sweeney and Wilbourn 1992; Cunningham *et al.* 2004).

Local Wound Complications

Local complications are rare and include infection; hematoma or, rarely, major hemorrhage from leakage or rupture of the arteriotomy or patch, which can be life-threatening if it causes tracheal compression; aneurysm formation weeks or years later; and malignant tumor in the scar (Graver and Mulcare 1986; Martin-Negrier *et al.* 1996; Bond *et al.* 2002c). Although surgeons often notice the hemostatic defect caused by preoperative aspirin, this probably does not increase the rate of reoperation for bleeding (Lindblad *et al.* 1993). Very rarely, the thoracic duct can be damaged and cause a chyle fistula.

Headache and Facial Pain

Headache ipsilateral to the operation may herald cerebral hyperperfusion (van Mook *et al.* 2005; Adhiyaman and Alexander 2007), but it may also be due to something akin to cluster headache and caused by subtle damage to the sympathetic plexus around the carotid artery (De Marinis *et al.* 1991; Ille *et al.* 1995). Very rarely, focal epileptic seizures occur as well as headache (Youkey *et al.* 1984; Naylor *et al.* 2003). Facial pain ipsilateral to surgery and related to eating is unusual and may in some way be caused by disturbed innervation of the parotid gland (Truax 1989).

Potential Benefits of Carotid Endarterectomy

As a result of the large randomized controlled trials, it is now clear that endarterectomy of recently symptomatic severe carotid stenosis almost completely abolishes the high risk of ischemic stroke ipsilateral to the operated artery over the subsequent 2 or 3 years (see Chapter 27 for detailed discussion of the selection of patients for surgery). Moreover, this effect is durable over at least 10 years (European Carotid Surgery Trialists' Collaborative Group 1991, 1998; Mayberg *et al.* 1991; North American Symptomatic Carotid Endarterectomy Trial Collaborators 1991; Barnett *et al.* 1998; Rothwell *et al.* 2003). Indeed, the ipsilateral stroke risk becomes so low that presumably both embolic and low-flow strokes are being prevented (Fig. 25.1).

On average, there is an advantage to surgery when the symptomatic stenosis exceeds 80% diameter reduction of the arterial lumen using the European Carotid Surgery Trial (ECST) method, which is about the same as 70% using the North American Symptomatic

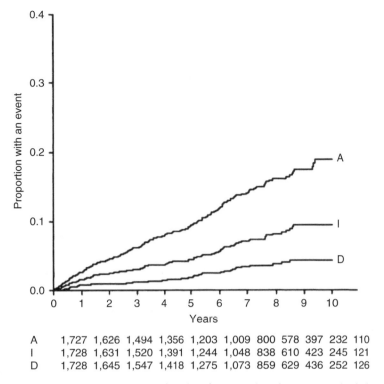

A	1,727	1,626	1,494	1,356	1,203	1,009	800	578	397	232	110
I	1,728	1,631	1,520	1,391	1,244	1,048	838	610	423	245	121
D	1,728	1,645	1,547	1,418	1,275	1,073	859	629	436	252	126

Fig. 25.1 Kaplan–Meier curves showing risks of stroke after carotid endarterectomy (excluding the 30-day immediate postoperative period). A, any stroke; I, any ipsilateral ischemic stroke; D, disabling ipsilateral ischemic stroke.

Carotid Endarterectomy Trial (NASCET) method (see Chapter 27). The risk of surgery is much the same at all degrees of stenosis, and so because the unoperated risk of stroke in patients with less than 60% stenosis (in ECST) is so low, the risk of surgery is not worthwhile for them. Because the risk of stroke in patients with moderate stenosis remains low for several years, there is no point in duplex follow-up to see if the stenosis becomes more severe. No doubt severe stenosis does sometimes develop, but unless there are further symptoms, the stenosis by this time is essentially asymptomatic and carries such a low risk of stroke that there is no overall advantage for surgery. It is preferable to ask the patient to return if there are any further cerebrovascular symptoms and *then*, if the stenosis is 80% (ECST) or more, it is reasonable to recommend carotid endarterectomy.

Carotid endarterectomy may also improve cognitive performance, perhaps by increasing cerebral blood flow or by reducing the frequency of subclinical emboli, which declines after surgery (Markus *et al.* 1995; van Zuilen *et al.* 1995; Watanabe *et al.* 2014). However, subtle cognitive difficulties may complicate the procedure itself (Lloyd *et al.* 2004; Bossema *et al.* 2005; Lal 2007), and there is some evidence that previous carotid endarterectomy is associated with more rapid cognitive decline in the longer term (Bo *et al.* 2006). Unfortunately, studies addressing this issue have been beset with methodological difficulties (Lunn *et al.* 1999), and it is difficult to imagine that this balance of cognitive benefit and risk will ever be resolved because further randomized trials will probably never be done, at least not in patients with symptomatic stenosis.

It is conceivable that patients with impaired cerebral reactivity and raised oxygen extraction fraction are at particular risk of stroke without surgery and that this impairment can be corrected by carotid endarterectomy, but the studies have been too small to be sure (Schroeder 1988; Naylor *et al.* 1993b; Yonas *et al.* 1993; Hartl *et al.* 1994; Yamauchi *et al.* 1996; Visser *et al.* 1997; Silvestrini *et al.* 2000; Markus and Cullinane 2001). Also, we do not know what proportion of strokes in patients with recently symptomatic severe carotid stenosis are actually caused by impaired cerebral reactivity, either as a direct result of low flow or perhaps indirectly as a result of an inadequate collateral circulation to compensate for acute arterial occlusion if it should occur. Nor do we know whether the risk of surgery is higher in these patients and so whether, on balance, carotid endarterectomy will indeed reduce stroke risk any more than in those without impaired reactivity.

References

Adhiyaman V, Alexander S (2007). Cerebral hyperperfusion syndrome following carotid endarterectomy. *Quarterly Journal of Medicine* **100**:239–244

Andrews BT, Levy ML, Dillon W *et al.* (1987). Unilateral normal perfusion pressure breakthrough after carotid endarterectomy: Case report. *Neurosurgery* **21**:568–571

Babu MA, Meissner I, Meyer FB (2013). The durability of carotid endarterectomy: Long-term results for restenosis and stroke. *Neurosurgery* **72**:835–838

Barnett HJM, Plum F, Walton JN (1984). Carotid endarterectomy: An expression of concern. *Stroke* **15**:941–943

Barnett HJM, Taylor DW, Eliasziw M for the North American Symptomatic Carotid Endarterectomy Trial Collaborators (1998). Benefit of carotid endarterectomy in patients with symptomatic moderate or severe stenosis. *New England Journal of Medicine* **339**:1415–1425

Belardi P, Lucertini G, Ermirio D (2003). Stump pressure and transcranial Doppler for predicting shunting in carotid endarterectomy. *European Journal of Vascular Endovascular Surgery* **25**:164–167

Bo M, Massaia M, Speme S *et al.* (2006). Risk of cognitive decline in older patients after carotid endarterectomy: An observational study. *Journal of the American Geriatric Society* **54**:932–936

Bond R, Warlow CP, Naylor R *et al.* (2002a). Variation in surgical and anaesthetic technique and associations with operative risk in the European Carotid Surgery Trial: Implications for trials of ancillary techniques. *European Journal of Vascular Endovascular Surgery* **23**:117–126

Bond R, Rerkasem K, Rothwell PM (2002b). Routine or selective carotid artery shunting for carotid endarterectomy. *Cochrane Database of Systematic Reviews* **2**:CD000190

Bond R, Narayan S, Rothwell PM *et al.* (2002c). Clinical and radiological risk factors for operative stroke and death in the European Carotid Surgery Trial. *European Journal of Vascular Endovascular Surgery* **23**:108–116

Bond R, Rerkasem K, Rothwell PM (2003a). A systematic review of the risks of carotid endarterectomy in relation to the clinical indication and the timing of surgery. *Stroke* **34**:2290–2301

Bond R, Rerkasem K, Rothwell PM (2003b). High morbidity due to endarterectomy for asymptomatic carotid stenosis. *Cerebrovascular Diseases* **16**(Suppl 4):65

Bond R, Rerkasem K, Shearman CP *et al.* (2004). Time trends in the published risks of stroke and death due to endarterectomy for symptomatic carotid stenosis. *Cerebrovascular Diseases* **18**:37–46

Bossema ER, Brand N, Moll FL *et al.* (2005). Perioperative microembolism is not associated with cognitive outcome three months after carotid endarterectomy. *European Journal of Vascular Endovascular Surgery* **29**:262–268

Breen JC, Caplan LR, Dewitt LD *et al.* (1996). Brain oedema after carotid surgery. *Neurology* **46**:175–181

Brothers TE (2005). Initial experience with eversion carotid endarterectomy: Absence of a learning curve for the first 100 patients. *Journal of Vascular Surgery* 42:429–434

Campbell WB (1993). Can reported carotid surgical results be misleading?. In *Surgery for Stroke*. Greenhalgh GM and Hollier LH (eds.), pp. 331–337. London: Saunders

Cao P, Giordano G, De Rango P for the Collaborators of the EVEREST Study Group (1998). A randomised study on eversion versus standard carotid endarterectomy: Study design and preliminary results: The Everest Trial. *Journal of Vascular Surgery* 27:595–605

Cao PG, De Rango P, Zannetti S et al. (2001). Eversion versus conventional carotid endarterectomy for preventing stroke. *Cochrane Database of Systematic Reviews*, 2:CD001921

Cao P, De Rango P, Zannetti S (2002). Eversion versus conventional carotid endarterectomy: A systematic review. *European Journal of Vascular and Endovascular Surgery* 23:195–201

Carrea R, Molins M, Murphy G (1955). Surgical treatment of spontaneous thrombosis of the internal carotid artery in the neck. Carotid–carotideal anastomosis. Report of a case. *Acta Neurologica Latin America* 1:71–78

Chambers BR, Norris J (1984). The case against surgery for asymptomatic carotid stenosis. *Stroke* 15:964–967

Chambers BR, Smidt V, Koh P (1994). Hyperfusion post-endarterectomy. *Cerebrovascular Diseases* 4:32–37

Chiari H (1905). Uber des verhalten des teilungswinkels der carotis communis bei der endarteritis chronica deformans. *Verhandlungen der Deutschen Gesellschaft für Pathologie* 9:326–330

Chongruksut W, Vaniyapong T, Rerkasem K (2014). Routine or selective carotid artery shunting for carotid endarterectomy (and different methods of monitoring in selective shunting). *Cochrane Database of Systematic Reviews* 23:CD000190

Cooper A (1836). Account of the first successful operation performed on the common carotid artery for aneurysm in the year 1808 with the post-mortem examination in the year 1821. *Guy's Hospital Report* 1:53–59

Cunningham E, Bond R, Mehta Z et al. (2002). Long-term durability of carotid endarterectomy in the European Carotid Surgery Trial. *Stroke* 33:2658–2663

Cunningham EJ, Bond R, Mayberg MR et al. (2004). Risk of persistent cranial nerve injury after carotid endarterectomy. *Journal of Neurosurgery* 101:455–458

Darling RC, Paty PSK, Shah DM et al. (1996). Eversion endarterectomy of the internal carotid artery: Technique and results in 449 procedures. *Surgery* 120:635–639

DeBakey ME (1975). Successful carotid endarterectomy for cerebrovascular insufficiency. Nineteen-year follow-up. *Journal of the American Medical Association* 233:1083–1085

Demirel S, Attigah N, Bruijnen H et al. (2012). Multicenter experience on eversion versus conventional carotid endarterectomy in symptomatic carotid artery stenosis. *Stroke* 43:1865–1871

De Marinis M, Zaccaria A, Faraglia V et al. (1991). Post-endarterectomy headache and the role of the oculosympathetic system. *Journal of Neurology, Neurosurgery and Psychiatry* 54:314–317

Dos Santos JC (1976). From embolectomy to endarterectomy or the fall of a myth. *Journal of Cardiovascular Surgery* 17:113–128

Eastcott HHG, Pickering GW, Rob CG (1954). Reconstruction of internal carotid artery in a patient with intermittent attacks of hemiplegia. *Lancet* ii, 994–996

Eliasziw M, Spence JD, Barnett HM for the North American Symptomatic Carotid Endarterectomy Trial (1998). Carotid endarterectomy does not affect long term blood pressure: Observations from the NASCET. *Cerebrovascular Diseases* 8:20–24

European Carotid Surgery Trialists' Collaborative Group (1991). MRC European Carotid Surgery Trial: Interim results for symptomatic patients with severe (70–99%) or with mild (0–29%) carotid stenosis. *Lancet* 337:1235–1243

European Carotid Surgery Trialists' Collaborative Group (1998). Randomised trial of endarterectomy for recently symptomatic carotid stenosis: Final results of the MRC European Carotid Surgery Trial (ECST). *Lancet* 351:1379–1387

Ferguson GG (1986). Carotid endarterectomy. To shunt or not to shunt? *Archives of Neurology* 43:615–618

Ferguson GG, Eliasziw M, Barr HWK for the North American Symptomatic Carotid Endarterectomy Trial (NASCET) Collaborators (1999). The North American Symptomatic Carotid Endarterectomy Trial: surgical results in 1415 patients. *Stroke* 30:1751–1758

Fields WS, Maslenikov V, Meyer JS *et al.* (1970). Joint study of extracranial arterial occlusion. V. Progress report of prognosis following surgery or nonsurgical treatment for transient cerebral ischaemic attacks and cervical carotid artery lesions. *Journal of the American Medical Association* 211:1993–2003

Fisher M (1951). Occlusion of the internal carotid artery. *Archives of Neurology and Psychiatry* 65:346–377

Fisher M (1954). Occlusion of the carotid arteries. *Archives of Neurology and Psychiatry* 72:187–204

Frericks H, Kievit J, van Baalen JM *et al.* (1998). Carotid recurrent stenosis and risk of ipsilateral stroke: A systematic review of the literature. *Stroke* 29:244–250

GALA Trial Collaborative Group (2008). General anesthesia versus local anesthesia for carotid surgery (GALA): A multicenter, randomized controlled trial. *Lancet* 9656:2132–2142

Gaunt ME, Naylor AR, Sayers RD *et al.* (1993). Sources of air embolisation during carotid surgery: The role of transcranial Doppler ultrasonography. *British Journal of Surgery* 80:1121

Gillum RF (1995). Epidemiology of carotid endarterectomy and cerebral arteriography in the United States. *Stroke* 26:1724–1728

Graver LM, Mulcare RJ (1986). Pseudoaneurysm after carotid endarterectomy. *Journal of Cardiovascular Surgery* 27:294–297

Gurdjian ES (1979). History of occlusive cerebrovascular disease, I: From Wepfer to Moniz. *Archives of Neurology* 36:340–343

Gutrecht JA, Jones HR (1988). Bilateral hypoglossal nerve injury after bilateral carotid endarterectomy. *Stroke* 19:261–262

Hafner DH, Smith RB, King OW *et al.* (1987). Massive intracerebral haemorrhage following carotid endarterectomy. *Archives of Surgery* 122:305–307

Hamby WB (1952). *Intracranial Aneurysms.* Springfield, IL: Charles C Thomas

Hartl WH, Janssen I, Furst H (1994). Effect of carotid endarterectomy on patterns of cerebrovascular reactivity in patients with unilateral carotid artery stenosis. *Stroke* 25:1952–1957

Hunter GC, Palmaz JC, Hayashi HH *et al.* (1987). The aetiology of symptoms in patients with recurrent carotid stenosis. *Archives of Surgery* 122:311–315

Ille O, Woimant F, Pruna A *et al.* (1995). Hypertensive encephalopathy after bilateral carotid endarterectomy. *Stroke* 26:488–491

Jansen C, Ramos LMP, van Heesewijk JPM *et al.* (1994a). Impact of microembolism and hemodynamic changes in the brain during carotid endarterectomy. *Stroke* 25:992–997

Jansen C, Sprengers AM, Moll FL *et al.* (1994b). Prediction of intracerebral haemorrhage after carotid endarterectomy by clinical criteria and intraoperative transcranial Doppler monitoring. *European Journal of Vascular Surgery* 8:303–308

Jonas S (1987). Can carotid endarterectomy be justified? No. *Archives of Neurology* 44:652–654

Keevil JJ (1949). David Fleming and the operation for ligation of the carotid artery. *British Journal of Surgery* 37:92–95

Krul JMJ, van Gijn J, Ackerstaff RGA *et al.* (1989). Site and pathogenesis of infarcts associated with carotid endarterectomy. *Stroke* 20:324–328

Kumamaru H, Jalbert JJ, Nguyen LL *et al.* (2015). Surgeon case volume and 30-day mortality after carotid endarterectomy among contemporary Medicare beneficiaries: Before and after national coverage determination for carotid artery stenting. *Stroke* 46:1288–1294

Lal BK (2007). Cognitive function after carotid artery revascularization. *Vascular and Endovascular Surgery* 41:5–13

Levi CR, O'Malley HM, Fell G et al. (1997). Transcranial Doppler detected cerebral microembolism following carotid endarterectomy. High microembolic signal loads predict postoperative cerebral ischaemia. *Brain* **120**:621–629

Lindblad B, Persson NH, Takolander R et al. (1993). Does low-dose acetylsalicylic acid prevent stroke after carotid surgery? A double-blind, placebo-controlled randomised trial. *Stroke* **24**:1125–1128

Lloyd AJ, Hayes PD, London NJ et al. (2004). Does carotid endarterectomy lead to a decline in cognitive function or health related quality of life? *Journal of Clinical and Experimental Neuropsychology* **26**:817–825

Loftus CM, Quest DO (1987). Technical controversies in carotid artery surgery. *Neurosurgery* **20**:490–495

Lopez-Valdes E, Chang HM, Pessin MS et al. (1997). Cerebral vasoconstriction after carotid surgery. *Neurology* **49**:303–304

Lunn S, Crawley F, Harrison MJG et al. (1999). Impact of carotid endarterectomy upon cognitive functioning. A systematic review of the literature. *Cerebrovascular Diseases* **9**:74–81

Maniglia AJ, Han DP (1991). Cranial nerve injuries following carotid endarterectomy: An analysis of 336 procedures. *Head and Neck* **13**:121–124

Markus H, Cullinane M (2001). Severely impaired cerebrovascular reactivity predicts stroke and TIA risk in patients with carotid artery stenosis and occlusion. *Brain* **124**:457–467

Markus HS, Thomson ND, Brown MM (1995). Asymptomatic cerebral embolic signals in symptomatic and asymptomatic carotid artery disease. *Brain* **118**:1005–1011

Martin-Negrier ML, Belleannee G, Vital C et al. (1996) Primitive malignant fibrous histiocytoma of the neck with carotid occlusion and multiple cerebral ischemic lesions. *Stroke* **27**:536–537

Mayberg MR, Wilson E, Yatsu F for the Veterans Affairs Cooperative Studies Programe 309 Trialist Group (1991). Carotid endarterectomy and prevention of cerebral ischaemia in symptomatic carotid stenosis. *Journal of the American Medical Association* **266**:3289–3294

Moniz E (1927). L'encephalographic arterielle: son importance dans la localisation des tumeurs cerebrales. *Revue de Neurologie* **2**:72–90

Moniz E, Lima A, de Lacerda R (1937). Hemiplegies par thrombose de la carotide interne. *Presse Medicine* **45**:977–980

Naylor AR, Ruckley CV (1996). Complications after carotid surgery. In *Complications in Arterial Surgery. A Practical Approach to Management*, Campbell (ed.), pp. 73–88. Oxford: Butterworth-Heinemann

Naylor AR, Bell PRF, Ruckley CV (1992). Monitoring and cerebral protection during carotid endarterectomy. *British Journal of Surgery* **79**:735–741

Naylor AR, Merrick MV, Sandercock PAG et al. (1993a). Serial imaging of the carotid bifurcation and cerebrovascular reserve after carotid endarterectomy. *British Journal of Surgery* **80**:1278–1282

Naylor AR, Whyman MR, Wildsmith JAW et al. (1993b). Factors influencing the hyperaemic response after carotid endarterectomy. *British Journal of Surgery* **80**:1523–1527

Naylor AR, Evans J, Thompson MM et al. (2003). Seizures after carotid endarterectomy: Hyperperfusion, dysautoregulation or hypertensive encephalopathy? *European Journal of Vascular Endovascular Surgery* **26**:39–44

North American Symptomatic Carotid Endarterectomy Trial Collaborators (1991). Beneficial effect of carotid endarterectomy in symptomatic patients with high-grade carotid stenosis. *New England Journal of Medicine* **325**:445–453

Ojemann RG, Heros RC (1986). Carotid endarterectomy. *To shunt or not to shunt? Archives of Neurology* **43**:617–618

Ouriel K, Shortell CK, Illig KA et al. (1999). Intracerebral haemorrhage after carotid endarterectomy: Incidence, contribution to neurologic morbidity, and predictive factors. *Journal of Vascular Surgery* **29**:82–89

Paciaroni M, Eliasziw M, Kappelle LJ for the North American Symptomatic Carotid Endarterectomy Trial (NASCET) Collaborators (1999). Medical complications associated with carotid endarterectomy. *Stroke* 30:1759–1763

Penzoldt F (1891). Uber thrombose (autochtone oder embolische) der carotis. *Deutschen Archir Für Klinische Medizin* 28:80–93

Piepgras DG, Morgan MK, Sundt TM *et al.* (1988). Intracerebral haemorrhage after carotid endarterectomy. *Journal of Neurosurgery* 68:532–536

Pokras R, Dyken ML (1988). Dramatic changes in the performance of endarterectomy for diseases of the extracranial arteries of the head. *Stroke* 19:1289–1290

Rerkasem K and Rothwell PM (2009). Patch angioplasty versus primary closure for carotid endarterectomy. *Cochrane Database of Systematic Reviews* 4:CD000160

Rerkasem K and Rothwell PM (2010). Patches of different types for carotid patch angioplasty. *Cochrane Database of Systematic Reviews* 3: CD000071

Riles TS, Kopelman I, Imparato AM (1979). Myocardial infarction following carotid endarterectomy. A review of 683 operations. *Surgery* 85:249–252

Riles TS, Imparato AM, Jacobowitz GR *et al.* (1994). The cause of perioperative stroke after carotid endarterectomy. *Journal of Vascular Surgery* 19:206–216

Rothwell PM, Warlow CP (1995). Is self-audit reliable? *Lancet* 346:1623

Rothwell PM, Slattery J, Warlow CP (1996a). A systematic comparison of the risk of stroke and death due to carotid endarterectomy for symptomatic and asymptomatic stenosis. *Stroke* 27:266–269

Rothwell PM, Slattery J, Warlow CP (1996b). A systematic review of the risk of stroke and death due to carotid endarterectomy. *Stroke* 27:260–265

Rothwell PM, Warlow CP on behalf of the European Carotid Surgery Trialists' Collaborative Group (1999). Interpretation of operative risks of individual surgeons. *Lancet* 353:1325

Rothwell PM, Gutnikov SA, Warlow CP for the ECST (2003). Re-analysis of the final results of the European Carotid Surgery Trial. *Stroke* 34:514–523

Schroeder T (1988). Hemodynamic significance of internal carotid artery disease. *Acta Neurologica Scandinavica* 77:353–372

Schroeder T, Sillesen H, Sorensen O *et al.* (1987). Cerebral hyperfusion following carotid endarterectomy. *Journal of Neurosurgery* 66:824–829

Shaw DA, Venables GS, Cartlidge NEF *et al.* (1984). Carotid endarterectomy in patients with transient cerebral ischaemia. *Journal of Neurological Sciences* 64:45–53

Silvestrini M, Vernieri F, Pasqualetti P *et al.* (2000). Impaired cerebral vasoreactivity and risk of stroke in patients with asymptomatic carotid artery stenosis. *Journal of American Medical Association* 283:2122–2127

Solomon RA, Loftus CM, Quest DO *et al.* (1986). Incidence and etiology of intracerebral haemorrhage following carotid endarterectomy. *Journal of Neurosurgery* 64:29–34

Spencer MP (1997). Transcranial Doppler monitoring and causes of stroke from carotid endarterectomy. *Stroke* 28:685–691

Steed DL, Peitzman AB, Grundy BL *et al.* (1982). Causes of stroke in carotid endarterectomy. *Surgery* 92:634–639

Sweeney PJ Wilbourn AJ (1992). Spinal accessory (11th) nerve palsy following carotid endarterectomy. *Neurology* 42:674–675

Thompson JE (1996). The evolution of surgery for the treatment and prevention of stroke. The Willis Lecture. *Stroke* 27:1427–1434

Truax BT (1989). Gustatory pain: A complication of carotid endarterectomy. *Neurology* 39:1258–1260

Tu JV, Hannan EL, Anderson GM *et al.* (1998). The fall and rise of carotid endarterectomy in the United States and Canada. *New England Journal of Medicine* 339:1441–1447

Urbinati S, di Pasquale G, Andreoli A *et al.* (1994). Preoperative noninvasive coronary risk stratification in candidates for carotid endarterectomy. *Stroke* 25:2022–2027

van Mook WN, Rennenberg RJ, Schurink GW *et al.* (2005). Cerebral hyperperfusion syndrome. *Lancet Neurology* 4:877–888 van Zuilen EV, Moll FL, Vermeulen FEE *et al.* (1995). Detection of cerebral microemboli by means of transcranial Doppler monitoring before and after carotid endarterectomy. *Stroke* **26**:210–213

Vaniyapong T, Chongruksut W, Rerkasem K (2013). Local versus general anesthesia for carotid endarterectomy. *Cochrane Database of Systematic Reviews* 12:CD000126

Visser GH, van Huffelen AC, Wieneke GH *et al.* (1997). Bilateral increase in CO reactivity after unilateral carotid endarterectomy. *Stroke* **28**:899–905

Warlow CP (1984). Carotid endarterectomy: Does it work? *Stroke* **15**:1068–1076

Watanabe J, Ogata T, Hamada O *et al.* (2014). Improvement of cognitive function after carotid endarterectomy: A new strategy for the evaluation of cognitive function. *Journal of Stroke and Cerebrovascular Diseases* **23**:1332–1336

Wennberg DE, Lucas FL, Birkmeyer JD *et al.* (1998). Variation in carotid endarterectomy mortality in the Medicare population: Trial hospitals, volume, and patient characteristics. *Journal of the American Medical Association* **279**:1278–1281

Wilson PV, Ammar AD (2005). The incidence of ischemic stroke versus intracerebral hemorrhage after carotid endarterectomy: A review of 2452 cases. *Annals of Vascular Surgery* **19**:1–4

Winslow CM, Solomon DH, Chassin MR (1988). The appropriateness of carotid endarterectomy. *New England Journal of Medicine* **318**:721–727

Wood JR (1857). Early history of the operation of ligature of the primitive carotid artery. *New York Journal of Medicine* **July**:1–59

Wyeth JA (1878). Prize essay: Essays upon the surgical anatomy and history of the common, external and internal carotid arteries and the surgical anatomy of the innominate and subclavian arteries. *Appendix to Transactions of the American Medical Association (AMA) Philadelphia* **29**:1–245

Yadav JS, Roubin GS, King P *et al.* (1996). Angioplasty and stenting for restenosis after carotid endarterectomy. Initial experience. *Stroke* **27**:2075–2079

Yamauchi H, Fukuyama H, Nagahama Y *et al.* (1996). Evidence of misery perfusion and risk of recurrent stroke in major cerebral arterial occlusive diseases from PET. *Journal of Neurology, Neurosurgery and Psychiatry* **61**:18–25

Yonas H, Smith HA, Durham SR *et al.* (1993). Increased stroke risk predicted by compromised cerebral blood flow reactivity. *Journal of Neurosurgery* **79**:483–489

Youkey JR, Clagett GP, Jaffin JH *et al.* (1984). Focal motor seizures complicating carotid endarterectomy. *Archives of Surgery* **119**:1080–1084

Chapter 26

Carotid Stenting and Other Interventions

Endovascular treatment was first used in the limbs in the 1960s and subsequently in the renal and coronary arteries (Dotter *et al.* 1967), but it was introduced more cautiously for treatment of stenosis of the cerebral, carotid, and vertebral arteries because of the perception of a likely high procedural risk of stroke.

Carotid Stenting

If endarterectomy of a recently symptomatic severe carotid stenosis largely abolishes the risk of ipsilateral ischemic stroke (see Chapters 25 and 27), then percutaneous transluminal balloon angioplasty, particularly with stenting to maintain arterial patency, might be expected to be similarly effective (Mathur *et al.* 1998) (Fig. 26.1 and Table 26.1). The endovascular approach is now widely used in patients with challenging technical or anatomic factors that make endarterectomy difficult (e.g., high bifurcation, post-radiation stenosis, history of neck operation, contralateral carotid occlusion, concomitant intracranial disease, contralateral vocal cord palsy, or presence of a tracheostomy). However, carotid stenting may not always be feasible because of contrast allergy, difficult vascular anatomy, or lumen thrombus.

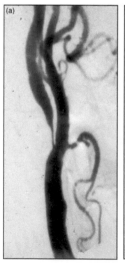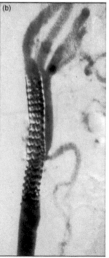

Fig. 26.1 Carotid stenosis before (a) and after (b) carotid angioplasty and stenting.

Table 26.1 Potential advantages and disadvantages of carotid stenting compared with carotid endarterectomy

Advantages	Disadvantages
Faster, less-invasive procedure	Increased risk of embolization of debris from atherothrombotic plaque
Procedure carried out under local anesthetic with consequent better neurological monitoring and reduced anesthetic complications	Risk of arterial wall dissection
Reduced procedural blood pressure variability	Carotid sinus stimulation
Reduced local wound complications	Local groin injury at arterial cannulation site
Reduced local nerve damage	(Inferior long-term evidence base)
Reduced length of stay in hospital	

Angioplasty and stenting are usually less unpleasant and less invasive than carotid endarterectomy, and it is generally more convenient and quicker. As it is carried out under local anesthesia there may be less perioperative hypertension, although cerebral hemorrhage and hyperperfusion have been reported (McCabe *et al.* 1999; Qureshi *et al.* 1999). It is less likely to cause nerve injuries, wound infection, venous thromboembolism, or myocardial infarction, and the hospital stay may be shorter. However, there are also some potential disadvantages of stenting. The angioplasty balloon may dislodge atherothrombotic debris, which then embolizes to the brain or eye, although use of protection devices might help to reduce the risk of stroke from periprocedural embolization (Reimers *et al.* 2001). The procedure may cause arterial wall dissection at the time or afterward, and late embolization might occur from thrombus formation on the damaged plaque. The angioplasty balloon may obstruct carotid blood flow for long enough to cause low-flow ischemic stroke, and dilatation of the balloon may cause bradycardia or hypotension through carotid sinus stimulation or aneurysm formation and even arterial rupture if the arterial wall is over-distended. Hematoma and aneurysm formation may also occur at the site of arterial cannulation in the groin. Rarely, the stent may erode through the arterial wall or fracture.

Data on the complication rates of carotid angioplasty/stenting are available from published case series and registries, but as was demonstrated for endarterectomy (see Chapters 25 and 27), such studies tend to underestimate risks. Formal randomized comparisons of endarterectomy and angioplasty/stenting are, therefore, required for reliable determination of the overall balance of risks and benefits. Prior to 2006, only five relatively small randomized controlled trials (1,269 patients) had been reported (Naylor *et al.* 1998; Alberts 2001; Brooks *et al.* 2001; CAVATAS Investigators 2001; Yadav *et al.* 2004). The largest of these trials suggested that the procedural stroke complication rate of angioplasty and stenting was similar to that of carotid endarterectomy (both 6%) (albeit with wide confidence intervals [CI]) and that there are few strokes in the long term (with even wider CI values) (CAVATAS Investigators 2001). Taken together, the five trials suggested that angioplasty/stenting might have a higher procedural risk of stroke and death than endarterectomy (odds ratio 1.33; 95% CI, 0.86–2.04) and a higher rate of restenosis (Coward *et al.* 2005).

However, improvements in endovascular techniques and embolic protection devices might have reduced the procedural risks (Reimers *et al.* 2001), and so several larger trials were initiated, including Stenting and Angioplasty with Protection in Patients with High Risk for Endarterectomy (SAPPHIRE), Endarterectomy Versus Angioplasty in Patients with Symptomatic Severe Carotid Stenosis (EVA-3S), Stent-Supported Percutaneous Angioplasty of the Carotid Artery versus Endarterectomy (SPACE), International Carotid Stenting Study (ICSS), and Carotid Revascularization Endarterectomy versus Stenting Trial (CREST) (Yadav *et.* 2004; Mas *et al.* 2006; SPACE Collaborative Group 2006; Brott *et al.* 2010; International Carotid Stenting Study Investigators 2010).

Subsequently, a meta-analysis of 16 trials (7,572 patients) showed that, compared with endarterectomy, carotid artery stenting was associated with a 70–80% greater risk of periprocedural death or stroke at 30 days after randomization ($p = 0.0003$) (Bonati *et al.* 2012). An interaction with age was present, such that the increased risk with stenting was mainly observed in patients of age $\geq$ 70 years but not in those age < 70. In contrast, carotid artery stenting was associated with a 55% lower risk of myocardial infarction ($p = 0.02$), 90% lower risk of cranial nerve palsy ($p < 0.00001$), and 65% lower risk of access site hematomas ($p = 0.008$) during the perioperative period (Bonati *et al.* 2012). After the perioperative period, there were no differences in long-term functional outcome and risk of stroke, myocardial infarction, or death between patients who underwent carotid artery stenting or endarterectomy (Bonati *et al.* 2012). These findings were similar in the long-term follow-up findings of CREST and ICSS (Bonati *et al.* 2015; Brott *et al.* 2016). At 10 years after intervention, risk of restenosis in patients who received carotid artery stenting and endarterectomy was also not significantly different (12.2% versus 9.7%) (Brott *et al.* 2016).

Carotid artery stenting can therefore be considered as an alternative to endarterectomy in patients with symptomatic carotid stenosis, particularly those < 70 years of age or those with technical or anatomic factors (noted earlier) that would render endarterectomy difficult. In view of the low long-term risk of restenosis, routine follow-up imaging of the extra-cranial carotid circulation with carotid Doppler ultrasound is not recommended unless patients present with a recurrent TIA/ischemic stroke and restenosis is suspected.

Surgery, Angioplasty, and Stenting for Vertebrobasilar Ischemia

There is no evidence that surgery or stenting improves the prognosis of patients with vertebrobasilar ischemia. There is, however, no shortage of ingenious, if technically demanding, techniques, which are far from risk-free (Box 26.1).

There are no randomized trials of open surgical procedures for posterior circulation disease, and therefore, data are only available from case series. For proximal vertebral reconstruction, perioperative mortality in published case series is 0–4%, with rates of stroke and death of 2.5–25% (Eberhardt *et al.* 2006). For distal vertebral reconstruction, a 2–8% mortality rate has been reported.

In patients with extracranial vertebral artery stenosis (Figs. 26.2 and 26.3; see also Fig. 12.4), whether stenting plus best medical treatment is superior to best medical treatment alone remains uncertain (Feng *et al.* 2017; Markus *et al.* 2017). Many of the previous trials were small in sample size and were underpowered (Feng *et al.* 2017). Recently, the Vertebral Artery Ischemia Stenting Trial (VIST) randomized 182 patients

---

BOX 26.1 Interventional Procedures for Vertebrobasilar Ischemia

Endarterectomy of severe carotid stenosis to improve collateral blood flow, via the circle of Willis, to the basilar artery distal to vertebral or basilar artery stenosis or occlusion

Resection and anastomosis

Resection and reimplantation

Bypass or endarterectomy of proximal vertebral artery stenosis

Release of the vertebral artery from compressive fibrous bands or osteophytes

Extracranial-to-intracranial procedures to bypass vertebral artery stenosis or occlusion

Angioplasty and stenting of the vertebral and basilar arteries

Sources: From Diaz *et al.* (1984), Harward *et al.* (1984), Thevenet and Ruotolo (1984), Hopkins *et al.* (1987), Spetzler *et al.* (1987), Terada *et al.* (1996), and Malek *et al.* (1999).

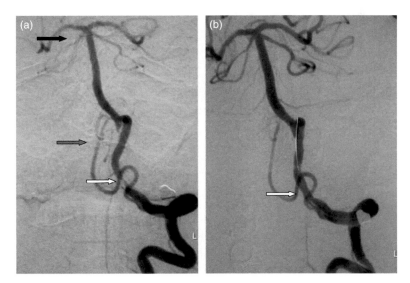

Fig. 26.2 (a) Cerebral angiogram showing proximal left vertebral stenosis (white arrow) with hypoplastic right vertebral artery (gray arrow) and poorly perfused posterior circulation owing to absence of posterior communicating arteries (black arrow). (b) Repeat angiogram after angioplasty and stenting of the left vertebral artery, showing improved perfusion of the distal posterior circulation territory (arrow).

with symptomatic vertebral artery stenosis to stenting plus best medical treatment versus best medical treatment alone (Markus *et al.* 2017). The rate of periprocedural complications in patients receiving stenting to the extracranial vertebral arteries was low. After a median of 3.5 years of follow-up, those who received stenting were at 60% lower risk of fatal and non-fatal stroke, although this did not reach statistical significance (Markus *et al.* 2017). Further, larger trials are therefore required to confirm the benefit of stenting in patients with symptomatic extracranial vertebral stenosis over medical treatment.

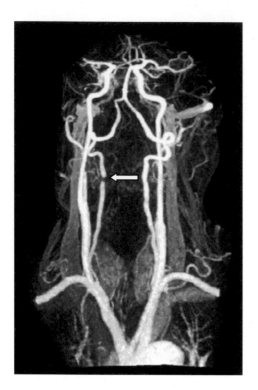

Fig. 26.3 A distal right vertebral artery stenosis (arrow) seen in MR angiography.

Intracranial Atherosclerosis

The Stenting and Aggressive Medical Management for Preventing Recurrent Stroke in Intracranial Stenosis (SAMMPRIS) trial was the first randomized controlled trial that compared the efficacy of aggressive medical treatment alone versus percutaneous transluminal angioplasty and stenting (PTAS) combined with aggressive medical treatment in patients with a recent symptomatic (TIA/minor ischemic stroke within 30 days) 70–99% intracranial atherosclerosis (Chimowitz *et al.* 2011; Derdeyn *et al.* 2014). Aggressive medical treatment was composed of aspirin 325 mg daily and clopidogrel 75 mg daily for 90 days followed by aspirin alone, blood pressure control to a systolic blood pressure target of < 140 mmHg (< 130 mmHg if diabetic), and rosuvastatin (LDL-cholesterol target ≤ 1.8 mmol/L) as well as other lifestyle modifications (smoking cessation, weight reduction and exercise, etc.). The Wingspan stent system was used in patients who received PTAS. SAMMPRIS was stopped prematurely after enrollment of 451 patients as patients in the PTAS arm had a significantly greater 30-day risk of stroke or death compared with patients who received aggressive medical treatment alone (14.7% versus 5.8%, $p = 0.002$) (Chimowitz *et al.* 2011). At 3 years, the absolute risk reduction with medical therapy alone remained the same at 9%, suggesting that PTAS did not provide further benefit in prevention of recurrent events beyond the periprocedural period (Derdeyn *et al.* 2014).

The high 30-day risk of PTAS (twofold than estimated) seen in SAMMPRIS could be explained by several factors (Abou-Chebl and Steinmetz 2012). First, the average time between event and randomization was 7 days (range 4–19 days). This may have resulted in selection bias, as very high-risk patients may have developed recurrent ischemic events before recruitment into SAMMPRIS and received PTAS outside of the trial setting. Patients recruited into SAMMPRIS are therefore possibly of lower risk and may partially account for the very good outcome of patients who received medical treatment only. Second, patients were enrolled based on lesion severity rather than lesion site or nature of TIA/ischemic stroke event. PTAS in patients presenting with perforator ischemia may therefore result in a high risk of perioperative ischemic stroke, as although PTAS restores luminal diameter, by displacing the atherosclerotic plaque against the vessel wall, it can result in further occlusion of stenosed perforators, causing a complete infarction in the territory supplied by the perforating blood vessel. Indeed, out of the 33 periprocedural strokes, 23 were ischemic strokes of which 12 were perforator infarcts. Excluding these periprocedural perforator infarcts would have significantly reduced the 30-day stroke/death rate from 14.7% to 9.4% in the PTAS arm. Similarly, plaque morphology and composition would have bearings on plaque stability and vulnerability of recurrent ischemic events. Third, 25 of recurrent strokes in SAMMPRIS occurred within 24 hours of PTAS. In SAMMPRIS, intracranial arteries between 2 to 4.5 mm in diameter were stented. However, treatment of very small arteries < 2.75 mm is notoriously risky as small vessels are prone to injury with PTAS due to a higher risk of oversizing of balloons and stents, thus increasing the risk of vessel injury and intracerebral hemorrhage. The Wingspan stent system also requires an over-the-wire exchange technique that may further add to the risks. In SAMMPRIS, there were four immediate periprocedural subarachnoid hemorrhages due to wire perforation of the vessels, and the remaining cases of intracerebral hemorrhage all occurred shortly after PTAS. These were attributed to cerebral hyperperfusion syndrome, possibly secondary to a slightly higher target postoperative systolic blood pressure < 150 mmHg than usual. Previous studies have shown that aggressive systolic blood pressure lowering < 120 mmHg greatly reduces the risk of ICH due to carotid angioplasty or stenting-associated cerebral reperfusion syndrome (Abou-Chebl et al. 2007). Fourth, all patients receiving PTAS in SAMMPRIS underwent general anesthesia, and this would have led to an increased difficulty in examination of patients during the procedure, hindering the early detection of procedure-related complications. Often, patients may experience pain due to severe vasospasm, intimal injury, or excessive balloon dilation, prompting the neuro-interventionalist to react quickly to prevent further neurological injury. Fifth, as discussed in Chapter 25, operator experience is crucial in determining the outcome of vascular surgery. In SAMMPRIS, there was a marked difference in complication rate based on the volume of enrollment with an 8% intracerebral hemorrhage rate at sites that enrolled < 12 patients compared with a 2% intracerebral hemorrhage rate at sites that enrolled ≥ 12 patients. SAMMPRIS has also been criticized for the fact that neuro-interventionalists may not have had adequate experience with use of the Wingspan stent in patients with intracranial atherosclerosis. This was reflected in the higher-than-expected rate of angiographic stroke as well as the high number of patients who received two stents, which suggests that the original stent was incorrectly placed, the lesion length was underestimated, or the initial procedure resulted in vessel dissection.

In view of the potential procedural risks associated with use of the Wingspan stent, the Vitesse Intracranial Stent Study for Ischemic Stroke Therapy (VISSIT) was conducted (Zaidat et al. 2015). In VISSIT, a balloon-mounted stent was used instead of the Wingspan stent, which is theoretically associated with a lower risk of wire perforation and residual post-procedure stenosis. VISSIT similarly compared the use of aggressive medical treatment alone with PTAS plus medical treatment in patients with ischemic stroke. Enrollment in VISSIT was however, stopped early after randomization of 112 patients due to a higher-than-expected rate of stroke in the stenting group – 30-day TIA/stroke rate was 24.1% in the PTAS group versus 9.4% in the medical treatment alone arm ($p = 0.05$).

In SAMMPRIS, 60 patients had a symptomatic 70–99% intracranial vertebral artery stenosis and 100 had significant basilar artery stenosis (Chimowitz *et al.* 2011; Derdeyn *et al.* 2014). However, PTAS was associated with a twofold higher risk of stroke or death at 2 years compared to patients who received medical treatment alone (Derdeyn *et al.* 2014). Similar high rates of periprocedural complications in patients receiving stenting to the intracranial vertebral arteries have been noted in the Vertebral Artery Stenting Trial (VAST) and VIST (Compter *et al.* 2015; Markus et al. 2017).

Therefore, before PTAS could be recommended in patients with intracranial cerebral or vertebrobasilar artery stenosis, further trials are required to identify the best stent system as well as patient and lesion selection criteria. Like carotid endarterectomy, trials to determine the feasibility of performing PTAS under general versus loco-regional anesthesia would be required.

Subclavian Steal Syndrome

Subclavian (and innominate) steal, although commonly detected with ultrasonography, very rarely causes neurological symptoms and does not seem to lead to ischemic stroke (Potter and Pinto 2014). However, incapacitatingly frequent vertebrobasilar TIAs in the presence of demonstrated unilateral or bilateral retrograde vertebral artery flow distal to severe subclavian or innominate disease may sometimes be relieved by angioplasty or stenting of the subclavian artery (Potter and Pinto 2014). Other surgical revascularization procedures that have been tried include carotid-to-subclavian or femoral-to-subclavian bypass, transposition of the subclavian artery to the common carotid artery, transposition of the vertebral artery to the common carotid artery, and axillary-to-axillary artery bypass grafting (Potter and Pinto 2014). All these procedures probably carry a significant risk of complications. Irrespective of the neurological situation, some kind of interventional procedure may be needed if the hand and arm become ischemic distal to subclavian or innominate artery disease.

Extracranial-to-Intracranial Bypass Surgery

Approximately 5–10% of patients with carotid territory TIA or minor ischemic stroke have occlusion of the internal carotid artery, stenosis of the internal carotid artery wall distal to the bifurcation, or middle cerebral artery occlusion or stenosis. Neither endarterectomy nor stenting is possible once a vessel has occluded, but many of these lesions can be bypassed by anastomosing a branch of the external carotid artery (usually the superficial temporal) via a skull burr hole to a cortical branch of the middle cerebral artery. This "surgical collateral" aims to improve the blood supply in the distal middle cerebral artery bed and so reduce the risk of stroke and to reduce the severity of any stroke that might occur. However, there are several reasons why the procedure might not work: The artery feeding the anastomosis can take months to dilate into an effective collateral channel; many patients have good collateral flow already from orbital collaterals or via the circle of Willis; not all strokes distal to internal carotid artery/middle cerebral artery occlusion or inaccessible stenosis are caused by low flow; the risk of stroke in patients with internal carotid artery occlusion is not that high compared with severe and recently symptomatic internal carotid artery stenosis (less than 10%/year) and, anyway, not all of these strokes are ipsilateral to the occlusion; neither resting cerebral blood flow nor cerebral reactivity is necessarily depressed in these patients; and the risk of surgery may outweigh the benefit (Latchaw *et al.* 1979; Hankey and Warlow 1991; Karnik *et al.* 1992; Klijn *et al.* 1997; Powers *et al.* 2000).

The risk–benefit relationship has been evaluated in only one completed randomized trial, and this failed to show any benefit from routine surgery (EC–IC Bypass Study Group 1985). However, it has been argued that patients with impaired cerebrovascular reactivity or with maximal oxygen extraction were not identified, and perhaps it is these patients who might benefit from surgery (Warlow 1986; Derdeyn *et al.* 2005), but proof of this hypothesis would require a further randomized trial in this specific subgroup (Karnik *et al.* 1992).

The Carotid Occlusion Surgery Study (COSS) determined whether superficial temporal artery-middle cerebral artery anastomosis, when combined with best medical therapy, would reduce subsequent risk of ipsilateral ischemic stroke in patients with symptomatic internal carotid artery occlusion and increased oxygen extraction fraction demonstrated by positron emission tomography (Grubb *et al.* 2013). Ninety-seven patients were randomized to the surgical group and 98 to the medical group. However, superficial temporal artery-middle cerebral artery anastomosis was not superior to medical treatment alone in prevention of recurrent ischemic stroke.

Other Surgical Procedures

Innominate or proximal common carotid artery stenosis or occlusion is quite often seen on angiograms in symptomatic patients but, unless very severe, does not influence the decision about endarterectomy for any internal carotid artery stenosis. Although it is possible to bypass such lesions, it is highly doubtful whether this reduces the risk of stroke unless, perhaps, several major neck vessels are involved and the patient has low-flow cerebral or ocular symptoms. This very rare situation can be caused by atheroma, Takayasu's disease, or aortic dissection. Clearly, close consultation between physicians and vascular surgeons is needed to sort out, on an individual patient basis, what to do for the best outcome.

Coronary artery bypass surgery (or angioplasty) may, of course, be indicated in patients presenting with cerebrovascular events who also happen to have cardiac symptoms. However, because asymptomatic coronary artery disease is so often associated with symptomatic cerebrovascular disease, would coronary intervention also be worthwhile even if there were no cardiac symptoms or signs? Given the high risk of cardiac events that might be reduced in the long term, this is a perfectly reasonable question but one that can only be answered by a randomized controlled trial, perhaps first in patients who are thought to be at particularly high risk of coronary events on the basis of clinical features or noninvasive cardiac investigation.

Aortic arch atheroma is now increasingly diagnosed by transesophageal echocardiography in patients with TIAs or ischemic stroke, but so far there are no surgical, or indeed medical, treatment options over and above controlling vascular risk factors and antiplatelet drugs. The Aortic Arch Related Cerebral Hazard (ARCH) trial randomized 172 patients with a thoracic aortic plaque > 4 mm with TIA, ischemic stroke, or peripheral embolism to aspirin and clopidogrel and 177 patients to warfarin (Amarenco *et al.* 2014). After a median follow-up of 3.4 years, there were no significant differences in risk of stroke, myocardial infarction, or vascular death between the two groups ($p = 0.2$). However, the trial had to terminate prematurely due to lack of funding and hence was underpowered to detect any significant effects between the two treatment arms.

References

Abou-Chebl A, Reginelli J, Bajzer CT *et al.* (2007). Intensive treatment of hypertension decreases the risk of hyperperfusion and intracerebral hemorrhage following carotid artery stenting. *Catheterization and Cardiovascular Interventions* **69**:690–696

Abou-Chebl A, Steinmetz H (2012). Critique of "Stenting Versus Aggressive Medical Therapy for Intracranial Arterial Stenosis" by Chimowitz *et al.* in the *New England Journal of Medicine*. *Stroke* **43**:616–620

Alberts MJ for the Publications Committee of the WALLSTENT (2001). Results of a multicentre prospective randomised trial of carotid artery stenting vs. carotid endarterectomy. *Stroke* **32**:325

Amarenco P, Davis S, Jones EF *et al.* (2014). Clopidogrel plus aspirin versus warfarin in patients with stroke and aortic arch plaques. *Stroke* **45**:1248–1257

Bonati LH, Lyrer P, Ederle J *et al.* (2012). Percutaneous transluminal balloon angioplasty and stenting for carotid artery stenosis. *Cochrane Database of Systematic Reviews* **9**: CD000515

Bonati LH, Dobson J, Feathersone RL *et al.* (2015). Long-term outcomes after stenting versus endarterectomy for treatment of symptomatic carotid stenosis: The International Carotid Stenting Study (ICSS) randomized trial. *Lancet* **385**:529–538

Brooks WH, McClure RR, Jones MR *et al.* (2001). Carotid angioplasty and stenting versus carotid endarterectomy: Randomized trial in a community hospital. *Journal of the American College of Cardiologists* **38**:1589–1595

Brott TG, Hobson RW II, Howard G *et al.* (2010). Stenting versus Endarterectomy for Treatment of Carotid-Artery Stenosis. *New England Journal of Medicine* **363**:11–23

Brott TG, Howard G, Roubin GS *et al.* (2016). Long-term results of stenting versus endarterectomy for carotid-artery stenosis. *New England Journal of Medicine* **374**:1021–1031

CAVATAS investigators (2001). Endovascular versus surgical treatment in patients with carotid stenosis in the Carotid and Vertebral Artery Transluminal Angioplasty Study (CAVATAS): A randomized trial. *Lancet* **357**:1729–1737

Chimowitz MI, Lynn MJ, Derdeyn CP *et al.* (2011). Stenting versus aggressive medical therapy for intracranial arterial stenosis. *New England Journal of Medicine* **365**:993–1003

Compter A, van der Worp HB, Schonewille WJ *et al.* (2015). Stenting versus medical treatment in patients with symptomatic vertebral artery stenosis: A randomized open-label phase 2 trial. *Lancet Neurology* **14**:606–614

Coward LJ, Featherstone RL, Brown MM (2005). Safety and efficacy of endovascular treatment of carotid artery stenosis compared with carotid endarterectomy: A Cochrane systematic review of the randomized evidence. *Stroke* **36**:905–911

Derdeyn CP, Grubb RL Jr., Powers WJ (2005). Indications for cerebral revascularization for patients with atherosclerotic carotid occlusion. *Skull Base* **15**:7–14

Derdeyn CP, Chimowitz MI, Lynn MJ *et al.* (2014). Aggressive medical treatment with or without stenting in high-risk patients with intracranial artery stenosis (SAMMPRIS): The final results of a randomised trial. *Lancet* **383**:333–341

Diaz FG, Ausman JI, de los Reyes RA *et al.* (1984). Surgical reconstruction of the proximal vertebral artery. *Journal of Neurosurgery* **61**:874–881

Dotter CT, Judkins MP, Rosch J (1967). Nonoperative treatment of arterial occlusive disease: A radiologically facilitated technique. *Radiology Clinics of North America* **5**:531–542

Eberhardt O, Naegele T, Raygrotzki S *et al.* (2006) Stenting of vertebrobasilar arteries in symptomatic atherosclerotic disease and acute occlusion: Case series and review of the literature. *Journal of Vascular Surgery* **43**:1145–1154

EC–IC Bypass Study Group (1985). Failure of extracranial–intracranial arterial bypass to reduce the risk of ischaemic stroke: Results of an international randomised trial. *New England Journal of Medicine* **313**:1191–1200

Feng H, Xie Y, Mei B *et al.* (2017). Endovascular vs. medical therapy in symptomatic vertebral artery stenosis: A meta-analysis. *Journal of Neurology* **264**:829–838

Grubb RL Jr., Powers WJ, Clarke WR *et al.* (2013). Surgical results of the Carotid Occlusion Surgery Study. *Journal of Neurosurgery* 118:25–33

Hankey GJ, Warlow CP (1991). Prognosis of symptomatic carotid artery occlusion. An overview. *Cerebrovascular Diseases* 1:245–256

Harward TRS, Wickbom IG, Otis SM *et al.* (1984). Posterior communicating artery visualization in predicting results of carotid endarterectomy for vertebrobasilar insufficiency. *American Journal of Surgery* 148:43–48

Hopkins LN, Martin NA, Hadley MN *et al.* (1987). Vertebrobasilar insufficiency. Part 2: microsurgical treatment of intracranial vertebrobasilar disease. *Journal of Neurosurgery* 66:662–674

International Carotid Stenting Study Investigators (2010). Carotid artery stenting compared with endarterectomy in patients with symptomatic carotid stenosis (International Carotid Stenting Study): An interim analysis of a randomized controlled trial. *Lancet* 375:985–997

Karnik R, Valentin A, Ammerer HP *et al.* (1992). Evaluation of vasomotor reactivity by transcranial Doppler and acetazolamide test before and after extracranial–intracranial bypass in patients with internal carotid artery occlusion. *Stroke* 23:812–817

Klijn CJM, Kappelle LJ, Tulleken CAF *et al.* (1997). Symptomatic carotid artery occlusion. A reappraisal of haemodynamic factors. *Stroke* 28:2084–2093

Latchaw RE, Ausman JI, Lee MC (1979). Superficial temporal–middle cerebral artery bypass. A detailed analysis of multiple pre- and postoperative angiograms in 40 consecutive patients. *Journal of Neurosurgery* 51:455–465

Malek AM, Higashida RT, Phatouros CC *et al.* (1999). Treatment of posterior circulation ischaemia with extracranial percutaneous balloon angioplasty and stent placement. *Stroke* 30:2073–2085

Markus HS, Larsson SC, Kuker W *et al.* (2017). Stenting for symptomatic vertebral artery stenosis: The Vertebral Artery Ischemia Stenting Trial. *Neurology* 89:1–8

Mas JL, Chatellier G, Beyssen B for the EVA-3S Investigators (2006). Endarterectomy versus stenting in patients with symptomatic severe carotid stenosis. *New England Journal of Medicine* 355:1660–1671

Mathur A, Roubin GS, Iyer SS *et al.* (1998). Predictors of stroke complicating carotid artery stenting. *Circulation* 97:1239–1245

McCabe DJH, Brown MM, Clifton A (1999). Fatal cerebral reperfusion haemorrhage after carotid stenting. *Stroke* 30:2483–2486

Naylor AR, Bolia A, Abbott RJ *et al.* (1998). Randomized study of carotid angioplasty and stenting versus carotid endarterectomy: A stopped trial. *Journal of Vascular Surgery* 28:326–334

Potter BJ, Pinto DS (2014). Subclavian steal syndrome. *Circulation* 129:2320–2323

Powers WJ, Derdeyn CP, Fritsch SM *et al.* (2000). Benign prognosis of never-symptomatic carotid occlusion. *Neurology* 54:878–882

Qureshi AI, Luft AR, Sharma M *et al.* (1999). Frequency and determinants of postprocedural haemodynamic instability after carotid angioplasty and stenting. *Stroke* 30:2086–2093

Reimers B, Corvaja N, Moshiri S *et al.* (2001). Cerebral protection with filter devices during carotid artery stenting. *Circulation* 104:12–15

SPACE Collaborative Group (2006). 30-day results from the SPACE trial of stent-protected angioplasty versus carotid endarterectomy in symptomatic patients: A randomised non-inferiority trial. *Lancet* 368:1239–1247

Spetzler RF, Hadley MN, Martin NA *et al.* (1987). Vertebrobasilar insufficiency. Part 1: Microsurgical treatment of extracranial vertebrobsilar disease. *Journal of Neurosurgery* 66:648–661

Terada T, Higashida RT, Halbach VV *et al.* (1996). Transluminal angioplasty for arteriosclerotic disease of the distal vertebral and basilar arteries. *Journal of Neurology, Neurosurgery and Psychiatry* 60:377–381

Thevenet A, Ruotolo C (1984). Surgical repair of vertebral artery stenoses. *Journal of Cardiovascular Surgery* 25:101–110

Warlow CP (1986). Extracranial to intracranial bypass and the prevention of stroke. *Journal of Neurology* 233:129–130

Yadav JS, Wholey MH, Kuntz RE *et al.* (2004). Protected carotid-artery stenting versus endarterectomy in high-risk patients. *New England Journal of Medicine* **351**:1493–1501

Zaidat OO, Fitzsimmons BF, Woodward BK *et al.* (2015). Effect of a balloon-expandable intracranial stent vs. medical therapy on risk of stroke in patients with symptomatic intracranial stenosis: The VISSIT randomized clinical trial. *JAMA* **313**:1240–1248

27

Selection of Patients for Carotid Intervention

Although only a minority of patients with TIA or ischemic stroke are potential candidates for carotid endarterectomy (CEA) or stenting, the decision to opt for interventional treatment rather than medical treatment alone can be difficult and is, therefore, given detailed consideration in this chapter. Most of the discussion relates to CEA because far more data are available on the risks and benefits of surgery than for stenting. However, most of the issues discussed are applicable to both procedures.

If the procedural risk of stroke from endarterectomy for symptomatic stenosis is, say, 7% in routine clinical practice rather than the more optimistic estimates of some surgeons; the unoperated risk of stroke is 20% after 2 years, which is, on average, the case for severe stenosis; and successful surgery reduces this risk of stroke to zero, which is not far from the truth, then doing about 15 operations would cause one stroke and avoid three. The net gain would be two strokes avoided. In order to reduce the number of patients who have to undergo surgery to prevent one having a stroke and, therefore, to maximize cost-effectiveness, we need to know who is at highest risk of surgical stroke and who will survive to be at highest risk of ipsilateral ischemic stroke if surgery is not done. In other words, safe surgery should be offered to those patients who have most to gain (those at highest risk of ipsilateral ischemic stroke without surgery) and who are most likely to survive for a number of years to enjoy that gain: surgery should be targeted to the small number of patients who will have a stroke without it, not to the larger number of patients who might have a stroke, because in the latter group there will be a lot of unnecessary operations.

The cost of identifying suitable patients for carotid surgery is high, with more than 30% of the cost attributed to the initial consultation at the neurovascular clinics. The cost of preventing one stroke by CEA in the UK in 1997–1998 was in the region of £100,000 if all the costs incurred in the workup of a cohort for potential CEA are included (Benade and Warlow 2002). Even excluding the cost of working up the very large number of patients with TIA and stroke to find the 5–10% or so suitable for surgery, surgery is not cheap: US$4,000 and $6,000 in a private and university hospital, respectively, in the USA in 1985 (Green and McNamara 1987), US$11,602 in Sweden in 1991 (Terent *et al.* 1994) and approximately US$7000 in Canada in 1996 (Smurawska *et al.* 1998). In the International Carotid Stenting Study, the mean cost per patient was US$10,477 in the stenting group and US$9,669 in the endarterectomy group (Morris *et al.* 2016).

Who Is at High (or Low) Risk of Surgery?

As well as being related to the skills of the surgeon and anesthetist and aspects of the surgical technique, the operative risk of stroke and death also depends on patient age and sex, the

Table 27.1 Factors predictive of operative risk of stroke or death at endarterectomy

Related to	Factors
Presenting event	Symptomatic versus asymptomatic Transient ischemic attack versus stroke Ocular versus cerebral events
Patient	Age Sex Vascular risk factors: previous stroke, hypertension, diabetes, contralateral internal cerebral artery occlusion, peripheral vascular disease
Operation	Side of surgery Nature of plaque (ulcerated versus non-ulcerated) Timing from event to surgery

nature of the presenting event, coexisting pathology such as coronary heart disease, and several other factors (Table 27.1).

Presenting Event

The operative risk of stroke and death is lower for patients with asymptomatic stenosis than for those with symptomatic stenosis (Rothwell *et al.* 1996; Bond *et al.* 2003). Not surprisingly, therefore, it also varies with the nature of the presenting symptoms. In a systematic review of all studies published from 1980 to 2000 inclusive that reported the risk of stroke and death from endartectomy (Bond *et al.* 2003), 103 of 383 studies stratified risk by the nature of the presenting symptoms (Table 27.2). As expected, the operative risk for symptomatic stenosis overall was higher than for asymptomatic stenosis (odds ratio [OR], 1.62; 95% confidence interval [CI], 1.45–1.81; $p < 0.00001$; 59 studies), but this depended on the nature of the symptoms, with the operative risk in patients with ocular events only tending to be lower than that for asymptomatic stenosis (OR, 0.75; 95% CI, 0.50–1.14; 15 studies). Operative risk was the same for stroke and cerebral TIA (OR, 1.16; 95% CI, 0.99–1.35; $p = 0.08$; 23 studies) but higher for cerebral TIA than for ocular events only (OR, 2.31; 95% CI, 1.72–3.12; $p < 0.00001$; 19 studies). Given that the operative risk of stroke is so highly dependent on the clinical indication, audits of risk should be stratified by the nature of any presenting symptoms, and patients should be informed of the risk that relates to their presenting event.

Age and Sex

In the randomized trials of CEA for both symptomatic and asymptomatic carotid stenosis, benefit was decreased in women (Rothwell 2004; Rothwell *et al.* 2004a), partly because of a higher operative risk than in men, but operative risk was independent of age. However, because these trial-based observations might not be generalizable to routine clinical practice (Chapter 18), a systematic review of all publications reporting data on the association between age and/or sex and procedural risk of stroke and/or death from 1980 to 2004 was carried out (Bond *et al.* 2005). Females had a higher rate of operative stroke and death (OR, 1.31; 95% CI, 1.17–1.47; $p < 0.001$; 25 studies) than males but no increase in operative

Table 27.2 A systematic review of the studies reporting the operative risks of stroke or death in carotid endarterectomy according to the nature of the presenting event and stratified according to year of publication

Presenting event	Time period	Number of studies	Number of operations	Absolute risk (% [95% CI])	p value (heterogeneity)
Symptomatic	< 1995	57	17,597	5.0 (4.4–5.5)	< 0.001
	≥ 1995	38	18,885	5.1 (4.7–5.6)	< 0.001
	Total	95	36,482	5.1 (4.6–5.6)	< 0.001
Urgent	< 1995	9	143	16.8 (8.0–25.5)	< 0.001
	≥ 1995	4	65	24.6 (17.6–31.6)	< 0.001
	Total	13	208	19.2 (10.7–27.8)	< 0.001
Stroke	< 1995	27	3,071	7.3 (6.1–8.5)	< 0.001
	≥ 1995	23	4,563	7.0 (6.2–7.9)	< 0.001
	Total	50	7,634	7.1 (6.1–8.1)	< 0.001
Cerebral TIA	< 1995	11	4,279	4.6 (3.9–5.2)	< 0.001
	≥ 1995	13	3,648	6.9 (6.2–7.5)	< 0.001
	Total	24	8,138	5.5 (4.7–6.3)	< 0.001
Ocular event	< 1995	9	1,050	3.0 (2.5–3.4)	0.9
	≥ 1995	9	734	2.7 (1.9–3.3)	< 0.001
	Total	18	1,784	2.8 (2.2–3.4)	< 0.001
Nonspecific	< 1995	16	1,275	4.2 (3.2–5.3)	< 0.001
	≥ 1995	8	476	4.3 (3.4–5.2)	< 0.001
	Total	24	1,751	4.2 (3.2–5.2)	< 0.001
Asymptomatic	< 1995	29	3,197	3.4 (2.5–4.4)	< 0.001
	≥ 1995	28	10,088	3.0 (2.5–3.5)	< 0.04
	Total	57	13,285	2.8 (2.4–3.2)	< 0.001
Redo surgery	< 1995	3	215	3.8 (2.7–4.9)	< 0.001
	≥ 1995	9	699	4.4 (3.1–5.8)	0.9
	Total	12	914	4.4 (2.4–6.4)	< 0.001

Notes: CI, confidence interval; TIA, transient ischemic attack.
Source: From Bond *et al.* (2003).

mortality (OR, 1.05; 95% CI, 0.81–0.86; p = 0.78; 15 studies). Compared with younger patients, operative mortality was increased at ≥ 75 years (OR, 1.36; 95% CI, 1.07–1.68; p = 0.02; 20 studies), at age ≥ 80 years (OR, 1.80; 95% CI, 1.26–2.45; p < 0.001; 15 studies), and in older patients overall (OR, 1.50; 95% CI, 1.26–1.78; p < 0.001; 35 studies). In contrast, however, operative risk of non-fatal stroke alone was not increased: ≥ 75 years (OR, 1.01; 95% CI, 0.8–1.3; p = 0.99; 16 studies) and ≥ 80 years (OR, 0.95; 95% CI, 0.61–1.20; p = 0.43; 15 studies). Consequently, the overall perioperative risk of stroke and death was only slightly increased at age ≥ 75 years (OR, 1.18; 95% CI, 0.94–1.44; p = 0.06; 21 studies), at age ≥ 80 years (OR, 1.14; 95% CI, 0.92–1.36; p = 0.34; 10 studies), and in older patients overall (OR, 1.17; 95% CI, 1.04–1.31; p = 0.01; 36 studies). Therefore, the effects of age and sex on the operative risk in published case series are broadly consistent with those observed in the trials. Operative risk of stroke is increased in women and operative mortality in patients aged ≥ 75 years, but the risk of stroke is not increased in patients aged ≥ 75 years.

Other Patient Factors

Only a few serious attempts have been made to sort out which other patient-related factors affect perioperative stroke risk and then which factors are independent from each other so they can be used in combination to predict surgical risk in individuals (Sundt *et al.* 1975; McCrory *et al.* 1993; Goldstein *et al.* 1994; Riles *et al.* 1994; Golledge *et al.* 1996; Kucey *et al.* 1998; Ferguson *et al.* 1999). Risk factors almost certainly include hypertension, peripheral vascular disease, contralateral internal carotid occlusion, and stenosis of the ipsilateral external carotid artery and carotid siphon (Rothwell *et al.* 1997). Operating on the left carotid artery being more risky than on the right clearly needs confirmation and, if true, might have to do with the easier detection of verbal than nonverbal cognitive deficits or with the surgical feeling that it is more difficult operating on the left side (Barnett *et al.* 1998; Kucey *et al.* 1998; Ferguson *et al.* 1999). The independent surgical risk factors for patients in the pooled analysis of data from European Carotid Surgery Trial (ECST) and the North American Symptomatic Carotid Endarterectomy Trial (NASCET) were female sex, presenting event, diabetes, ulcerated plaque, and previous stroke (Rothwell *et al.* 2004a). Other predictors in the ECST that were not available from NASCET included systolic blood pressure and peripheral vascular disease (Bond *et al.* 2002), but the predictive model derived from the ECST patients must be validated in an independent dataset.

Timing of Surgery

The optimal timing of surgery was a highly controversial topic (Pritz 1997; Eckstein *et al.* 1999). However, it is increasingly clear that surgery should be performed as soon as it is reasonably safe to do so, given the very high early risk of stroke during the first few days and weeks after the presenting TIA or stroke in patients with symptomatic carotid stenosis (Lovett *et al.* 2004; Fairhead and Rothwell 2005). Any increased operative risk from early surgery must be balanced against the substantial risk of stroke occurring prior to delayed surgery (Blaser *et al.* 2002; Fairhead and Rothwell 2005). If the operative risk is unrelated to the timing of surgery, then urgent surgery would, of course, be indicated. The pooled analyses of data from the randomized trials of CEA for symptomatic carotid stenosis showed that benefit from surgery was greatest in patients randomized within 2 weeks after their last ischemic event and fell rapidly with increasing delay (Rothwell *et al.* 2004a) For patients with ≥ 50% stenosis, the number needed to undergo surgery (NNT) to prevent one ipsilateral stroke in 5 years was five for patients randomized within 2 weeks after their last ischemic event versus 125 for patients randomized > 12 weeks. This trend was a result, in part, of the fact that the operative risk of endarterectomy in the trials was not increased in patients operated on within a week of their last event (Rothwell *et al.* 2004a, b).

A systematic review of all published surgical case series that reported data on operative risk by time since presenting event also found that there was no difference between early (first 3 to 4 weeks) and later surgery in stable patients (OR, 1.13; 95% CI, 0.79–1.62; $p = 0.62$; 11 studies). For neurologically stable patients with TIA and minor stroke, benefit from endarterectomy is greatest if performed within a week of the event. However, in the same systematic review (Bond *et al.* 2003; Fairhead and Rothwell 2005), emergency CEA for patients with evolving symptoms (stroke in evolution, crescendo TIA, "urgent cases") had a high operative risk of stroke and death (19.2%; 95% CI, 10.7–27.8), which was much greater than that for surgery in patients with stable symptoms in the same studies (OR, 3.9; 95% CI, 2.7–5.7; $p < 0.001$; 13 studies). Some uncertainty does exist, therefore, in relation to the balance of risk and benefit of surgery within perhaps 24–72 hours of the presenting event, particularly in patients with stroke, and a randomized trial of early versus delayed surgery during this time scale would be ethical (Welsh *et al.* 2004; Fairhead and Rothwell 2005; Rantner *et al.* 2005). However, delays to surgery in routine clinical practice in many countries can currently be measured in months (Rodgers *et al.* 2000; Turnbull *et al.* 2000; Pell *et al.* 2003; Fairhead and Rothwell 2005), and so the question of by how many hours should surgery be delayed is of somewhat theoretical interest in these healthcare systems.

Audit and Monitoring of Surgical Results

It is very difficult to compare surgical morbidity between surgeons or institutions in the same place at different times or before and after the introduction of a particular change in the technique without adjusting adequately for case mix: in other words, for the patient's inherent surgical risk. In addition, large enough numbers have to be collected to avoid random error (Rothwell *et al.* 1999a). This level of sophistication has never been achieved, and nor probably have adequate methods of routine data collection to support it, in normal clinical practice. It is clearly important, however, to have some idea of the risk of surgery in one's own hospital. Risks reported in the literature are irrelevant because they are not generalizable to one's own institution.

Which Patients Have Most to Gain from Surgery for Symptomatic Carotid Stenosis?

Not all patients with even extremely severe symptomatic stenosis go on to have an ipsilateral ischemic stroke. In the ECST, although approximately 30% with 90–99% stenosis had a stroke in 3 years, 70% did not, and these 70% could only have been harmed by surgery. Both the ECST and NASCET have shown very clearly the importance of increasing severity of carotid stenosis ipsilateral to the cerebral or ocular symptoms in the prediction of ischemic stroke in the same arterial distribution, although even this relationship is not straightforward in that if the internal carotid artery "collapses" distal to an extreme stenosis, the risk of stroke is substantially reduced (Morgenstern *et al.* 1997; Rothwell *et al.* 2000a) (Fig. 27.1). Angiographically demonstrated "ulceration" or "irregularity" increases the stroke risk even more, but it is unclear whether this can be translated to the appearances on ultrasound (Eliasziw *et al.* 1994; Rothwell *et al.* 2000b). These and other determinants of benefit are reviewed later. To complicate matters further, one also must avoid offering surgery to patients unlikely to survive long enough to enjoy any benefit of stroke prevention and so for whom the immediate surgical risks would not be worthwhile. These include the very elderly and patients with advanced cancer. It would also seem sensible to avoid surgery in patients with severe symptomatic cardiac disease who are likely to die from a cardiac death within a year or two.

Which Range of Stenosis?

To target CEA appropriately, it is first necessary to determine as precisely as possible how the overall average benefit from surgery relates to the degree of carotid stenosis. The analyses of each of the main trials of endarterectomy for symptomatic carotid stenosis were stratified by the severity of stenosis of the symptomatic carotid artery, but different methods of measurement of the degree of stenosis on pre-randomization angiograms were

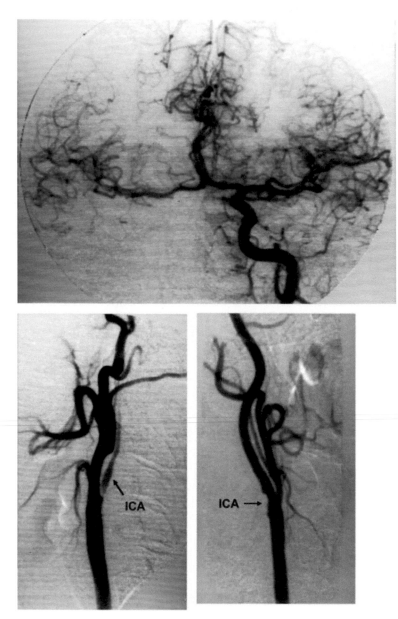

Fig. 27.1 Selective arterial angiograms of both carotid circulations in a patient with a recently symptomatic carotid "near occlusion" (lower left) and a mild stenosis at the contralateral carotid bifurcation (lower right). The near-occluded internal carotid artery (ICA) is markedly narrowed, and flow of contrast into the distal ICA is delayed. After selective injection of contrast into the contralateral carotid artery, significant collateral flow can be seen across the anterior communicating arteries with filling of the middle cerebral artery of the symptomatic hemisphere (top).

used, the NASCET method underestimating stenosis compared with the ECST method (Fig. 27.2) (Rothwell *et al.* 1994). Stenoses reported to be 70–99% in the NASCET were equivalent to 82–99% by the ECST method, and stenoses reported to be 70–99% by the ECST were 55–99% by the NASCET method (Rothwell *et al.* 1994).

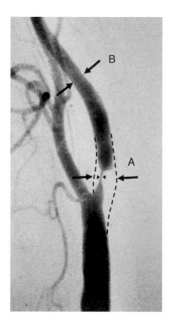

Fig. 27.2 A selective catheter angiogram of the carotid bifurcation showing a 90% stenosis. To calculate the degree of stenosis, the lumen diameter at the point of maximum stenosis (A) was measured as the numerator in both the European Carotid Surgery Trial (ECST) method and the North American Symptomatic Carotid Endarterectomy Trial (NASCET) method. However, the NASCET used the lumen diameter of the distal internal carotid artery (B) as the denominator, whereas the ECST used the estimated normal lumen diameter (dotted lines) at the point of maximum stenosis.

In 1998, the ECST (European Carotid Surgery Trialists' Collaborative Group 1998) showed that there was no benefit from surgery in patients with 30–49% stenosis or 50–69% stenosis (defined by their method) but that there was major benefit in patients with 70–99% stenosis. When the results of the ECST were stratified by decile of stenosis, endarterectomy was only beneficial in patients with 80–99% stenosis. The 11.6% absolute reduction in risk of major stroke or death at 3 years was consistent with the 10.1% reduction in major stroke or death at 2 years reported in the NASCET (Barnett *et al.* 1998) in patients with 70–99% stenosis, as defined by NASCET. However, in contrast to the ECST, the NASCET reported a 6.9% ($p = 0.03$) absolute reduction in risk of disabling stroke or death in patients with 50–69% stenosis (equivalent to 65–82% stenosis in ECST).

Given this apparent disparity between the results of the trials, the ECST group reanalyzed its results such that they were comparable with the results of the NASCET (Rothwell *et al.* 2003a). To do so, the original ECST angiograms were remeasured by the method used in the NASCET, and the outcome events were redefined. Reanalysis of the ECST showed that endarterectomy had reduced the 5-year risk of *any stroke or surgical death* by 5.7% (95% CI, 0–11.6) in patients with 50–69% stenosis as defined by NASCET ($n = 646$; $p = 0.05$) and by 21.2% (95% CI, 12.9–29.4) in patients with NASCET-defined 70–99% stenosis without "near occlusion" ($n = 429$; $p < 0.0001$). Surgery was harmful in patients with < 30% stenosis ($n = 1321$; $p = 0.007$) and of no benefit in patients with 30–49% stenosis ($n = 478$; $p = 0.6$). Therefore, the results of the two trials were consistent when analyzed in the same way. This allowed a pooled analysis of data from the ECST, NASCET, and the Veterans Affairs Cooperative Study Program 309 (VA 309) trials (Mayberg *et al.* 1991), which included more than 95% of patients with symptomatic carotid stenosis ever randomized to endarterectomy versus medical treatment (Rothwell *et al.* 2003b).

The pooled analysis showed that there was no statistically significant heterogeneity between the trials in the effect of the randomized treatment allocation on the relative

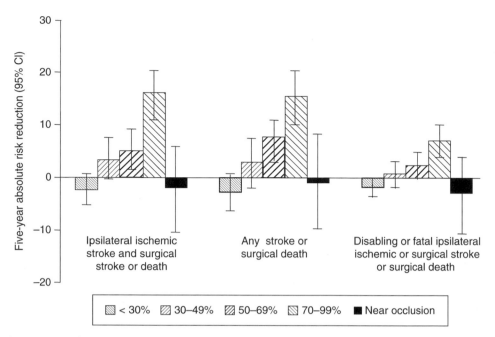

Fig. 27.3 The effect of endarterectomy on the 5-year risks of each of the main trial outcomes in patients with varying degrees of stenosis (< 30%, 30–49%, ≥ 70% without near occlusion, and near occlusion) in an analysis of pooled data from the three main randomized trials of endarterectomy versus medical treatment for recently symptomatic carotid stenosis (Rothwell *et al.* 2003b).

risks of any of the main outcomes in any of the stenosis groups. Data were, therefore, merged on 6,092 patients with 35,000 patient-years of follow-up (Rothwell *et al.* 2003b). The overall operative mortality was 1.1% (95% CI, 0.8–1.5), and the operative risk of stroke and death was 7.1% (95% CI, 6.3–8.1). The effect of surgery on the risks of the main trial outcomes is shown by stenosis group in Fig. 27.3. Endarterectomy reduced the 5-year absolute risk of any stroke or death in patients with NASCET-defined 50–69% stenosis (absolute risk reduction [ARR], 7.8%; 95% CI, 3.1–12.5) and was highly beneficial in patients with 70–99% stenosis (ARR, 15.3%; 95% CI, 9.8–20.7) but was of no benefit in patients with near occlusion. The CI values around the estimates of treatment effect in the near occlusions were wide, but the difference in the effect of surgery between this group and patients with ≥ 70% stenosis without near occlusion was statistically highly significant for each of the outcomes. Qualitatively similar results were seen for disabling stroke.

The results of these pooled analyses show that, with the exception of near occlusions, the degree of stenosis above which surgery is beneficial is 50% as defined by NASCET (equivalent to approximately 65% stenosis as defined by ECST). Given the confusion generated by the use of different methods of measurement of stenosis in the original trials, it has been suggested that the NASCET method be adopted as the standard in future (Rothwell *et al.* 2003b). There are several arguments in favor of the continued use of selective arterial angiography in the selection of patients for endarterectomy (Johnston and Goldstein 2001; Norris and Rothwell 2001). However, if noninvasive techniques are used to select patients for surgery, then they must be properly validated against catheter angiography within individual centers (Rothwell *et al.* 2000c). More work is also required to assess the accuracy of noninvasive methods of carotid imaging in detecting near occlusion (Bermann *et al.* 1995; Ascher *et al.* 2002).

What about Near Occlusions?

Near occlusions (Fig. 27.1) as a group were identified in the NASCET because it is not possible to measure the degree of stenosis using the NASCET method in situations where the post-stenotic internal carotid artery is narrowed or collapsed as a result of markedly reduced post-stenotic blood flow. Patients with "abnormal post-stenotic narrowing" of the internal carotid artery were also identified in the ECST (Rothwell *et al.* 2000a). In both trials, these patients had a paradoxically low risk of stroke on medical treatment. The low risk of stroke most likely reflects the presence of a good collateral circulation, which is visible on angiography in the vast majority of the patients with narrowing of the internal carotid artery distal to a severe stenosis. The benefit from surgery in the near occlusion group in the NASCET had been minimal, and both the reanalysis of the ECST (Rothwell *et al.* 2003a) and the pooled analysis (Rothwell *et al.* 2003b) suggested no benefit at all in this group in terms of preventing stroke (Fig. 27.3). Some patients with near occlusion may still wish to undergo surgery, particularly if they experience recurrent TIAs. In the reanalysis of the ECST (Rothwell *et al.* 2003a), CEA did reduce the risk of recurrent TIA in patients with near occlusion (ARR, 15%; $p = 0.007$). However, patients should be informed that endarterectomy does not prevent stroke.

Which Subgroups Benefit Most?

The overall trial results are of only limited help to patients and clinicians in making decisions about surgery. Although endarterectomy reduces the relative risk of stroke by approximately 30% over the next 3 years in patients with a recently symptomatic severe stenosis, only 20% of such patients have a stroke on medical treatment alone. The operation is of no value in the other 80% of patients, who, despite having a symptomatic stenosis, are destined to remain stroke-free without surgery and can only be harmed by it. It would, therefore, be useful to be able to identify in advance and operate on only those patients with a high risk of stroke on medical treatment alone but a relatively low operative risk. The degree of stenosis is a major determinant of benefit from endarterectomy, but there are several other clinical and angiographic characteristics that might influence the risks and benefits of surgery.

Eleven reports of different univariate subgroup analyses were published by NASCET, which have been summarized elsewhere (Rothwell 2005). Although interesting, the results are difficult to interpret because several of the subgroups contain only a few tens of patients, with some of the estimates of the effect of surgery based on only one or two outcome events in each treatment group; the 95% CI values around the ARRs in each subgroup have generally not been given; and there have been no formal tests of the interaction between the subgroup variable and the treatment effect. It is, therefore, impossible to be certain whether differences in the effect of surgery between subgroups are real or occur by chance.

Subgroup analyses of pooled data from ECST and NASCET have greater power to determine subgroup–treatment interactions reliably, and several clinically important interactions have been reported (Rothwell *et al.* 2004a). Sex ($p = 0.003$), age ($p = 0.03$), and time from the last symptomatic event to randomization ($p = 0.009$) modify the effectiveness of surgery (Fig. 27.4). Benefit from surgery was greatest in men, patients aged ≥ 75 years, and patients randomized within 2 weeks after their last ischemic event, and it fell rapidly with increasing delay. For patients with ≥ 50% stenosis, the number of patients needed to undergo surgery (NNT) to prevent one ipsilateral stroke in 5 years was 9 for men versus 36 for women, 5 for age ≥ 75 versus 18 for age < 65 years, and 5 for patients randomized within 2 weeks after their last ischemic event versus 125 for patients randomized > 12 weeks. The corresponding ARR values are shown separately for patients with 50–69% stenosis and 70–99% stenosis in Fig. 27.5. These observations were consistent across the 50–69% and ≥ 70% stenosis groups, and similar trends were present in both ECST and NASCET.

Women had a lower risk of ipsilateral ischemic stroke on medical treatment and a higher operative risk in comparison with men. For recently symptomatic carotid stenosis, surgery is very clearly beneficial in women with ≥ 70% stenosis but not in women with 50–69% stenosis (Fig. 27.4). In contrast, surgery reduced the 5-year absolute risk of stroke by 8.0% (95% CI, 3.4–12.5) in men with 50–69% stenosis. This sex difference was statistically significant even when the analysis of the interaction was confined to the 50–69% stenosis group. These same patterns were also shown in both of the large published trials of CEA for asymptomatic carotid stenosis (Rothwell 2004).

Benefit from CEA increased with age in the pooled analysis of trials in patients with recently symptomatic stenosis, particularly in patients aged > 75 years (Fig. 27.4). Although patients randomized in trials generally have a good prognosis and there is some evidence of an increased operative mortality in elderly patients in routine clinical practice, as discussed previously, a systematic review of all published surgical case series reported no increase in the operative risk of stroke and death in older age groups. There is, therefore, no justification for withholding CEA in patients aged > 75 years who are deemed to be medically fit to undergo surgery. The evidence suggests that benefit is likely to be greatest in this group because of their high risk of stroke on medical treatment.

Benefit from surgery is probably also greatest in patients with stroke, intermediate in those with cerebral TIA, and lowest in those with retinal events. There was also a trend in the trials toward greater benefit in patients with irregular plaque than a smooth plaque.

Which Individuals Benefit Most?

There are some clinically useful subgroup observations in the pooled analysis of the endarterectomy trials, but the results of univariate subgroup analysis are often of only limited use in clinical practice. Individual patients frequently have several important risk factors, each of which interacts in a way that cannot be described using univariate subgroup analysis and all of which should be taken into account in order to determine the likely balance of risk and benefit from surgery (Rothwell *et al.* 1999b). For example, what would be the likely benefit from surgery in a 78-year-old (increased benefit) female (reduced benefit) with 70% stenosis who presented within 2 weeks (increased benefit) of an ocular ischemic event (reduced benefit) and was found to have an ulcerated carotid plaque (increased benefit)?

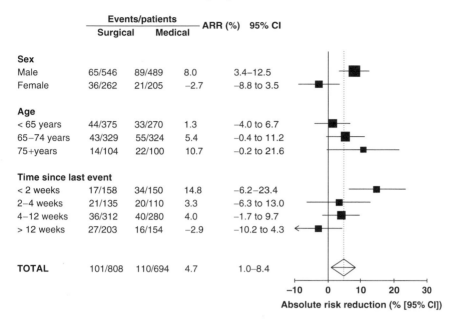

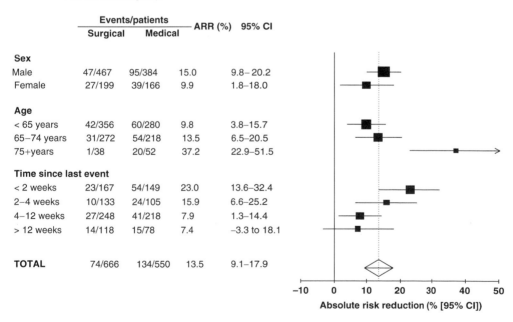

Fig. 27.4 Absolute risk reduction (ARR) with surgery in the 5-year risk of ipsilateral carotid territory ischemic stroke and any stroke or death within 30 days after trial surgery according to predefined subgroup variables in an analysis of pooled data from the two largest randomized trials of endarterectomy versus medical treatment for recently symptomatic carotid stenosis (derived form Rothwell *et al.* 2004b). CI, confidence interval.

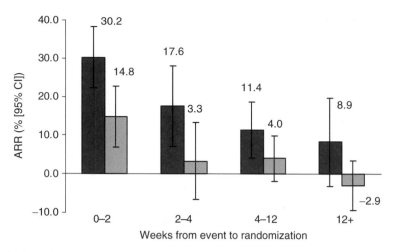

Fig. 27.5 Absolute risk reduction (ARR) with surgery in the five-year risk of ipsilateral carotid territory ischemic stroke and any stroke or death within 30 days after trial surgery in patients with 50–69% stenosis (white columns) and ≥ 70% stenosis (black columns) without near occlusion stratified by the time from last symptomatic event to randomization. This is an analysis of pooled data from the two largest randomized trials of endarterectomy versus medical treatment for recently symptomatic carotid stenosis (Rothwell *et al.* 2004a). The numbers above the bars indicate the actual absolute risk reduction. CI, confidence interval.

One way in which clinicians can weigh the often-conflicting effects of the important characteristics of an individual patient on the likely benefit from treatment is to base decisions on the predicted absolute risks of a poor outcome with each treatment option using prognostic models (see Chapter 14). A model for prediction of the risk of stroke on medical treatment in patients with recently symptomatic carotid stenosis has been derived from the ECST (Rothwell *et al.* 1999b, 2005) (Table 27.3). The model was validated using data from the NASCET and showed very good agreement between predicted and observed medical risk (Mantel–Haenszel χ^2_{trend} = 41.3 [degrees of freedom, 1]; p < 0.0001), reliably distinguishing between individuals with a 10% risk of ipsilateral ischemic stroke after 5 years of follow-up and individuals with a risk of more than 40% (Fig. 27.6). Importantly, Fig. 27.6 also shows that the operative risk of stroke and death in patients who were randomized to surgery in NASCET was unrelated to the medical risk (Mantel–Haenszel χ^2_{trend} = 0.98 [degrees of freedom, 1]; p = 0.32). Therefore, when the operative risk and the small additional residual risk of stroke following successful endarterectomy were taken into account, benefit from endarterectomy at 5 years varied significantly across the quintiles (p = 0.001), with no benefit in patients in the lower three quintiles of predicted medical risk (ARR, 0–2%), moderate benefit in the fourth quintile (ARR, 10.8%; 95% CI, 1.0–20.6), and substantial benefit in the highest quintile (ARR, 32.0%; 95% CI, 21.9–42.1).

Prediction of risk using models requires a computer, a pocket calculator with an exponential function, or internet access (the ECST model can be found at www.ndcn .ox.ac.uk/divisions/cpsd). As an alternative, a simplified risk score based on the hazard ratios derived from the relevant risk model can be derived. Table 27.3 shows a score for the 5-year risk of stroke (derived from the ECST model) in patients with recently symptomatic carotid stenosis treated medically. As is shown in the example, the total

Table 27.3 A predictive model for 5-year risk of ipsilateral ischemic stroke on medical treatment in patients with recently symptomatic carotid stenosis[a]

Model			Scoring system		
Risk factor	Hazard ratio (95% CI)	p value	Risk factor	Score	Example
Stenosis (per 10%)	1.18 (1.10–1.25)	< 0.0001	Stenosis (%)		
			50–59	2.4	2.4
			60–69	2.8	
			70–79	3.3	
			80–89	3.9	
			90–99	4.6	
Near occlusion[b]	0.49 (0.19–1.24)	0.1309	Near occlusion	0.5	No
Male sex	1.19 (0.81–1.75)	0.3687	Male sex	1.2	No
Age (per 10 years)	1.12 (0.89–1.39)	0.3343	Age (years)		
			31–40	1.1	
			41–50	1.2	
			51–60	1.3	
			61–70	1.5	1.5
			71–80	1.6	
			81–90	1.8	
Time since last event (per 7 days)	0.96 (0.93–0.99)	0.0039	Time since last event (days)		
			0–13	8.7	8.7
			14–28	8.0	
			29–89	6.3	
			90–365	2.3	
Presenting event[c]		0.0067	Presenting event		
Ocular	1.000		Ocular	1.0	
Single TIA	1.41 (0.75–2.66)		Single TIA	1.4	
Multiple TIAs	2.05 (1.16–3.60)		Multiple TIAs	2.0	
Minor stroke	1.82 (0.99–3.34)		Minor stroke	1.8	
Major stroke[d]	2.54 (1.48–4.35)		Major stroke	2.5	2.5
Diabetes	1.35 (0.86–2.11)	0.1881	Diabetes	1.4	1.4
Previous MI	1.57 (1.01–2.45)	0.0471	Previous MI	1.6	No
PVD	1.18 (0.78–1.77)	0.4368	PVD	1.2	No
Treated hypertension[e]	1.24 (0.88–1.75)	0.2137	Treated hypertension	1.2	1.2
Irregular/ ulcerated plaque	2.03 (1.31–3.14)	0.0015	Irregular/ ulcerated plaque	2.0	2.0
Total risk score					263

Table 27.3 (cont.)

	Model			Scoring system		
Risk factor	Hazard ratio (95% CI)	p value		Risk factor	Score	Example
Predicted medical risk using nomogram						37

[a] TIA, transient ischemic attack; MI, myocardial infarction; PVD, peripheral vascular disease; CI, confidence interval. Hazard ratios derived from the model are used for the scoring system. The score for the 5-year risk of stroke is the product of the individual scores for each of the risk factors present. The score is converted into a risk using Fig. 27.6.

[b] In cases of near occlusion, enter degree of stenosis as 85%.

[c] Presenting event is coded as the most severe ipsilateral symptomatic event in the past 6 months (severity is as ordered: ocular events are least severe, and major stroke is most severe).

[d] Major stroke is defined as stroke with symptoms persisting for at least 7 days.

[e] Treated hypertension includes previously treated or newly diagnosed hypertension.

Source: From Rothwell *et al.* (2005).

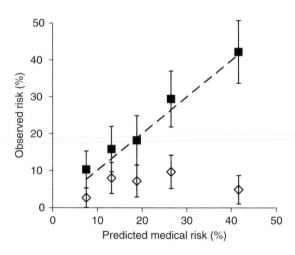

Fig. 27.6 A model derived from the data from the European Carotid Surgery Trial (ESCT) for the 5-year risk of ipsilateral risk of ischemic stroke on medical treatment tested on data from the North American Symptomatic Carotid Endarterectomy Trial (NASCET). The closed squares show the risk of stroke in the medical treatment group in NASCET stratified into quintiles on the basis of predicted risk. The open diamonds show the operative risk of stroke and death in the surgical group in NASCET stratified by their predicted medical risk.

risk score is the product of the scores for each risk factor. Fig. 27.7 shows a plot of the total risk score against the 5-year predicted risk of ipsilateral carotid territory ischemic stroke derived from the full model and is used as a nomogram for the conversion of the score into a risk prediction.

Alternatively, risk tables allow a relatively small number of important variables to be considered and have the major advantage that they do not require the calculation of any score by the clinician or patient. Fig. 27.8 shows a risk table for the 5-year risk of ipsilateral ischemic stroke in patients with recently symptomatic carotid stenosis on medical treatment, derived from the ECST model. The table is based on the five variables that were significant predictors of risk in the ECST model (Table 27.3) and yielded clinically important subgroup–treatment effect interactions in the analysis of pooled data from the relevant

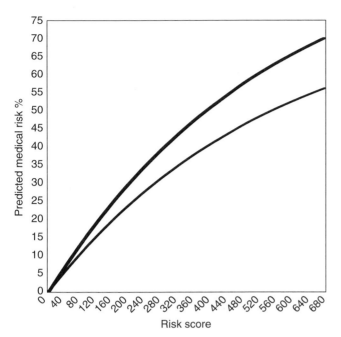

Fig. 27.7 A plot of the total risk score derived in the European Carotid Surgery Trial (ECST; see Table 27.3) against the 5-year predicted risk of ipsilateral carotid territory ischemic stroke derived from the full model. This graph is used to convert the score from Table 27.3 into a risk prediction. The finer line on the graph is the predicted risk if one assumes a 20% reduction in risk with newer secondary preventive therapies compared with those available when the model was developed.

trials (sex, age, time since last symptomatic event, type of presenting event(s), and carotid plaque surface morphology).

One potential problem with the ECST risk model is that it might overestimate risk in current patients because of improvements in medical treatment, such as the increased use of statins. However, such improvements in treatment pose more problems for interpretation of the overall trial results than for the risk-modeling approach. For example, it would take only a relatively modest improvement in the effectiveness of medical treatment to erode the overall benefit of endarterectomy in patients with 50–69% stenosis. In contrast, very major improvements in medical treatment would be required in order to significantly reduce the benefit from surgery in patients in the high predicted-risk quintile in Fig. 27.6. Therefore, the likelihood that ancillary treatments have improved, and are likely to continue to improve, is an argument in favor of a risk-based approach to targeting treatment. However, it would be reasonable in a patient on treatment with a statin, for example, to reduce the risks derived from the risk model by 20% in relative terms.

Other prognostic tools, such as measurements of cerebral reactivity and emboli load on transcranial Doppler (Molloy and Markus 1999; MacKinnon et al. 2005; Markus and MacKinnon 2005), are not widely used in clinical practice, and it is unclear to what extent they are likely to add to the predictive value of the ECST model.

Patients with Multiple Potential Causes of Stroke

Patients often have multiple possible causes for their TIA or stroke. For example, patients with a lacunar ischemic stroke or TIA may have ipsilateral severe carotid stenosis. The question then arises whether the stenosis is "symptomatic" (i.e., a small deep lacunar infarct

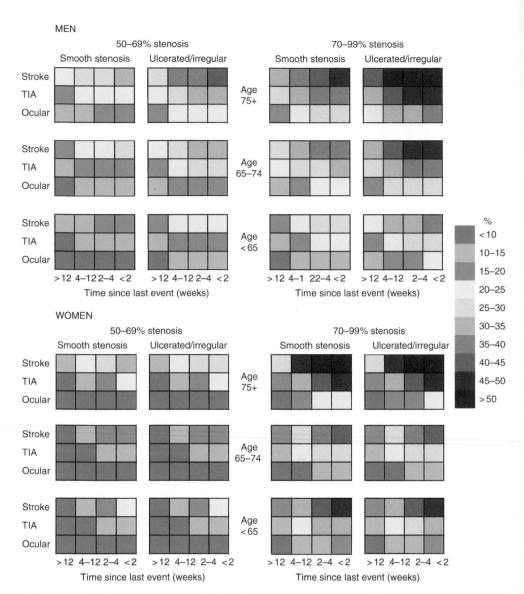

Fig. 27.8 A risk table for the 5-year risk of ipsilateral ischemic stroke in patients with recently symptomatic carotid stenosis on medical treatment derived from the ECST model. European Carotid Surgery Trial (ECST) method. TIA, transient ischemic attack.

has, unusually, been caused by artery-to-artery embolism or low flow) or "asymptomatic" (i.e., the stenosis is a coincidental bystander and the infarct was really caused by intracranial small vessel disease). Unsurprisingly, the number of such patients in the randomized trials is very small, and there are only limited published data (Boiten *et al.* 1996; Inzitari *et al.* 2000), but pooled analysis of the individual patient data shows that surgery is beneficial for patients with severe stenosis ipsilateral to a lacunar TIA or stroke (PM Rothwell, unpublished data). The observational studies mostly show that severe stenosis is about equally rare in the symptomatic and contralateral carotid arteries, which supports the notion of the stenosis being coincidental (Mead *et al.* 2000), but it does not mean that surgery would not still be beneficial. In practice, most clinicians would recommend surgery, particularly if the stenosis is very severe, because even if the artery was in truth asymptomatic there is some evidence that the risk of ipsilateral ischemic stroke is high enough to justify the risk of surgery. The same arguments probably apply if there is also a major coexisting source of embolism from the heart (such as non-rheumatic atrial fibrillation), in which case the patient may reasonably be offered surgery as well as anticoagulation. With the more widespread use of diffusion-weighted imaging, it is now often possible to infer the likely etiology of stroke from the distribution of acute ischemic lesions (see Chapters 10 and 11).

References

Ascher E, Markevich N, Hingorani A *et al.* (2002). Pseudo-occlusions of the internal carotid artery: A rationale for treatment on the basis of a modified duplex scan protocol. *Journal of Vascular Surgery* **35**:340–350

Barnett HJM, Taylor DW, Eliasziw M for the North American Symptomatic Carotid Endarterectomy Trial Collaborators (1998). Benefit of carotid endarterectomy in patients with symptomatic moderate or severe stenosis. *New England Journal of Medicine* **339**:1415–1425

Benade MM, Warlow CP (2002). Cost of identifying patients for carotid endarterectomy. *Stroke* **33**:435–439

Bermann SS, Devine JJ, Erdos LS *et al.* (1995). Distinguishing carotid artery pseudo-occlusion with colour-flow Doppler. *Stroke* **26**:434–438

Blaser T, Hofmann K, Buerger T *et al.* (2002). Risk of stroke, transient ischaemic attack, and vessel occlusion before endarterectomy in patients with symptomatic severe carotid stenosis. *Stroke* **33**:1057–1062

Boiten J, Rothwell PM, Slattery J for the European Carotid Surgery Trialists' Collaborative Group (1996). Lacunar stroke in the European Carotid Surgery Trial: Risk factors, distribution of carotid stenosis, effect of surgery and type of recurrent stroke. *Cerebrovascular Diseases* **6**:281–287

Bond R, Narayan S, Rothwell PM *et al.* (2002). Clinical and radiological risk factors for operative stroke and death in the European Carotid Surgery Trial. *European Journal of Vascular Endovascular Surgery* **23**:108–116

Bond R, Rerkasem K, Rothwell PM (2003). A systematic review of the risks of carotid endarterectomy in relation to the clinical indication and the timing of surgery. *Stroke* **34**:2290–2301

Bond R, Rerkasem K, Cuffe R *et al.* (2005). A systematic review of the associations between age and sex and the operative risks of carotid endarterectomy. *Cerebrovascular Diseases* **20**:69–77

Eckstein H, Schumacher H, Klemm K *et al.* (1999). Emergency carotid endarterectomy. *Cerebrovascular Diseases* **9**:270–281

Eliasziw M, Streifler JY, Fox AJ for the North American Symptomatic Carotid Endarterectomy Trial (1994). Significance of plaque ulceration in symptomatic patients with high-grade carotid stenosis. *Stroke* **25**:304–308

European Carotid Surgery Trialists' Collaborative Group (1998). Randomised trial of endarterectomy for recently symptomatic carotid stenosis: Final results of the MRC European Carotid Surgery Trial (ECST). *Lancet* **351**:1379–1387

Fairhead JF, Rothwell PM (2005). The need for urgency in identification and treatment of symptomatic carotid stenosis is already established. *Cerebrovascular Diseases* **19**:355–358

Ferguson GG, Eliasziw M, Barr HWK for the North American Symptomatic Carotid Endarterectomy Trial (NASCET) Collaborators (1999). The North American Symptomatic Carotid Endarterectomy Trial: Surgical results in 1415 patients. *Stroke* **30**:1751–1758

Goldstein LB, McCrory DC, Landsman PB et al. (1994). Multicenter review of preoperative risk factors for carotid endarterectomy in patients with ipsilateral symptoms. *Stroke* **25**:1116–1121

Golledge J, Cuming R, Beattie DK et al. (1996). Influence of patient-related variables on the outcome of carotid endarterectomy. *Journal of Vascular Surgery* **24**:120–126

Green RM, McNamara J (1987). Optimal resources for carotid endarterectomy. *Surgery* **102**:743–748

Inzitari D, Eliasziw M, Gates P for the North American Symptomatic Carotid Endarterectomy Trial Group (2000). The causes and risk of stroke in patients with asymptomatic internal-carotid-artery stenosis. *New England Journal of Medicine* **342**:1693–1700

Johnston DC, Goldstein LB (2001). Clinical carotid endarterectomy decision making: Non-invasive vascular imaging versus angiography. *Neurology* **56**: 1009–1015

Kucey DS, Bowyer B, Iron K et al. (1998). Determinants of outcome after carotid endarterectomy. *Journal of Vascular Surgery* **28**:1051–1058

Lovett JK, Coull A, Rothwell PM on behalf of the Oxford Vascular Study (2004). Early risk of recurrent stroke by aetiological subtype: Implications for stroke prevention. *Neurology* **62**:569–574

MacKinnon AD, Aaslid R, Markus HS (2005). Ambulatory transcranial Doppler cerebral embolic signal detection in symptomatic and asymptomatic carotid stenosis. *Stroke* **36**:1726–1730

Markus HS, MacKinnon A (2005). Asymptomatic embolization detected by Doppler ultrasound predicts stroke risk in symptomatic carotid artery stenosis. *Stroke* **36**:971–975

Mayberg MR, Wilson E, Yatsu F for the Veterans Affairs Cooperative Studies Program 309 Trialist Group (1991). Carotid endarterectomy and prevention of cerebral ischaemia in symptomatic carotid stenosis. *Journal of the American Medical Association* **266**:3289–3294

McCrory DC, Goldstein LB, Samsa GP et al. (1993). Predicting complications of carotid endarterectomy. *Stroke* **24**:1285–1291

Mead GE, Lewis SC, Wardlaw JM, Dennis MS, Warlow CP (2000). Severe ipsilateral carotid stenosis in lacunar ischaemic stroke: Innocent bystanders? *Journal of Neurology* **249**:266–271

Molloy J, Markus HS (1999). Asymptomatic embolization predicts stroke and TIA risk in patients with carotid artery stenosis. *Stroke* **30**:1440–1443

Morgenstern LB, Fox AJ, Sharpe BL et al. for the North American Symptomatic Carotid Endarterectomy Trial (NASCET) Group (1997). The risks and benefits of carotid endarterectomy in patients with near occlusion of the carotid artery. *Neurology* **48**:911–915

Morris S, Patel NV, Dobson J et al. (2016). Cost-utility analysis of stenting versus endarterectomy in the International Carotid Stenting Study. *International Journal of Stroke* **11**:446–453

Norris J, Rothwell PM (2001). Noninvasive carotid imaging to select patients for endarterectomy: Is it really safer than conventional angiography? *Neurology* **56**:990–991

Pell JP, Slack R, Dennis M et al. (2003). Improvements in carotid endarterectomy in Scotland: Results of a national prospective survey. *Scottish Medical Journal* **49**:53–56

Pritz MB (1997). Timing of carotid endarterectomy after stroke. *Stroke* **28**:2563–2567

Rantner B, Pavelka M, Posch L, Schmidauer C, Fraedrich G (2005). Carotid endarterectomy after ischemic stroke: Is there a justification for delayed surgery? *European Journal of Vascular Endovascular Surgery* **30**:36–40

Riles TS, Imparato AM, Jacobowitz GR et al. (1994). The cause of perioperative stroke after carotid endarterectomy. *Journal of Vascular Surgery* **19**:206–216

Rodgers H, Oliver SE, Dobson R et al. (2000). A regional collaborative audit of the practice and outcome of carotid endarterectomy in the United Kingdom. Northern Regional

Carotid Endarterectomy Audit Group. *European Journal of Vascular Endovascular Surgery* **19**:362–369

Rothwell PM (2004). ACST: Which subgroups will benefit most from carotid endarterectomy? *Lancet* **364**:1122–1123

Rothwell PM (2005). Risk modelling to identify patients with symptomatic carotid stenosis most at risk of stroke. *Neurology Research* **27**(Suppl 1): S18–S28

Rothwell PM, Gibson RJ, Slattery J et al. (1994). Equivalence of measurements of carotid stenosis: A comparison of three methods on 1001 angiograms. *Stroke* **25**:2435–2439

Rothwell PM, Slattery J, Warlow CP (1996). A systematic comparison of the risk of stroke and death due to carotid endarterectomy for symptomatic and asymptomatic stenosis. *Stroke* **27**:266–269

Rothwell PM, Slattery J, Warlow CP (1997). Clinical and angiographic predictors of stroke and death from carotid endarterectomy: Systematic review. *British Medical Journal* **315**:1571–1577

Rothwell PM, Warlow CP on behalf of the European Carotid Surgery Trialists' Collaborative Group (1999a). Interpretation of operative risks of individual surgeons. *Lancet* **353**:1325

Rothwell PM, Warlow CP on behalf of the European Carotid Surgery Trialists' Collaborative Group (1999b). Prediction of benefit from carotid endarterectomy in individual patients: A risk modelling study. *Lancet* **353**:2105–2110

Rothwell PM, Warlow CP on behalf of the European Carotid Surgery Trialists' Collaborative Group (2000a). Low risk of ischaemic stroke in patients with reduced internal carotid artery lumen diameter distal to severe symptomatic carotid stenosis. *Stroke* **31**:622–630

Rothwell PM, Gibson R, Warlow CP on behalf of the European Carotid Surgery Trialists' Collaborative Group (2000b). Interrelation between plaque surface morphology and degree of stenosis on carotid angiograms and the risk of ischaemic stroke in patients with symptomatic carotid stenosis. *Stroke* **31**:615–621

Rothwell PM, Pendlebury ST, Wardlaw J et al. (2000c). Critical appraisal of the design and reporting of studies of imaging and measurement of carotid stenosis. *Stroke* **31**:1444–1450

Rothwell PM, Gutnikov SA, Warlow CP for the ECST (2003a). Re-analysis of the final results of the European Carotid Surgery Trial. *Stroke* **34**:514–523

Rothwell PM, Gutnikov SA, Eliasziw M et al. for the Carotid Endarterectomy Trialists' Collaboration (2003b). Pooled analysis of individual patient data from randomised controlled trials of endarterectomy for symptomatic carotid stenosis. *Lancet* **361**:107–116

Rothwell PM, Eliasziw M, Gutnikov SA for the Carotid Endarterectomy Trialists Collaboration (2004a). Effect of endarterectomy for symptomatic carotid stenosis in relation to clinical subgroups and to the timing of surgery. *Lancet* **363**:915–924

Rothwell PM, Gutnikov SA, Eliasziw M et al. (2004b). Sex difference in effect of time from symptoms to surgery on benefit from endarterectomy for transient ischaemic attack and non-disabling stroke. *Stroke* **35**:2855–2861

Rothwell PM, Mehta Z, Howard SC et al. (2005). From subgroups to individuals: General principles and the example of carotid endartectomy. *Lancet* **365**: 256–265

Smurawska LT, Bowyer B, Rowed D et al. (1998). Changing practice and costs of carotid endarterectomy in Toronto, Canada. *Stroke* **29**:2014–2017

Sundt TM, Sandok BA, Whisnant JP (1975). Carotid endarterectomy. Complications and preoperative assessment of risk. *Mayo Clinic Proceedings* **50**:301–306

Terent A, Marke LA, Asplund K et al. (1994). Costs of stroke in Sweden. A national perspective. *Stroke* **25**:2363–2369

Turnbull RG, Taylor DC, Hsiang YN *et al.* (2000). Assessment of patient waiting times for vascular surgery. *Canadian Journal of Surgery* **43**:105–111

Welsh S, Mead G, Chant H *et al.* (2004). Early carotid surgery in acute stroke: A multicentre randomized pilot study. *Cerebrovascular Disease* **18**:200–205

Intervention for Asymptomatic Carotid Stenosis

Although asymptomatic carotid stenosis can be identified during screening programs of apparently healthy people (i.e., in a primary prevention setting); it is also often identified in a secondary prevention setting, such as when a carotid bruit is heard in patients with angina, claudication, or non-focal neurological symptoms; when bilateral carotid imaging is done in patients with unilateral carotid symptoms (i.e., the patient is symptomatic but one carotid artery is asymptomatic); and when patients are being assessed for major surgery below the neck.

When asymptomatic carotid stenosis is discovered, four questions arise.

• What is the risk of operating?
• What is the risk (of stroke) if the stenosis is left unoperated?
• Does surgery reduce the risk of stroke?
• What is the balance of immediate surgical risk versus long-term benefit?

The answers to these questions are different for asymptomatic carotid stenosis than for symptomatic stenosis because the risk of stroke on medical treatment alone is lower distal to an asymptomatic stenosis (Fig. 28.1).

Is There Evidence of Benefit from Surgery or Stenting?

For many years, guidelines have recommended carotid endarterectomy or carotid artery stenting for patients of average surgical risk with ~50–99% asymptomatic

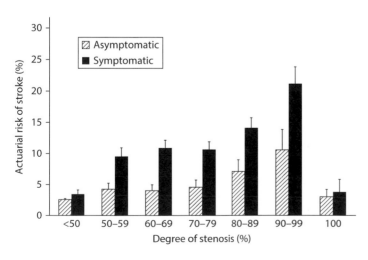

Fig. 28.1 The 3-year risk of carotid territory ipsilateral ischemic stroke distal to symptomatic carotid stenosis versus that distal to contralateral asymptomatic carotid stenosis in patients with a recent transient ischemic attack or ischemic stroke in the Carotid Endarterectomy Trialists' Collaboration (PM Rothwell, unpublished data).

carotid artery stenosis or carotid artery stenting in patients of high surgical risk due to comorbidities or vascular anatomy (Abbott *et al.* 2015). These guidelines were based predominantly on three large multicenter randomized trials in patients with asymptomatic ≥ 60% carotid artery stenosis – the Asymptomatic Carotid Atherosclerosis Study (ACAS), Asymptomatic Carotid Surgery Trial (ACST), and Carotid Revascularization Endarterectomy versus Stenting Trial (CREST) (Executive Committee for the Asymptomatic Carotid Atherosclerosis Study 1995; Halliday *et al.* 2004, 2010; Brott *et al.* 2010, 2016).

The ACAS was performed between 1987 and 1993 and randomized 1,662 subjects with ≥ 60% asymptomatic carotid artery stenosis to either carotid endarterectomy with optimal medical treatment or optimal medical treatment alone (Executive Committee for the Asymptomatic Carotid Atherosclerosis Study 1995). All subjects received aspirin. The ACAS reported a 47% relative reduction in the risk of ipsilateral stroke and perioperative death in the surgical arm despite a 5-year risk of ipsilateral stroke without the operation of only 11%. However, even in this optimal trial environment, the absolute reduction in risk of stroke with endarterectomy was only about 1% per year. In addition, the very low operative risks in ACAS may not be matched in routine clinical practice. This study only accepted surgeons with an excellent safety record, rejecting 40% of initial applicants and subsequently barring from further participation some surgeons who had adverse operative outcomes during the trial (Moore *et al.* 1996).

ACST was a more pragmatic trial and probably produced more widely generalizable results (Halliday *et al.* 2004). Between 1993 and 2003, ACST randomized 3,120 patients with ≥ 60% mainly asymptomatic carotid stenosis (12% had symptoms at least 6 months previously) to immediate endarterectomy plus medical treatment versus medical treatment alone or until the operation became necessary. Surgeons were required to provide evidence of an operative risk of 6% or less for their last 50 patients having an endarterectomy for asymptomatic stenosis, but none was excluded on the basis of his/her operative risk during the trial. Selection of patients was based on the "uncertainty principle" with very few exclusion criteria.

Despite the differences in methods of ACST and ACAS, the absolute reductions in 5-year risk of stroke with surgery were similar: 5.3% (95% confidence interval [CI], 3.0–7.8) and 5.1% (95% CI, 0.9–9.1), respectively. Absolute reduction in 10-year risk of stroke or perioperative death with surgery was also reported in ACST to be 4.6% (95% CI, 1.2–7.9) (Halliday *et al.* 2010). In addition, whereas ACAS had reported only a nonsignificant 2.7% reduction ($p = 0.26$) in the absolute risk of disabling or fatal stroke with surgery, ACST reported a significant 2.5% (95% CI, 0.8–4.3; $p = 0.004$) absolute reduction, although the number needed to treat to prevent one disabling or fatal stroke after 5 years remained about 40. The main differences between the trials were in the 30-day operative risks of death (0.14% [95% CI, 0–0.4] in ACAS and 1.11% [95% CI, 0.6–1.8] in ACST; $p = 0.02$) and in the combined operative risk of stroke and death (1.5% [95% CI, 0.6–2.4] in ACAS and 3.0% [95% CI, 2.1–4.0] in ACST; $p = 0.04$).

In CREST, 1,181 patients with asymptomatic carotid artery stenosis were randomized to either carotid endarterectomy or carotid artery stenting (Brott *et al.* 2010, 2016). During the 10-year study period, 9.9% (95% CI, 7.9–12.2) of patients randomized to receive endarterectomy developed a periprocedural vascular event or death or post-procedural ipsilateral stroke compared with 11.8% (95% CI, 9.1–14.8) of patients randomized to receiving carotid artery stenting ($p = 0.51$) (Brott *et al.* 2016).

Selection of Patients for Endarterectomy for Asymptomatic Stenosis

The decision to perform carotid endarterectomy or stenting for asymptomatic stenosis should not be taken lightly, given the inevitable anxiety and procedural risks faced by the patient. If the procedural risk of stroke is, say, 4% in routine clinical practice, the risk of stroke on intensive medical treatment alone is 10% after 5 years (based on ACAS and ACST), and successful surgery reduces this risk of stroke to almost zero, then doing about 100 operations would cause 4 strokes and avoid up to 10. To maximize cost-effectiveness, it is essential that we know who is at highest risk of surgical stroke and who will survive to be at highest risk of ipsilateral ischemic stroke if surgery is not done. Furthermore, given the high cost of intervention for symptomatic carotid stenosis (Benade and Warlow 2002a, b), we need to be aware of the health-economic and public health issues related to intervention for asymptomatic stenosis.

It should be noted, however, that risk estimates of stroke in patients with asymptomatic carotid stenosis on best medical treatment were based on subjects that were managed during the period 1983–2003 (Executive Committee for the Asymptomatic Carotid Atherosclerosis Study 1995; Halliday *et al.* 2004). Since then, patients with asymptomatic carotid artery stenosis have been much more aggressively managed with more liberal use of antiplatelet agents, statins, and perhaps anti-hypertensive agents as well. Data from the Oxford Vascular Study subsequently revealed a much lower risk of stroke in patients with asymptomatic carotid artery stenosis (Marquardt *et al.* 2010). In 1,153 consecutively imaged patients presenting with stroke or TIA during 2002–2009, 101 had ≥ 50% asymptomatic stenosis (mean age 75 years). More than 95% of all subjects were prescribed with an antiplatelet agent or oral anticoagulant, > 85% were on a statin, and > 80% were on one or more anti-hypertensive agents. During a mean 3-year follow-up, there were only six ischemic events in the territory of an asymptomatic stenosis (one minor stroke and five TIAs). The average annual event rates on medical treatment were 0.34% (95% CI, 0.01–1.87) for any ispsilateral ischemic stroke and 0% (95% CI, 0.00–0.99) for a disabling ipsilateral stroke (Marquardt *et al.* 2010). Similar annual stroke rates of ~0.4% were noted in other cohorts (den Hartog *et al.* 2013). In other words, the 5-year risk of ipsilateral TIA or stroke in patients with asymptomatic carotid stenosis managed with intensive contemporary medical treatment is much lower compared with those noted in ACAS or ACST and estimated to be ~1.7–2%.

Risk of Carotid Endarterectomy for Asymptomatic Carotid Stenosis

There are a large number of case series with very different reported surgical stroke risks, for the same reasons as in symptomatic carotid stenosis (Chapter 27). Overall, the risk is about half that for symptomatic carotid stenosis (Rothwell *et al.* 1996; Bond *et al.* 2003a), but the risk may not necessarily be low in all patients – for example, patients with angina whose carotid stenosis was discovered during preparation for coronary artery surgery or patients who have already had an endarterectomy on one side and are at risk of bilateral vagal or hypoglossal nerve palsies if both sides are operated on.

As for symptomatic stenosis, the risk of surgery cannot be generalized from the literature to one's own institution, a risk that should be known locally. For example, ACAS reported an operative mortality of 0.14% and a risk of stroke and death of 1.5%. However, a systematic review of all studies published during 1990–2000 inclusive that

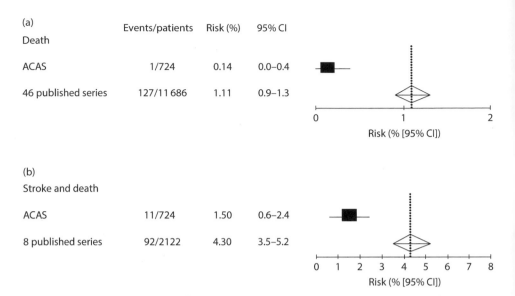

Fig. 28.2 The overall results of a meta-analysis of the operative risk of death (a) and stroke and death (b) from all studies published between 1990 and 2000 inclusive that reported risks from carotid endarterectomy for asymptomatic stenosis (Bond *et al.* 2003a) compared with the same risks in the ACAS Trial (Executive Committee for the Asymptomatic Carotid Atherosclerosis Study 1995). Studies in the analysis of risk of stroke and death are confined to those in which patients were assessed by neurologists. CI, confidence interval; OR, odds ratio.

reported the risks of stroke and death from endarterectomy for asymptomatic stenosis found much higher risks (Bond *et al.* 2003b). The overall risk of stroke and death was 3.0% (95% CI, 2.5–3.5) in 28 studies published post-ACAS (1995–2000). The risk in 12 studies in which outcome was assessed by a neurologist (4.6%; 95% CI, 3.6–5.7) was three times higher than in ACAS (odds ratio [OR], 3.1; 95% CI, 1.7–5.6; $p = 0.0001$). Operative mortality during 1995–2000 (1.1% 95% CI, 0.9–1.4) was eight times higher than in ACAS (OR, 8.1; 95% CI, 1.3–58; $p = 0.01$; Fig. 28.2). In studies that reported outcome after endarterectomy for symptomatic and asymptomatic stenosis in the same institution, operative mortality was no lower for asymptomatic stenosis (OR, 0.80; 95% CI, 0.6–1.1). The proportion of patients operated on for asymptomatic stenosis in these studies increased from 16% during 1990–1994 to 45% during 1995–2000. Therefore, published risks of stroke and death from surgery for asymptomatic stenosis are considerably higher than in ACAS, particularly if outcome was assessed by a neurologist. If operative mortality is eight times higher than in ACAS, then endarterectomy for asymptomatic carotid stenosis in routine clinical practice might even increase population mortality through stroke. Even after community-wide performance measurement and feedback, the overall risk for stroke or death after endarterectomy performed for asymptomatic stenosis in 10 US states was 3.8% (including 1% mortality) (Kresowik *et al.* 2004).

Who Benefits Most from Surgery for Asymptomatic Carotid Stenosis?

Given the surgical risk (which depends on the type of patient under consideration as well as surgical skill), the added risk of any preceding catheter angiography, and what appears to be a remarkably low risk of stroke in unoperated patients (Marquardt *et al.* 2010; den Hartog *et al.* 2013), there is clearly no reason to recommend routine carotid endarterectomy or carotid artery stenting for asymptomatic stenosis. It follows that deliberately screening apparently healthy people for carotid stenosis is unwarranted. A prognostic model (Chapter 14) is required to identify those very few patients whose asymptomatic stenosis is particularly likely to cause stroke to whom surgery may be offered.

Which Range of Stenosis?

Although there is evidence that the risk of ipsilateral ischemic stroke on medical treatment increases with degree of angiographic asymptomatic carotid stenosis (Fig. 28.1), in contrast to trials of endarterectomy in patients with symptomatic carotid stenosis (Chapter 27), neither ACST nor ACAS showed increasing benefit from surgery with increasing degree of stenosis within the 60–99% range. There are several possible explanations for this.

First, ultrasound may be less accurate than catheter angiography in measuring the degree of stenosis. In ACAS, only patients randomized to surgery underwent catheter angiography, and in ACST all imaging was by Doppler ultrasound without any centralized audit (Halliday *et al.* 1994). The importance of the precise methods used to measure stenosis was highlighted in a study of patients randomized to the medical arm of the European Carotid Surgery Trial (ECST), which demonstrated that angiographic measures of stenosis were most reliable in predicting recurrent stroke when selective carotid contrast injections had been given, when biplane views were available, and when the mean of measurements made by two independent observers was used (Cuffe and Rothwell 2006).

Second, patients with carotid near occlusion, which is not readily detectable on ultrasound, were not identified in the randomized trials of endarterectomy for asymptomatic stenosis. In ECST, for example, the proportion of near occlusions was 0.6% at 60–69% stenosis, 2.3% at 70–79% stenosis, 9.2% at 80–89% stenosis, and 29.5% at 90–99% stenosis (Rothwell *et al.* 2000), and only when near occlusions were removed was the increased benefit of endarterectomy with increasing stenosis between 70% and 99% clearly apparent (Rothwell *et al.* 2003). This issue is further complicated by the findings of a study of 1,115 patients with asymptomatic stenosis, in which increasing stenosis on ultrasound was positively associated with risk of ipsilateral hemispheric ischemic events at a mean of 38 months of follow-up when stenosis was measured using ECST criteria but not when North American Symptomatic Carotid Endarterectomy Trial (NASCET) criteria were used (Nicolaides *et al.* 2005).

Third, the rate of stenosis progression may determine the risk of stroke in patients with asymptomatic stenosis, which is potentially very important considering the longer time frame over which strokes occur in patients with asymptomatic compared with symptomatic stenosis. In the ECST, a strong association between the risk of ipsilateral stroke and the degree of carotid stenosis was only seen for strokes that occurred during the first year after randomization, and no relationship was seen between initial stenosis and strokes occurring more than 2 years later (European Carotid Surgery Trialists' Collaborative Group 1998; Rothwell *et al.* 2000). While this could have been partly a consequence of plaque "healing," it is conceivable that in some patients the degree of stenosis had progressed and the rate of this progression, rather than the degree of stenosis at baseline, was the important determinant of stroke risk.

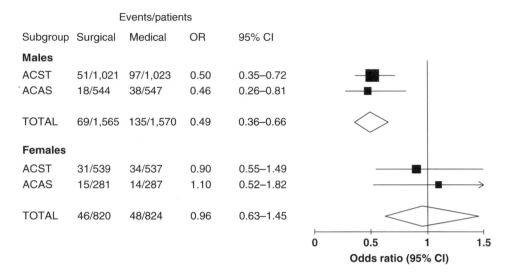

Events/patients

Subgroup	Surgical	Medical	OR	95% CI
Males				
ACST	51/1,021	97/1,023	0.50	0.35–0.72
ACAS	18/544	38/547	0.46	0.26–0.81
TOTAL	69/1,565	135/1,570	0.49	0.36–0.66
Females				
ACST	31/539	34/537	0.90	0.55–1.49
ACAS	15/281	14/287	1.10	0.52–1.82
TOTAL	46/820	48/824	0.96	0.63–1.45

Odds ratio (95% CI)

Fig. 28.3 The effect of endarterectomy for asymptomatic carotid stenosis on the risk of any stroke and operative death by sex (Rothwell 2004) in the Asymptomatic Carotid Surgery Trial (ACST; Halliday *et al.* 2004) and the ACAS Trial (Executive Committee for the Asymptomatic Carotid Atherosclerosis Study 1995). CI, confidence interval; OR, odds ratio.

Which Subgroups Benefit Most?

Although some subgroup analyses were reported in ACAS, the trial had insufficient power to analyze subgroup–treatment effect interactions reliably. Because of its larger sample size, ACST had greater power to evaluate subgroups, although no analyses were prespecified in the trial protocol (Halliday *et al.* 1994). Although ACST did perform some subgroup analyses, the trial only reported results separately for the reduction in risk of non-perioperative stroke (i.e., the benefit) and the perioperative risk (i.e., the harm) (Halliday *et al.* 2004). The overall balance of hazard and benefit, which is of most importance to patients and clinicians, was not reported, although the data could be extracted from the web tables that accompanied the ACST report (Halliday *et al.* 2004).

The ACAS reported a statistically borderline sex–treatment effect interaction, with no benefit from endarterectomy in women (Executive Committee for the Asymptomatic Carotid Atherosclerosis Study 1995). The same trend was seen in ACST (Halliday *et al.* 2004). A meta-analysis of the effect of endarterectomy on the 5-year risk of any stroke and perioperative death in ACAS and ACST (Rothwell 2004) (Fig. 28.3) showed that benefit from surgery was greater in men than in women (pooled interaction, $p = 0.01$). However, 10-year follow-up data from ACST subsequently revealed that a sex–treatment effect interaction was absent and that men and women < 75 years of age both benefited equally from endarterectomy, while no benefit was seen in men or women aged ≥ 75 years (Halliday *et al.* 2010).

In patients with symptomatic 70–99% carotid stenosis, the surgical complication rate is higher in the presence of contralateral occlusion, although the evidence still favors endarterectomy in these patients (Rothwell *et al.* 2004). However, a post-hoc analysis from ACAS found that patients with contralateral occlusion derived no long-term benefit from endarterectomy, largely because of the lower long-term risk on medical treatment (Baker *et al.*

2000), but this analysis was underpowered (163 patients), and there was no significant heterogeneity according to presence of contralateral occlusion in ACST (Halliday *et al.* 2010).

Which Individuals Benefit Most?

Given the small absolute reductions in the risk of stroke with endarterectomy in ACST and ACAS, there is an urgent need to identify which individual patients are at highest risk of stroke and which individuals are at such low risk of stroke that the risks of surgery cannot be justified. A risk-modeling approach similar to that used in symptomatic carotid stenosis is required (Chapters 14 and 27), perhaps combining patient clinical features with the results of potentially prognostic investigations, such as transcranial Doppler-detected emboli, impaired cerebral reactivity, the nature of the stenotic plaque on imaging, and the rate of plaque progression.

Rates of microembolic signals detected on transcranial Doppler ultrasound scanning have been shown to provide prognostically useful information (Markus and MacKinnon 2005; Spence *et al.* 2005; Markus *et al.* 2010). The Asymptomatic Carotid Emboli Study (ACES) studied 467 patients with asymptomatic carotid stenosis of at least 70% (Markus *et al.* 2010). Presence of microembolic signals was significantly associated with a higher risk of ipsilateral stroke and TIA at 2 years (hazard ratio 2.54, 95% CI, 1.20–5.36, $p = 0.015$). The absolute annual risk of ipsilateral stroke or TIA at 2 years was 7.13% in patients with embolic signals and 3.04% in those without and for ipsilateral stroke was 3.62% in patients with embolic signals and 0.70% in those without (Markus *et al.* 2010). Detection of asymptomatic embolization on transcranial Doppler ultrasound can hence be used to risk-stratify patients with asymptomatic carotid stenosis and identify individuals at higher risk of stroke and TIA who would more likely benefit from carotid endarterectomy or stenting.

Several observational studies have suggested that increased plaque echolucency (a marker of plaque lipid and hemorrhage content) on ultrasound is associated with higher risks of stroke and TIA distal to a carotid stenosis. A meta-analysis of seven studies (7,557 subjects) with mean follow-up of 3 years identified 23% of subjects to have a positive ultrasound test for echolucency (Gupta *et al.* 2015). A significant positive relationship between predominantly echolucent (compared with predominantly echogenic) plaques with risk of future ipsilateral stroke across all stenosis severities (relative risk 2.31, 95% CI, 1.47–4.63, $p = 0.001$) and in subjects with $\geq$ 50% stenosis (relative risk 2.61, 95% CI, 1.46–4.63, $p = 0.001$) was noted (Gupta *et al.* 2015). Cumulative incidence of ipsilateral stroke in the echolucent plaque group was 5.7% compared with 2.4% in the non-echolucent plaque group (Gupta *et al.* 2015).

Other methods of plaque imaging might also be of prognostic value. In a meta-analysis of nine studies (779 patients) where MRI was used to delineate carotid plaque composition, presence of intraplaque hemorrhage, lipid-rich necrotic core and thinning, or rupture of the fibrous cap were all noted to be significant predictors of subsequent stroke and TIA risk with hazard ratios of 4.59 (95% CI, 2.91–7.24), 3.00 (1.51–5.95), and 5.93 (2.65–13.20), respectively (Gupta *et al.* 2013).

There is also good evidence that inflammation has a causal role in carotid plaque instability (van der Wal *et al.* 1994; Redgrave *et al.* 2006). Visualization of plaque macrophages by MRI after their uptake of ultra-small particles of iron oxide is now possible (Trivedi *et al.* 2004; Tang *et al.* 2006). However, large prospective studies are required to determine whether these imaging characteristics predict the risk of stroke.

Carotid Intervention before or during Coronary Artery Surgery

If patients with recently symptomatic carotid stenosis who also have symptomatic coronary heart disease requiring surgery, it is unclear whether coronary artery bypass (CABG) should be done before the carotid endarterectomy (and risk a stroke during the procedure), after the carotid endarterectomy (and risk cardiac complications during carotid endarterectomy), or simultaneously under the same general anesthetic (and risk both stroke and cardiac complications all at once) (Graor and Hertzer 1988; Akins 1995; Davenport et al. 1995). The apparently high risk of the last option may well be unacceptable, although a small quasi-randomized trial suggests otherwise (Hertzer et al. 1989; Borger et al. 1999).

Although carotid endarterectomy or stenting is increasingly recommended before coronary surgery, there is little evidence to support this practice. In an attempt to determine the role of carotid artery disease in the etiology of stroke after CABG, Naylor et al. (2002) performed a systematic review of published case series. The risk of stroke during the first few weeks after CABG was approximately 2% and remained unchanged from 1970 to 2000. Two-thirds of strokes occurred after day 1, and 23% of patients died. There was no significant carotid disease in 91% of screened CABG patients. Stroke risk was approximately 3% in predominantly asymptomatic patients with a unilateral 50–99% stenosis, 5% in those with bilateral 50–99% stenoses, and 7–11% in patients with carotid occlusion. Significant predictive factors for post-CABG stroke included carotid bruit (OR 3.6, 95% CI 2.8–4.6), prior stroke/TIA (OR, 3.6, 95% CI 2.7–4.9), and severe carotid stenosis/occlusion (OR 4.3, 95% CI 3.2–5.7). However, the systematic review indicated that 50% of stroke sufferers did not have significant carotid disease and 60% of territorial infarctions on CT scan/autopsy could not be attributed to carotid disease alone. Therefore, although carotid disease is an important etiological factor in the pathophysiology of post-CABG stroke, carotid endarterectomy could only ever prevent approximately 40% of procedural strokes at most, even assuming that prophylactic carotid endarterectomy carried no additional risk.

In a subsequent systematic review, Naylor et al. (2003) aimed to determine the overall cardiovascular risk for patients with coronary and carotid artery disease undergoing synchronous CABG and carotid endarterectomy, staged endarterectomy then CABG, and reverse staged CABG then endarterectomy. In a systematic review of 97 published studies following 8,972 staged or synchronous operations, mortality was highest in patients undergoing synchronous endarterectomy plus CABG (4.6%, 95% CI 4.1–5.2). The risk of death or stroke was also highest in patients undergoing this approach (8.7%, 95% CI 7.7–9.8) and lowest following staged endarterectomy then CABG (6.1%, 95% CI 2.9–9.3). The risk of death/stroke or myocardial infarction was 11.5% (95% CI 10.1–12.9) following synchronous procedures. Therefore, approximately 10–12% of patients undergoing staged or synchronous procedures suffer death or major cardiovascular morbidity (stroke, myocardial infarction) within 30 days of surgery.

In summary, the available data suggest that only approximately 40% of strokes complicating CABG could be attributable to ipsilateral carotid artery disease. The rate of death and stroke following staged or synchronous carotid surgery in published series is high, but a large randomized trial is necessary to determine whether a policy of prophylactic carotid endarterectomy or stenting reduces the risk of stroke after cardiac surgery. However, in the absence of any randomized evidence of benefit, the available data do not support a policy of routine intervention for carotid stenosis in patients undergoing CABG (Naylor, 2004).

References

Abbott AL, Paraskevas KI, Kakkos SK et al. (2015). Systematic review of guidelines for the management of asymptomatic and symptomatic carotid stenosis. Stroke 46:3288–3301

Akins CW (1995). The case for concomitant carotid and coronary artery surgery. British Heart Journal 74:97–98

Baker WH, Howard VJ, Howard G et al. (2000). Effect of contralateral occlusion on long-term efficacy of endarterectomy in the asymptomatic carotid atherosclerosis study (ACAS). ACAS Investigators. Stroke 31:2330–2334

Benade MM, Warlow CP (2002a). Cost of identifying patients for carotid endarterectomy. Stroke 33:435–439

Benade MM, Warlow CP (2002b). Costs and benefits of carotid endarterectomy and associated preoperative arterial imaging: A systematic review of health economic literature. Stroke 33:629–638

Bond R, Rerkasem K, Rothwell PM (2003a). A systematic review of the risks of carotid endarterectomy in relation to the clinical indication and the timing of surgery. Stroke 34:2290–2301

Bond R, Rerkasem K, Rothwell PM (2003b). High morbidity due to endarterectomy for asymptomatic carotid stenosis. Cerebrovascular Diseases 16(Suppl 4):65

Borger MA, Fremes SE, Weisel RD et al. (1999). Coronary bypass and carotid endartertomy: A combined approach increases risk? A meta-analysis. Annals of Thoracic Surgery 68:14–21

Brott TG, Hobson RW II, Howard G et al. (2010). Stenting versus endarterectomy for treatment of carotid-artery stenosis. New England Journal of Medicine 363:11–23

Brott TG, Howard G, Roubin GS et al. (2016). Long-term results of stenting verus endarterectomy for carotid-artery stenosis. New England Journal of Medicine 374:1021–1031

Cuffe RL, Rothwell PM (2006). Effect of non-optimal imaging on the relationship between the measured degree of symptomatic carotid stenosis and risk of ischemic stroke. Stroke 37:1785–1791

Davenport RJ, Dennis MS, Sandercock PA et al. (1995). How should a patient presenting with unstable angina and a recent stroke be managed? British Medical Journal 310:1449–1452

den Hartog AG, Achterberg S, Moll FL et al. (2013). Asymptomatic carotid artery stenosis and the risk of ischemic stroke according to subtype in patients with clinical manifest arterial disease. Stroke 44:1002–1007

European Carotid Surgery Trialists' Collaborative Group (1998). Randomised trial of endarterectomy for recently symptomatic carotid stenosis: Final results of the MRC European Carotid Surgery Trial (ECST). Lancet 351:1379–1387

Executive Committee for the Asymptomatic Carotid Atherosclerosis Study (1995). Endarterectomy for asymptomatic carotid artery stenosis. Journal of the American Medical Association 273:1421–1428

Graor RA, Hertzer NR (1988). Management of coexistent carotid artery and coronary artery disease. Stroke 19:1441–1443

Gupta A, Baradaran H, Schweitzer AD et al. (2013). Carotid plaque MRI and stroke risk: A systematic review and meta-analysis. Stroke 44:3071–3077

Gupta A, Kesavabhotla K, Baradaran H et al. (2015). Plaque echolucency and stroke risk in asymptomatic carotid stenosis: A systematic review and meta-analysis. Stroke 46:91–97

Halliday AW, Thomas D, Mansfield A (1994). The Asymptomatic Carotid Surgery Trial (ACST). Rationale and design. Steering Committee. European Journal of Vascular Surgery 8:703–710

Halliday A, Mansfield A, Marro J et al. (2004). Prevention of disabling and fatal strokes by successful carotid endarterectomy in patients without recent neurological symptoms: Randomised controlled trial. Lancet 363:1491–1502

Halliday A, Harrison M, Hayter E et al. (2010). 10-year stroke prevention after successful carotid endarterectomy for asymptomatic stenosis (ACST-1): A multicenter randomized trial. Lancet 376:1074–1084

Hertzer NR, Loop FD, Beven EG et al. (1989). Surgical staging for simultaneous coronary and carotid disease: A study including prospective randomisation. *Journal of Vascular Surgery* 9:455–463

Kresowik TF, Bratzler DW, Kresowik RA *et al.* (2004). Multistate improvement in process and outcomes of carotid endarterectomy. *Journal of Vascular Surgery* 39:372–380

Markus HS, MacKinnon A (2005). Asymptomatic embolization detected by Doppler ultrasound predicts stroke risk in symptomatic carotid artery stenosis. *Stroke* 36:971–975

Markus HS, King A, Shipley M *et al.* (2010). Asymptomatic embolization for prediction of stroke in the Asymptomatic Carotid Emboli Study (ACES): A prospective observational study. *Lancet Neurology* 9:663–671

Marquardt L, Geraghty OC, Mehta Z *et al.* (2010). Low risk of ipsilateral stroke in patients with asymptomatic carotid stenosis on best medical treatment: A prospective, population-based study. *Stroke* 41:e11–e17

Moore WS, Young B, Baker WH *et al.* (1996). Surgical results: A justification of the surgeon selection process for the ACAS trial. The ACAS Investigators. *Journal of Vascular Surgery* 23:323–328

Naylor AR (2004). A critical review of the role of carotid disease and the outcomes of staged and synchronous carotid surgery. *Seminars in Cardiothoracic Vascular Anesthesia* 8:37–42

Naylor AR, Mehta Z, Rothwell PM *et al.* (2002). Carotid artery disease and stroke during coronary artery bypass: A critical review of the literature. *European Journal of Vascular Endovascular Surgery* 23:283–294

Naylor AR, Cuffe RL, Rothwell PM *et al.* (2003). A systematic review of outcomes following staged and synchronous carotid endarterectomy and coronary artery bypass. *European Journal of Vascular Endovascular Surgery* 25:380–389

Nicolaides AN, Kakkos SK, Griffin M *et al.* (2005). Severity of asymptomatic carotid stenosis and risk of ipsilateral hemispheric ischaemic events: Results from the ACSRS study. *European Journal of Vascular Endovascular Surgery* 30:275–284

Redgrave JN, Lovett JK, Gallagher PJ *et al.* (2006). Histological assessment of 526 symptomatic carotid plaques in relation to the nature and timing of ischemic symptoms: The Oxford plaque study. *Circulation* 113:2320–2328

Rothwell PM (2004). ACST: Which subgroups will benefit most from carotid endarterectomy? *Lancet* 364:1122–1123

Rothwell PM, Slattery J, Warlow CP (1996). A systematic review of the risk of stroke and death due to carotid endarterectomy. *Stroke* 27:260–265

Rothwell PM, Warlow CP on behalf of the European Carotid Surgery Trialists' Collaborative Group (2000). Low risk of ischaemic stroke in patients with reduced internal carotid artery lumen diameter distal to severe symptomatic carotid stenosis. *Stroke* 31:622–630

Rothwell PM, Gutnikov SA, Eliasziw M for the Carotid Endarterectomy Trialists' Collaboration (2003). Pooled analysis of individual patient data from randomised controlled trials of endarterectomy for symptomatic carotid stenosis. *Lancet* 361:107–116

Rothwell PM, Eliasziw M, Gutnikov SA *et al.* for the Carotid Endarterectomy Trialists Collaboration (2004). Effect of endarterectomy for symptomatic carotid stenosis in relation to clinical subgroups and to the timing of surgery. *Lancet* 363:915–924

Spence JD, Tamayo A, Lownie SP *et al.* (2005). Absence of microemboli on transcranial Doppler identifies low-risk patients with asymptomatic carotid stenosis. *Stroke* 36:2373–2378

Tang T, Howarth SP, Miller SR *et al.* (2006). Assessment of inflammatory burden contralateral to the symptomatic carotid stenosis using high-resolution ultrasmall, superparamagnetic iron oxide-enhanced MRI. *Stroke* 37:2266–2270

Trivedi RA, King-Im JM, Graves MJ *et al.* (2004). In vivo detection of macrophages in human carotid atheroma: Temporal dependence of ultrasmall superparamagnetic particles of iron oxide-enhanced MRI. *Stroke* 35:1631–1635

van der Wal AC, Becker AE, van der Loos CM *et al.* (1994). Site of intimal rupture or erosion of thrombosed coronary atherosclerotic plaques is characterized by an inflammatory process irrespective of the dominant plaque morphology. *Circulation* 89:36–44

Cerebral Venous Thrombosis

Thrombosis in the dural sinuses or cerebral veins is much less common than cerebral arterial thromboembolism and accounts for 0.5% of all strokes (Bousser and Ferro 2007). Although previous studies have estimated the incidence of cerebral venous thrombosis to be between two to five cases per million population per year (Stam 2005; Bousser and Ferro 2007), recent studies have reported a much higher incidence at 13 to 16 cases per million population per year (Coutinho *et al.* 2012; Devasagayam *et al.* 2016), possibly due to more accurate coding and advances in neuroimaging.

The median age of onset is approximately 37 years (Ferro *et al.* 2004). It causes a variety of clinical syndromes that often do not resemble stroke (Bousser and Ferro 2007). While arterial ischemic stroke and cerebral venous thrombosis share some causes (Southwick *et al.* 1986), others are specific to cerebral venous thrombosis (Table 29.1). A particularly high index of suspicion is required in women on the oral contraceptive pill (especially those who are obese) (Saadatnia and Tajmirriahi 2007; Zuurbier *et al.* 2016), and in the puerperium. Cerebral venous thrombosis is typically multifactorial. Approximately 45% of cases have more than one cause or predisposing factor, the most common of which include genetic or acquired thrombophilias, pregnancy and puerperium, oral contraceptives, parameningeal infections, hematological disorders, and malignancy (Ferro *et al.* 2004). No cause is found in around 12.5% of cases (Ferro *et al.* 2004).

Clinical Features

In cerebral venous thrombosis, the superior sagittal sinus (Fig. 29.1) and the transverse sinuses are those most commonly affected. These are followed by the straight sinuses and the cavernous sinuses (Stam 2005; Girot *et al.* 2007) (see Fig. 4.4 [p. 58] for anatomy). Thrombosis of the galenic system or isolated involvement of the cortical veins is infrequent. Cerebral sinus thrombosis causes a rise in venous pressure, leading to venous distension and edema. This is often accompanied by raised intracranial pressure secondary to impaired absorption of cerebrospinal fluid, since the dural sinuses contain most of the arachnoid villi and granulations in which cerebrospinal fluid absorption takes place. Occlusion of one of the larger venous sinuses is not likely to cause localized tissue damage unless there is involvement of cortical veins or the galenic venous system, since alternative drainage routes will suffice. Thrombosis in cerebral veins, with or without dural sinus thrombosis, causes multiple "venous" infarcts, which are congested, edematous, and often hemorrhagic. Subarachnoid bleeding may occur. Transient neurological deficits may be caused by temporary ischemia and edema.

The incidence of cerebral venous thrombosis is uncertain since it has a wide range of clinical manifestations (Bousser and Ferro 2007), which may sometimes be obscured by the

Table 29.1 Causes of intracranial venous thrombosis

Disorder	Examples
Conditions affecting the cerebral veins and sinuses directly	Infection – bacterial meningitis, subdural empyema, local sepsis (sinus, ears, mastoid, nasopharynx) Tumor invasion of dural sinus (malignant meningitis, lymphoma, skull base secondary, etc.) Trauma – lumbar puncture, cranial trauma, jugular venous catheterization, neurosurgical procedures Dural arteriovenous fistula
Systemic disorders	Genetic and acquired thrombophilias – deficiencies of antithrombin, protein C and protein S; Factor V Leidin mutation; prothrombin gene mutation 20210; antiphospholipid syndrome; hyperhomocysteinemia; nephrotic syndrome Obesity Pregnancy and the puerperium Hematological disorders – anemia, polycythemia, essential thrombocytosis, paroxysmal nocturnal hemoglobinuria Non-metastatic effect of extracranial malignancy Chronic inflammatory disorders – vasculitis, inflammatory bowel disease Drugs, e.g., oral contraceptives, hormone replacement therapy, steroid, chemotherapy (e.g., tamoxifen, L-asparginase) Dehydration

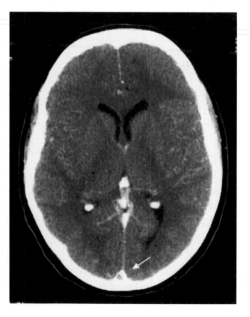

Fig. 29.1 A CT brain scan from a young woman with superior sagittal sinus thrombosis showing the "empty delta sign" – a triangular pattern of enhancement surrounding a central relatively hypodense area of thrombosis (arrow).

BOX 29.1 Clinical Features of Cerebral Venous Thrombosis

Headache

Seizure

Reduced conscious level

Focal neurological deficit

Cranial nerve palsies

Features of raised intracranial pressure:

- papilledema.
- vomiting.

underlying disease process, such as meningitis. It may be asymptomatic, and diagnosis depends on access to cerebral imaging. Cerebral venous thrombosis should be suspected when a patient develops signs of raised intracranial pressure with or without focal neurological deficits, papilledema, and seizures, particularly when the CT brain scan is normal (Box 29.1). Headache, which is often the presenting complaint, is present in nearly 90% of those affected. It is typically diffuse and often progresses in severity over days to weeks. A minority of patients may present with a thunderclap headache. Papilledema occurs in approximately 30% and visual loss in about 15%. Seizures occur in approximately 40%, focal deficits in 20%, and alterations in consciousness in about 15%. Isolated cranial nerve palsies have been described with transverse sinus thrombosis (Kuehnen *et al.* 1998). Cerebral venous thrombosis may be the underlying cause in patients with features suggestive of diffuse encephalopathy, stroke, and, rarely, subarachnoid hemorrhage (de Bruijn *et al.* 1996), psychosis, or migraine (Jacobs *et al.* 1996). It should be considered in all cases of apparent idiopathic intracranial hypertension, particularly when the patient is male or a non-obese female (Tehindrazanarivelo *et al.* 1992).

The progression of symptoms and signs in cerebral venous thrombosis is highly variable, ranging from less than 48 hours to greater than 30 days. A gradual onset over days or weeks of headache, papilledema, and, less frequently, cranial nerve VI palsy, tinnitus, and transient visual obscurations may occur. The prognosis of cerebral venous thrombosis is also variable and difficult to predict for an individual patient: A comatose patient may go on to make a complete recovery, whereas a patient with few signs may gradually deteriorate and die. The current 30-day mortality rate is 5–6% (Dentali *et al.* 2006), which is mainly due to transtentorial herniation secondary to a large hemorrhagic lesion, multiple lesions, or diffuse cerebral edema (Canhao *et al.* 2005). Other causes of death include status epilepticus, medical complications, and pulmonary embolism. Ten percent of patients have permanent neurological deficits at 12 months follow-up (Dentali *et al.* 2006). Independent predictors of death or disability include old age, male sex, coma, mental disturbance, motor disturbances, deep cerebral vein thrombosis, intracerebral hemorrhage, and posterior fossa lesions (Canhao *et al.* 2005; Girot *et al.* 2007).

Cavernous sinus thrombosis is a restricted form of cerebral venous thrombosis, usually associated with sepsis spreading from the veins in the face, nose, orbits, or sinuses (Ebright *et al.* 2001). In diabetics and immunocompromised hosts, fungal infection can be responsible, particularly mucormycosis. The presentation is with unilateral orbital pain, periorbital edema, chemosis, proptosis, reduced visual acuity, and papilledema. Cranial nerves III, IV,

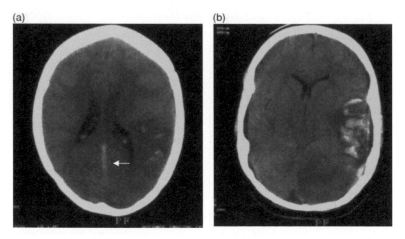

Fig. 29.2 Non-contrast CT brain scans showing fresh thrombus in the straight sinus ("cord sign") (a; arrow) and a hemorrhagic left temporal lobe infarct (b).

and VI and the upper two divisions of V may be involved. Thrombus may propagate to the other cavernous sinus to cause bilateral signs. Septic meningitis and epidural empyema are occasional complications. The patients are generally severely toxic and ill. The differential diagnosis includes severe facial and orbital infection and caroticocavernous fistula.

Diagnosis

Headache, papilledema, and a normal computed tomography (CT) scan should raise the possibility of cerebral venous thrombosis. Often cerebral venous thrombosis is not considered until other diagnoses have been excluded, particularly when the presentation is atypical. However, it is not a diagnosis of exclusion – it must be confirmed on imaging.

A non-contrast CT scan has poor sensitivity in detecting cerebral venous thrombosis and is abnormal in only ~ 30% of cases (Saposnik *et al.* 2011). In these instances, the acutely thrombosed cortical veins or dural sinuses may appear hyperdense relative to the gray matter. Two signs that may be encountered include the "filled delta sign," which is a dense triangle as a result of thrombosis within the posterior superior saggital sinus, and the "cord sign," which refers to a cord-like hyper-attenuation seen on a single slice in which fresh thrombus appears as increased density relative to gray matter in structures parallel to the scanning plane such as the straight sinus (Fig. 29.2) (Saposnik *et al.* 2011). Venous infarcts, with or without hemorrhagic transformation and cerebral edema, may also be present (Saposnik *et al.* 2011). Compared with arterial strokes, venous infarcts cross the arterial boundary and are often in close proximity to a venous sinus. Small non-traumatic juxta-cortical hemorrhages are also specific features of cerebral venous thrombosis, in particular those involving the superior sagittal sinus, and are rarely encountered in other conditions (Coutinho *et al.* 2014). Sometimes there is subarachnoid blood, which is most unusual following either arterial infarcts or primary intracerebral hemorrhage (Bakac and Wardlaw 1997).

Contrast-enhanced CT and CT venography provides up to 95% sensitivity and 91% specificity (as compared with digital subtraction angiography) for detection of cerebral

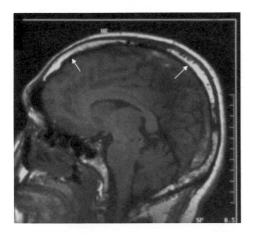

Fig. 29.3 Saggital T_1-weighted MRI showing hyperintensity in the saggital sinus indicating subacute thrombosis (arrows).

venous thrombosis (Wetzel *et al.* 1999). Filling defects within major venous sinuses may be visualized. In patients with superior sagittal sinus cerebral venous thrombosis, the "empty delta sign" may be present, which is a triangular pattern of enhancement from dilated venous collateral channels surrounding a central relatively hypodense area of thrombus (Fig 29.1). Intense contrast enhancement of the falx and tentorium may also be seen. Although brain CT with contrast is normal in up to 25% of patients with proven cerebral venous thrombosis, it is an appropriate first-line investigation, particularly in sick patients in whom magnetic resonance imaging (MRI) is difficult to undertake. Disadvantages of CT, however, include exposure to ionizing radiation, risk of contrast reactions or iodinated contrast nephropathy, and poor detection of deep venous thrombosis (Saposnik *et al.* 2011).

MRI and MR venography have greater sensitivity than CT for detecting changes due to cerebral venous thrombosis, in particular relating to pathologies involving the superficial and deep venous systems (Ferro *et al.* 2007, Saposnik *et al.* 2011). In the acute phase, at less than 7 days, the thrombus is isointense on T_1 and hypointense on T_2-weighted sequences due to increased deoxyhemoglobin. Subsequently, the thrombus becomes hyperintense due to methemoglobin (Fig. 29.3). After 2 to 3 weeks, findings depend on whether the sinus remains occluded or whether it is partly or completely recanalized. Hemosiderin-sensitive sequences such as T_2 gradient echo or susceptibility-weighted images may also help improve the accuracy of diagnosing cerebral venous thrombosis as thrombosed dural sinuses or veins would be of low signal in these sequences (Selim *et al.* 2002)

The imaging changes in patients with deep cerebral venous thrombosis are particularly striking, with bilateral deep hemorrhagic infarction (Fig. 29.4). MRI and MR venography can now provide a definitive diagnosis in most patients, although care must be taken to exclude artifacts.

Cerebral angiography or direct cerebral venography with late venous views is the "gold standard" for the diagnosis of cerebral venous thrombosis. Nowadays, this should only be performed in cases where the diagnosis remains in doubt after CT or MRI. There should be total or partial occlusion of at least one dural sinus on two projections. Often, there is also occlusion of cerebral veins, late venous emptying, and evidence of venous collateral circulation. In subacute encephalopathies of uncertain cause, cerebral angiography or MR

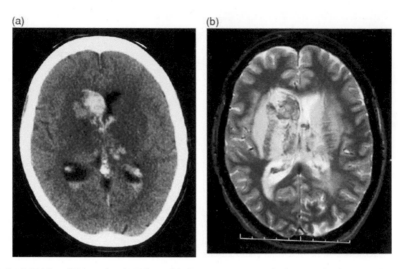

Fig. 29.4 Axial CT (a) and T_2-weighted MR brain (b) slices in a patient with deep cerebral venous thrombosis with bilateral deep hemorrhagic infarction.

venography should always be carried out to exclude cerebral venous thrombosis before resorting to brain biopsy.

In view of the high frequency of thrombophilias among patients who develop cerebral venous thrombosis, screening for hypercoagulable conditions should be performed (Piazza 2012). Serum D-dimer levels, which are a product of fibrin degradation, may be elevated in patients with cerebral venous thrombosis. However, caution needs to be exercised in patients presenting with isolated headache as the false negative rate of D-dimer is particularly high (Crassard *et al.* 2005). D-dimer levels also decline with time from onset of symptoms, and hence patients with subacute or chronic symptoms are more likely to have negative D-dimer levels (Kosinski *et al.* 2004). Patients with a less severe cerebral venous thrombosis may also have a false negative D-dimer result (Kosinski *et al.* 2004). Hence, if there is a strong suspicion of cerebral venous thrombosis, a negative D-dimer level should not preclude further investigations (Saposnik *et al.* 2011).

Cerebrospinal fluid is often abnormal in cerebral venous thrombosis: The pressure is usually raised, and there may be elevated protein and pleocytosis, especially in patients with focal signs. Lumbar puncture may be indicated in patients with isolated intracranial hypertension in order to lower cerebrospinal fluid pressure when vision is threatened and to exclude meningeal infection.

The electroencephalogram is abnormal in approximately 75% of patients with cerebral venous thrombosis, but findings are nonspecific, e.g., generalized slowing (often asymmetrical) with superimposed epileptic activity.

Treatment

The general principles of stroke treatment apply. Current guidelines recommend initial anticoagulation with adjusted-dose unfractionated heparin or low-molecular-weight heparin followed by vitamin K antagonists (target international normalized ratio 2–3), regardless of presence of intracerebral hemorrhage (Saposnik *et al.* 2011). These have been supported by studies that have shown a reduction in poor outcome in patients with cerebral venous thrombosis who have been anticoagulated versus patients who were assigned a placebo. Although it may be difficult to accept for some to use anticoagulation in the presence of preexisting venous infarcts that may have been complicated with hemorrhage, use of anticoagulation appears to improve venous outflow obstruction and hence decreases venular and capillary pressure, all in all reducing the risk of further hemorrhage (Piazza 2012). The duration of anticoagulation for patients with provoked cerebral venous thrombosis is suggested to be 3–6 months and 6–12 months for unprovoked cases (Piazza 2012). Patients with recurrent cerebral venous thrombosis, severe thrombophilia, or extracranial thrombosis complicating cerebral venous thrombosis should be considered for lifelong anticoagulation (Piazza 2012). The use of non-vitamin K antagonist oral anticoagulants in patients with cerebral venous thrombosis has not yet been approved, but clinical trials are currently under way. The Thrombolysis Or Anticoagulation for Cerebral Venous Thrombosis (TO-ACT) trial showed that, compared with standard treatment, endovascular therapy does not seem to improve clinical outcome in patients with severe cerebral venous thrombosis (Coutinho *et al.* 2017).

Intracranial hypertension resulting from cerebral venous thrombosis may result in seizures, visual impairment, focal neurological deficits, or even death due to cerebral herniation. Treatments to reduce intracranial pressure include acetazolamide and lumbar puncture (Saposnik *et al.* 2011). A minority of patients may require optic nerve decompression or shunts to preserve optic nerve function (Saposnik *et al.* 2011). Those who have progressive neurological deterioration due to a severe mass effect may require decompressive hemicraniectomy (Saposnik *et al.* 2011; Aaron *et al.* 2013; Ferro *et al.* 2017). Steroids are not recommended, as they have been shown to enhance hypercoaguloability and increase the risk of death and dependence (Saposnik *et al.* 2011, Ferro *et al.* 2017). In patients who develop seizures, early use of anti-epileptic medications is recommended to prevent recurrent seizures (Saposnik *et al.* 2011; Ferro *et al.* 2017). However, in the absence of seizures, the routine use of anti-epileptic medications is not recommended (Saposnik *et al.* 2011).

An underlying cause resulting in the cerebral venous thrombosis should be addressed. The cumulative venous thrombosis recurrence rate is estimated to be approximately 18% at 10 years (Palazzo *et al.* 2017). Patients with a previous venous thrombotic event, history of malignancy, or cerebral venous thrombosis due to an unknown cause are at a higher risk of recurrence (Palazzo *et al.* 2017). Women who develop cerebral venous thrombosis during pregnancy or during the postpartum period are also at an increased risk of recurrent venous thrombotic events during subsequent pregnancies (de Sousa *et al.* 2016). Prophylactic anticoagulation with low-molecular-weight heparin in future pregnancies and the postpartum period is recommended (Saposnik *et al.* 2011), and rate of miscarriage is not significantly different from that of the general population (de Sousa *et al.* 2016). As for those who develop cerebral venous thrombosis while on the combined oral contraceptive pill, alternative non-estrogen-based methods of contraception should be sought.

References

Aaron S, Alexander M, Moorthy RK *et al.* (2013). Decompressive craniectomy in cerebral venous thrombosis: A single center experience. *Journal of Neurology, Neurosurgery and Psychiatry* **84**:995–1000

Bakac G, Wardlaw JM (1997). Problems in the diagnosis of intracranial venous infarction. *Neuroradiology* **39**:566–570

Bousser MG, Ferro JM (2007). Cerebral venous thrombosis: An update. *Lancet Neurology* **6**:162–170

Canhao P, Ferro JM, Lindgren AG *et al.* (2005). Causes and predictors of death in cerebral venous thrombosis. *Stroke* **36**:1720–1725

Coutinho JM, Zuurbier SM, Aramideh M *et al.* (2012). The incidence of cerebral venous thrombosis: A cross-sectional study. *Stroke* **43**:3375–3377

Coutinho JM, van den Berg R, Zuurbier SM *et al.* (2014). Small juxtacortical hemorrhages in cerebral venous thrombosis. *Annals of Neurology* **75**:908–916

Coutinho J, Ferro J, Zuurbier S *et al.* (2017). Thrombolysis or Anticoagulation for Cerebral Venous Thrombosis (TO-ACT): A randomized controlled trial. *European Stroke Journal* **2** (IS):479

Crassard I, Soria C, Tzourio C *et al.* (2005). A negative D-dimer assay does not rule out cerebral venous thrombosis: A series of seventy-three patients. *Stroke* **36**:1716–1719

de Bruijn SFTM, Stam J, Kappelle LJ (1996). Thunderclap headache as first symptom of cerebral venous sinus thrombosis. *Lancet* **348**:1623–1625

de Sousa DA, Canhao P, Ferro JM (2016). Safety of pregnancy after cerebral venous thrombosis: A systematic review. *Stroke* **47**:713–718

Dentali F, Gianni M, Crowther MA *et al.* (2006). Natural history of cerebral vein thrombosis: A systematic review. *Blood* **108**:1129–1134

Devasagayam S, Wyatt B, Leyden J *et al.* (2016). Cerebral venous sinus thrombosis incidence is higher than previously thought: A retrospective population-based study. *Stroke* **47**:2180–2182

Ebright JR, Pace MT, Niazi AF (2001). Septic thrombosis of the cavernous sinuses. *Archives of Internal Medicine* **161**:2671–2676

Ferro JM, Canhao P, Stam J *et al.* (2004). Prognosis of cerebral vein and dural sinus thrombosis: Results from the International Study on Cerebral Vein and Dural Sinus Thrombosis (ISCVT). *Stroke* **35**:664–670

Ferro JM, Morgado C, Sousa R *et al.* (2007). Interobserver agreement in the magnetic resonance location of cerebral vein and dural sinus thrombosis. *European Journal of Neurology* **14**:353–356

Ferro JM, Bousser MG, Canhão *et al.* (2017). European Stroke Organization guideline for the diagnosis and treatment of cerebral venous thrombosis – Endorsed by the European Academy of Neurology. *European Stroke Journal* **2**:195–221

Girot M, Ferro JM, Canhao P *et al.* (2007). Predictors of outcome in patients with cerebral venous thrombosis and intracerebral hemorrhage. *Stroke* **38**:337–342

Jacobs K, Moulin T, Bogousslavsky J *et al.* (1996). The stroke syndrome of cortical vein thrombosis. *Neurology* **47**:376–382

Kosinski CM, Mull M, Schwarz M *et al.* (2004). Do normal D-dimer levels reliably exclude cerebral sinus thrombosis? *Stroke* **35**:2820–2825

Kuehnen J, Schwartz A, Neff W *et al.* (1998). Cranial nerve syndrome in thrombosis of the transverse/sigmoid sinuses. *Brain* **121**:381–388

Piazza G (2012). Cerebral venous thrombosis. *Circulation* **125**:1704–1709

Palazzo P, Agius P, Ingrand P *et al.* (2017). Venous thrombotic recurrence after cerebral venous thrombosis: A long-term follow-up study. *Stroke* **48**:321–326

Saadatnia M, Tajmirriahi M (2007). Hormonal contraceptives as a risk factor for cerebral venous and sinus thrombosis. *Acta Neurology Scandinavica* **115**:295–300

Saposnik G, Barinagarrementeria F, Brown RD Jr. *et al.* (2011). Diagnosis and management of cerebral venous thrombosis: A statement for healthcare professionals from the American Heart Association/American Stroke Association. *Stroke* **42**:1158–1192

Selim M, Fink J, Linfante I *et al.* (2002). Diagnosis of cerebral venous thromobosis with echo-planar T_2*-weighted magnetic resonance imaging. *Archives of Neurology* **59**:1021–1026

Southwick FS, Richardson EP, Swartz MN (1986). Septic thrombosis of the dural venous sinuses. *Medicine (Baltimore)* **65**:82–106

Stam J (2005). Thrombosis of the cerebral veins and sinuses. *New England Journal of Medicine* **352**:1791–1798

Tehindrazanarivelo A, Evrard S, Schaison M *et al.* (1992). Prospective study of cerebral sinus venous thrombosis in patients presenting with benign intracranial hypertension. *Cerebrovascular Diseases* **2**:22–27

Wetzel SG, Kirsch E, Stock KW *et al.* (1999). Cerebral veins: Comparative study of CT venography with intraarterial digital subtraction angiography. *American Journal of Neuroradiology* **20**:249–255

Zuurbier SM, Arnold M, Middeldorp S *et al.* (2016). Risk of cerebral venous thrombosis in obese women. *JAMA Neurology* **73**:579–584

Chapter 30

Spontaneous Subarachnoid Hemorrhage

Subarachnoid hemorrhage (SAH) accounts for approximately 5% of all strokes (Feigin *et al.* 2009), but it is relatively more common in younger people than other forms of cerebrovascular disease. Although the prognosis is grave, there has been a fall in mortality over recent decades, which suggests improvements in management of the condition. The presentation is usually dramatic, with sudden-onset severe headache, but diagnostic difficulty may arise in atypical cases or with other conditions that can mimic SAH.

Epidemiology

The incidence of subarachnoid hemorrhage increases with age and is approximately 9 per 100,000 population per annum (de Rooij *et al.* 2007). Nonetheless, about 40% of cases occur in those younger than 55 years (Lovelock *et al.* 2010). Data from the Oxford Community Stroke Project (OCSP), the Oxford Vascular Study (OXVASC), and other population-based studies show that there has been no change in the incidence of SAH since the late 1980s but there has been a fall in mortality by ~0.8% per annum, suggesting improved management of the condition (de Rooij *et al.* 2007; Nieuwkamp *et al.* 2009; Lovelock *et al.* 2010). Risk factors include hypertension, smoking, and heavy alcohol consumption (Andreasen *et al.* 2013). Together, these three factors account for two-thirds of the population-attributable risk of SAH (Andreasen *et al.* 2013). The overall prognosis is poor: Approximately one-quarter of patients die, and one-fifth are left dependent (Nieuwkamp *et al.* 2009; Macdonald and Schweizer 2017). Old age, history of hypertension, worse admission neurological condition, more severe SAH on CT scan, large aneurysm, posterior circulation aneurysm, and aneurysm repair by clipping rather than coiling are all associated with a worse prognosis (Jaja *et al.* 2013; Macdonald and Schweizer 2017). Focal neurological deficits and, more commonly, cognitive deficits, behavioral disorders, seizures, mood disorders, fatigue, sleep disturbances, and poor quality of life are frequent long-term sequelae (Al-Khindi *et al.* 2010). Chronic or repeated subarachnoid bleeding can produce the rare syndrome of superficial hemosiderosis of the central nervous system (CNS), with sensorineural deafness, cerebellar ataxia, pyramidal signs, dementia, and bladder disturbance (Fearnley *et al.* 1995).

Causes

Approximately 85% of spontaneous SAHs are caused by ruptured aneurysm, 10% are perimesencephalic, and the remainder are caused by rare disorders (van Gijn and Rinkel 2001). The pattern of bleeding on CT scan is a clue to the underlying cause. Blood in the interhemispheric fissure suggests an anterior communicating artery aneurysm and in the sylvian fissure suggests internal carotid artery or middle cerebral artery aneurysm (Fig. 30.1).

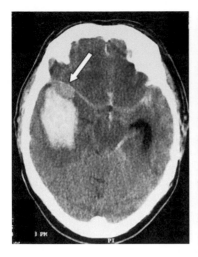 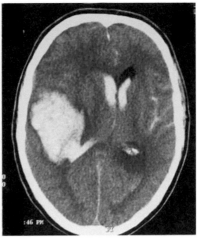

Fig. 30.1 These CT brain scans from a patient with a ruptured right middle cerebral artery aneurysm (arrow) show widespread subarachnoid blood and extension into the right cerebral hemisphere and the ventricular system.

Intracranial aneurysms are not congenital but develop over the course of life. Approximately 10% of aneurysms are familial, and candidate genes identified thus far include those coding for the extracellular matrix. Saccular aneurysms tend to occur at branching points on the circle of Willis and proximal cerebral arteries: approximately 40% on the anterior communicating artery complex, 30% on the posterior communicating artery or distal internal carotid artery, 20% on the middle cerebral artery, and 10% in the posterior circulation (Fig. 30.2). Approximately 25% occur at multiple sites. Aneurysms vary from a few millimeters to several centimeters in diameter and can enlarge with time. The prevalence of unruptured aneurysms is 3.2% (Brown and Broderick 2014), and the average size of a ruptured aneurysm is 6–7 mm (Beck *et al.* 2006).

Aneurysms may present with various clinical features:

- most commonly in middle life with subarachnoid hemorrhage.
- with primary intracerebral hemorrhage.
- with compression of adjacent structures, such as the optic nerve by an anterior communicating artery aneurysm; III, IV, and V cranial nerves by a distal internal carotid artery or posterior communicating artery aneurysm; or brainstem by a basilar artery aneurysm.
- with seizures.
- with TIA or ischemic stroke through embolism of intra-aneurysmal thrombus (Chapters 6, 8, and 9).
- with caroticocavernous fistula from rupture of an intracavernous internal carotid artery aneurysm (Raps *et al.* 1993).

Clinical Features

Subarachnoid hemorrhage may be provoked by exertion and rarely occurs during sleep (Ferro and Pinto 1994; Vermeer *et al.* 1997). The cardinal symptom is sudden severe headache, usually generalized, but other modes of presentation are possible. It is described as of instantaneous onset in about 50% of patients, but it may develop subacutely over 5 minutes or more (Linn *et al.* 1998) and may persist for weeks (Vermeulen *et al.* 1992;

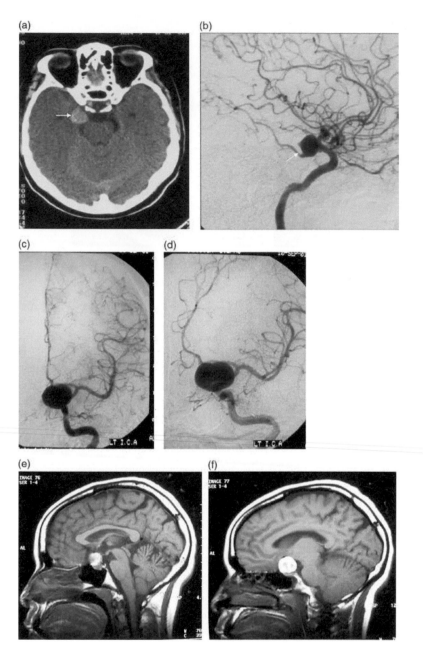

Fig. 30.2 Unruptured aneurysm of posterior communicating artery on CT brain imaging (a) and catheter angiography (b). (c, d) Cerebral angiogram showing a large aneurysm at the origin of the left internal carotid artery. (e, f) Sagittal T1-weighted MRI showing a large thrombosed aneurysm.

Warlow *et al.* 1996a; Schievink 1997). Headaches preceding SAH, thought to be caused by so-called "warning leaks" or "sentinel bleeds", are rare, and overestimation of their importance is likely to have resulted from recall bias in hospital studies. Therefore, the presence or

Table 30.1 World Federation of Neurological Surgeons Scale for grading subarachnoid hemorrhage

Grade	Glasgow Coma Scale	Motor or language deficit
I	15	Absent
II	14–13	Absent
III	14–13	Present
IV	12–7	Present or absent
V	6–3	Present or absent

absence of previous headache has no bearing on the diagnosis of SAH. About a quarter of patients presenting with sudden severe headache will have SAH; a further 40% will have benign thunderclap headache, and about an eighth have some other serious neurological disorder. The remainder have other headache syndromes (Linn *et al.* 1998).

Headache may be the only symptom in SAH, or there may be accompanying symptoms that may also be seen with other causes of sudden-onset headache and so are not diagnostic. Patients are often irritable and photophobic. Loss of consciousness occurs in around half the patients but may only be brief. Nausea and vomiting are less common. Partial or generalized seizures occasionally occur at the onset period; since these do not occur in perimesencephalic hemorrhage or in thunderclap headache, their presence is a strong indicator of aneurysmal rupture (Pinto *et al.* 1996). Early development of focal symptoms and signs suggest:

- an associated intracerebral hematoma.
- local pressure from an aneurysm, such as posterior communicating artery aneurysm causing a third nerve palsy.

Later on, focal symptoms are more likely to result from delayed cerebral ischemia. Meningism develops over a few hours, and pain may radiate down the legs, mimicking sciatica, but neck stiffness may be absent in unconscious patients. Preretinal and subhyaloid hemorrhages occur in a seventh of patients. There may be a mild fever and raised blood pressure and electrocardiographic changes that may be mistaken for myocardial infarction. Cardiac arrest occurs at onset of hemorrhage in approximately 3% of patients, half of whom survive to independent existence with resuscitation (Toussaint *et al.* 2005). Approximately 10% of SAHs results in sudden death, and approximately 15% of patients die before receiving medical attention (Huang and van Gelder 2002). The patient's state can be graded using the World Federation of Neurological Surgeons Scale (Table 30.1).

Diagnosis

Since no clinical feature is specific to SAH, the diagnosis must be excluded in anyone presenting with sudden-onset severe headache (thunderclap headache) lasting more than an hour and for which there is no alternative explanation. However, the differential diagnosis is wide (Table 30.2).

Brain Imaging

Unenhanced CT scan is the quickest, most informative, and most cost-effective confirmatory investigation to detect blood in the subarachnoid space (Warlow *et al.* 1996b). The sensitivity of

Table 30.2 Differential diagnosis of thunderclap headache (Ducros 2012)

Usually detected by non-contrast CT
Subarachnoid hemorrhage
Intracerebral and intraventricular hemorrhage
Acute subdural hematoma
Cerebral infarcts
Tumors (e.g., third ventricle colloid cyst)
Acute obstructive hydrocephalus
Usually detected by analysis of CSF after normal CT
Subarachnoid hemorrhage
Meningitis/encephalitis
Possibly presenting with normal CT results with normal or near-normal CSF
Intracranial venous thrombosis
Carotid or vertebral artery dissection (extra or intracranial)
Reversible cerebral vasoconstriction syndrome
Pituitary apoplexy
Expanding intracranial aneurysm
Intracranial hypotension
Benign headache
Migraine
Postcoital headache

CSF, cerebrospinal fluid; CT, computed tomography.

CT for detecting subarachnoid blood depends on the amount of subarachnoid blood, the interval after symptom onset, the resolution of the scanner, and the skills of the radiologist. In patients who are scanned with a multi-detector CT within 6 hours of thunderclap headache onset and imaging interpreted by qualified radiologists, CT has a sensitivity of 100% in detecting SAH (Perry *et al.* 2011). Scanning with CT misses approximately 2% of SAHs within 12 hours; this rises to 7% at 24 hours, 20% at 3 days, and 50% at 7 days (Suarez *et al.* 2006). Blood is almost completely reabsorbed within 10 days and probably sooner with very mild SAHs (Brouwers *et al.* 1992). A false-positive diagnosis of SAH may be made in diffuse brain swelling when congested subarachnoid blood vessels cause a hyperdense appearance in the subarachnoid space.

Use of CT provides a baseline for the diagnosis of later rebleeding; reveals any intra-cerebral, ventricular, or subdural hematoma or complicating hydrocephalus; and may show calcification in the rim of an aneurysm. The pattern of bleeding may indicate the culprit aneurysm if

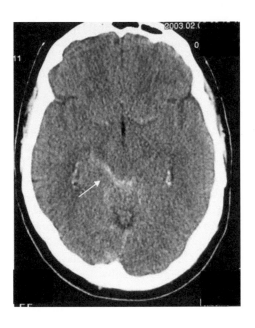

Fig. 30.3 A CT brain scan showing a perimesencephalic subarachnoid hemorrhage with blood in the basal cisterns only (arrow).

multiple aneurysms are found on later angiography (Adams *et al.* 1983; Vermeulen and van Gijn 1990), or it may show benign perimesencephalic hemorrhage (Rinkel *et al.* 1991) (Fig. 30.3). Evidence of primary or secondary head injury – including brain contusion, soft tissue swelling of the scalp, and skull fracture – may be present.

Lumbar Puncture

In patients who present beyond 6 hours of symptoms and have a normal CT, lumbar puncture is recommended (Perry *et al.* 2011; Backes *et al.* 2012). The lumbar puncture should be delayed until at least 12 hours after the onset of the headache, unless CNS infection is suspected, to allow hemoglobin to degrade into oxyhemoglobin and bilirubin (Cruickshank *et al.* 2008; Backes *et al.* 2012). Bilirubin signifies SAH since it is only synthesized in vivo, whereas oxyhemoglobin may result from a traumatic spinal tap. Acutely, the cerebrospinal fluid (CSF) glucose may be low and the protein slightly raised with mild pleocytosis. The presence of "xanthochromia", the yellow bilirubin pigment present in CSF following SAH, may be seen when the CSF is examined with the naked eye against a white background (Linn *et al.* 2005). However, samples of CSF should also be sent for spectrophotometry to detect bilirubin (Cruickshank *et al.* 2008). The least blood-stained sample of CSF should be taken to the laboratory and centrifuged immediately. The sample should be protected from light to prevent degradation of bilirubin. The estimation of red blood cell counts in serial samples does not reliably distinguish SAH from traumatic tap (van Gijn and Rinkel 2001).

Subarachnoid Hemorrhage Presenting More Than Two Weeks after Onset

If CT and CSF examination are normal within 2 weeks of headache onset, then SAH has been excluded. However, since xanthochromia is only detected in 70% of patients after 3 weeks and only 40% after 4 weeks, patients presenting beyond 2 weeks require investigation with CT, MR, or digital subtraction angiography. Hemosiderin-sensitive MRI sequences, such as T2* gradient echo and susceptibility weighted imaging, are also useful in detection of subarachnoid blood in patients who present weeks after a possible SAH (Lummel *et al.* 2015).

Angiography

Once the diagnosis of SAH is confirmed, vascular imaging should be performed to identify the source of bleeding. Vascular imaging could be in the form of CT, MR, or digital subtraction angiography (DSA). While DSA with 3D reconstruction remains the gold standard for identifying the cause of bleeding and for planning treatment, it is invasive and carries a small but potential risk of stroke (0.14%), death (0.06%), and aneurysm rebleeding (Kaufmann *et al.* 2007). Nowadays, multislice CT angiography with or without 3D reconstruction is considered as the first-line imaging modality in patients with SAH due to its high sensitivity (~98%) and specificity (~100%) in detection of intracranial aneurysms (Westerlaan *et al.* 2011). CT angiography can also be performed very quickly and is well tolerated with a good safety profile. In instances where CT angiography is unavailable or when the cause of bleeding could not be identified via CT angiography, DSA should be performed (Macdonald and Schweizer 2017). DSA may also be arranged as part of endovascular treatment or for surgical planning in patients where an aneurysm is identified on CT angiography and deemed suitable for surgery (Macdonald and Schweizer 2017).

Compared with CT angiography, MR angiography has a slightly lower sensitivity (~95%) and specificity (~89%) for detection of intracranial aneurysms (Sailer *et al.* 2014). MR angiography is also less convenient, especially in sick patients.

Perimesencephalic Subarachnoid Hemorrhage

Idiopathic perimesencephalic SAH is restricted to the perimesencephalic cistern surrounding the midbrain (Fig. 30.3) (Schwartz and Solomon 1996). Patients present with acute headache, which may be more gradual in onset than in aneurysmal rupture (Linn *et al.* 1998), but loss of consciousness, focal symptoms, and seizures are rare. The cause of perimesencephalic SAH is usually unknown and is suspected to be due to rupture of a dilated vein or a venous malformation in the prepontine or interpeduncular cistern (Rinkel *et al.* 1993). The prognosis is nevertheless extremely good since rebleeding and vasospasm are unlikely (Rinkel *et al.* 1993). Perimesecenpahalic SAH accounts for approximately 10% of all patients with SAH (Rinkel *et al.* 1993), and approximately 10% of perimesencephalic SAH are due to posterior circulation aneurysms (Macdonald and Schweizer 2017). Such aneurysms may be excluded by performing high-quality CT angiography (Agid *et al.* 2010, Kumar *et al.* 2014), and follow-up imaging is not required if initial imaging studies are normal (Agid *et al.* 2010; Kumar *et al.* 2014).

Angiogram-Negative Subarachnoid Hemorrhage

In up to 20% of CT- or CSF-positive SAH, the cerebral angiogram shows no aneurysm, so-called "angiogram-negative SAH" (Rinkel *et al.* 1993). It should be noted that a traumatic lumbar puncture may be misdiagnosed as xanthochromic. Angiogram-negative SAH results when there is a false-negative angiogram (~2%). Other causes include SAH due to an occult (non-visualized) aneurysm, intracranial artery dissection, dural or cervical arteriovenous malformation, mycotic aneurysm, trauma, coagulation disorder, substance abuse, or cortical superficial siderosis (Rinkel *et al.* 1993; Charidimou *et al.* 2015). The pattern of subarachnoid bleeding is an important clue as to whether the bleed is likely to have been caused by an underlying aneurysm. In two-thirds of patients with angiogram-negative SAH, the CT shows perimesencephalic blood (Fig. 30.3). These are associated with a good prognosis (Rinkel *et al.* 1993), and repeat angiogram is not necessary (Kumar *et al.* 2014). Patients with diffuse or anteriorly located blood on CT that represents an aneurysmal pattern of hemorrhage are at risk of rebleeding, and repeat angiography should be performed, unless other causes such as trauma, coagulation disorders, or substance abuse (e.g., cocaine) are obvious from the history. Repeat angiography is also required where the previous angiogram was technically inadequate or if views of the cerebral vasculature were incomplete owing to vasospasm or hemorrhage. Patients with cortical superficial siderosis may present with acute convexity SAH with hyperdensity along sulci on CT (Charidimou *et al.* 2015). They have a characteristic bilinear "track-like" appearance on hemosiderin-sensitive MRI sequences and have been associated with cerebral amyloid angiopathy (Charidimou *et al.* 2015).

Spinal Subarachnoid Hemorrhage

Spinal subarachnoid hemorrhage is very rare. It is caused by a vascular malformation, hemostatic failure, coarctation of the aorta, inflammatory vascular disease, mycotic aneurysm, or a vascular tumor such as ependymoma. Accumulating hematoma may compress the spinal cord. Suspicion is raised if the cerebral angiogram is negative and the patient develops spinal cord signs.

Treatment

The aims of management are to identify the cause of the SAH, to treat the source of the bleeding to prevent recurrence, to prevent the general complications of stroke, and to manage the complications of SAH (Vermeulen *et al.* 1992; Wijdicks 1995). Close monitoring using the Glasgow Coma Score, pupillary responses as well as for the development of focal deficits is required.

General Measures and Medical Treatment

The patient should be nursed in a quiet, darkened room. As with other stroke types, the management of raised blood pressure is controversial.

Secondary ischemia is a frequent complication after SAH and is responsible for a substantial proportion of patients with poor outcome. The cause of secondary ischemia is postulated to be a combination of vasospasm, impaired autoregulation, microthrombosis, and cortical spreading ischemia (Macdonald 2014). The neurological status of patients should be monitored closely, and their body temperature, body fluid volume, hemoglobin, glucose, electrolytes (in particular sodium and magnesium) should be maintained as much as possible (Macdonald and Schweizer 2017). Hypovolemia should be avoided. However, treatments such as inducing hypervolemia, hypertension, hypermagnesemia, and hypothermia have not been shown to be beneficial and are currently not recommended by international guidelines (Connolly *et al.* 2012; Steiner *et al.* 2013).

The risk of delayed cerebral ischemia is also thought to be reduced and the overall outcome improved by prophylactic calcium blockers, specifically nimodipine, 60 mg every

4 hours, administered orally or by nasogastric tube for 21 days (Dorhout Mees *et al.* 2007). If this causes hypotension, then the dose should be reduced. There is no good evidence to support intravenous nimodipine, which is particularly likely to cause hypotension. Evidence is inconclusive for other potentially neuroprotective drugs, such as nicardipine and magnesium (Dorhout Mees *et al.* 2007). There is also no evidence of benefit from corticosteroids in patients with either SAH or primary intracerebral hemorrhage (Feigin *et al.* 2005).

Cardiac arrhythmias are common in the first few days but seldom need treatment (Andreoli *et al.* 1987; Brouwers *et al.* 1989), although electrocardiographic monitoring is advisable. Neurogenic pulmonary edema is rare but can occur very early, causing diagnostic confusion. The mechanism is unclear, but intensive cardiovascular monitoring and treatment are required (Parr *et al.* 1996). The patient can be mobilized when the headache has resolved (Warlow *et al.* 1996b).

Surgical Treatments for Certain Patients

Intracerebral extension of the hemorrhage occurs in at least a third of patients. Patients with a large hematoma and depressed consciousness might require immediate evacuation of the hematoma, preferably preceded by occlusion of the aneurysm (Niemann *et al.* 2003). Alternatively, extensive craniectomy can be employed to allow expansion of the brain, as for malignant middle cerebral artery infarction (Smith *et al.* 2002). Subdural hematomas are rare but life-threatening and should be removed.

Rebleeding Risk

Approximately 8–23% of untreated aneurysms rebleed within 72 hours of SAH, most of which occur during the first 6 hours (Larsen and Astrup 2013). Thereafter, the rebleeding rate is approximately 3% per annum (Macdonald and Schweizer 2017). Deterioration is usually sudden, with reduced conscious level or fixed dilatation of the pupils in ventilated patients. Mortality from rebleeding is high, with reported figures of up to 60% in patients who are hospitalized (Larsen and Astrup 2013). Risk factors for rebleeding include poor neurological status, hypertension during admission, large aneurysms, and possibly use of antiplatelet agents (Larsen and Astrup 2013). In view of the high morbidity and mortality due to rebleeding, current guidelines recommend that SAH patients due to aneurysm should be treated within 72 hours of symptom onset, unless in severe cases or in patients with significant underlying comorbidity (Larsen and Astrup 2013; Steiner *et al.* 2013). Antifibrinolytic agents such as tranexamic acid reduce rebleeding but are not associated with an improvement in clinical outcome (Hillman *et al.* 2002). They may however, increase the risk of thromboembolic complications (Foreman *et al.* 2015) and seizures (Lecker *et al.* 2012).

Ruptured arteriovenous malformations have a lower mortality than aneurysmal SAH (Mast *et al.* 1997). They are also less likely to rebleed (~6–16% rebleeding risk in the first year and reducing to 2–8% per annum thereafter) (Gross and Du 2012). Children, females, and patients with deep-seated arteriovenous malformations are at approximately threefold increased risk of rebleeding after an initial cerebral arteriovenous malformation (Yamada *et al.* 2007).

Endovascular and Surgical Treatment

The purpose of occluding the source of SAH is to prevent rebleeding. Occlusion may not be appropriate in severe cases or where there is significant comorbidity. Neurosurgical

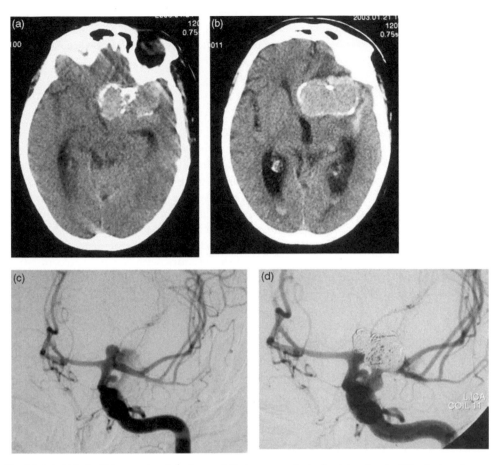

Fig. 30.4 (a, b) Brain CT images showing a large calcified aneurysm in the frontal region. (c, d) Cerebral angiograms show a small area of filling within the aneurysm owing to occlusion of a large part of the aneurysm with thrombus, making the aneurysm appear relatively small (c); this is then completely occluded by endovascular coiling (d).

"clipping" was used routinely for ruptured saccular aneurysms, but endovascular occlusion using detachable electrically released thrombogenic platinum coils ("coiling") is now the method of choice (Fig. 30.4). For aneurysms suitable for either treatment, coiling is recommended. A recent meta-analysis of randomized controlled trials revealed that coiling reduced the risk of unfavorable outcome (death or dependency) at 1 year to 23% compared with 31% with clipping (Li *et al.* 2013). Long-term follow-up data from the International Subarachnoid Aneurysm Trial (ISAT) also demonstrated that patients receiving endovascular coiling were at 34% increased odds of being alive or independent at 10 years compared with patients who received clipping (Molyneux *et al.* 2015). The risk of epilepsy was also substantially lower in patients allocated to endovascular treatment (Molyneux *et al.* 2005), and vasospasm was more common in patients who received clipping (Li *et al.* 2013). Risk of rebleeding is low in both groups but about twice as frequent in patients receiving coiling (21 per 8,351 and 12 per 8,228 patient-years) (Molyneux *et al.* 2015). Risk of ischemic infarct, shunt-dependent hydrocephalus, and procedural complications rates did not differ between the two techniques (Li *et al.* 2013).

Treatment of arteriovenous malformations and cavernomas is discussed in Chapter 22.

Complications

Hydrocephalus

Hydrocephalus is caused by blood obstructing CSF flow and occurs within days of SAH onset in approximately 20–30% of patients (Germanwala *et al.* 2010). It may cause clinical deterioration, including a gradual reduction in conscious level. Patients with intraventricular blood or with extensive hemorrhage in the perimesencephalic cisterns are particularly predisposed to developing acute hydrocephalus. The diagnosis is confirmed with CT scanning. Temporary external ventricular drainage may lead to dramatic improvement, but complications may occur. These include infections (e.g., meningitis or ventriculitis) and hemorrhage, both with a prevalence of ~8% (Dey *et al.* 2015). Symptomatic hemorrhage is, however, rare with a prevalence of ~0.7% (Dey *et al.* 2015). Risk of rebleeding from an untreated aneurysm may be slightly increased (Hellingman *et al.* 2007), although many believe that the rebleeding is unlikely to be due to ventricular drainage itself (Gigante *et al.* 2010). Lumbar puncture may be performed in patients without an intracranial space-occupying lesion or gross intraventricular hemorrhage, but this requires certainty that the site of obstruction is in the subarachnoid space and not the ventricular system. In addition, it is not clear whether lumbar puncture increases the risk of rebleeding (Ruijs *et al.* 2005). Months or years after SAH, organized thrombus and fibrosis in the CSF pathways can lead to the syndrome of normal pressure hydrocephalus.

Delayed Cerebral Ischemia

Delayed ischemia secondary to vasospasm appears 3–14 days after onset in approximately 25% of patients. It is associated with a bad prognosis, and there is currently lack of an effective treatment (Beseoglu *et al.* 2013). Loss of consciousness at onset, large quantities of subarachnoid or intraventricular blood on CT, and history of smoking are strong predictors of delayed cerebral ischemia (Macdonald 2014). Clinical onset is usually gradual, with deteriorating conscious level and evolving focal neurological signs. Currently, nimodipine is the only drug that has been shown to reduce the risk of delayed ischemia and poor outcome (Dorhout Mees *et al.* 2007), and current guidelines recommend initiation of nimodipine within 96 hours of SAH (Connolly *et al.* 2012; Steiner *et al.* 2013).

Hyponatremia

Hyponatremia occurs in approximately a third of patients in the first week or two after SAH and is related to the severity of the initial presentation. It is not usually caused by inappropriate antidiuretic hormone secretion but by "salt wasting," in which there is excessive loss of salt and water by the kidneys with a decrease in plasma volume. Correction with plasma volume expansion is necessary in patients with a plasma sodium of less than 125 mmol/L (Berendes *et al.* 1997).

Intracerebral Hematoma

Intracerebral hematoma may cause a focal deficit and should be considered for removal if there is associated coma, clinical deterioration, and brain shift.

Long-Term Complications

In the ISAT study, long-term follow-up data over 18 years showed that late rebleeding from the initial treated aneurysm occurs in ~2% of patients who received clipping of aneurysm and in ~0.6% of patients who received endovascular coiling (Molyneux *et al.* 2015).

Epilepsy develops in 2% of all patients with SAH (Macdonald and Schweizer 2017). However, the risk is up to 25% in patients with severe SAH (Macdonald and Schweizer 2017). Risk factors include young age, loss of consciousness at onset, history of hypertension, middle cerebral artery aneurysm, severe SAH on CT, intracerebral and/or subdural hematoma, aneurysm repair by clipping compared with coiling, and delayed cerebral ischemia (Ibrahim *et al.* 2013).

Anosmia is a sequela in almost 30% of patients, particularly after surgery and in patients with anterior communicating artery aneurysms. Cognitive deficits and psychosocial dysfunction are common in patients who otherwise make a good recovery (Al-Khindi *et al.* 2010). They persist for years. In one study, a quarter of previously employed patients had stopped working, and another quarter worked shorter hours or in a position with reduced responsibility (Wermer *et al.* 2007a). Changes in personality included increased irritability and emotionality. Overall, only 25% of those living independently reported a complete absence of psychosocial problems.

Unruptured Aneurysms

Unruptured intracranial aneurysms are present in 2–3% of the general population (Vlak *et al.* 2011). They are more common in the elderly, in women, in patients with a positive family history of aneurysm and SAH, and in patients with autosomal polycystic kidney disease (Box 30.1) (Vlak *et al.* 2011; Brown and Broderick 2014). In patients with unruptured aneurysms ≥ 2 mm, the annual rupture risk is 0.7% (Wiebers *et al.* 2003). Size (especially ≥ 7 mm), location (posterior circulation and anterior communicating arteries), and presence of a daughter sac are important determinants of aneurysm rupture (Table 30.3) (Wiebers *et al.* 2003; Wermer *et al.* 2007b; UCAS Japan Investigators 2012). Other risks factors for rupture include age > 60 years and female sex (Wermer *et al.* 2007b).

The decision whether to treat unruptured aneurysms (by surgical clipping or endovascular coiling) depends on a balance of the risks of aneurysm rupture and also the benefits and risks of intervention (Raaymakers *et al.* 1998; Williams and Brown 2013; Brown and Broderick 2014). A summary of recommendations is shown in Box 30.2. Small aneurysms with lack of high-risk features that do not require intervention should be monitored regularly by MR or CT angiography, e.g., on a yearly basis for 3 years and then on several more occasions at a reduced frequency (Brown and Broderick 2014). Patients with aneurysm growth should be considered for interventional treatment.

Individuals with an affected first-degree relative have a 5 to 12 times greater lifetime risk of SAH than the general population, representing a lifetime risk of 2–5%. However, the chances of finding an aneurysm by screening in an individual with a single affected relative

Table 30.3 Five-year cumulative aneurysm rupture rates according to size and location of unruptured aneurysm (Wiebers *et al.* 2003)

	< 7 mm		7–12 mm	13–24 mm	≥ 25 mm
	Without SAH	With SAH			
Cavernous carotid artery	0	0	0	3.0	6.4
ACA/ACOM/MCA/ICA (excluding cavernous segment)	0	1.5	2.6	14.5	40
VB/PCA/PCOM	2.5	3.4	14.5	18.4	50

Notes: ACA, anterior cerebral artery; ACOM, anterior communicating artery; ICA, internal carotid artery; MCA, middle cerebral artery; PCA, posterior cerebral artery; PCOM, posterior communicating artery; VB, vertebrobasilar artery.

BOX 30.1 Associations of Intracranial Saccular Aneurysms

Autosomal dominant polycystic kidney disease[a]

Fibromuscular dysplasia

Cervical artery dissection[a]

Coarctation of the aorta

Intracranial arteriovenous malformations[a]

Marfan's syndrome[a]

Ehlers–Danlos syndrome type IV[a]

Pseudoxanthoma elasticum[a]

Neurofibromatosis type I[a]

α_1-Antitrypsin deficiency[a]

Hereditary hemorrhagic telangiectasia[a]

Moyamoya disease

Multiple endocrine neoplasia[a]

Sickle cell disease[a]

Systemic lupus erythematosus

Klinefelter's syndrome

Progeria

[a] These can be familial.

---

is only 1.7 times higher than in the general population. This suggests that familial aneurysms have a higher rupture rate or grow faster than others. Currently, screening for aneurysms is recommended for patients who have (1) two or more family members who have a history of unruptured intracranial aneurysm or SAH, (2) autosomal dominant polycystic kidney disease with a family history of unruptured intracranial aneurysm or SAH, and (3) patients with coarctation of the aorta (Williams and Brown 2013; Brown and

BOX 30.2 Recommendations for Intervention of Unruptured Intracranial Aneurysm (Williams and Brown 2013; Brown and Broderick 2014)

Strongly consider intervention with clipping or coiling	Possibly consider intervention	Do not recommend intervention

• ≥ 12 mm in diameter
• Symptomatic aneurysm
• Enlarging aneurysm
	• 7–11 mm AND
	   • Age < 60 OR
	   • High-risk location (posterior circulation or posterior communicating artery) OR
	   • Aneurysm with daughter sac OR
	   • Family history of SAH
	• < 7 mm in age < 60 AND
	   • High-risk location (posterior circulation or posterior communicating artery) OR
	   • Aneurysm with daughter sac OR
	   • Family history of SAH
		• < 7 mm in anterior circulation without high-risk features such as family history of SAH or presence of daughter sac
		• Asymptomatic cavernous internal carotid artery aneurysms

Broderick 2014). In patients with autosomal dominant polycystic kidney disease without family history of aneurysm or in patients who have only one family member with unruptured intracranial aneurysm or SAH, screening may be considered (Williams and Brown 2013). If initial screening is negative, high-risk individuals may need repeat screening once every 5 years (Rinkel 2005) as the risk of finding a de-novo aneurysm in individuals with a family history of SAH is approximately 5% at each follow-up screen during two decades of follow-up (Bor *et al.* 2014). Patients should be referred to specialist clinics where an informed decision can be made on the basis of that individual's risks and benefits and their preferences. Screening for new aneurysms in those who have survived SAH is not thought to be beneficial except in those with multiple aneurysms or who are very young at presentation.

References

Adams HP, Kassell NF, Torner JC *et al.* (1983). CT and clinical correlations in recent aneurysmal subarachnoid haemorrhage: A preliminary report of the Cooperative Aneurysm Study. *Neurology* **33**:981–988

Agid R, Andersson T, Almqvist H *et al.* (2010) Negative CT angiography findings in patients with spontaneous subarachnoid hemorrhage: When is digital subtraction angiography still needed? *American Journal of Neuroradiology* **31**:696–705

Al-Khindi T, Macdonald RL, Schweizer TA. (2010) Cognitive and functional outcome after aneurysmal subarachnoid haemorrhage. *Stroke* **41**:e519–536

Andreasen TH, Bartek J Jr., Andresen M *et al.* (2013). Modifiable risk factors for aneurysmal subarachnoid hemorrhage. *Stroke* **44**:3607–3612

Andreoli A, di Pasquale G, Pinelli G *et al.* (1987). Subarachnoid haemorrhage: Frequency and severity of cardiac arrhythmias. A survey of 70 cases studied in the acute phase. *Stroke* **18**:558–564

Backes D, Rinkel GJ, Kemperman H *et al.* (2012) Time-dependent test characteristics of head computed tomography in patients suspected of nontraumatic subarachnoid hemorrhage. *Stroke* **43**:2115–2119

Beck J, Rohde S, Berkefeld J *et al.* (2006). Size and location of ruptured and unruptured intracranial aneurysms measured by 3-dimentsional rotational angiography. *Surgical Neurology* **65**:18–25

Berendes E, Walter M, Cullen P *et al.* (1997). Secretion of brain natriuretic peptide in patients with aneurysmal subarachnoid haemorrhage. *Lancet* **349**:245–249

Beseoglu K, Holtkamp K, Steiger HJ *et al.* (2013). Fatal aneurysmal subarachnoid haemorrhage: Causes of 30-day in-hospital case fatalities in a large single-centre historical patient cohort. *Clinical Neurology and Neurosurgery* **115**:77–81

Bor AS, Rinkel GJ, van Norden J *et al.* (2014). Long-term, serial screening for intracranial aneurysms in individuals with a family history of aneurysmal subarachnoid haemorrhage: A cohort study. *Lancet Neurology* **13**:385–392

Brouwers PJ, Wijdicks EF, Hasan D *et al.* (1989). Serial electrocardiographic recording in aneurysmal subarachnoid hemorrhage. *Stroke* **20**:1162–1167

Brouwers PJ, Wijdicks EF, van Gijn J (1992). Infarction after aneurysm rupture does not depend on distribution or clearance rate of blood. *Stroke* **23**:374–379

Brown RD Jr., Broderick JP (2014). Unruptured intracranial aneurysms: Epidemiology, natural history, management options, and familial screening. *Lancet Neurology* **13**:393–404

Charidimou A, Linn J, Vernooij MW *et al.* (2015). Cortical superficial siderosis: Detection and clinical significance in cerebral amyloid angiopathy and related conditions. *Brain* **138** (8):2126–2139

Connolly ES Jr., Rabinstein AA, Carhuapoma JR *et al.* (2012) Guidelines for the management of aneurysmal subarachnoid hemorrhage: A guideline for healthcare professional from the American Heart Association/American Stroke Association. *Stroke* **43**:1711–1737

Cruickshank A, Auld P, Beetham R *et al.* (2008). Revised national guidelines for analysis of cerebrospinal fluid for bilirubin in suspected subarachnoid haemorrhage. *Annals of Clinical Biochemistry* **45**:238–244

de Rooij NK, Linn FH, van der Plas JA *et al.* (2007). Incidence of subarachnoid haemorrhage: A systematic review with emphasis on region, age, gender and time trends. *Journal of Neurology Neurosurgery and Psychiatry* **78**:1365–1372

Dey M, Stadnik A, Riad F *et al.* (2015). Bleeding and infection with external ventricular drainage: A systematic review in comparison with adjudicated adverse events in the ongoing Clot Lysis Evaluating Accelerated Resolution of Intraventricular Hemorrhage Phase III (CLEAR-III LVH) trial. *Neurosurgery* **76**:291–300

Dorhout Mees SM, Rinkel GJ, Feigin VL *et al.* (2007) Calcium antagonists for aneurysmal subarachnoid haemorrhage. *Cochrane Database of Systematic Reviews* **3**:CD000277

Ducros A (2012). Reversible cerebral vasoconstriction syndrome. *Lancet Neurology* **11**:906–917

Fearnley JM, Stevens JM, Rudge P (1995). Superficial siderosis of the central nervous system. *Brain* **118**:1051–1066

Feigin VL, Anderson N, Rinkel GJ (2005). Corticosteroids for aneurysmal subarachnoid haemorrhage and primary intracerebral haemorrhage. *Cochrane Database of Systematic Reviews* **3**:CD004583

Feigin VL, Lawes CM, Bennett DA *et al.* (2009). Worldwide stroke incidence and early case fatality reported in 56 population-based studies: A systematic review. *Lancet Neurology* **8**:355–369

Ferro JM, Pinto AN (1994). Sexual activity is a common precipitant of subarachnoid haemorrhage. *Cerebrovascular Diseases* **4**:375

Foreman PM, Chua M, Harrigan MR et al. (2015). Antifibrinolytic therapy in aneurysmal subarachnoid hemorrhage increases the risk for deep vein thrombosis: A case-control study. *Clinical Neurology and Neurosurgery* **139**:66–69

Gigante P, Hwang BY, Appelboom G *et al.* (2010) External ventricular drainage following aneurysmal subarachnoid haemorrhage. *British Journal of Neurosurgery* **24**:625–632

Germanwala AV, Huang J and Tamargo RJ (2010). Hydrocephalus after aneurysmal subarachnoid hemorrhage. *Neurosurgery Clinics of North America* **21**:263–270

Gross BA and Du R (2012). Rate of re-bleeding of arteriovenous malformations in the first year after rupture. *Journal of Clinical Neuroscience* **19**:1087–1088

Hellingman CA, van den Bergh WM, Beijer IS *et al.* (2007). Risk of rebleeding after treatment of acute hydrocephalus in patients with aneurysmal subarachnoid hemorrhage. *Stroke* **38**:96–99

Hillman J, Fridriksson S, Nilsson O *et al.* (2002). Immediate administration of tranexamic acid and reduced incidence of early rebleeding after aneurysmal subarachnoid hemorrhage: A prospective randomized study. *Journal of Neurosurgery* **97**:771–778

Huang J, van Gelder JM (2002). The probability of sudden death from rupture of intracranial aneurysms: A meta-analysis. *Neurosurgery* **51**:1101–1107

Ibrahim GM, Fallah A, Macdonald RL (2013). Clinical, laboratory, and radiographic predictors of the occurrence of seizures following aneurysmal subarachnoid haemorrhage. *Journal of Neurosurgery* **119**:347–352

Jaja BN, Cusimano MD, Etminan N *et al.* (2013). Clinical prediction models for aneurysmal subarachnoid hemorrhage: A systematic review. *Neurocritical Care* **18**:143–153

Kaufmann TJ, Houston J III, Mandrekar JN *et al.* (2007). Complications of diagnostic cerebral angiography: Evaluation of 19,826 consecutive patients. *Radiology* **243**:812–819

Kumar R, Das KK, Sahu RK *et al.* (2014). Angio negative spontaneous subarachnoid hemorrhage: Is repeat angiogram required in all cases? *Surgical Neurology International* **5**:125

Larsen CC, Astrup J (2013). Rebleeding after aneurysmal subarachnoid hemorrhage: A literature review. *World Neurosurgery* **79**:307–312

Lecker I, Wang DS, Romaschin AD *et al.* (2012) Tranexamic acid concentrations associated with human seizures inhibit glycine receptors. *The Journal of Clinical Investigation* **122**:4654–4666

Li H, Pan R, Wang H *et al.* (2013). Clipping versus coiling for ruptured intracranial aneurysms: A systematic review and meta-analysis. *Stroke* **44**:29–37

Linn FH, Rinkel GJ, Algra A *et al.* (1998). Headache characteristics in subarachnoid haemorrhage and benign thunderclap headache. *Journal of Neurology, Neurosurgery and Psychiatry* **65**:791–793

Linn FH, Voorbij HA, Rinkel GJ *et al.* (2005). Visual inspection versus spectrophotometry in detecting bilirubin in cerebrospinal fluid. *Journal of Neurology, Neurosurgery and Psychiatry.* **76**:1452–1454

Lovelock CE, Rinkel GJ, Rothwell PM (2010). Time trends in outcome of subarachnoid hemorrhage: Population-based study and systematic review. *Neurology* **74**:1494–1501

Lummel N, Bernau C, Thon N *et al.* (2015). Prevalence of superficial siderosis following singular, acute aneurysmal subarachnoid hemorrhage. *Neuroradiology* **57**:349–356

Macdonald RL (2014). Delayed neurological deterioration after subarachnoid haemorrhage. *Nature Reviews Neurology* **10**:44–58

Macdonald RL, Schweizer TA (2017). Spontaneous subarachnoid haemorrhage. *Lancet* **389**:655–666

Mast H, Young WL, Koennecke HC *et al.* (1997). Risk of spontaneous haemorrhage after diagnosis of cerebral arteriovenous malformation. *Lancet* **350**:1065–1068

Molyneux AJ, Kerr RS, Yu LM *et al.* (2005). International subarachnoid aneurysm trial (ISAT) of neurosurgical clipping versus endovascular coiling in 2143 patients with ruptured intracranial aneurysms: A randomised comparison of effects on survival, dependency, seizures, rebleeding subgroups and aneurysm occlusion. *Lancet* **366**:809–817

Molyneux AJ, Birks J, Clarke A *et al.* (2015). The durability of endovascular coiling versus neurosurgical clipping of ruptured cerebral aneurysms: 18 year follow-up of the UK cohort of the International Subarachnoid Aneurysm Trial (ISAT). *Lancet* **385**:691–697

Niemann DB, Wills AD, Maartens NF *et al.* (2003). Treatment of intracerebral hematomas caused by aneurysm rupture: Coil placement followed by clot evacuation. *Journal of Neurosurgery* **99**:843–847

Nieuwkamp DJ, Setz LE, Algra A *et al.* (2009). Changes in case fatality of aneurysmal subarachnoid haemorrhage over time, according to age, sex, and region: A meta-analysis. *Lancet Neurology* **8**:635–642

Parr MJA, Finfer SR, Morgan MK (1996). Reversible cardiogenic shock complicating subarachnoid haemorrhage. *British Medical Journal* **313**:681–683

Perry JJ, Stiell IG, Sivilotti ML (2011). Sensitivity of computed tomography performed within six hours of onset of headache for diagnosis of subarachnoid haemorrhage: Prospective cohort study. *British Medical Journal* **343**:d4277

Pinto AN, Canhao P, Ferro JM (1996). Seizures at the onset of subarachnoid haemorrhage. *Journal of Neurology* **243**:161–164

Raaymakers TWM, Rinkel GJE, Limburg M *et al.* (1998). Mortality and morbidity of surgery for unruptured intracranial aneurysms: A meta-analysis. *Stroke* **29**:1531–1538

Raps EC, Rogers JD, Galetta SL *et al.* (1993). The clinical spectrum of unruptured intracranial aneurysms. *Archives of Neurology* **50**:265–268

Rinkel GJE. (2005). Intracranial aneurysm screening: Indications and advice for practice. *Lancet Neurology* **4**:122–128

Rinkel GJE, van Gijn J, Wijdicks EFM (1993). Subarachnoid haemorrhage without detectable aneurysm. A review of the causes. *Stroke* **24**:1403–1409

Rinkel GJE, Wijdicks EFM, Hasan D *et al.* (1991). Outcome in patients with subarachnoid haemorrhage and negative angiography according to pattern of haemorrhage on computed tomography. *Lancet* **338**:964–968

Ruijs AC, Dirven CM, Algra A *et al.* (2005). The risk of rebleeding after external lumbar drainage in patients with untreated ruptured cerebral aneurysms. *Acta Neurochirurgie* **147**:1157–1161

Sailer AM, Wagemans BA, Nelemans PJ *et al.* (2014). Diagnosing intracranial aneurysms with MR angiography: A systematic review and meta-analysis. *Stroke* **45**:119–126

Schievink WI (1997). Intracranial aneurysms. *New England Journal of Medicine* **336**:28–40

Schwartz TH, Solomon RA (1996). Perimesencephalic nonaneurysmal subarachnoid hemorrhage: Review of the literature. *Neurosurgery* **39**:433–440

Steiner T, Juvela S, Unterberg A *et al.* (2013). European Stroke Organization guidelines for the management of intracranial aneurysms and subarachnoid haemorrhage. *Cerebrovascular Diseases* **35**:93–112

Suarez JI, Tarr RW and Selman WR (2006). Aneurysmal subarachnoid hemorrhage. *New England Journal of Medicine* **354**:387–396

Smith ER, Carter BS, Ogilvy CS (2002). Proposed use of prophylactic decompressive craniectomy in poor-grade aneurismal subarachnoid hemorrhage patients presenting with associated large sylvian haematomas. *Neurosurgery* **51**:117–124

Toussaint LG III, Friedman JA, Wijdicks EF *et al.* (2005). Survival of cardiac arrest after aneurysmal subarachnoid hemorrhage. *Neurosurgery* **57**:25–31

UCAS Japan Investigators (2012). The natural course of unruptured cerebral aneurysms in a Japanese cohort. *New England Journal of Medicine* **366**:2474–2482

van Gijn J, Rinkel GJ (2001). Subarachnoid haemorrhage: Diagnosis, causes and management. *Brain* **124**:249–278

Vermeer SE, Rinkel GJE, Algra A (1997). Circadian fluctuations in onset of subarachnoid haemorrhage. New data on aneurysmal and perimesencephalic haemorrhage and a systematic review. *Stroke* **28**:805–808

Vermeulen M, van Gijn J (1990). The diagnosis of subarachnoid haemorrhage. *Journal of Neurology, Neurosurgery and Psychiatry* **53**:365–372

Vermeulen M, Lindsay KW, van Gijn J (1992). *Subarachnoid Haemorrhage*. London: Saunders

Vlak MH, Algra A, Brandenburg R *et al.* (2011). Prevalence of unruptured intracranial aneurysms, with emphasis on sex, age, comorbiditiy, country, and time period: A systematic review and meta-analysis. *Lancet Neurology* **10**:626–636

Warlow CP, Dennis MS, van Gijn J *et al.* (1996a). What pathological type of stroke is it? *Stroke: A Practical Guide to Management*, pp. 146–189. Oxford: Blackwell Scientific

Warlow CP, Dennis MS, van Gijn J *et al.* (1996b). Specific treatment of aneurysmal subarachnoid haemorrhage. In *Stroke: A Practical Guide to Management*, pp. 438–468. Oxford: Blackwell Scientific

Wermer MJ, Kool H, Albrecht KW *et al.* (2007a). Aneurysm Screening after Treatment for Ruptured Aneurysms Study Group. Subarachnoid hemorrhage treated with clipping: Long-term effects on employment, relationships, personality and mood. *Neurosurgery* **60**:91–97

Wermer MJ, van der Schaaf IC, Algra A *et al.* (2007a). Risk of rupture of unruptured intracranial aneurysms in relation to patient and aneurysm characteristics: An updated meta-analysis. *Stroke* **38**:1404–1410

Westerlaan HE, van Dijk JM, Jansen-van der Weider MC *et al.* (2011). Intracranial aneurysms in patients with subarachnoid hemorrhage: CT angiography as a primary examination tool for diagnosis – systematic review and meta-analysis. *Radiology* **258**:134–145

Wiebers DO, Whisnant JP, Huston J III *et al.* (2003). Unruptured intracranial aneurysms: Natural history, clinical outcome and risks of surgical and endovascular treatment. *Lancet* **362**:103–110

Wijdicks EFM (1995). Worse-case scenario: Management in poor-grade aneurysmal subarachnoid haemorrhage. *Cerebrovascular Diseases* **5**:163–169

Williams LN, Brown RD Jr. (2013). Management of unruptured intracranial aneurysms. *Neurology: Clinical Practice* **3**:99–108

Yamada S, Takagi Y, Nozaki K *et al.* (2007). Risk factors for subsequent hemorrhage in patients with cerebral arteriovenous malformations. *Journal of Neurosurgery* **107**:965–972

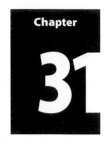

Chapter 31

Vascular Cognitive Impairment: Epidemiology, Definitions, Stroke-Associated Dementia, and Delirium

Stroke is associated with a high risk of future dementia. Dementia with an underlying vascular etiology, "vascular dementia," may also occur in patients without a history of clinically eloquent stroke as a result of silent large or small vessel disease and/or widespread white matter disease. The term *vascular cognitive impairment* is used here to include both vascular dementia and cognitive impairment not severe enough to cause dementia. Vascular cognitive impairment may coexist with Alzheimer's pathology or other neurodegenerative disorders. The incidence of all types of dementia rises with age, and cognitive impairment is likely to become an increasing problem as more people survive into old age. Interest in potential therapeutic strategies for vascular cognitive impairment is growing partly driven by the lack of progress in treatments for neurodegeneration.

Epidemiology

Vascular dementia is the second most common cause of dementia in later life in white populations and the most common cause in Far Eastern countries (Jorm and Jolley 1998; Lobo *et al.* 2000; Neuropathology Group of the Medical Research Council Cognitive Function and Aging Study 2001). However, vascular pathology is present in the majority of older people (> 75 years) dying with dementia, making it difficult to quantify prevalence and incidence specifically of "vascular" dementia (see later). The incidence of all-cause dementia rises exponentially from the age of ~75 years and is overall slightly higher in women who have a higher incidence of Alzheimer's disease whereas vascular dementia is more common in men. Importantly, several recent studies have shown a fall in the age-specific prevalence and incidence of all-cause dementia over the past few decades (Wu *et al.* 2017), suggesting that previous projections of future dementia burden with population aging may have been overly pessimistic. The reasons for the fall in dementia incidence and prevalence are unclear, but it is likely that multiple factors including better education, living conditions, and health care are important. There are few data specifically on changes in vascular dementia rates (and determining changes in dementia subtypes is challenging because of classification difficulties), but in the United Kingdom, the reduction in dementia has occurred largely in men and may be linked to lower vascular event rates including stroke and better control of vascular risk factors (Matthews *et al.* 2013, 2016).

Since stroke and dementia are common, they often coexist. Further, epidemiological studies have shown that stroke and dementia share reciprocal risks: Stroke increases the risk of dementia, and dementia increases the risk of stroke and of more severe stroke (Appelros *et al.* 2002; Jin *et al.* 2006; Rostamian *et al.* 2014; Pendlebury and Rothwell 2009; Pendlebury *et al.* 2017a). Vascular risk factors in midlife, particularly hypertension but also high cholesterol, are associated with increased risk of dementia in later life (Skoog *et al.* 1996; Freitag *et al.* 2006; Solomon *et al.* 2007; Gorelick *et al.* 2011). It has been proposed that the development of neurofibrillary tangles and amyloid plaques may, in part, be secondary to ischemia (de la Torre 2002; Gorelick *et al.* 2011). The overlap of risk factors and the coexistence of vascular and Alzheimer's type pathology means that vascular cognitive impairment cannot be considered in isolation and there may be important synergistic relationships between the two syndromes (see later).

Studies of the speed of cognitive progression in Alzheimer's disease versus vascular cognitive impairment have shown conflicting results: Similar rates have been reported in observational studies (Chui and Gonthier 1999) with comparable rates of serial atrophy on MRI over a 1-year period (O'Brien *et al.* 2001). However, patients selected for clinical trials with probable vascular dementia appear to have a more stable course than those with Alzheimer's disease (Black *et al.* 2003) in keeping with diagnostic criteria for vascular dementia that include stepwise progression and the high early versus later risk of dementia after stroke (Pendlebury and Rothwell 2009; Pendlebury *et al.* 2017b). The discrepancy between rates of progression of cognitive impairment seen in trials and in observational studies is probably explained by selection bias and the fact that cognitive trajectories in vascular cognitive impairment are likely to vary with the heterogeneous underlying pathology.

Definitions and Clinical Features of Vascular Cognitive Impairment

Vascular cognitive impairment is a heterogeneous syndrome encompassing cognitive impairment associated with large cortical infarcts, single strategically sited infarcts, multiple small infarcts, cerebral hemorrhage, white matter disease and vasculopathies including cerebral autosomal dominant arteriopathy with silent infarcts and leukoaraiosis (CADSIL), lipohyalinosis, and cerebral amyloid angiopathy (Table 31.1). Different subtypes of vascular pathology may coexist in an individual patient as well as with neurodegenerative disease.

There is no universally accepted definition for the clinical diagnosis of dementia, and the various definitions available (e.g., the *International Classification of Diseases*, 10th revision [ICD-10; World Health Organization 1987] and the Diagnostic and *Statistical Manual of Mental Disorders*, 4th and 5th editions [DSM-IV, 5; American Psychiatric Association 1994, 2013]) use different diagnostic criteria: Both DSM-IV and ICD-10 (but not DSM 5) require the presence of memory impairment together with one or more (DSM-IV) or two or more (ICD-10) other cognitive domains to be affected. In DSM 5, the term *dementia* has been replaced with *major neurocognitive disorder* with *mild neurocognitive disorder* being used for milder cognitive impairments. Since patients with vascular cognitive impairment may have severe impairment of cognitive function but relatively well-preserved memory, they may not be classified as having dementia by the DSM-IV and ICD-10 criteria but would meet DSM 5 criteria for major neurocognitive disorder.

Definitions for less severe cognitive impairment, i.e., cognitive decline greater than expected for an individual's age and education level but not impacting on activities of daily living, arc similarly diverse and include cognitive impairment, no dementia (CIND) and mild cognitive impairment (MCI) as well as mild neurocognitive disorder. Even within a given definition, e.g., for MCI, there is no consensus on how to operationalize the criteria, and widely differing rates of MCI may result (Pendlebury *et al.* 2013, Fig. 31.1). Patients with

Table 31.1 Subtypes of vascular cognitive impairment

Type	Causes
Cortical	Primarily from cortical infarcts
Small vessel (subcortical)	Primarily from subcortical lacunes, white and/or deep gray matter lesions
Cortical-subcortical	Cortical infarcts coexistent with white matter disease or subcortical infarcts
Strategic infarct	Unilateral or bilateral infarction in a strategic area (e.g., thalamus, hippocampus)
Hypoperfusion	Hypoperfusion-induced brain damage, e.g., caused by systemic hypotension or cardiac arrest
Hemorrhagic	Intracerebral hemorrhage including from cerebral amyloid angiopathy
Alzheimer's disease with cerebrovascular disease (mixed)	Coexistent degenerative and vascular pathology
Hereditary vascular dementia (CADASIL)	Autosomal dominant arteriopathy (with silent infarcts and leukoaraiosis)

MCI/CIND of Alzheimer's type have an increased risk of progression to frank Alzheimer's disease, and the risk of (vascular) dementia also appears higher in those with mild vascular cognitive impairment, although risks vary with case mix and criteria used to define cognitive impairment (Wentzel *et al.* 2001; Narasimhalu 2009).

The earliest attempt to improve the definition of vascular dementia as a distinct subtype of dementia was made by Hachinski and colleagues (1975), who proposed an ischemic score derived from the multi-infarct model of dementia. The Hachinski score requires a history of stroke and the presence of focal neurological signs, and it separates vascular dementia secondary to multi-infarct dementia from Alzheimer's disease effectively. However, it is rather insensitive for other subtypes of vascular dementia. Both ICD-10 and DSM-IV and 5 contain diagnostic criteria for vascular dementia, but the Neuroepidemiology Branch of the National Institute of Neurological Disorders and Stroke–Association Internationale pour la Recherche et l'Enseignement en Neurosciences (NINDS/AIREN) consensus criteria based on ICD-10 (Román *et al.* 1993) have been the most commonly used. Diagnostic criteria have also been proposed for subtypes of vascular dementia, including subcortical ischemic vascular dementia (Erkinjuntti *et al.* 2002). Not surprisingly, different sets of criteria identify different groups of patients (Pohjasvaara *et al.* 2000; Lopez *et al.* 2005), although in post-stroke dementia this effect is small in comparison to the impact of differences in case mix/study methodology (Pendlebury and Rothwell 2009). More recently, consensus criteria have been developed by the International Society of Vascular Behavioural and Cognitive Disorders (VasCog) to classify mild and major vascular cognitive disorders that are aligned with the DSM 5 criteria (Sachdev *et al.* 2014). New guidelines have also been proposed according to a Delphi exercise involving participants in 27 countries but have yet to be evaluated in clinical/research studies (Skrobot *et al.* 2016).

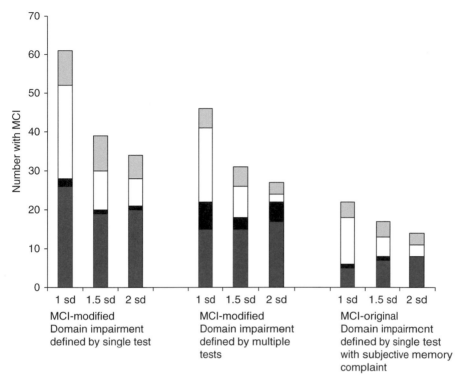

Fig. 31.1 Total numbers with MCI and with the different MCI subtypes (dark gray = non-amnestic single-domain, black = amnestic single-domain, white = non-amnestic multiple-domain, light gray = amnestic multiple-domain) for the different operational definitions of MCI. MCI, mild cognitive impairment; SD, standard deviation. From Pendlebury *et al.* (2013).

The NINDS/AIREN (and VasCog) criteria divide cases into probable and possible vascular dementia along the lines of the NINCDS/ADRDA criteria for Alzheimer's disease (McKhann *et al.* 1984). In the NINDS/AIREN, probable vascular dementia requires the presence of dementia, defined as memory and at least one other cognitive domain being affected, and the presence of cerebrovascular disease (focal neurological signs and evidence of relevant cerebrovascular disease on brain imaging). The onset of cognitive impairment must occur within 3 months of the cerebrovascular disease or must be abrupt with a stepwise/fluctuating course. The less-certain diagnosis of possible vascular dementia can be made if brain imaging criteria are not met or if the relationship between cerebrovascular disease and dementia is not clear. The NINDS/AIREN criteria were among the first to propose clear neuroimaging criteria for the diagnosis of vascular dementia, requiring a combination of topography (lesion location) and severity (Table 31.2). In the VasCog criteria, as for DSM 5, impairment of memory is not a prerequisite for the diagnosis of major vascular cognitive disorder, and the difficulties in defining thresholds for neuroimaging abnormalities including white matter disease are acknowledged (Sachdev *et al.* 2014).

Autopsy confirmation of the diagnostic accuracy of the various criteria for vascular dementia (Gold *et al.* 2002) has not been well studied in comparison to Alzheimer's disease, and there is variability in methods to identify and quantify vascular neuropathological changes (Foster *et al.* 2014; Chen *et al.* 2016). Neuropathological criteria include the relative

Table 31.2 NINDS/AIREN imaging criteria for vascular cognitive impairment

Criterion	Features
Topography	Large vessel strokes Extensive white matter changes Lacunes (frontal/basal ganglia) Bilateral thalamic lesions
Severity	Large vessel lesion of dominant hemisphere Bilateral strokes White matter lesion affecting ~ 25% white matter

Note: NINDS/AIREN, Neuroepidemiology Branch of the National Institute of Neurological Disorders and Stroke–Association Internationale pour la Recherche et l'Enseignement en Neurosciences.

absence of Alzheimer's-type pathology and the presence of some vascular change, both of which are subjective. However, recent attempts to harmonize approaches have resulted in better agreement and standardization of criteria among neuropathologists (Skrobot *et al.* 2016).

The neuropsychological deficits seen in vascular cognitive impairment are qualitatively different from those of Alzheimer's disease, certainly in the early stages (Pendlebury *et al.* 2012a; Figs. 31.2 and 31.3). The different underlying pathologies causing vascular cognitive impairment have different disease mechanisms and cognitive profiles (Bastos-Leite *et al.* 2007) with contributions from lesion location, medial temporal lobe atrophy, and large vessel and small vessel disease. Deficits in attentional, motivational, and executive domains (Desmond 2004; Prins *et al.* 2005; Bastos-Leite *et al.* 2007; Hachinski *et al.* 2006) are prominent in contrast to Alzheimer's disease, in which memory deficits predominate.

Further support for a distinctive pattern of cognitive deficits in vascular disease comes from studies of CADASIL (Chapter 3) patients in which multiple subcortical infarcts occur at a young age before the onset of neurodegenerative changes (Buffon *et al.* 2006). Patients with CADASIL show early impairment of executive function that is frequently associated with a decline in attention and memory performance compatible with some degree of dysfunction in subcortico-frontal networks (Buffon *et al.* 2006). Later in the course of the disease, there is extension of cognitive deficits to involve multiple cognitive domains. However, even late in the disease, memory impairment does not involve the encoding process, and retrieval is significantly improved with cues in contrast to Alzheimer's disease, in which early impairment of memory encoding is characteristic. Cholinergic neuronal impairment occurs in CADASIL and provides a rationale for therapies to enhance cholinergic function in subcortical vascular cognitive impairment (Mesulam *et al.* 2003). Similarly, lesion load within the cholinergic pathways has been shown to correlate with cognitive impairment in patients post-stroke (Lim *et al.* 2014).

Commonly used screening instruments for dementia such as the Mini-Mental State Examination (MMSE) (Folstein *et al.* 1983) and the Alzheimer's Disease Assessment Scale – Cognitive subscale (ADAS-cog) (Rosen *et al.* 1984) were primarily developed for assessing cognition in Alzheimer's disease and are relatively insensitive to executive and attentional function and milder cognitive deficits (Fig. 31.3), although they are reliable

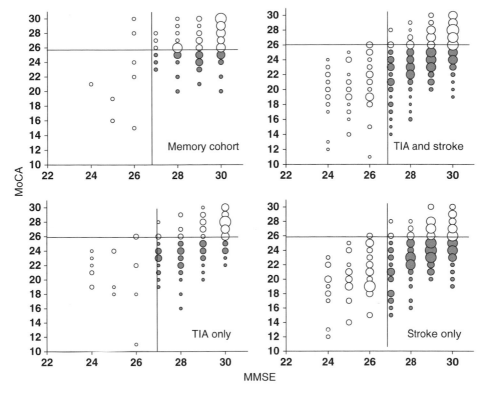

Fig. 31.2 Bubble plots of MMSE versus MoCA score for a memory research cohort and OXVASC patients: TIA and stroke combined, TIA only, and stroke only. Shaded bubbles indicate subjects who had MMSE ≥ 27 but MoCA < 26. MMSE, Mini-Mental State Examination; MoCA, Montreal Cognitive Assessment; TIA, transient ischemic attack; OXVASC, Oxford Vascular Study. From Pendlebury *et al.* (2010, 2012a).

in identifying moderate/severe cognitive impairment in vascular patients (Lees *et al.* 2014). The more recent 30-point Montreal Cognitive Assessment (MoCA), along with the Addenbrooke's Cognitive examination (Hsieh *et al.* 2013), is more sensitive, although neither incorporates timed tests necessary to measure impaired processing speed (Pendlebury *et al.* 2010, 2012b; Dong *et al.* 2010, 2012; Mai *et al.* 2016). The Harmonisation Standards consensus paper (Hachinski *et al.* 2006) recommends the MoCA (Nasreddine *et al.* 2005) to screen for vascular cognitive impairment, and more detailed quantification of frontal/executive deficits can be made using a neuropsychological battery including verbal fluency, trail making, digit span, and symbol digit test (Hachinski *et al.* 2006). Such tests may be also incorporated into the ADAS-cog to create the Vascular Dementia Assessment Scale cognitive subscale (VADAS-cog) for use in vascular cognitive impairment (Mohs *et al.* 1997).

Behavioral changes are common in patients with vascular cognitive impairment, with high rates of depression and apathy, particularly in those with small vessel disease. For example, in the Cache County Study, significantly more participants with vascular dementia (32%) than Alzheimer's disease (20%) suffered from depression, the reverse being true for the presence of delusions (Lyketsos *et al.* 2000). Depression may be a result of the neuropathological processes, and this is supported by the observation that depression is a risk factor for vascular cognitive impairment (Barnes *et al.* 2006). Vascular cognitive

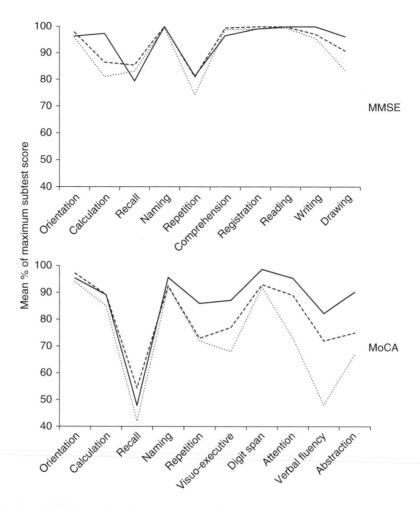

Fig. 31.3 Mean MMSE (upper figure) and MoCA (lower figure) subtest scores shown as a percentage of the maximum subtest score for memory research subjects (solid gray line), TIA patients (dashed line), and stroke patients (dotted line). MMSE, Mini-Mental State Examination; MoCA, Montreal Cognitive Assessment; TIA, transient ischemic attack. From Pendlebury *et al.* (2012a).

impairment may also be associated with agitation, disinhibition, aggression, aberrant motor behavior, and hallucinations (Lyketsos *et al.* 2000).

Overlap between Vascular Cognitive Impairment and Alzheimer's Disease

In clinical practice, distinguishing between Alzheimer's disease and vascular cognitive impairment is often difficult, and many patients are likely to have coexistent pathology as stated earlier. In a large community-based study of unselected older people who were followed longitudinally and underwent autopsy, mixed Alzheimer's and vascular pathology was found to be the most common cause of cognitive impairment (Neuropathology Group of the Medical Research Council Cognitive Function and

Aging Study 2001). This is consistent with other studies showing mixed pathology to be at least as common as "pure" vascular dementia (Knopman *et al.* 2003). There is also poor correlation between clinical diagnosis of dementia subtype and neuropathological findings: Up to 30% of patients diagnosed with Alzheimer's disease have evidence of vascular pathology at autopsy. Deep white matter lesions can also be demonstrated on MRI in approximately 50% of those with Alzheimer's disease, with periventricular lesions found in more than 90%.

The widespread coexistence of cerebral infarcts and Alzheimer's pathology is accompanied by interactions between the two pathologies: Patients with Alzheimer's pathology and cerebrovascular disease have a greater severity of cognitive impairment than those with similar severity of either pathology (Snowdon *et al.* 1997; Esiri *et al.* 1999; Schneider *et al.* 2007). After controlling for severity of cortical infarcts and Alzheimer's pathology, subcortical infarcts increase the risk of dementia by almost four times (Schneider *et al.* 2007). However, the synergistic effect between cerebrovascular disease and Alzheimer's pathology is only seen in those with mild neurodegenerative change. In patients with severe neurodegenerative disease, associated vascular pathology becomes less important.

Vascular mechanisms may be important in the expression and development of Alzheimer's pathology. Vascular risk factors are risk factors for Alzheimer's disease, and cerebral hypoperfusion and microcirculatory changes may precede the neuropathological and clinical changes of Alzheimer's disease, making it, in effect, a vascular disorder (Kalaria 2000; de la Torre 2002; Gorelick *et al.* 2011). Further evidence for a vascular mechanism comes from the observation that biochemical and structural changes occur in cerebral vessel walls in patients with early Alzheimer's disease, leading to altered vasoreactivity, impaired autoregulation, and a greater degree of arterial pressure transmittal to the capillary circulation, thus predisposing to microvessel damage (Stopa *et al.* 2008).

Stroke-Associated Cognitive Impairment and Dementia

Dementia/cognitive impairment occurring as a result of stroke is a subtype of vascular cognitive impairment (Leys *et al.* 2005). The reciprocal risks of stroke and dementia (Rostamian *et al.* 2014; Pendlebury and Rothwell 2009) suggest that there may be a shared susceptibility to the two syndromes (Pendlebury *et al.* 2017b).

Most studies of stroke-associated dementia are cross-sectional hospital series with a focus on major strokes; very few include patients with TIA, and many studies may have been affected by selection (Pendlebury *et al.* 2015a) and attritional biases (Pendlebury *et al.* 2015b). Although rates are overall heterogeneous, this is largely explained by variations in case mix and methodology that far exceed the small effects of the use of different criteria to define dementia (Rasquin *et al.* 2005a; Pendlebury and Rothwell 2009). Pre-stroke dementia ranges from 7% to 16% with the lowest prevalence in population-based studies of first-ever stroke and highest prevalence in hospital-based series of any stroke (Fig. 31.4). Similarly, post-stroke dementia cumulative incidence to 1-year post-stroke ranges from 7% to 41% with lowest risk in first-ever stroke and highest risk in hospital studies of recurrent stroke (Fig. 31.5). Overall about 1 in 10 patients have dementia before their stroke and 1 in 10 develop new dementia after a first-ever stroke. The risk of new-incident dementia following stroke is non-linear, being high in the first few months and relatively low thereafter in the absence of recurrent stroke, although the risk remains elevated above the background in the long term (Pendlebury and Rothwell 2009; Fig. 31.6). Data from the population-based

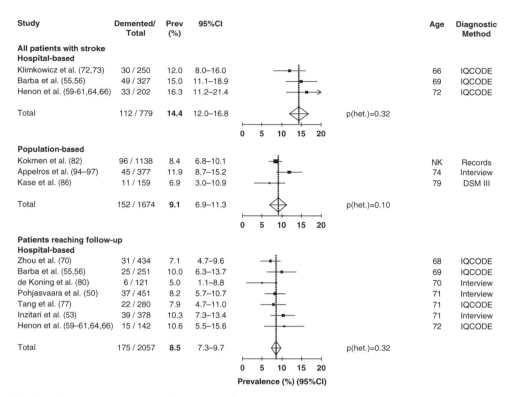

Fig. 31.4 Pooled prevalence (%) of pre-stroke dementia stratified by study setting (hospital- versus population-based) and time of assessment (at the time of stroke or at follow-up some months after stroke) together with the mean age of the patients in each study and the method of dementia diagnosis (Records = retrospective review of medical records, Interview = interview of informant without IQCODE questionnaire). Numbers in brackets refer to individual studies included in the source publication. From Pendlebury and Rothwell (2009).

Oxford Vascular Study (OXVASC) have shown that the prevalence of dementia pre-TIA is similar to the UK age-matched population rate at ~5%, whereas it is ~20% (about four times the background rate) in patients presenting with stroke NIHSS > 10. Post-event dementia incidence relative to the background incidence rate in the first year after the event is ~3 times after TIA and ~40 times greater after a stroke with NIHSS >10, with a stepwise relationship with event severity (Pendlebury *et al.* 2017b; Fig. 31.7).

Factors associated with post-stroke dementia include those related to brain vulnerability (age, education, prior cognitive impairment, white matter disease) and stroke factors including severity, previous/recurrent stroke, and multiple strokes (Moulin *et al.* 2016; Mok *et al.* 2017; Pendlebury *et al.* 2017a). Vascular risk factors are not associated with dementia. In hemorrhagic stroke, superficial/lobar versus deep bleeding is associated with a higher dementia risk owing to its association with cerebral amyloid angiopathy (Moulin *et al.* 2016).

The exact mechanisms underlying post-stroke dementia are unclear, although both immediate lesion impact and preexisting brain vulnerability are important as suggested by the independent associates (Pendlebury *et al.* 2017a). Therefore, risk of dementia after

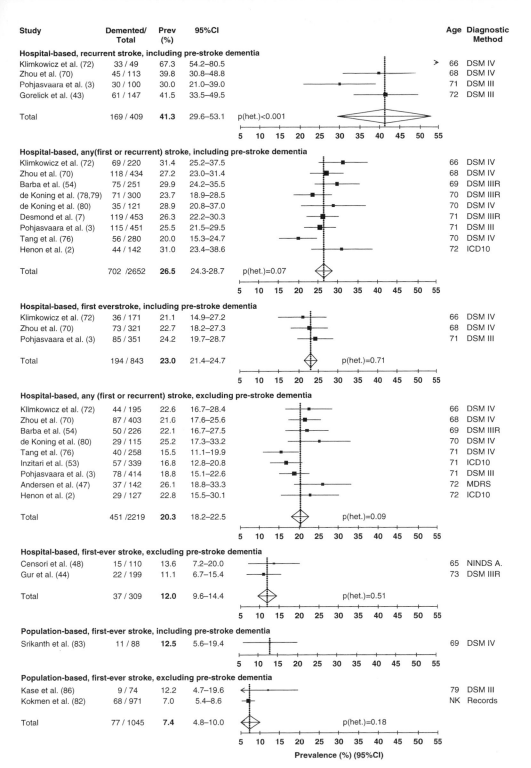

Fig. 31.5 Pooled prevalence (%) of post-stroke dementia up to 1 year after stroke stratified by study setting (hospital versus population-based), inclusion or exclusion of pre-stroke dementia, and first-ever versus any (first ever or recurrent) versus recurrent stroke. Mean age of the patients in each study is shown in the right column together with method of dementia diagnosis (NINDS A.= NINDS AIREN). Numbers in brackets refer to individual studies included in the source publication. NK, not known. From Pendlebury and Rothwell (2009).

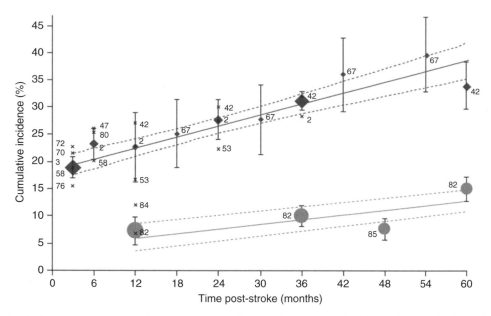

Fig. 31.6 Pooled cumulative incidence (linear regression-solid line, 95% CI-dashed lines) of post-stroke dementia excluding pre-stroke dementia in hospital-based cohorts of any (first-ever or recurrent) stroke (diamonds) and population-based cohorts of first-ever stroke (circles) (symbol size is proportional to the inverse of the variance for each time point; error bars indicate 95% CI at each point). Individual studies denoted by crosses with corresponding article reference. Population data only shown to month 60, but regression line calculated to 25 years post-stroke. From Pendlebury and Rothwell (2009).

TIA is low in patients with otherwise healthy brains but is much higher in patients with poor brain health (Pendlebury *et al.* 2017a). Brain vulnerability may be revealed by transient cognitive impairment associated with the cerebrovascular event that identifies a group at high risk of subsequent dementia (Nys *et al.* 2005; Pendlebury *et al.* 2011; Mazzucco *et al.* 2016). Similarly, a low score on cognitive testing at baseline is strongly predictive of future dementia risk (Allan *et al.* 2011; Salvadori *et al.* 2013; Dong *et al.* 2016; Pendlebury *et al.* 2017a) as is overt delirium (Oldenbeuving *et al.* 2011).

Early post-stroke dementia may occur in patients with a high burden of Alzheimer pathology, even where the precipitating stroke is mild, whereas later post-stroke dementia may be more related to accrual of vascular pathology and worsening white matter disease (Henon *et al.* 2001; Allan *et al.* 2011; Mok *et al.* 2017). PET amyloid imaging using amyloid markers such as PiB or flutemetamol (Ye *et al.* 2015; Liu *et al.* 2015; Wollenweber *et al.* 2016) has been used in an attempt to identify coexistent Alzheimer pathology in patients post-stroke (Fig. 31.8) and has been reported to be associated with increased risk of cognitive decline but lack of specificity for Alzheimer's pathology, particularly in older patients, limits its utility. Inflammatory effects of the stroke lesion and coexistent systemic illness such as pneumonia may also play a role in post-stroke dementia (Govan *et al.* 2007; Pendlebury and Rothwell 2009; van Gool *et al.* 2010).

The risk of cognitive impairment without dementia is also increased post-stroke and also in younger patients with TIA versus controls (van Rooij *et al.* 2014), although lack of consensus in definitions makes reliable estimates problematic (Pendlebury *et al.* 2011).

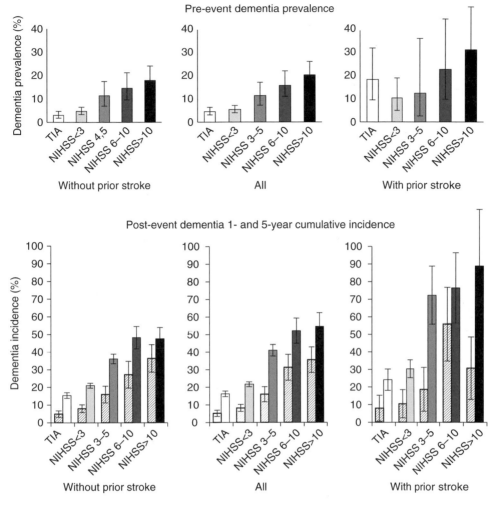

Fig. 31.7 Results from the Oxford Vascular Study, a population-based study covering the full spectrum of cerebrovascular events, showing a stepwise association between event severity and dementia that is modified by previous/recurrent events: Pre-event dementia prevalence and post-event 1-year (stippled bars) and 5-year (solid bars) cumulative incidence of dementia. From Pendlebury *et al.* (2017b).

Further, as stated earlier in relation to transient cognitive impairment, many patients improve after the event, and individual patient cognitive trajectories are heterogeneous and difficult to predict (del Ser *et al.* 2005; Rasquin *et al.* 2005a; Srikanth *et al.* 2006). Diabetic patients appear less likely to improve, and initial attentional and executive deficits may be more persistent than memory deficits.

Because of the high risk of dementia after cerebrovascular events and patient concerns, assessment of cognitive function after stroke is recommended. To date, there is no single recommended test, and choice of test will depend on time available and patient factors (see earlier). Short screening tests may be more practical for routine use than extensive neuropsychological batteries. Importantly, it should be noted that more than half of patients

(a) PIB negative

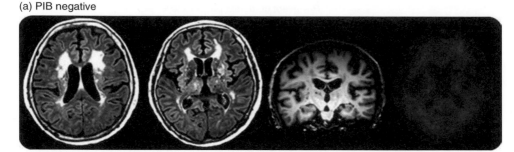

(b) PIB positive

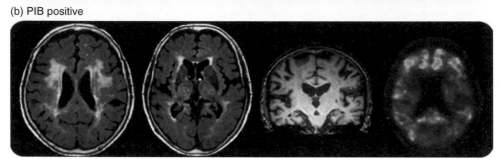

Fig. 31.8 PET amyloid imaging post-stroke. From Mok *et al.* (2017)

with major stroke have problems with completing short cognitive tests or may be untestable in the immediate post-stroke phase because of stroke effects (e.g., aphasia, delirium) or other problems such as poor vision (Pasi *et al.* 2013; Horstmann *et al.* 2014; Pendlebury *et al.* 2015c). While testability rates rise with time after stroke, this is largely because of high mortality rates in untestable patients. Testability issues are likely higher with lengthy neuropsychological batteries, but there are few data.

While both primary and secondary prevention of stroke will reduce the overall burden of cognitive impairment and dementia, available data suggest that treatment of vascular risk factors after stroke may not be effective in reducing post-stroke cognitive decline beyond preventing recurrent events. Treatment of vascular dementia as a whole is discussed in Chapter 32.

Delirium

Delirium (acute confusional state) is characterized by acute change in cognition with fluctuation, attentional, and other cognitive deficits and altered conscious level (hyper- or hypo-arousal) secondary to underlying physiological disturbance. Delirium occurs in up to one-fifth of hospitalized acute stroke patients. It is more common with increasing age, stroke severity, and complications including infection. Some studies have also linked stroke location to delirium risk. As for delirium occurring in the context of acute illness (Pendlebury *et al.* 2015d), delirium associated with stroke carries an increased risk of mortality, longer length of stay, institutionalization, and dementia (Oldenbeuving *et al.* 2011; Shi *et al.* 2012; Carin-Levy *et al.* 2012). Delirium may also occur on a background of established vascular dementia often as a result of systemic illness especially infection.

Table 31.3 Distinguishing between dementia and delirium

Feature	Delirium	Dementia
Onset	Acute, often at night	Insidious
Course	Fluctuating, lucid times	Stable
Duration	Hours/weeks	Months/years
Awareness	Reduced	Clear
Alertness	Abnormal (low/high)	Usually normal
Attention	Impaired, distractible	Usually unaffected
Orientation	Impaired	Impaired in later stages
Short-term memory	Always impaired	Normal at first
Episodic memory	Impaired	Impaired
Thinking	Disorganized, delusions	Impoverished
Perception	Illusions/hallucinations	Absent early, common later
Sleep cycle	Always disrupted	Usually normal

It may be difficult to distinguish between dementia and delirium in older confused patients in the hospital setting where the patient's premorbid state is unknown and collateral history is unavailable. Factors distinguishing between dementia and delirium are shown in Table 31.3, although in practice, the two conditions frequently coexist. In a person with established preexisting cognitive decline, relatives are often aware that a change in behavior may indicate underlying illness. A number of screening tools for delirium are available, including for delirium associated with stroke, although the presence of focal deficits may complicate assessment (Lees *et al.* 2013).

References

Allan LM, Rowan EN, Firbank MJ, Thomas AJ, Parry SW, Polvikoski TM, O'Brien JT, Kalaria RN (2011). Long term incidence of dementia, predictors of mortality and pathological diagnosis in older stroke survivors. *Brain* **134**(12):3716–3727

American Psychiatric Association (1994). *Diagnostic and Statistical Manual of Mental Disorders*, 4th edn. Washington, DC: American Psychiatric Press

American Psychiatric Association (2013). *Diagnostic and Statistical Manual of Mental Disorders*, 5th edn. Washington, DC: American Psychiatric Press

Appelros P, Nydevik I, Seiger A, Terent A (2002). Predictors of severe stroke: Influence of preexisting dementia and cardiac disorders. *Stroke* **33**(10):2357–2362

Barnes DE, Alexopoulos GS, Lopez OL *et al.* (2006). Depressive symptoms, vascular disease, and mild cognitive impairment: Findings from the Cardiovascular Health Study. *Archives of General Psychiatry* **63**:273–279

Bastos-Leite AJ, van der Flier WM, van Straaten EC *et al.* (2007). The contribution of medial temporal lobe atrophy and vascular pathology to cognitive impairment in vascular dementia. *Stroke* **38**:3182–3185

Black S, Roman GC, Geldmacher DS *et al.* (2003). Efficacy and tolerability of donepezil in vascular dementia: Positive results of a 24-week, multicenter, international, randomized, placebo-controlled clinical trial. *Stroke* **34**:2323–2330

Buffon F, Porcher R, Hernandez K *et al.* (2006). Cognitive profile in CADASIL. *Journal of Neurology, Neurosurgery and Psychiatry* 77:175–180

Carin-Levy G, Mead GE, Nicol K, Rush R, van Wijck F (2012). Delirium in acute stroke: Screening tools, incidence rates and predictors: A systematic review. *J Neurol* 259(8):1590–1599

Chen A, Akinyemi RO, Hase Y, Firbank MJ, Ndung'u MN, Foster V, Craggs LJ, Washida K, Okamoto Y, Thomas AJ, Polvikoski TM, Allan LM, Oakley AE, O'Brien JT, Horsburgh K, Ihara M, Kalaria RN (2016). Frontal white matter hyperintensities, clasmatodendrosis and gliovascular abnormalities in ageing and post-stroke dementia. *Brain.* 139(Pt 1):242–258

Chui H, Gonthier R (1999). Natural history of vascular dementia. *Alzheimer Disease Association Disorders* 13(Suppl 3):S124–S130

de la Torre JC (2002). Alzheimer disease as a vascular disorder: Nosological evidence. *Stroke* 33:1152–1162

del Ser T, Barba R, Morin MM *et al.* (2005). Evolution of cognitive impairment after stroke and risk factors for delayed progression. *Stroke* 36:2670–2675

Desmond DW (2004). The neuropsychology of vascular cognitive impairment: Is there a specific cognitive deficit? *Journal of Neurology Science* 226:3–7

Dong Y, Sharma VK, Chan BP, Venketasubramanian N, Teoh HL, Seet RC, Tanicala S, Chan YH, Chen C. (2010). The Montreal Cognitive Assessment (MoCA) is superior to the Mini-Mental State Examination (MMSE) for the detection of vascular cognitive impairment after acute stroke. *J Neurol Sci* 299 (1–2):15–18

Dong Y, Lee WY, Basri NA, Collinson SL, Merchant RA, Venketasubramanian N, Chen CL (2012). The Montreal Cognitive Assessment is superior to the Mini-Mental State Examination in detecting patients at higher risk of dementia. *Int Psychogeriatr* 24(11):1749–1755

Dong Y, Xu J, Chan BP, Seet RC, Venketasubramanian N, Teoh HL, Sharma VK, Chen CL (2016). The Montreal Cognitive Assessment is superior to National Institute of Neurological Disease and Stroke-Canadian Stroke Network 5-minute protocol in predicting vascular cognitive impairment at 1 year. *BMC Neurol.* 12(16):46

Esiri MM, Nagy Z, Smith MZ *et al.* (1999). Cerebrovascular disease and threshold for dementia in the early stages of Alzheimer's disease. *Lancet* 354:919–920

Folstein MF, Robins LN, Helzer JE (1983). The Mini-Mental State Examination. *Archives of General Psychiatry* 40:812

Foster V, Oakley AE, Slade JY, Hall R, Polvikoski TM, Burke M, Thomas AJ, Khundakar A, Allan LM, Kalaria RN. (2014). Pyramidal neurons of the prefrontal cortex in post-stroke, vascular and other ageing-related dementias. *Brain* 137(9):2509–2521

Freitag MH, Peila R, Masaki K *et al.* (2006). Midlife pulse pressure and incidence of dementia: The Honolulu–Asia Aging Study. *Stroke* 37:33–37

Gold G, Bouras C, Canuto A *et al.* (2002). Clinicopathological validation study of four sets of clinical criteria for vascular dementia. *American Journal of Psychiatry* 159:82–87

Gorelick PB, Scuteri A, Black SE, *et al.* on behalf of the American Heart Association Stroke Council, Council on Epidemiology and Prevention, Council on Cardiovascular Nursing, Council on Cardiovascular Radiology and Intervention, Council on Cardiovascular Surgery and Anesthesia Stroke. (2011). Vascular contributions to cognitive impairment and dementia: A statement for healthcare professionals from the American Heart Association/American Stroke Association. *Stroke* 42(9):2672–2713

Gorelick PB, Scuteri A, Black SE, Decarli C, Greenberg SM, Iadecola C *et al.* (2011). Vascular contributions to cognitive impairment and dementia: A statement for healthcare professionals from the American Heart Association/American Stroke Association. *Stroke* 42:2672–2713

Govan L, Langhorne P, Weir CJ (2007). Stroke Unit Trialists Collaboration. Does the prevention of complications explain the survival benefit of organized inpatient (stroke unit) care?: Further analysis of a systematic review. *Stroke* 38:2536–2540

Hachinski VC, Iliff LD, Zilhka E *et al.* (1975). Cerebral blood flow in dementia. *Archives of Neurology* 32:632–637

Hachinski V, Iadecola C, Petersen RC *et al.* (2006). National Institute of Neurological Disorders and Stroke-Canadian Stroke Network vascular cognitive impairment harmonization standards. *Stroke* 37:2220–2241

Henon H, Durieu I, Guerouaou D, Lebert F, Pasquier F, Leys D (2001). Poststroke dementia: Incidence and relationship to prestroke cognitive decline. *Neurology* 57(7):1216–1222

Horstmann S, Rizos T, Rauch G, Arden C, Veltkamp R (2014). Feasibility of the Montreal Cognitive Assessment in acute stroke patients. *Eur J Neurol* 21(11):1387–1393

Hsieh S, Schubert S, Hoon C, Mioshi E, Hodges JR (2013). Validation of the Addenbrooke's Cognitive Examination III in frontotemporal dementia and Alzheimer's disease. *Dement Geriatr Cogn Disord* 36(3–4):242–250

Jin YP, Di Legge S, Ostbye T, Feightner JW, Hachinski V. (2006). The reciprocal risks of stroke and cognitive impairment in an elderly population. *Alzheimers Dement* 2(3):171–178

Jorm AF, Jolley D (1998). The incidence of dementia: A meta-analysis. *Neurology* 51:728–733

Kalaria RN (2000). The role of cerebral ischemia in Alzheimer's disease. *Neurobiology Aging* 21:321–330

Knopman DS, Parisi JE, Boeve BF *et al.* (2003). Vascular dementia in a population-based autopsy study. *Archives of Neurology* 60:569–575

Lees R, Corbet S, Johnston C, Moffitt E, Shaw G, Quinn TJ (2013). Test accuracy of short screening tests for diagnosis of delirium or cognitive impairment in an acute stroke unit setting. *Stroke* 44(11):3078–3083

Lees R, Selvarajah J, Fenton C, Pendlebury ST, Langhorne P, Stott DJ, Quinn TJ (2014). Test accuracy of cognitive screening tests for diagnosis of dementia and multidomain cognitive impairment in stroke. *Stroke* 45 (10):3008–3018

Leys D, Hénon H, Mackowiak-Cordoliani MA, Pasquier F (2005). Poststroke dementia. *Lancet Neurol* 4(11):752–759

Lim JS, Kim N, Jang MU, Han MK, Kim S, Baek MJ, Jang MS, Ban B, Kang Y, Kim DE, Lee JS, Lee J, Lee BC, Yu KH, Black SE, Bae HJ (2014). Cortical hubs and subcortical

cholinergic pathways as neural substrates of poststroke dementia. *Stroke* 45(4):1069–1076

Liu W, Wong A, Au L, Yang J, Wang Z, Leung EY, Chen S, Ho CL, Mok VC (2015). Influence of amyloid-β on cognitive decline after stroke/transient ischemic attack: Three-year longitudinal study. *Stroke* 46(11):3074–3080

Lobo A, Launer LJ, Fratiglioni L, Andersen K, Di Carlo A, Breteler MM, Copeland JR, Dartigues JF, Jagger C, Martinez-Lage J, Soininen H, Hofman A (2000). Prevalence of dementia and major subtypes in Europe: A collaborative study of population-based cohorts. Neurologic Diseases in the Elderly Research Group. *Neurology* 54(11 Suppl 5):S4–9

Lopez OL, Kuller LH, Becker JT *et al.* (2005). Classification of vascular dementia in the Cardiovascular Health Study Cognition Study. *Neurology* 64:1539–1547

Lyketsos CG, Steinberg M, Tschanz JT *et al.* (2000). Mental and behavioral disturbances in dementia: Findings from the Cache County Study on Memory in Aging. *American Journal of Psychiatry* 157:708–714

Mai LM, Sposato LA, Rothwell PM, Hachinski V, Pendlebury ST (2016). A comparison between the MoCA and the MMSE visuoexecutive sub-tests in detecting abnormalities in TIA/stroke patients. *Int J Stroke* 11(4):420–424

McKhann G, Drachman D, Folstein M *et al.* (1984). Clinical diagnosis of Alzheimer's disease: Report of the NINCDS–ADRDA Work Group under the auspices of Department of Health and Human Services Task Force on Alzheimer's Disease. *Neurology* 34:939–944

Matthews, FE *et al.* (2013). A two-decade comparison of prevalence of dementia in individuals aged 65 years and older from three geographical areas of England: Results of the Cognitive Function and Ageing Study I and II. *Lancet* 382:1405–1412

Matthews, FE *et al.* (2016). A two decade dementia incidence comparison from the Cognitive Function and Ageing Studies I and II. *Nat Commun* 7:11398

Mazzucco S, Li L, Tuna MA, *et al.* Oxford Vascular Study. (2016). Hemodynamic correlates of transient cognitive impairment after transient ischemic attack and minor stroke:

A transcranial Doppler study. *Int J Stroke* 11:978–986

Mesulam M, Siddique T, Cohen B (2003). Cholinergic denervation in a pure multi-infarct state: Observations on CADASIL. *Neurology* 60:1183–1185

Mohs RC, Knopman D, Petersen RC *et al.* (1997). Development of cognitive instruments for use in clinical trials of antidementia drugs: Additions to the Alzheimer's Disease Assessment Scale that broaden its scope. The Alzheimer's Disease Cooperative Study. *Alzheimer Disease Association Disorders* 11 (Suppl 2):S13–S21

Neuropathology Group Medical Research Council Cognitive Function and Aging Study (2001). Pathological correlates of late-onset dementia in a multicentre, community-based population in England and Wales. *Lancet* 357:169–175

Mok VC, Lam BY, Wong A, Ko H, Markus HS, Wong LK (2017). Early-onset and delayed-onset poststroke dementia – revisiting the mechanisms. *Nat Rev Neurol* 13(3):148–159

Narasimhalu K, Ang S, De Silva DA, Wong MC, Chang HM, Chia KS, Auchus AP, Chen C (2009). Severity of CIND and MCI predict incidence of dementia in an ischemic stroke cohort. *Neurology* 73(22):1866–1872

Nasreddine ZS, Phillips NA, Bedirian V *et al.* (2005). The Montreal cognitive assessment, MOCA: A brief screening tool for mild cognitive impairment. *J Am Geriatr Soc* 53:695–699

Nys GM, van Zandvoort MJ, de Kort PL, van der Worp HB, Jansen BP, Algra A, de Haan EH, Kappelle LJ (2005). The prognostic value of domain-specific cognitive abilities in acute first-ever stroke. *Neurology* 64(5):821–827

Oldenbeuving AW, de Kort PL, Jansen BP, Algra A, Kappelle LJ, Roks G (2011). Delirium in the acute phase after stroke: Incidence, risk factors, and outcome. *Neurology* 76(11):993–999

O'Brien JT, Paling S, Barber R *et al.* (2001). Progressive brain atrophy on serial MRI in dementia with Lewy bodies, AD, and vascular dementia. *Neurology* 56:1386–1388

Pasi M, Salvadori E, Poggesi A, Inzitari D, Pantoni L (2013). Factors predicting the Montreal cognitive assessment (MoCA) applicability and performances in a stroke unit. *J Neurol* 260(6):1518–1526

Pendlebury ST, Rothwell PM (2009). Prevalence, incidence, and factors associated with pre-stroke and post-stroke dementia: A systematic review and meta-analysis. *Lancet Neurol* 8 (11):1006–1018

Pendlebury ST, Cuthbertson FC, Welch SJ, Mehta Z, Rothwell PM (2010). Underestimation of cognitive impairment by Mini-Mental State Examination versus the Montreal Cognitive Assessment in patients with transient ischemic attack and stroke: A population-based study. *Stroke* 41(6):1290–1293

Pendlebury ST, Wadling S, Silver LE, Mehta Z, Rothwell PM (2011). Transient cognitive impairment in TIA and minor stroke. *Stroke* 42 (11):3116–3121

Pendlebury ST, Markwick A, de Jager CA, Zamboni G, Wilcock GK, Rothwell PM (2012a). Differences in cognitive profile between TIA, stroke and elderly memory research subjects: A comparison of the MMSE and MoCA. *Cerebrovasc Dis* 34(1):48–54

Pendlebury ST, Mariz J, Bull L, Mehta Z, Rothwell PM (2012b). MoCA, ACE-R, and MMSE versus the National Institute of Neurological Disorders and Stroke-Canadian Stroke Network Vascular Cognitive Impairment Harmonization Standards Neuropsychological Battery after TIA and stroke. *Stroke* 43(2):464–469

Pendlebury ST, Mariz J, Bull L, Mehta Z, Rothwell PM (2013). Impact of different operational definitions on mild cognitive impairment rate and MMSE and MoCA performance in transient ischaemic attack and stroke. *Cerebrovasc Dis* 36(5–6):355–362

Pendlebury ST, Chen PJ, Bull L, Silver L, Mehta Z, Rothwell PM (2015a). Oxford Vascular Study. Methodological factors in determining rates of dementia in transient ischemic attack and stroke: (I) impact of baseline selection bias. *Stroke* 46(3):641–646

Pendlebury ST, Chen PJ, Welch SJ, Cuthbertson FC, Wharton RM, Mehta Z, Rothwell PM (2015b). Oxford Vascular Study. Methodological factors in determining risk of dementia after transient ischemic attack and stroke: (II) Effect of attrition on follow-up. *Stroke* 46(6):1494–1500

Pendlebury ST, Klaus SP, Thomson RJ *et al.* Oxford Vascular Study. (2015c) Methodological factors in determining risk of dementia after transient ischemic attack and stroke: (III) Applicability of cognitive tests. *Stroke* **46** (11):3067–3073

Pendlebury ST, Lovett NG, Smith SC *et al.* (2015d). Observational, longitudinal study of delirium in consecutive unselected acute medical admissions: Age-specific rates and associated factors, mortality and re-admission. *BMJ Open* **5**(11):e007808

Pendlebury ST, Wharton RM, Rothwell PM (2017a). Predictors of dementia after TIA/ stroke: 15-year population-based follow-up study. *J Eur Stroke* **2**(suppl 1):AS11–003

Pendlebury ST, Wharton RM, Rothwell PM (2017b). Stepwise relationship between severity of acute cerebrovascular events and pre-post-event dementia: Population-based study of TIA and stroke. *J Eur Stroke* **2**(suppl 1):AS11–010

Pohjasvaara T, Mäntylä R, Ylikoski R, Kaste M, Erkinjuntti T (2000). Comparison of different clinical criteria (DSM-III, ADDTC, ICD-10, NINDS-AIREN, DSM-IV) for the diagnosis of vascular dementia. National Institute of Neurological Disorders and Stroke-Association Internationale pour la Recherche et l'Enseignement en Neurosciences. *Stroke* **31** (12):2952–2957

Prins ND, van Dijk EJ, den Heijer T *et al.* (2005). Cerebral small-vessel disease and decline in information processing speed, executive function and memory. *Brain* **128**:2034–2041

Rasquin SM, Lodder J, Verhey FR (2005a). Predictors of reversible mild cognitive impairment after stroke: A 2-year follow-up study. *Journal of Neurology Science* **15**:21–25

Rasquin SM, Lodder J, Verhey FR (2005b). The effect of different diagnostic criteria on the prevalence and incidence of post-stroke dementia. *Neuroepidemiology* **24**:189–195

Román GC, Tatemichi TK, Erkinjuntti T *et al.* (1993). Vascular dementia: Diagnostic criteria for research studies. Report of the NINDS–AIREN International Workshop. *Neurology* **43**:250–260

Rosen WG, Mohs RC, Davis KL (1984). A new rating scale for Alzheimer's disease. *American Journal of Psychiatry* **141**:1356–1364

Rostamian S, Mahinrad S, Stijnen T, Sabayan B, de Craen AJ (2014). Cognitive impairment and risk of stroke: A systematic review and meta-analysis of prospective cohort studies. *Stroke* **45**:1342–1348

Sachdev P, Kalaria R, O'Brien J *et al.* (2014). International Society for Vascular Behavioral and Cognitive Disorders. Diagnostic criteria for vascular cognitive disorders: A VASCOG statement. *Alzheimer Dis Assoc Disord* **28** (3):206–218

Salvadori E, Pasi M, Poggesi A, Chiti G, Inzitari D, Pantoni L (2013). Predictive value of MoCA in the acute phase of stroke on the diagnosis of mid-term cognitive impairment. *J Neurol* **260**(9):2220–2227

Schneider JA, Boyle PA, Arvanitakis Z *et al.* (2007). Subcortical infarcts, Alzheimer's disease pathology, and memory function in older persons. *Annals of Neurology* **62**:59–66

Shi Q, Presutti R, Selchen D, Saposnik G (2012). Delirium in acute stroke: A systematic review and meta-analysis. *Stroke* **43**(3):645–649

Skoog I, Lernfelt B, Landahl S *et al.* (1996). 15-year longitudinal study of blood pressure and dementia. *Lancet* **27**:1141–1145

Skrobot OA, Attems J, Esiri M, Hortobagyi T, Ironside JW, Kalaria RN, King A, Lammie GA, Mann D, Neal JW *et al.* (2016). Cognitive Impairment Neuropathology Guidelines (VCING) – a multi-centre study of the contribution of cerebrovascular pathology to cognitive impairment. *Brain* **139**(11):2957–2969

Snowdon DA, Greiner LH, Mortimer JA *et al.* (1997). Brain infarction and the clinical expression of Alzheimer disease. The Nun Study. *Journal of American Medical Association* **277**:813–817

Solomon A, Kåreholt I, Ngandu T *et al.* (2007). Serum cholesterol changes after midlife and late-life cognition: Twenty-one-year follow-up study. *Neurology* **68**:751–756

Srikanth VK, Quinn SJ, Donnan GA *et al.* (2006). Long-term cognitive transitions, rates of cognitive change, and predictors of incident dementia in a population-based first-ever stroke cohort. *Stroke* **37**:2479–2483

Stopa EG, Butala P, Salloway S *et al.* (2008). Cerebral cortical arteriolar angiopathy, vascular

[beta]-amyloid, smooth muscle actin, Braak stage and APOE genotype. *Stroke* **39**:814–821

van Gool WA, van de Beek D, Eikelenboom P (2010). Systemic infection and delirium: When cytokines and acetylcholine collide. *Lancet* **375**:773–775

van Rooij FG, Schaapsmeerders P, Maaijwee NA et al. (2014). Persistent cognitive impairment after transient ischemic attack. *Stroke* **45**:2270–2274

Wentzel C, Rockwood K, MacKnight C et al. (2001). Progression of impairment in patients with vascular cognitive impairment without dementia. *Neurology* **57**:714–716

Wollenweber FA, Därr S, Müller C, Duering M, Buerger K, Zietemann V, Malik R, Brendel M, Ertl-Wagner B, Bartenstein P, Rominger A, Dichgans M (2016). Prevalence of amyloid positron emission tomographic positivity in poststroke mild cognitive impairment. *Stroke* **47**(10):2645–2648

World Health Organization (1987). *International Classification of Diseases, 10th revision*. Geneva: World Health Organization

Wu YT, Beiser AS, Breteler MMB, Fratiglioni L, Helmer C, Hendrie HC, Honda H, Ikram MA, Langa KM, Lobo A, Matthews FE, Ohara T, Pérès K, Qiu C, Seshadri S, Sjölund BM, Skoog I, Brayne C (2017). The changing prevalence and incidence of dementia over time – current evidence. *Nat Rev Neurol* **13**(6):327–339

Ye BS, Seo SW, Kim JH, Kim GH, Cho H, Noh Y, Kim HJ, Yoon CW, Woo SY, Kim SH, Park HK, Kim ST, Choe YS, Lee KH, Kim JS, Oh SJ, Kim C, Weiner M, Lee JH, Na DL (2015). Effects of amyloid and vascular markers on cognitive decline in subcortical vascular dementia. *Neurology* **85**(19): 1687–1693

Chapter 32

Vascular Cognitive Impairment: Investigation and Treatment

When assessing a patient with cognitive impairment, it is important to rule out treatable causes including metabolic and endocrine disorders and to establish the time course including whether the onset was sudden or insidious. At first assessment of confused patients, in TIA and stroke or in acute systemic illness, it may be difficult to be certain whether cognitive impairment is preexisting or has occurred as a result of the event. Often, a sudden deterioration in cognition occurs on a background of preexisting cognitive decline, and time is required to allow for recovery of physical and cognitive deficits before a more stable cognitive state is reached. In patients with TIA and stroke, the etiology of the cognitive impairment will be at least partly vascular, but there will be variable contributions from neurodegenerative or other disorders. In the memory clinic setting, many patients will not have a clinical history of overt cerebrovascular event, but vascular disease is nevertheless prevalent. The subtype of cognitive impairment may be difficult to determine, especially in older patients or those with more advanced dementia, but in other patients, the subtype is easier to define, and this can help guide prognosis and treatment.

Routine Investigations

Routine blood tests for the investigation of cognitive impairment are shown in Table 32.1. In cases of suspected autoimmune encephalopathy (fluctuating cognition/arousal often with seizures), autoantibodies including voltage gated K channel antibodies should be sent (Varley *et al.* 2017). Current UK guidelines recommend structural brain imaging to exclude pathologies such as space-occupying lesion or subdural hematoma and to aid in dementia subtype identification. Although MRI has better spatial resolution and sensitivity than CT, for the majority of memory clinic patients, CT is adequate and the increased cost of MRI is not justified. For patients post-stroke or TIA, brain imaging will be performed as part of usual TIA/stroke clinical workup and will usually include MRI/DWI or CT/CT angiogram.

Perfusion hexamethylpropyleneamine oxime (HMPAO) single-photon emission computed tomography (SPECT) or 2-[^{18}F]fluoro-2-deoxy-D-glucose positron emission tomography (FDG PET) can be used to help to differentiate between Alzheimer's disease, vascular dementia, and frontotemporal dementia, although findings may be inconclusive. PET imaging using amyloid markers (e.g., PiB, flutemetamol) has been proposed to identify Alzheimer-type pathology but is not in routine clinical use since high rates of amyloid positivity occur in older people without cognitive decline, resulting in lack of specificity.

Cerebrospinal fluid examination and electroencephalography are not required routinely in the investigation of dementia. Lumbar puncture is indicated in suspected

Table 32.1 Routine tests for the investigation of cognitive impairment

Test	Comments
Full blood count	
Electrolytes, creatinine	
Glucose	
Calcium	
Liver function	
Thyroid function	
Vitamin B$_{12}$	Cognitive impairment may occur in the absence of other symptoms
Folate	
Erythrocyte sedimentation rate	Temporal arteritis may cause strokes and cognitive impairment
Midstream urine	If delirium suspected
Syphilis serology	Only if clinical picture is suggestive
Human immunodeficiency virus	Only if clinical picture is suggestive

Creutzfeldt–Jakob disease, paraneoplastic syndromes, or other forms of rapidly progressive dementia. Recently, biomarkers including CSF levels of tau and amyloid-beta have been proposed as adjuncts in the diagnosis of (Alzheimer's) dementia, but their clinical utility is unproven (Ritchie *et al.* 2017), and they appear to have high sensitivity but low specificity, raising the risk of overdiagnosis. Electroencephalography is not routine but may be useful in Creutzfeldt–Jakob disease or suspected non-convulsive status epilepticus or in the assessment of suspected seizure disorder in those with dementia.

Silent Infarcts, White Matter Changes, and Microbleeds

As stated in Chapter 31, vascular changes on brain imaging are included in most diagnostic criteria for vascular cognitive disorder including the Neuroepidemiology Branch of the National Institute of Neurological Disorders and Stroke–Association Internationale pour la Recherche et l'Enseignement en Neurosciences (NINDS/AIREN) criteria (Roman *et al.* 1993) and the Vascular Behavioral and Cognitive Disorders (VASCOG) criteria (Sachdev *et al.* 2014). However, the link between imaging abnormalities, dementia subtype, and cognition is not straightforward. Frequent findings on brain imaging in patients with cognitive impairment include (silent) infarcts, white matter changes, microbleeds and hemorrhage, and sometimes superficial siderosis (Fig. 32.1) suggestive of cerebral amyloid angiopathy (Barber *et al.*1999; Won Seo *et al.* 2007; Moulin *et al.* 2016; Banerjee *et al.* 2017) (Chapters 7 and 10).

Silent infarcts and white matter disease may exist in the presence of normal cognition (Smith *et al.* 2000), but clinical, epidemiological, and pathological studies suggest that, in general, people with white matter change and silent infarcts are more likely to have cognitive impairment than those with normal brains (Frisoni *et al.* 2007; Vermeer *et al.* 2007) and to develop cognitive and functional decline (Pantoni *et al.* 2015) and dementia after stroke

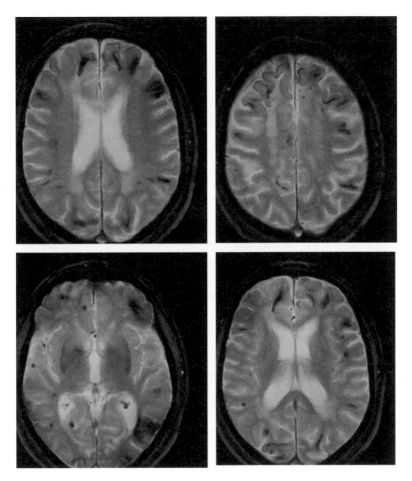

Fig. 32.1 Superficial siderosis in a patient with cerebral amyloid angiopathy and cognitive decline.

(Leys *et al.* 1998; Pendlebury and Rothwell 2009; Chen *et al.* 2016; Mok *et al.* 2017; Pendlebury *et al.* 2017). Severity of white matter change, brain atrophy, and the presence of infarction are associated with decline in information-processing speed and executive function (Prins *et al.* 2005). Presence of subcortical hyperintensities is associated with cognitive impairment following clinical stroke secondary to lacunar infarction (Mok *et al.* 2005; Grau-Olivares *et al.* 2007).

The neuropathology of white matter changes seen on brain imaging is variable and includes partial neuronal loss, axonal loss, demyelination, and gliosis (Jagust *et al.* 2008). The mechanisms underlying such changes are uncertain but there are associations with age, hypertension and diabetes. White matter changes are thought to contribute to cognitive impairment through circuit interruption and disconnection particularly of fronto-subcortical circuits linking the frontal lobes to the striatum, globus pallidus and ventral anterior and mediodorsal thalamus (Liang *et al.* 2016; Kim *et al.* 2015a, b). Interruption of specific parts of the fronto-subcortical circuit causes specific deficits: executive dysfunction and impaired recall (dorsolateral circuit), behavioral and emotional change (orbitofrontal circuit), and abulia and akinetic mutism (anterior cingulate circuit) (Cummings 1993; Tekin and Cummings 2002). The extent and location of white matter changes affect the neuropsychological profile in unimpaired control subjects, patients with stroke, and patients with cognitive impairment and dementia (Delano-Wood et al. 2008; Libon et al. 2008; Swartz et al. 2008; Wright et al. 2008). Several studies highlight the critical role of the thalamus in cognitive function: Patients with thalamic dysfunction secondary to thalamic lesions or to subcortical diaschisis perform poorly in cognitive tests involving frontal and temporal lobe function (Stebbins et al. 2008; Swartz et al. 2008; Wright et al. 2008). There is some evidence that early network disruption in small vessel disease is indicative of dementia risk (Tuladhar et al. 2016).

Cerebral microbleeds seen on $T2^*$-weighted MRI (see Chapter 7) are associated with lacunar infarcts, hemorrhages, white matter changes, hypertension, and cognitive impairment. At present, it is unclear whether the presence and number of microbleeds are independent predictors of cognitive impairment over and above other measures of cerebrovascular pathology (Charimidou and Werring 2012). Location of microbleeds may indicate underlying pathology: Deep microbleeds are associated with hypertensive small vessel disease, whereas lobar microbleeds are associated with cerebral amyloid angiopathy (Chapter 7) in which there is often coexisting leukoaraiosis and cognitive impairment. Recently, consensus criteria have been developed for the quantification of small vessel disease changes on imaging (STandards for ReportIng Vascular changes on nEuroimaging [STRIVE]; Wardlaw et al. 2013), which should aid comparison between studies of small vessel disease and cognitive impairment.

Brain Atrophy and Temporal Lobe Atrophy

Generalized brain atrophy is associated with cognitive impairment in small vessel disease (Mungas et al. 2001; O'Sullivan et al. 2004; Mok et al. 2005) and after stroke (Pendlebury and Rothwell 2009). This may be related to white matter tract degeneration and disconnection (Fein et al. 2000), a process supported by recent diffusion tensor imaging studies (O'Sullivan et al. 2005) (discussed later). However, a primary mechanism cannot be excluded. Loss of brain volume in the syndrome of cerebral autosomal dominant arteriopathy with silent infarcts and leukoaraiosis (CADASIL) is predicted by age, apparent diffusion coefficient, and volume of lacunar lesion, suggesting that brain atrophy is related to both the consequences of lacunar lesions and the widespread microstructural changes beyond the lacunar lesions including in normal appearing white matter (Jouvent et al. 2007).

Temporal lobe atrophy is a well-recognized association of Alzheimer's disease, and early loss of temporal lobe volume occurs in people who are cognitively intact but who go on to develop Alzheimer's disease (Jobst et al. 1992; de Leon et al. 1993). Neuropathological studies have confirmed that the medial temporal lobes are affected very early on in the course of the disease and the resultant impairment of temporal lobe function causes early memory loss. Medial temporal lobe atrophy is also associated with vascular cognitive impairment (Bastos-Leite et al. 2007; Kalaria and Ihara 2017) including post-stroke dementia (Pendlebury and Rothwell 2009) and is not necessarily caused by coexistent neurodegenerative pathology (Fein et al. 2000). Therefore, medial temporal lobe atrophy is not specific to Alzheimer's dementia (Laakso et al. 1996). However, it may be of some discriminatory value in early disease (Jobst et al. 1998; O'Brien et al. 2000), although this may be less so in older patients in whom medial temporal lobe atrophy may simply reflect age-related cerebral atrophy.

Medial temporal lobe atrophy is associated with a greater risk of developing post-stroke dementia in patients who were not demented prior to stroke (Cordoliani-Mackowiak *et al.* 2003; Firbank *et al.* 2007). In a study of delayed cognitive impairment after stroke, medial temporal lobe atrophy, but not white matter hyperintensity volume, was associated with delayed (more than 3 months after stroke) cognitive decline (Firbank *et al.* 2007). The authors suggested that this indicated a greater role for Alzheimer's rather than vascular pathology in delayed post-stroke cognitive impairment. However, given the lack of specificity of medial temporal lobe atrophy for Alzheimer's disease, this may be oversimplistic, and other studies have suggested that progression of white matter disease and multiple vascular risk factors are more important (Allan *et al.* 2011; Mok *et al.* 2017).

Diffusion Tensor, Multimodal, and Functional MR Imaging

Although there is a strong association between stroke severity and risk of post-stroke dementia, lesion location is also important as seen for motor deficits (Chapter 24). While the effect of a lesion on well-defined white matter tracts such as the descending motor pathways can be estimated with some accuracy (Pendlebury *et al.* 1999; Pineiro *et al.* 2000) (Chapter 23), it is almost impossible to do this for tracts passing through the deep white matter since the anatomy and connections of these tracts are not well known. Even if the anatomy of the deep white matter tracts was better understood, it would be impossible to define the exact intersections between multiple tracts and multiple white matter lesions (which in any case are neuropathologically heterogeneous) using standard structural imaging.

Recently, diffusion tensor imaging has been used to perform tractography (the imaging of defined fiber tracts), including of the thalamocortical projections and the limbic network. Tractography has been used quantitatively to correlate stroke severity and outcome from lenticulostriate infarcts with damage to the corticospinal tract (Konishi *et al.* 2005). Studies of cognitive change and tractography are few, but in the future, imaging of deep white matter tract damage may aid in defining the prognosis and response to treatment in patients with vascular cognitive impairment.

Diffusion tensor imaging may also be used to measure fractional anisotropy, a marker of the degree of disruption of fiber tracts. Decreased fractional anisotropy has been shown in leukoaraiosis and also in normal-appearing white matter in patients with leukoraiosis, the latter correlating with the degree of executive impairment (O'Sullivan *et al.* 2001; Altamura *et al.* 2016) and in older people with normal brain imaging (Taylor *et al.* 2007). Fractional anisotropy is therefore a more sensitive tool for the detection of white matter damage than standard structural MRI, including FLAIR. Changes in fractional anisotropy correlate with N-acetyl aspartate measured using MR spectroscopy (Charlton *et al.* 2006). Since decreased fractional anisotropy is seen in normal-appearing white matter, it may prove useful in identifying those at risk of subsequent cognitive decline (Xu *et al.* 2010). Multimodal MRI may detect early white matter changes and define a group at high risk of cognitive decline (Jokinen *et al.* 2015; Liang *et al.* 2016). Brain network changes measured using functional MRI may also identify increased dementia risk (Kim *et al.* 2015a, b; Liang *et al.* 2016; Tuladhar *et al.* 2016).

Treatments for Vascular Cognitive Impairment

Therapy can be divided into primary prevention (preventing cerebrovascular disease), secondary prevention (slowing progression of established disease and preventing recurrent cerebrovascular events), symptomatic treatments and disease-modifying treatments. Effective primary prevention of vascular disease will reduce vascular cognitive impairment caused by stroke and help maintain overall brain health and cognitive reserve. However, it is important to note that although epidemiological studies have shown a clear link between midlife vascular factors and dementia, the relationship with risk factors that arise later in life is less clear and therefore primary prevention interventions might be expected to be more effective in younger versus older subjects.

Regarding specific primary preventive therapies, a meta-analysis of four randomized, controlled trials of antihypertensive drugs including more than 20,000 subjects found a non-significant trend (relative risk, 0.80; 95% confidence interval, 0.63–1.02; $p = 0.07$) toward reduction in cognitive decline with blood pressure–lowering treatment (Feigin et al. 2005). One observational study of statin use and cognitive function in the elderly found a slight reduction in cognitive decline in those using statins that could not be completely explained by the effect of statins on lowering of serum cholesterol (Bernick et al. 2005). However, no favorable effect of statins was seen in two large randomized trials (Heart Protection Study Collaborative Group 2002; Shepherd et al. 2002). Other studies have recruited subjects defined as at high risk of dementia using risk scores focused on vascular factors. In the Finnish Geriatric Intervention Study to Prevent Cognitive Impairment and Disability (FINGER) trial (Ngandu et al. 2015), participants aged 60–77 years were randomized to multicomponent intervention including diet, exercise, cognitive training, and vascular risk monitoring versus usual care. After 2 years, the intervention group performed better on a neuropsychological battery than the control group, suggesting that such interventions might help maintain brain health in younger old patients at risk of dementia. More effective treatment of vascular risk factors including hypertension and lifestyle changes may be linked to the recent observed reductions in age-specific incidence and prevalence of dementia (Matthews et al. 2013, 2016; see Chapter 31).

Secondary preventive interventions have included exercise in subjects with mild vascular impairment of subcortical origin (Liu-Ambrose et al. 2016) with a suggestion of possible benefit. In the Perindopril Protection Against Recurrent Stroke Study (PROGRESS) of blood pressure lowering after stroke (PROGRESS Collaborative Group 2001), the incidence of dementia was less in the treatment group in those who suffered a recurrent stroke than in the placebo group. However, three recent trials of vascular risk factor interventions in patients post-stroke showed no clear evidence of benefit (Ihle-Hansen et al. 2014; Matz et al. 2015; Bath et al. 2017), although follow-up was short (≤ 2 years) and included patients were likely to have been at low overall risk of dementia. Given the lack of relationship between vascular risk factors at the time of the event and post-stroke dementia seen in observational studies (see Chapter 31), it is unlikely that aggressive risk factor management will be effective in reducing post-stroke dementia, particularly in the era of robust secondary prevention. Trials of putative neuroprotective agents to reduce cognitive decline post-stroke are currently under way (Guekht et al. 2017).

Regarding symptomatic treatment, several randomized, double-blind, placebo-controlled trials have been undertaken in vascular dementia, although they have been criticized for using design and outcomes designed for Alzheimer's disease. Early studies concentrated on agents such as vasodilators and antioxidants but were disappointing. Only one study of aspirin in 70 people with multi-infarct dementia has been undertaken (Meyer *et al.* 1989), which showed that those taking 325 mg aspirin (compared with no treatment) had significantly higher cognitive performance at the end of 3 years, although dropout rates were high (61 percent by 3 years).

There have been two studies of memantine, an NMDA receptor antagonist, in vascular dementia, both of which showed significant effects on cognition compared with placebo over a 6-month period. However, there was no effect on global outcome measure, making the results of uncertain clinical relevance (Orgogozo *et al.* 2002; Wilcock *et al.* 2002). Similar improvement in cognition without consistent changes in activities of daily living, behavior, and global assessment were seen in studies of cholinesterase inhibitors: three studies of donepezil and two of galantamine, of which two remain unpublished (Erkinjuntti *et al.* 2002; Black *et al.* 2003; Wilkinson *et al.* 2003). Therefore, the use of cholinesterase inhibitors in patients with probable vascular dementia is not recommended, although they may be effective in patients with mixed Alzheimer's disease and vascular dementia. In practice, because of the difficulties in excluding coexistent neurodegenerative pathology particularly in older patients, a pragmatic trial of cholinesterase inhibitors is often undertaken.

There is a high incidence of depression in patients with vascular cognitive impairment, and late-life depression is a risk factor for dementia, particularly of the vascular subtype (Diniz *et al.* 2013). Treatment of depression may improve function as well as improve the patient's quality of life, although pharmacological treatments appear less effective in those with vascular cognitive impairment (Sheline *et al.* 2010), and there is no evidence to support the use of any particular type of antidepressant. Behavioral disturbance is common in vascular cognitive impairment as it is in Alzheimer's disease and should be managed with non-pharmacological interventions in the first instance, e.g., stimulating activity, increased carer attention, cognitive behavioral therapy, provision of a calm and quiet environment, and search for exacerbating factors such as pain or constipation. Patients and carers should be informed of the risk of delirium and cognitive decompensation in the context of acute illness, surgery, or new environments (Chapter 31). Severe behavioral disturbance resulting in risks to the patient or others or patient distress may require neuroleptic treatment, but the risks and benefits of such medications should be carefully considered owing to the adverse effects of such drugs, which include an increased risk of stroke.

References

Altamura C, Scrascia F, Quattrocchi CC, Errante Y, Gangemi E, Curcio G, Ursini F, Silvestrini M, Maggio P, Beomonte Zobel B, Rossini PM, Pasqualetti P, Falsetti L, Vernieri F (2016). Regional MRI diffusion, white-matter hyperintensities, and cognitive function in Alzheimer's disease and vascular dementia. *J Clin Neurol* **12** (2):201–208

Banerjee G, Carare R, Cordonnier C, Greenberg SM, Schneider JA, Smith EE, Buchem MV, Grond JV, Verbeek MM, Werring DJ (2017). The increasing impact of cerebral amyloid angiopathy: Essential new insights for clinical practice. *J Neurol Neurosurg Psychiatry* **88**(11):982–994

Barber R, Scheltens P, Gholkar A *et al.* (1999). White matter lesions on magnetic resonance imaging in dementia with Lewy bodies, Alzheimer's disease, vascular dementia, and normal aging. *Journal of Neurology, Neurosurgery and Psychiatry* **67**:66–72

Bastos-Leite AJ, van der Flier WM, van Straaten EC *et al.* (2007). The contribution of medial temporal lobe atrophy and vascular pathology to cognitive impairment in vascular dementia. *Stroke* **38**:3182–3185

Bath PM, Scutt P, Blackburn DJ *et al.* PODCAST Trial Investigators. (2017). Intensive versus guideline blood pressure and lipid lowering in patients with previous stroke: Main results from the pilot "Prevention of Decline in Cognition after Stroke Trial" (PODCAST) randomised controlled trial. PLoS One 12(1):e0164608

Bernick C, Katz R, Smith NL et al. (2005). Statins and cognitive function in the elderly: The Cardiovascular Health Study. Neurology 65:1388–1394

Black S, Roman GC, Geldmacher DS et al. (2003). Efficacy and tolerability of donepezil in vascular dementia: Positive results of a 24-week, multicenter, international, randomized, placebo-controlled clinical trial. Stroke 34:2323–2330

Charidimou A, Werring DJ (2012). Cerebral microbleeds and cognition in cerebrovascular disease: An update. J Neurol Sci 322(1–2):50–55

Charlton RA, Barrick TR, McIntyre DJ et al. (2006). White matter damage on diffusion tensor imaging correlates with age-related cognitive decline. Neurology 66:217–222

Chen A, Akinyemi RO, Hase Y, Firbank MJ, Ndung'u MN, Foster V, Craggs LJ, Washida K, Okamoto Y, Thomas AJ, Polvikoski TM, Allan LM, Oakley AE, O'Brien JT, Horsburgh K, Ihara M, Kalaria RN (2016). Frontal white matter hyperintensities, clasmatodendrosis and gliovascular abnormalities in ageing and post-stroke dementia. Brain 139(1):242–258

Cordoliani-Mackowiak M, Hénon H, Pruvo J et al. (2003). Post stroke dementia: Influence of hippocampal atrophy. Archives of Neurology 60:585–590

Cummings JL (1993). Frontal-subcortical circuits and human behavior. Archives of Neurology 50:873–880

Delano-Wood L, Abeles N, Sacco JM et al. (2008). Regional white matter pathology in mild cognitive impairment: Differential influence of lesion type on neuropsychological functioning. Stroke 39:794–799

de Leon MJ, Golomb J, George AE et al. (1993). The radiologic prediction of Alzheimer disease: the atrophic hippocampal formation. American Journal of Neuroradiology 14:897–906

Diniz BS, Butters MA, Albert SM, Dew MA, Reynolds CF III (2013). Late-life depression and risk of vascular dementia and Alzheimer's disease:

Systematic review and meta-analysis of community-based cohort studies. Br J Psychiatry 202:329–335

Erkinjuntti T, Kurz A, Gauthier S et al. (2002). Efficacy of galanthamine in probable vascular dementia and Alzheimer's disease combined with cerebrovascular disease: A randomised trial. Lancet 359:1283–1290

Feigin V, Ratnasabapathy Y, Anderson C (2005). Does blood pressure lowering treatment prevent dementia or cognitive decline in patients with cardiovascular and cerebrovascular disease? Journal of Neurology Science 15:151–155

Fein G, Di Sclafani V, Tanabe J et al. (2000). Hippocampal and cortical atrophy predict dementia in subcortical ischemic vascular disease. Neurology 55:1626–1635

Firbank MJ, Burton EJ, Barber R et al. (2007). Medial temporal atrophy rather than white matter hyperintensities predict cognitive decline in stroke survivors. Neurobiology Aging 28:1664–1669

Frisoni GB, Galluzzi S, Pantoni L et al. (2007). The effect of white matter lesions on cognition in the elderly – small but detectable. Nature Clinical and Practical Neurology 3:620–627

Guekht A, Skoog I, Edmundson S, Zakharov V, Korczyn AD (2017). ARTEMIDA trial (a randomized trial of efficacy, 12 months international double-blind actovegin): A randomized controlled trial to assess the efficacy of actovegin in poststroke cognitive impairment. Stroke 48:1262–1270

Grau-Olivares M, Bartrés-Faz D, Arboix A et al. (2007). Mild cognitive impairment after lacunar infarction: Voxel-based morphometry and neuropsychological assessment. Cerebrovascular Diseases 23:353–361

Heart Protection Study Collaborative Group (2002). MRC/BHF Heart Protection Study of cholesterol lowering with simvastatin in 20 536 high-risk individuals: A randomised placebo-controlled trial. Lancet 360:7–22

Ihle-Hansen H, Thommessen B, Fagerland MW, Øksengård AR, Wyller TB, Engedal K, Fure B (2014). Multifactorial vascular risk factor intervention to prevent cognitive impairment after stroke and TIA: A 12-month randomized controlled trial. Int J Stroke 9(7):932–938

Jagust WJ, Zheng L, Harvey DJ (2008). Neuropathological basis of magnetic resonance images in aging and dementia. *Annals of Neurology* **63**:72–82

Jobst KA, Smith AD, Szatmari M *et al.* (1992). Detection in life of confirmed Alzheimer's disease using a simple measurement of medial temporal lobe atrophy by computed tomography. *Lancet* **340**:1179–1183

Jobst KA, Barnetson LP, Shepstone BJ (1998). Accurate prediction of histologically confirmed Alzheimer's disease and the differential diagnosis of dementia: The use of NINCDS–ADRDA and DSM-III-R criteria, SPECT, X-ray CT, and Apo E4 in medial temporal lobe dementias. Oxford Project to Investigate Memory and Aging. *International Psychogeriatrics* **10**:271–302

Jokinen H, Gonçalves N, Vigário R, Lipsanen J, Fazekas F, Schmidt R, Barkhof F, Madureira S, Verdelho A, Inzitari D, Pantoni L, Erkinjuntti T (2015). LADIS Study Group. Early-stage white matter lesions detected by multispectral MRI segmentation predict progressive cognitive decline. *Front Neurosci* **2**(9):455

Jouvent E, Viswanathan A, Mangin JF *et al.* (2007). Brain atrophy is related to lacunar lesions and tissue microstructural changes in CADASIL. *Stroke* **38**:1786–1790

Kalaria RN, Ihara M (2017). Medial temporal lobe atrophy is the norm in cerebrovascular dementias. *Eur J Neurol* **24**(4):539–540

Kim HJ, Im K, Kwon H, Lee JM, Kim C, Kim YJ, Jung NY, Cho H, Ye BS, Noh Y, Kim GH, Ko ED, Kim JS, Choe YS, Lee KH, Kim ST, Lee JH, Ewers M, Weiner MW, Na DL, Seo SW (2015a). Clinical effect of white matter network disruption related to amyloid and small vessel disease. *Neurology* **85**(1):63–70

Kim HJ, Im K, Kwon H, Lee JM, Ye BS, Kim YJ, Cho H, Choe YS, Lee KH, Kim ST, Kim JS, Lee JH, Na DL, Seo SW (2015b). Effects of amyloid and small vessel disease on white matter network disruption. *J Alzheimers Dis* **44**(3):963–975

Konishi J, Yamada K, Kizu O *et al.* (2005). MR tractography for the evaluation of functional recovery from lenticulostriate infarcts. *Neurology* **64**:108–113

Laakso MP, Partanen K, Riekkinen P *et al.* (1996). Hippocampal volumes in Alzheimer's

disease, Parkinson's disease with and without dementia, and in vascular dementia: An MRI study. *Neurology* **46**:678–681

Leys D, Hénon H, Pasquier F (1998). White matter changes and poststroke dementia. *Dement Geriatr Cogn Disord* **9**(1):25–29

Liang Y, Sun X, Xu S, Liu Y, Huang R, Jia J, Zhang Z (2016). Preclinical Cerebral Network connectivity evidence of deficits in mild white matter lesions. *Front Aging Neurosci* **18**(8):27

Libon DJ, Price CC, Giovannetti T *et al.* (2008). Linking MRI hyperintensities with patterns of neuropsychological impairment: Evidence for a threshold effect. *Stroke* **39**:806–813

Liu-Ambrose T, Best JR, Davis JC *et al.* (2016). Aerobic exercise and vascular cognitive impairment: A randomized controlled trial. *Neurology* **87**:2082–2090.

Matthews, FE *et al.* (2013). A two-decade comparison of prevalence of dementia in individuals aged 65 years and older from three geographical areas of England: Results of the Cognitive Function and Ageing Study I and II. *Lancet* **382**:1405–1412

Matthews, FE *et al.* (2016). A two decade dementia incidence comparison from the Cognitive Function and Ageing Studies I and II. *Nat Commun* **7**:11398

Matz K, Teuschl Y, Firlinger B, Dachenhausen A, Keindl M, Seyfang L, Tuomilehto J, Brainin M, ASPIS Study Group (2015). Multidomain lifestyle interventions for the prevention of cognitive decline after ischemic stroke: Randomized trial. *Stroke* **46**(10):2874–2880

Meyer JS, Rogers RL, McClintic K *et al.* (1989). Randomized clinical trial of daily aspirin therapy in multi-infarct dementia. A pilot study. *Journal of the American Geriatric Society* **37**:549–555

Mok V, Wong A, Tang WK *et al.* (2005). Determinants of post stroke cognitive impairment in small vessel disease. *Dementia and Geriatric Cognitive Disorders* **20**:225–230

Mungas D, Jagust WJ, Reed BR *et al.* (2001). MRI predictors of cognition in subcortical ischemic vascular disease and Alzheimer's disease. *Neurology* **57**:2229–2235

Ngandu T, Lehtisalo J, Solomon A *et al.* (2015). A 2 year multidomain intervention of diet, exercise, cognitive training, and vascular risk monitoring versus control to prevent cognitive decline in at-risk elderly people (FINGER): A randomised controlled trial. *Lancet* **385** (9984):2255–2263

O'Brien JT, Metcalfe S, Swann A (2000). Medial temporal lobe width on CT scanning in Alzheimer's disease: Comparison with vascular dementia, depression and dementia with Lewy bodies. *Dementia and Geriatric Cognitive Disorders* **11**:114–118

Orgogozo JM, Rigaud AS, Stoffler A *et al.* (2002). Efficacy and safety of memantine in patients with mild to moderate vascular dementia: A randomized, placebo-controlled trial (MMM 300). *Stroke* **33**:1834–1839

O'Sullivan M, Summers PE, Jones DK *et al.* (2001). Normal-appearing white matter in ischemic leukoaraiosis: A diffusion tensor MRI study. *Neurology* **57**:2307–2310

O'Sullivan M, Morris RG, Huckstep B *et al.* (2004). Diffusion tensor MRI correlates with executive dysfunction in patients with ischaemic leukoaraiosis. *Journal of Neurology, Neurosurgery and Psychiatry* **75**:441–447

O'Sullivan M, Barrick TR, Morris RG *et al.* (2005). Damage within a network of white matter regions underlies executive dysfunction in CADASIL. *Neurology* **65**:1584–1590

Pantoni L, Fierini F, Poggesi A (2015). LADIS Study Group. Impact of cerebral white matter changes on functionality in older adults: An overview of the LADIS Study results and future directions. *Geriatr Gerontol Int.* **15** (1):10–16

Pendlebury ST, Blamire AM, Lee MA *et al.* (1999). Axonal injury in the internal capsule correlates with motor impairment after stroke. *Stroke* **30**:956–962

Pendlebury ST and Rothwell PM (2009). Prevalence, incidence, and factors associated with pre-stroke and post-stroke dementia: a systematic review and met-analysis. *Lancet Neurology* **8**:1006–1018

Pendlebury ST, Wharton RM, Rothwell PM (2017a). Predictors of dementia after TIA/ stroke: 15-year population-based follow-up study. *J Eur Stroke* **2**(suppl 1):AS11–003

Pineiro R, Pendlebury ST, Smith S *et al.* (2000). Relating MRI changes to motor deficit after ischemic stroke by segmentation of functional motor pathways. *Stroke* **31**:672–679

Prins ND, van Dijk EJ, den Heijer T *et al.* (2005). Cerebral small-vessel disease and decline in information processing speed, executive function and memory. *Brain* **128**:2034–2041

PROGRESS Collaborative Group (2001). Randomised trial of a perindopril-based blood-pressure-lowering regimen among 6105 individuals with previous stroke or transient ischaemic attack. *Lancet* **358**:1033–1041

Ritchie C, Smailagic N, Noel-Storr AH, Ukoumunne O, Ladds EC, Martin S (2017). CSF tau and the CSF tau/ABeta ratio for the diagnosis of Alzheimer's disease dementia and other dementias in people with mild cognitive impairment (MCI). Cochrane *Database Syst Rev.* 3:CD010803

Roman GC, Tatemichi TK, Erkinjuntti T *et al.* (1993). Vascular dementia: Diagnostic criteria for research studies. Report of the NINDS–AIREN International Workshop. *Neurology* **43**:250–260

Sachdev P, Kalaria R, O'Brien J *et al.* (2014). International Society for Vascular Behavioral and Cognitive Disorders. Diagnostic criteria for vascular cognitive disorders: A VASCOG statement. *Alzheimer Dis Assoc Disord.* 28 (3):206–218

Sheline YI, Pieper CF, Barch DM, Welsh-Bohmer K, McKinstry RC, MacFall JR, D'Angelo G, Garcia KS, Gersing K, Wilkins C *et al.* (2010). Support for the vascular depression hypothesis in late-life depression: Results of a 2-site, prospective, antidepressant treatment trial. *Arch Gen Psychiatry* **67**:277–285

Shepherd J, Blauw GJ, Murphy MB *et al.* (2002). PROspective Study of Pravastatin in the Elderly at Risk. Pravastatin in elderly individuals at risk of vascular disease (PROSPER): A randomised controlled trial. *Lancet* **360**:1623–1630

Smith CD, Snowdon DA, Wang H *et al.* (2000). White matter volumes and periventricular white matter hyperintensities in aging and dementia. *Neurology* **54**:838–842

Stebbins GT, Nyenhuis DL, Wang C *et al.* (2008). Gray matter atrophy in patients with ischemic stroke with cognitive impairment. *Stroke* 39:785–793

Swartz RH, Stuss DT, Gao F *et al.* (2008). Independent cognitive effects of atrophy, diffuse subcortical and thalamo-cortical cerebrovascular disease in dementia. *Stroke* 39:822–830

Taylor WD, Bae JN, MacFall JR *et al.* (2007). Widespread effects of hyperintense lesions on cerebral white matter structure. *American Journal of Roentgenology* 188:1695–1704

Tekin S, Cummings JL (2002). Frontal-subcortical neuronal circuits and clinical neuropsychiatry: An update. *Journal of Psychosomatic Research* 53:647–654

Tuladhar AM, van Uden IW, Rutten-Jacobs LC, Lawrence A, van der Holst H, van Norden A, de Laat K, van Dijk E, Claassen JA, Kessels RP, Markus HS, Norris DG, de Leeuw FE (2016). Structural network efficiency predicts conversion to dementia. *Neurology.* 86 (12):1112–1119

Varley J, Taylor J, Irani SR (2017). Autoantibody-mediated diseases of the CNS: Structure, dysfunction and therapy. *Neuropharmacology.* May 3. pii: S0028-3908(17) 30196–X

Vermeer SE, Longstreth WT Jr., Koudstaal PJ (2007). Silent brain infarcts: A systematic review. *Lancet Neurology* 6:611–619

Wardlaw JM, Smith EE, Biessels GJ *et al.* (2013). STandards for ReportIng Vascular changes on nEuroimaging (STRIVE v1). Neuroimaging standards for research into small vessel disease and its contribution to ageing and neurodegeneration. *Lancet Neurol.* 12 (8):822–838

Wilcock G, Mobius HJ, Stoffler A *et al.* (2002). A double-blind, placebo-controlled multicentre study of memantine in mild to moderate vascular dementia (MMM500). *International Clinical Psychopharmacology* 17:297–305

Wilkinson D, Doody R, Helme R *et al.* (2003). Donepezil in vascular dementia: A randomized placebo-controlled study. *Neurology* 61:479–486

Won Seo S, Hwa Lee B, Kim EJ *et al.* (2007). Clinical significance of microbleeds in subcortical vascular dementia. *Stroke* 38:1949–1951

Wright CB, Festa JR, Paik MC *et al.* (2008). White matter hyperintensities and subclinical infarction: Associations with psychomotor speed and cognitive flexibility. *Stroke* 39:800–805

Xu Q, Zhou Y, Li YS, Cao WW, Lin Y, Pan YM, Chen SD (2010). Diffusion tensor imaging changes correlate with cognition better than conventional MRI findings in patients with subcortical ischemic vascular disease. *Dement Geriatr Cogn Disord.* 30(4):317–326

Index